ALEX M WESTENFIELD, M.D.

Transitional Resident (6/97- 6/98)
Gundersen Lutheran Medical Center
LA CROSSE, WISCONSIN

Diagnostic Radiology Resident
Nebraska Health Systems
OMAHA, NE (7/98-

Body CT

Body CT
A Practical Approach

Editors

Richard M. Slone, MD, FCCP
Assistant Professor of Radiology
Thoracic Imaging Section
Mallinckrodt Institute of Radiology
Washington University School of Medicine
St. Louis, Missouri

Andrew J. Fisher, MD
Abdominal Imaging and Trauma Radiology
Radiology Imaging Associates
Denver, Colorado

Perry J. Pickhardt, MD
Mallinckrodt Institute of Radiology
Washington University School of Medicine
St. Louis, Missouri
Head, Radiology Department
U.S. Naval Hospital
Guantanamo Bay, Cuba

Fernando R. Gutierrez, MD
Associate Professor and Director of Cardiac Radiology
Mallinckrodt Institute of Radiology
Washington University School of Medicine
St. Louis, Missouri

Dennis M. Balfe, MD
Professor and Chief of Gastrointestinal Radiology
Mallinckrodt Institute of Radiology
Washington University School of Medicine
St. Louis, Missouri

McGRAW-HILL
Health Professions Division

New York St. Louis San Francisco Auckland Bogotá Caracas
Lisbon London Madrid Mexico City Milan Montreal
New Delhi San Juan Singapore Sydney Tokyo Toronto

McGraw-Hill
*A Division of The **McGraw-Hill** Companies*

Body CT
A Practical Approach

1234567890 DOCDOC 99

ISBN 0-07-058219-X

This book was set in Times Roman by Progressive Information Technologies.
The editors were Martin J. Wonsiewicz, Susan R. Noujaim, and Muza Navrozov.
The production supervisor was Catherine H. Saggese.
The index was prepared by Jerry Ralya.
R. R. Donnelley & Sons Company was printer and binder.

The book is printed on recycled, acid-free paper.

Library of Congress Cataloging-in-Publication Data
Body CT: a practical approach / editors, Richard M. Slone . . . [et al.].
p. cm.
Includes bibliographical references and index.
ISBN 0-07-058219-X
1. Tomography I. Slone, Richard M. /
[DNLM: 1. Tomography, X-Ray Computed—methods. 2. Diagnostic Imaging—methods. WN 206 B668 1999]
RC78.7.T6B63 2000
616.07'57—dc21
DNLM/DLC
for Library of Congress

To my parents (JHS, WMS), brothers (MCS, JCS), and son Logan

RMS

To JAF, MJF, RYK, and T: thanks for getting me through

AJF

To Mom, Dad, and Bethney—for their unconditional love and support

PJP

To my wife and children for their patience and endurance, and to my parents for pointing the way

FRG

To my wife, Marty, for her unfailing support

DMB

CONTENTS

Contributors		ix
Preface		xi
Acknowledgments		xiii
Chapter 1	**CT Techniques and Protocols** *Richard M. Slone*	1
Chapter 2	**Lungs** *Richard M. Slone*	9
Chapter 3	**Pleura and Diaphragm** *Richard M. Slone*	45
Chapter 4	**Mediastinum** *Fernando R. Gutierrez and Sanjeev Bhalla*	57
Chapter 5	**Cardiovascular CT** *Fernando R. Gutierrez*	75
Chapter 6	**Alimentary Tract** *Perry J. Pickhardt*	95
Chapter 7	**Liver and Biliary System** *Christopher J. Gordon*	113
Chapter 8	**Spleen** *Andrew J. Fisher*	135
Chapter 9	**Pancreas** *Andrea M. Fisher and Perry J. Pickhardt*	145
Chapter 10	**Peritoneum and Retroperitoneum** *Perry J. Pickhardt*	159

Chapter 11 **Adrenals** 179
Andrew J. Fisher

Chapter 12 **Kidneys** 189
Andrew J. Fisher

Chapter 13 **Pelvis** 205
Perry J. Pickhardt

Chapter 14 **Body Wall** 223
Richard Slone and Andrew J. Fisher

Chapter 15 **Trauma** 237
Andrew J. Fisher

Index *249*

CONTRIBUTORS*

Sanjeev Bhalla, MD [4]
Clinical Instructor, Thoracic Imaging and Body CT
Mallinckrodt Institute of Radiology
Washington University School of Medicine
St. Louis, Missouri

Andrea M. Fisher, MD [9]
Assistant Professor of Radiology
Division of Abdominal Imaging
New York Presbyterian Hospital
Cornell University
New York, New York

Andrew J. Fisher, MD [8, 11, 12, 14, 15]
Abdominal Imaging and Trauma Radiologist
Radiology Imaging Associates
Denver, Colorado

Christopher Gordon, MD [7]
Mallinckrodt Institute of Radiology
Washington University School of Medicine
St. Louis, Missouri
Staff Radiologist
Litton and Giddings Radiology Associates
Cox Health Systems
Springfield, Missouri

Fernando R. Gutierrez, MD [4, 5]
Associate Professor and Director of Cardiac Radiology
Mallinckrodt Institute of Radiology
Washington University School of Medicine
St. Louis, Missouri

Perry J. Pickhardt, MD [6, 9, 10, 13]
Mallinckrodt Institute of Radiology
Washington University School of Medicine
St. Louis, Missouri
Head, Radiology Department
U.S. Naval Hospital
Guantanamo Bay, Cuba

Richard M. Slone, MD [1, 2, 3, 14]
Assistant Professor of Radiology
Mallinckrodt Institute of Radiology
Washington University School of Medicine
St. Louis, Missouri

*Numbers in brackets refer to chapters authored or co-authored by the contributor.

PREFACE

Modern CT allows rapid, comprehensive, and detailed patient evaluation and is integral in diagnosis and follow-up of medical and surgical conditions. Wide availability and continued technological advances, including spiral imaging and most recently multiarray detectors, keep CT at the forefront of diagnostic imaging. In particular, CT plays a critical role in detecting malignancies and evaluating response to treatment. CT also plays an important role in assessing trauma victims and is becoming an important tool in vascular imaging. It is important to note that both image acquisition and interpretation are critical in addressing specific clinical questions and must be optimized to realize the full potential of information available from a CT examination. As with other radiologic studies, knowledge of the patient's clinical situation is important as is consultation with referring physicians.

Body CT: A Practical Approach is intended to provide radiologists with a comprehensive yet manageable guide to body CT techniques and interpretation. Chapter 1 introduces the principles of CT technology and provides detailed guidelines for tailoring examination protocols to specific clinical problems. Organized by organ system, subsequent chapters are divided into sections discussing technique, congenital, inflammatory, and neoplastic conditions. Anatomy and treatment options are introduced where relevant to image interpretation. Cardiovascular imaging and trauma are covered in separate chapters. The illustrations are from routine clinical examinations, and over 100 tables are included outlining the differential diagnosis for specific imaging findings. The most common differentials are set in boldface type, and rare conditions or manifestations are in italics. We hope you find this text valuable and the format refreshing as you further your skills in body CT interpretation.

R.M.S.

ACKNOWLEDGMENTS

We would like to gratefully acknowledge our thoughtful and experienced colleagues at Mallinckrodt with whom we have collaborated and learned from through the years. These include not only the Co-directors of Body CT, Jay Heiken, MD, and Stuart Sagel, MD, and faculty in the Chest and Abdominal Imaging Sections, but also our excellent residents and fellows who continue to both challenge and humble us in our daily practice. We would also like to thank Dr. Sagel for almost single-handedly developing and maintaining the resident teaching file, from which so many of our images originate. Tom Murry and Mickey Wynn, both expert photographers, prepared all the illustrations used in this textbook. They remain second to none in preparing the highest quality images expeditiously and cheerfully. We would also like to acknowledge the superb technical staff on the CT service, which is under the direction of Joe Lombardo, RT(R), Sue Gonzales, RT(R), and Michelle Onder, RT(R). Their skill and attention to detail result in consistently excellent quality examinations and patient care. Lynn Lammers, Anna Langenberg, and Linda Macker provided expert secretarial assistance in the myriad details of manuscript preparation. Susan Noujaim and Muza Navrozov at McGraw-Hill carefully coordinated the critical details of production as our book moved from conception, through editing, and into final publication. We are grateful to all these individuals for their contributions of skill, time, and enthusiasm.

Body CT

Chapter 1

CT Techniques and Protocols

Richard M. Slone

1.1 CT Physics
1.2 Contrast Agents
1.3 Protocols
1.4 Problem-Oriented Approach to Scanning

1.1 CT PHYSICS

- **Computed tomography (CT)** provides detailed anatomic information valuable in both diagnosis and disease management. Maximizing the diagnostic utility of each examination requires careful attention to selection of the acquisition parameters and display and interpretation of the images. Developed in the early 1970s, CT is a technique that mathematically constructs a digital cross-sectional image by assimilating tissue absorption information obtained from multiple transaxial x-ray projections. Gray-scale values are assigned to individual picture elements (pixels) based on the mean linear attenuation coefficients from individual volume elements (voxels). **Raw data** are collected as the x-ray tube in the gantry projects a fan beam through the patient. Each **projection** yields an array of data consisting of the transmitted radiation measured by detectors opposite the tube. The **ray sum** is the value measured by an individual detector during a single projection and is a result of the cumulative attenuation of all the tissues traversed by the beam. As the tube rotates around the patient, hundreds of projections and thousands of individual ray sums are obtained.
- **Image reconstruction** is the computerized process of converting the thousands of individual ray sums into image data for display. Filtered back-projection is the most commonly employed technique. **Back-projection** solves the thousands of equations required to calculate the attenuation value for each voxel based on the ray sum values collected. **Filtering** is a mathematical process that modifies the data to correct for image blur introduced by limitations in the data set.
- There are two general CT design types in common use. **Third-generation** scanners employ a coupled tube assembly and detector array that rotate in synchrony. **Fourth-generation** scanners have a rotating tube assembly and a fixed array of several thousand detectors. **Conventional CT** uses cables to connect the tube and detector assembly within the gantry with the power supply and electronics. Thus, following each image acquisition (which requires one full rotation), the tube assembly and cables must be unwound, requiring an interscan delay before the next scan is performed. During the interscan delay, the patient couch is advanced and the patient breathes. A 40-image study takes about 3 min.
- **Spiral CT** allows continuous data collection without interscan delay by utilizing slip-ring connectors (brushes and rings) that provide electrical contact. Without constraint by cables, the tube assembly rotates continuously and projectional data can be obtained during a single breath-hold. Depending on the equipment, the time for one rotation (**scan time**) can be varied from 0.5 to 2 s. During rotation, the couch is slowly moved through the gantry. The pathway projected by this combination of tube rotation and gantry translation is that of a helix, a specific form of a spiral. The rate at which the couch is advanced through the gantry is called the **table speed. Pitch,** a term unique to spiral CT, refers to the ratio of table movement per rotation to collimation. The greater the pitch, the greater the coverage for a given collimation; but as pitch increases, there is associated image degradation due to effective broadening of the slice profile. A pitch of 1 should be used when possible, and 2 is the upper limit for imaging.
- Eliminating the interscan delay allows examinations to be performed in less time and with less intravenous contrast. Continuous data acquisition through a single breath-hold also eliminates respiratory misregistration. Respiratory misregistration degrades examination quality by producing overlapping sections and gaps in coverage, allowing important pathology to be missed. The disadvantage of eliminating the interscan delay is the significant anode heating produced, which can limit scan duration and the milliamperes (mA) and kilovolts peak (kVp) that can be used.
- More recently, multiarray scanners have become available that allow simultaneous acquisition of up to four parallel projections, thus reducing total scan time while also allowing increased coverage and implementation of more complex protocols.
- **Reconstruction interval** is the spacing of images. Section thickness is always equal to the collimation used during data acquisition, but images can be reconstructed at any interval desired, including overlapping. Contiguous images are typically produced with a reconstruction interval equal to the collimation, but overlapping images (3×2 mm) or images separated by small spaces (5×8 mm) may be desired. For example, a useful tech-

nique when screening or following multiple small pulmonary nodules <5 mm is to perform a spiral examination with 8-mm collimation and reconstruct the image data set at 5-mm intervals, creating overlapping images, which increases sensitivity and measurement accuracy.

Image Display

- CT images are typically printed onto laser film, but they are increasingly being reviewed and interpreted on cathode ray tube (CRT) displays. Such soft-copy viewing coupled with picture archive and communication systems (PACS) allows simultaneous and remote viewing and image manipulation. The intensity values or CT numbers assigned to pixels are based on Hounsfield units (HU), where 1 HU = 1000 × (linear attenuation of voxel − linear attenuation of water)/(linear attenuation of water). On this scale, water is 0 HU and air is −1000 HU. Fat is about −90 HU, unenhanced soft tissue about 50 HU, and cortical bone 1000 to 2000 HU. The human visual system cannot distinguish between the subtle differences in attenuation CT can detect when the full range of values is displayed. Therefore contrast and brightness are altered when the image data is displayed to accentuate attenuation differences in the range of interest.
- **Window center** or **level** refers to the HU value assigned to middle gray and **window width** to the HU range between white and black. For example, with a center of 50 HU and a width of 500 HU, any pixel with a value less than −225 HU will be black and any pixel with a value above 275 HU will be white. Lung and air will both be black. With a center of −500 HU and a width of 1000 HU, pixels with values between −1000 and 0 HU will be assigned a gray scale and all pixels above 0 HU will be white. Thus, bone and all soft tissues other than fat will be white, but air-filled bullae (−1000) and lung (−800) can be distinguished. Specific window settings are often referred to by the tissue they are designed to display—for example, lung windows, soft tissue windows, liver windows, or bone windows.

Resolution

- **Spatial resolution** is the ability to discriminate adjacent high-contrast objects and is determined by pixel size, focal spot size, detector size, and detector separation. **Pixel size** is defined as the field of view (FOV) divided by the matrix size, typically 512 × 512 pixels (sometimes 1024 × 1024 on a few newer machines). The FOV is selected at the time of reconstruction, and if the raw data is saved, images can be produced with different FOVs. The smaller the FOV or larger the matrix, the greater the spatial resolution. For example, with a matrix of 512 and a field of view of 50 cm, each pixel is approximately 1 × 1 mm (500 mm/512), and with a FOV of 25 cm, each pixel is 0.5 × 0.5 mm. The height and width of the voxel are the same as the pixel dimensions, with depth determined by **collimation** (section thickness), ranging from 1 to 10 mm. Slice thickness limits the resolution of structures oblique to the z axis.
- The strength of CT is in **contrast resolution,** which is the ability to discriminate differences in attenuation. Compton scatter of x-rays within the patient degrades density resolution by artificially altering detector measurements. Scatter is reduced by the air gap between the patient and detectors and by detector collimation. The number of photons reaching the detectors affects the precision of the CT number assignments and therefore the contrast resolution. Image noise caused by **quantum mottle** is the result of relative photopenia and can obscure low-contrast detail, but it generally affects esthetics more than diagnosis. Image noise increases with increased patient thickness, and decreasing mA, kVp, detector efficiency, scan time, and voxel size (section thickness and FOV). Noise is more conspicuous in images reconstructed using a high-resolution algorithm. In general, factors that decrease radiation dose or increase spatial resolution also increase image noise. Depending on the amount of quantum mottle and the reconstruction filter chosen, CT can typically discriminate between tissues with linear attenuation values differing by 0.5 percent (5 HU).
- Filters used during image reconstruction that enhance spatial resolution or sharpness (small kernel size) by enhancing high-frequency information, increase image noise, and decrease density or contrast resolution. Filters that optimize contrast resolution and minimize image noise (large kernel size), introduce spatial smoothing that degrades spatial resolution. The filter chosen is determined by the task at hand **(Fig. 1.1).** Spatial resolution is more important for skeletal and high-resolution computed tomography (HRCT) studies and contrast resolution for soft tissue evaluation.
- **HRCT** involves obtaining representative sections with 1- to 2-mm collimation, a minimal field of view, and a high-spatial-frequency reconstruction algorithm to obtain detailed images of the lung comparable to gross tissue inspection. HRCT is valuable for detecting bronchiectasis, mild emphysema, and interstitial disease, particularly fibrosis and pneumoconiosis. Supine positioning often results in gravity-induced "dependent atelectasis," which can be mistaken for pulmonary fibrosis. Prone positioning reverses this distribution of microatelectasis and, when compared with supine images, allows distinction between gravity-related changes and inflammation or fibrosis. Imaging during suspended inspiration maximizes pulmonary aeration and minimizes dependent atelectasis, thus improving disease conspicuity. **Expiration** accentuates air trapping in emphysema and small airway disease such as bronchiolitis obliterans.

Artifacts

- Various artifacts may appear as a result of the image reconstruction process, equipment or electronics failure, and implants or monitoring devices on the patient. The **beam-hardening artifact** is a result of the preferential absorption of low-energy x-rays from a polychromatic source. This results in increased mean energy, and as a result, the x-ray beam is less attenuated by subsequent tissue it traverses and more radiation reaches the detector. The artifact is noticeable as focal areas of low attenuation adjacent to bone.
- **Partial-volume artifact:** Since the value assigned to each pixel is an average attenuation of the tissue in that voxel, when disparate tissues are in close proximity, the result is an artifactual value that can be misleading. For example, a voxel containing one-third fat (−90) and two-thirds soft tissue (50 HU) could result in an assigned value near 0 HU and mimic fluid.
- Motion can induce **streak artifacts** noticeable at the interface of tissues of different density, such as contrast and air in the gastrointestinal (GI) tract or bone and soft tissue. **Ring artifacts** are the result of a faulty detector and occur only in third-generation scanners, since the source and detectors are coupled. Peristalsis as well as respiratory, cardiac, and patient motion can degrade image quality. Images of the chest are routinely obtained during suspended inspiration to maximize aeration of the lung and images of the abdomen or pelvis during suspended end-expiration, which is more reproducible.

1.2 CONTRAST AGENTS

Intravenous Contrast

- **Intravenous (IV) contrast** greatly improves detection and characterization of solid-organ lesions, most importantly in the liver, pancreas, and kidneys. It also facilitates detection of blood vessels and vascular disease processes. It is almost universally utilized for examinations of the abdomen and pelvis. Common exceptions include evaluation for renal stones and retroperitoneal hematoma. In some cases, images are obtained both before and after IV contrast administration, in particular in assessing for aortic dissection, high-attenuation cysts, and potentially calcified lesions. In the chest, IV contrast is not needed when pulmonary nodules or interstitial lung disease is being evaluated, but it may help to identify lymph nodes, wall enhancement in empyemas and is necessary when evaluating vascular lesions, particularly pulmonary emboli.
- IV contrast material varies in its concentration and composition. Nonionic or low-osmolality contrast agents are associated with less discomfort and a lower incidence of allergic reactions but are more expensive than ionic contrast media. However, their cost has declined and some institutions use them exclusively. Nonionic contrast is preferred in patients with drug allergies, a prior contrast reaction, or a history of asthma, heart disease, or sickle cell disease, as well as in debilitated patients. IV contrast should be **avoided** in patients with a creatinine above 2.0. Diabetic patients taking Glucophage should discontinue that medication for 2 days and have close diabetic monitoring following IV contrast administration.
- Pretreatment with corticosteroids diminishes the risk of a reaction in patients with a history of prior mild contrast reactions, such as hives. Protocols vary, but 50 mg of oral prednisone 13, 7, and 1 h prior to examination is a typical regimen. This can be supplemented with an oral antihistamine 1 h prior to the examination. Contrast should not be used despite pretreatment in patients with prior serious contrast reactions such as bronchospasm, laryngeal edema, or anaphylaxis.

Oral Contrast

- **Oral contrast material** improves depiction of the GI tract. 700 to 800 mL usually provides adequate opacification when ingested over 1 h. This can be accomplished by providing the patient with three 250-mL cups of oral contrast to drink at half-hour intervals.

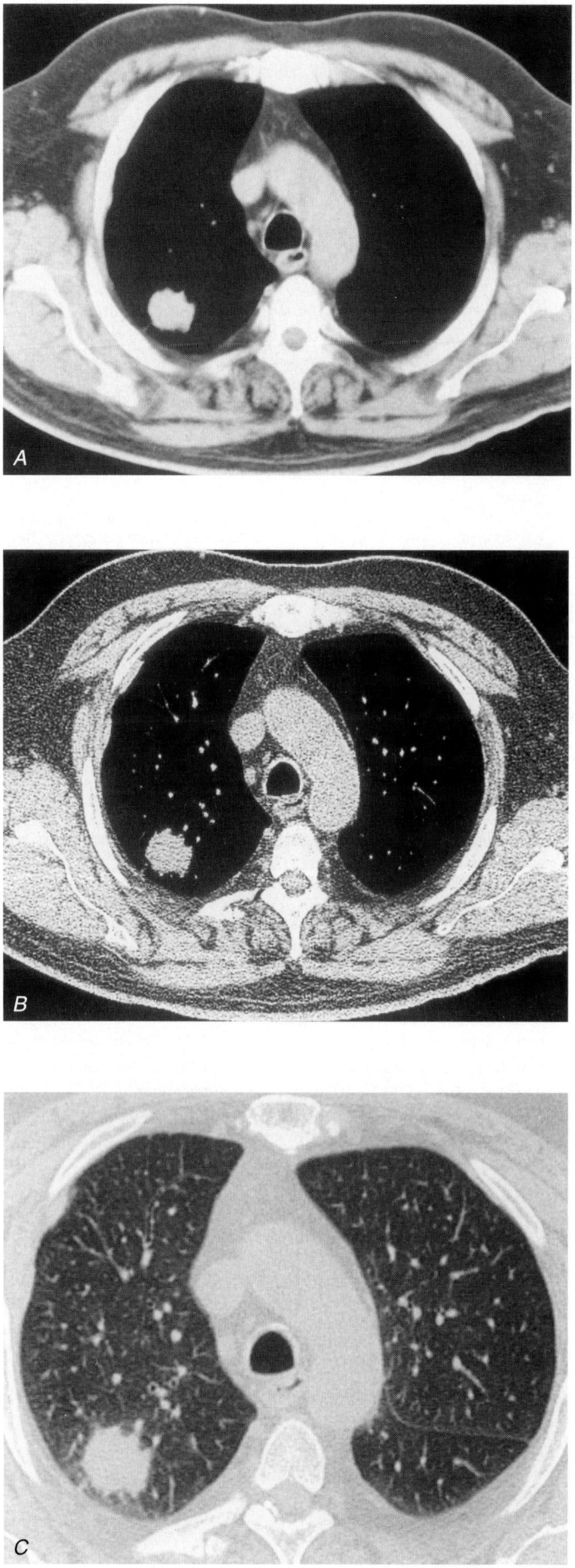

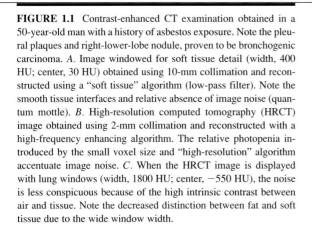

FIGURE 1.1 Contrast-enhanced CT examination obtained in a 50-year-old man with a history of asbestos exposure. Note the pleural plaques and right-lower-lobe nodule, proven to be bronchogenic carcinoma. *A*. Image windowed for soft tissue detail (width, 400 HU; center, 30 HU) obtained using 10-mm collimation and reconstructed using a "soft tissue" algorithm (low-pass filter). Note the smooth tissue interfaces and relative absence of image noise (quantum mottle). *B*. High-resolution computed tomography (HRCT) image obtained using 2-mm collimation and reconstructed with a high-frequency enhancing algorithm. The relative photopenia introduced by the small voxel size and "high-resolution" algorithm accentuate image noise. *C*. When the HRCT image is displayed with lung windows (width, 1800 HU; center, −550 HU), the noise is less conspicuous because of the high intrinsic contrast between air and tissue. Note the decreased distinction between fat and soft tissue due to the wide window width.

Negative contrast opacification of the stomach and duodenum is provided by 400 to 500 mL of water ingested just before scanning.

- Both water-soluble iodinated and barium-based suspensions are available. Iodinated contrast can be made by diluting a 60% concentration of water-soluble contrast 25:1 with water to produce a 2.5% solution. Iodine-based oral contrast stimulates bowel motility and is preferred in most patients, including surgical candidates and patients with suspected bowel obstruction or perforation.

1.3 PROTOCOLS

- The following protocols provide only a general guideline. Details will vary depending on the equipment and contrast used. Most examinations should be performed at 120 to 140 kVp with 210 to 320 mA.

Chest

- **Contrast:** If indicated, 100 mL IV at 2 mL/s with a 20- to 30-s delay.
- **Coverage:** Thoracic inlet (1 cm above lung apex) through lung bases (or adrenals depending on the clinical indication) in suspended inspiration.
- **Parameters:** 5- to 8-mm collimation and intervals with a pitch of 1 to 1.5.

Nodule Characterization

- **Contrast:** None.
- **Coverage:** 1 cm above to 1 cm below the lesion with targeted FOV in suspended inspiration.
- **Parameters:** 2- to 3-mm collimation and intervals with a pitch of 1 to 1.5.

HRCT

- **Contrast:** None.
- **Coverage:** Lung apex through base with FOV targeted to include ribs in suspended inspiration. An additional examination in suspended expiration may be indicated in some clinical situations to evaluate for air trapping. In cases of suspected fibrosis, the examination should be performed with the patient prone.
- **Parameters:** 1- or 2-mm collimation at 10-mm increments. High-spatial-frequency reconstruction algorithm. In most cases, HRCT is accompanied by a standard chest CT. Film with 1500-HU window width and −600-HU center.

Central Airway

- **Contrast:** None.
- **Coverage:** Vocal cords through bifurcation of bronchus intermedius with a 15-cm FOV in suspended inspiration.
- **Parameters:** 3-mm collimation at 3-mm intervals with a pitch of 1.5 to 2. Use 2-mm reconstruction intervals if three-dimensional processing or sagittal or coronal reformats are planned.

Aorta

- **Contrast:** Precontrast images in select cases, then 150 mL IV at 2 to 3 mL/s with 20-s delay.
- **Coverage:** Top of aortic arch through iliac bifurcation in suspended inspiration.
- **Parameters:** 5-mm collimation at 5-mm intervals with a pitch of 1.5.

Pulmonary Emboli

- **Contrast:** 150 mL IV at 3 mL/s. Use test injection or automated assessment to measure attenuation in pulmonary trunk to determine optimal delay (usually 15 to 20 s).
- **Coverage:** Lung base through top of aortic arch in suspended inspiration.
- **Parameters:** 3-mm collimation at 2-mm intervals with a pitch of 1.5. Review images on CRT display. Film alternating images.

Abdomen

- **Contrast:** 1000 mL oral and 100 to 150 mL IV at 2 mL/s with 60- to 80-s delay.
- **Coverage:** Dome of diaphragm to iliac crest in suspended end-expiration.
- **Parameters:** 5-mm collimation at 8-mm increments with a pitch of 1 to 1.5. In obese patients, consider contiguous 8- or 10-mm sections.

Pelvis

- **Contrast:** 1000 mL oral and 100 to 150 mL IV at 2 mL/s with 60- to 80-s delay.
- **Coverage:** Iliac crest to ischium in suspended end-expiration. Improved vascular depiction of ovarian and uterine malignancies can be obtained by scanning from ischium to iliac crest following a 20- to 30-s delay.
- **Parameters:** 5-mm collimation at 8-mm intervals with a pitch of 1 to 1.5. In cases of pelvic malignancies, consider scanning from caudal to cranial and using 5-mm reconstruction intervals in the pelvis. In obese patients, consider 8- or 10-mm collimation.

Abdomen and Pelvis

- **Contrast:** 800 mL oral and 125 to 150 mL IV at 2 mL/s with 60- to 80-s delay.
- **Coverage:** Dome of diaphragm to ischium in suspended end-expiration.
- **Parameters:** 5-mm collimation at 8-mm intervals with a pitch of 1 to 1.5. In cases of pelvic malignancies, consider scanning from caudal to cranial and using 5-mm reconstruction intervals in the pelvis. In obese patients, consider 8- or 10-mm collimation.

Adrenal Glands

- **Contrast:** None.
- **Coverage:** 1 cm above to 1 cm below adrenals with targeted FOV in suspended end-expiration.
- **Parameters:** 2- to 3-mm collimation and intervals targeted to adrenals with a pitch of 1 to 1.5.

Triple-Phase Liver

- **Contrast:** 800 mL oral and 150 mL IV at 3 to 5 mL/s.

- **(1)** Precontrast images, **(2)** arterial phase: 20-s delay, **(3)** portal venous phase: 50-s delay.
- **Coverage:** Dome of diaphragm to iliac crest in suspended end-expiration.
- **Parameters:** 5-mm collimation at 5-mm intervals with a pitch of 1 to 1.5.

Dual-Phase Pancreas

- **Contrast:** 800 mL water rather than positive contrast, 150 mL IV at 4 to 5 mL/s.
- **(1)** Precontrast to localize pancreas, **(2)** arterial phase: 30-s delay, **(3)** portal venous phase: 50-s delay.
- **Coverage:** Pancreas as localized on precontrast images in suspended end-expiration. Include entire duodenum during portal venous phase.
- **Parameters:** 3-mm collimation at 3-mm intervals with a pitch of 1.5.

Renal

- **Contrast:** 800 mL oral and 100 mL IV at 3 mL/s with 50-s delay.
- **Coverage:** Adrenals and kidneys in suspended end-expiration.
- **Parameters:** 5-mm collimation at 5-mm intervals with a pitch of 1 to 1.5 before and after IV contrast. Obtain ROI measurements in cystic lesions. To confidently characterize small lesions, 3-mm collimation and intervals may be needed.

Triple-Phase Renal

- **Contrast:** 800 mL oral and 100 mL IV at 3 mL/s.
- **(1)** Precontrast images, **(2)** corticomedullary phase: 30-s delay, **(3)** nephrographic phase: 60-s delay, **(4)** obtain delayed images at 5 to 10 min if ureteral tumor is suspected.
- **Coverage: (1 and 2)** Kidneys in suspended end-expiration, **(3)** abdomen.
- **Parameters:** 5-mm collimation at 5-mm intervals with a pitch of 1 to 1.5. Use 3-mm collimation and intervals in evaluating small lesions.

Renal Stone

- **Contrast:** None.
- **Coverage:** Upper pole of kidneys (T12) to pubic symphysis in suspended end-expiration.
- **Parameters:** 5-mm collimation and intervals with a pitch of 1.5. Rescan with 2-mm collimation and intervals and targeted FOV to clarify equivocal findings.

Chest, Abdomen, and Pelvis

- **Contrast:** 800 mL oral and 150 mL IV at 1.5 to 2 mL/s with 70-s delay.
- **Coverage:** Dome of diaphragm to ischium in suspended end-expiration using 100 mL IV contrast; then thoracic inlet through lung bases in suspended inspiration using remaining 50 mL IV contrast.
- **Parameters:** 5-mm collimation at 8-mm intervals with a pitch of 1 to 1.5 in the abdomen and pelvis and 8-mm collimation and intervals with a pitch of 1 to 1.5 in the chest. In obese patients, consider 8-mm collimation in the abdomen and pelvis and 10-mm in the chest.

1.4 PROBLEM-ORIENTED APPROACH TO SCANNING

- The optimal scanning parameters will vary depending on the specific clinical presentation and questions to be addressed by the examination. The following guidelines provide some suggested modifications to the general protocols listed above.

Lung and Mediastinum

- **Lung cancer staging or follow-up:** Routine chest protocol with IV contrast to include adrenals. Obtain additional targeted images with 2- to 3-mm collimation and intervals if lesion <3 cm.
- **Superior sulcus tumor:** Modified chest protocol using IV contrast with 3-mm sections at 3-mm intervals beginning 3 cm above apex and continuing through mass, then 8-mm contiguous sections through rest of lungs and adrenals. Save raw data for targeted reconstruction of images through apex with lung, soft tissue, and bone windows. Consider MRI as first-line imaging modality for better visualization of the brachial plexus and subclavian vessels.
- **Postobstructive pneumonia, consolidation, or abscess:** Chest protocol with additional targeted images using 3-mm collimation and intervals through the central airways. Use IV contrast if a mass is suspected.
- **Tracheal mass:** Central airway protocol. Save data for possible coronal and sagittal reformats or three-dimensional rendering.
- **Lymphoma:** General chest with IV contrast. Consider also scanning the neck if Hodgkin disease and the abdomen and pelvis if non-Hodgkin lymphoma.
- **Breast cancer:** General chest protocol with IV contrast to include adrenals. Inject arm opposite involved breast. It is important to have the arms symmetrically placed above head. The FOV should include the skin edge for radiation therapy planning.
- **Intensive care unit screening:** General chest protocol.

Mediastinum (see separate section on aorta)

- **Adenopathy or middle mediastinal mass:** General chest protocol with IV contrast. Give barium paste for middle mediastinal masses. Begin with 5-mm noncontrast images through the mass if duplication cyst suspected. Obtain ROI measurements in cystic lesions.
- **Posterior mediastinal mass:** General chest protocol with IV contrast and barium paste. Begin with 5-mm noncontrast images through the mass if duplication cyst suspected. Include bone windows to evaluate potential spine involvement. Consider MRI as primary modality. Obtain ROI measurements in cystic lesions.
- **Thymoma or anterior mediastinal mass:** General chest protocol with IV contrast beginning at cricoid to include thyroid.
- **Ectopic parathyroid:** General chest protocol with IV contrast using 5-mm collimation and intervals. Include neck.
- **Possible mediastinitis:** General chest protocol with IV contrast. Include bone windows.

- **Esophageal cancer:** General chest and abdomen protocols with IV contrast. Give barium paste on table before scan. Include adrenals and give 8 oz of oral contrast if chest only.

Pulmonary

- **Pulmonary metastases or multiple pulmonary nodules:** Chest protocol. Use 8-mm collimation with 5-mm reconstruction interval if small nodules (melanoma, thyroid) are suspected. Add HRCT imaging (2-mm collimation at 10-mm intervals) if lymphangitic spread suspected.
- **New pulmonary nodule:** General chest protocol without IV contrast, then targeted images with 2-mm collimation and intervals (not needed if clearly benign pattern of calcification).
- **Follow-up pulmonary nodule:** Duplicate previous examination parameters (FOV and collimation) to facilitate direct comparison.
- **Interstitial or occupational lung disease:** Chest protocol without IV contrast supine, then HRCT (1- to 2-mm collimation at 10-mm intervals) prone. Also perform HRCT in expiration in patients with pulmonary function test abnormalities disproportionate to chest radiograph findings, unexplained shortness of breath, or if bronchiolitis obliterans is suspected.
- **Lung transplant or evaluation for volume reduction surgery:** Chest protocol without IV contrast, then HRCT. Targeted spiral evaluation of indeterminate nodules in emphysema patients.
- **Bronchiectasis:** HRCT (2-mm collimation at 10-mm intervals) supine.
- **Arteriovenous malformation:** Chest protocol without contrast to localize lesion, then imaging through lesion every 10s during injection of 100 mL IV contrast.

Pleural

- **Empyema:** Chest protocol with IV contrast. Include the upper abdomen if the empyema is in the lung base.
- **Pleural mass:** Chest protocol with IV contrast. Additional images with targeted FOV and 2- to 3-mm collimation and intervals of the mass. Include bone windows if chest wall invasion suspected.
- **Pleural metastases or malignant effusion:** Chest protocol with IV contrast to include adrenals.
- **Pleural plaques:** Chest protocol without IV contrast. Add prone HRCT if asbestosis is suspected.

Aorta

- **Aortic dissection:** Precontrast images may help to detect thrombosed false lumen. Aorta protocol. Continue through abdomen and pelvis as needed.
- **Acute traumatic aortic injury:** Aorta protocol though chest.
- **Thoracic aortic aneurysm:** Chest and abdomen protocol with IV contrast. May need pelvis depending on extent.
- **Abdominal aortic aneurysm:** Abdomen and pelvis protocol. May also need chest, depending on extent. IV contrast may not be needed for routine follow-up of aneurysm size. Consider ultrasound for asymptomatic follow-up.
- **Possible aneurysm rupture:** Abdomen and pelvis protocol before and after IV contrast. May also need chest, depending on extent.

Abdomen and Pelvis

- **General survey** (pain, weight loss, trauma, intensive care unit): Abdomen and pelvis protocol with IV and oral contrast.
- **Abscess:** Abdomen and pelvis protocol with IV and oral contrast.
- **Bowel obstruction:** Abdomen and pelvis protocol with IV contrast. Oral contrast is usually not needed.
- **Ischemic bowel:** Abdomen and pelvis protocol with IV contrast. Administration of oral contrast may interfere with subsequent angiography in some cases.
- **Diverticulitis:** Abdomen and pelvis protocol with IV and oral contrast.
- **Cancer staging:** Abdomen and pelvis protocol with IV and oral contrast. Consider adding precontrast liver images for breast cancer and melanoma and triple-phase liver images for islet cell tumors and carcinoid. Include bone windows for prostate or breast cancer.
- **Lymphoma:** Abdomen and pelvis protocol with IV and oral contrast. May also need neck and chest.
- **Pelvic mass in a woman** (cervical, ovarian, or endometrial cancer): Abdomen and pelvis protocol with IV and oral contrast. Scan caudal to cephalad and consider 5-mm collimation with 5-mm intervals in the pelvis.
- **Postpartum fever** (possible ovarian vein thrombosis): Abdomen and pelvis protocol with IV and oral contrast. Add 30-s delay, or use test injection to optimize venous enhancement.
- **Retroperitoneal bleed:** Abdomen and pelvis protocol without oral or IV contrast. Consider contrast if there are other clinical questions.

Liver

- **Metastases:** Abdomen and pelvis protocol with IV and oral contrast. Consider adding precontrast images or using triple-phase protocol to detect hypervascular metastases such as breast cancer, melanoma, islet cell tumors, or carcinoid. Include bone windows for breast cancer.
- **Primary tumor** (focal nodular hyperplasia, hepatocellular carcinoma, adenoma): Triple-phase liver protocol.
- **Cirrhosis or pre–liver transplant:** Triple-phase liver protocol with delayed images at 5 min. Complete the abdomen and pelvis with 5-mm collimation at 8-mm intervals in the portal venous phase.
- **Sclerosing cholangitis or suspected cholangiocarcinoma:** Triple-phase liver protocol with delayed images at 15 min.
- **Common bile duct stones:** Obtain precontrast images through porta hepatis and pancreas with 5-mm collimation at 5-mm intervals, then routine abdomen protocol. Do not use positive oral contrast. Consider MRI pancreatography.
- **Possible Budd-Chiari:** Abdomen protocol with IV and oral contrast. Add 30-s delay to improve hepatic venous contrast. Consider ultrasound as first-line examination to better evaluate veins.
- **Hemangioma:** Triple-phase liver protocol with delayed images through lesion at 2-min intervals (locate lesion on precontrast images). Consider MRI or nuclear medicine tagged-red-cell scintigraphy.

Pancreas/Biliary

- **Pancreatitis:** Abdomen and pelvis protocol with IV and oral contrast.
- **New-onset jaundice:** Abdomen and pelvis protocol with IV and oral contrast. Begin with precontrast liver images using 5-mm collimation at 5-mm intervals and do not give positive oral contrast if stones in the common bile duct are suspected.
- **Pancreatic mass detection:** Dual-phase pancreas protocol. The scan delay should be shortened when an islet cell tumor is suspected.
- **Pancreatic cancer follow-up:** Abdomen and pelvis protocol with IV and oral contrast.

Adrenal Glands

- **Adrenal mass:** Adrenal protocol. Follow with abdomen and pelvis protocol with IV and oral contrast if indicated.

Urinary Tract

- **Renal mass:** Dual-phase renal protocol, then remainder of abdomen and pelvis with 5-mm collimation at 8-mm intervals. Add additional images following a 10-min delay (excretory phase) in patients with a suspected transitional-cell cancer.
- **Ureteral stone:** Renal stone protocol.
- **Hematuria or nephrolithiasis:** Renal protocol with precontrast images and additional images obtained following a 10-min delay to opacify the collecting system.
- **Nephrectomy follow-up:** Abdomen and pelvis protocol with IV and oral contrast.
- **Bladder cancer:** Abdomen and pelvis protocol with IV and oral contrast. Obtain delayed images through bladder. Consider 5-mm collimation with 5-mm intervals in pelvis.

Bibliography

Barnes GT, Lakshminarayanan AV. Conventional and spiral computed tomography: Physical principles and image quality considerations. In: Lee JKT, Stanley RL, Sagel SS, Heiken JP (eds.): *Computed Body Tomography with MRI Correlation*. Philadelphia: Lippincott-Raven, 1998, pp. 1–20.

Bushberg JT, Seibert JA, Leidholdt EM, Boone JM. X ray computed tomography. In: Passano III, WM (ed.): *The Essential Physics of Medical Imaging*. Baltimore: Williams & Wilkins, 1994, pp. 239–290.

Dowsett DJ, Kenny PA, Johnston RE. *The Physics of Diagnostic Imaging*. London: Chapman and Hall, 1998.

Sprawls P, Jr. *Pysical Principles of Medical Imaging*. Gaithersburg: Aspen Publishers, 1993, pp. 343–370.

Wiesen EJ, Miraldi F. Imaging principles in computed tomography. In: Gay SM (ed.): *Computed Tomography and Magnetic Resonance Imaging of the Whole Body*. St. Louis: Mosby-Year Book, 1994, pp. 3–25.

Wolbarst AB. Computed tomography II: Hardware and image quality. *Physics of Radiology*. Norwalk: Appleton & Lange, 1993, pp. 320–334.

Chapter 2

LUNGS

Richard M. Slone

2.1 Anatomy and Technique
2.2 Patterns of Disease
2.3 Atelectasis and Pulmonary Collapse
2.4 Pulmonary Infections
2.5 Interstitial Lung Disease
2.6 Pulmonary Nodules
2.7 Pulmonary Neoplasms
2.8 Bronchogenic Carcinoma
2.9 Congenital and Vascular Pulmonary Lesions
2.10 Large Airway Disease and Bronchiectasis
2.11 Small Airway and Obstructive Lung Disease
2.12 Environmental, Occupational, and Iatrogenic Lung Disease
2.13 Idiopathic Lung Disease
2.14 CT-Guided Biopsy and Thoracic Surgery

2.1 ANATOMY AND TECHNIQUE

Anatomy

- The lungs are divided into lobes by pleural fissures and subdivided into **bronchopulmonary segments** based on bronchial anatomy. The right upper lobe has three segments (apical, posterior, and anterior); the middle lobe two (medial and lateral); and the right lower lobe five (superior, anterior basal, posterior basal, medial basal, and lateral basal). The left upper lobe has four segments (apicoposterior, anterior, superior lingular, and inferior lingular), and the left lower lobe also has four (superior, anteromedial basal, lateral basal, and posterior basal).

  The **secondary pulmonary lobule,** the primary structural unit of the lung, is a polyhedron, measuring 1 to 2 cm on each side, formed by ***interlobular septa*** and containing veins, lymphatics, and connective tissue. The pulmonary lobule is subdivided by ***intralobular septa*** into acini, which are supplied by terminal bronchioles and pulmonary arterioles entering the lobule center. Acini are further divided into alveoli, each 0.3 mm in diameter.

- The **pulmonary arteries** travel with the bronchi, branching into a capillary network lining the alveolar walls. The **pulmonary veins** travel separately from the arteries and bronchi and converge into right and left superior and inferior pulmonary veins, draining into the left atrium. The **bronchial arteries** arise from the aorta and drain into the pulmonary veins and azygos system. They supply blood to the bronchial walls.

- The **lymphatic network** within the peribronchovascular and subpleural connective tissue and septa drains to bronchopulmonary, hilar, and then mediastinal lymph nodes. The American Thoracic Society mapping system is detailed in **Figure 4.3.** Small intrapulmonary lymph nodes are occasionally seen as 2- to 4-mm subpleural nodules.

Technique

- **The lung** is a common site of disease. Imaging, in conjunction with clinical history, is crucial in narrowing the differential diagnosis. **Chest radiography** is the initial imaging technique for evaluating lung disease, but abnormalities are often nonspecific and radiography is insensitive for detecting mild disease. **Computed tomography (CT)** provides excellent localization and characterization of lesions and allows identification of associated mediastinal disease and additional pulmonary lesions not visible on plain film. Contiguous sections should be obtained with 5- to 8-mm collimation through the entire chest, and include the adrenal glands when malignancy is suspected. **Intravenous contrast,** although seldom required for the evaluation of the lung, can help to determine or exclude the vascular nature of a lesion in selected cases.

- **High-resolution CT (HRCT)** is sensitive for detecting and characterizing interstitial and small airway disease. Expiratory HRCT can accentuate differences between normal and abnormal lung parenchyma in patients with air trapping, such as bronchiolitis obliterans.

2.2 PATTERNS OF DISEASE

- **Diffuse lung disease** encompasses a broad array of patterns and etiologies and can be divided into processes primarily involving the airspace, interstitium, airways, or a combination. Interstitial disease is the most frequent, although mixed patterns are common **(Fig. 2.1).** Some diseases have a particular pattern of distribution **(Differential 2.1).** The differential diagnosis can be further refined based on pulmonary volume, chronicity, associated findings, and symptoms. Imaging, clinical data, and pulmonary function testing are all useful in evaluation, but specific diagnosis may require pathologic evaluation.

- An **interstitial pattern** (infiltrate) can be caused by diverse diseases **(Differential 2.2)** which involve the supporting structures and tissue surrounding alveoli. Interstitial disease can present as thickened septa or nodules.

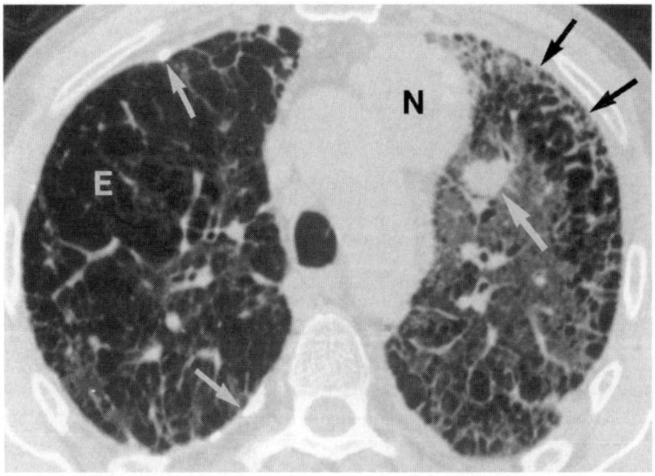

FIGURE 2.1 Asbestos exposure, emphysema, and lung cancer. HRCT in a 55-year-old man shows diffuse lung destruction primarily on the right, characteristic of emphysema (E). There are calcified pleural plaques *(small white arrows)* characteristic of prior asbestos exposure and peripheral fibrosis, seen best on the left, representing asbestosis (*black arrows*). The left upper lobe nodule *(large white arrow)* was proven to be bronchogenic carcinoma. Note massive mediastinal adenopathy (N).

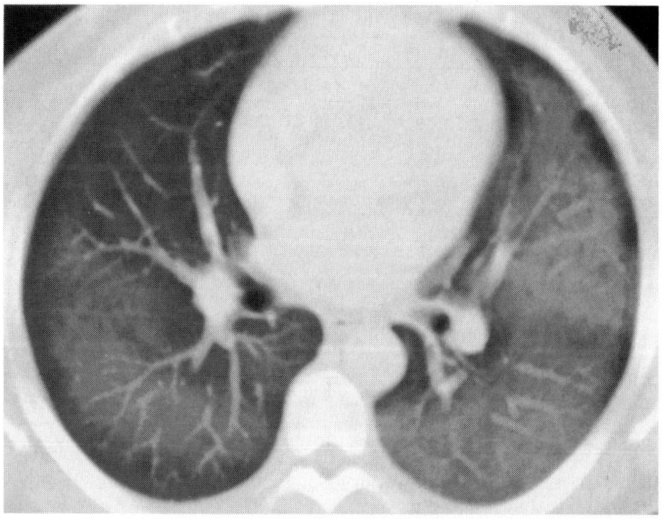

FIGURE 2.2 Noncardiogenic pulmonary edema. CT in a 26-year-old man shows diffuse ground-glass attenuation following cocaine overdose. Note sparing of the lung periphery.

- **Ground-glass** attenuation is an HRCT pattern simulating "frosted glass" and refers to increased parenchymal attenuation with preserved bronchovascular margins **(Fig. 2.2).** This pattern typically reflects an active, acute, and reversible although nonspecific disease process. The most common causes are alveolar inflammation (alveolitis), edema, partial filling of airspaces due to pneumonitis, or, rarely, subtle fibrosis **(Differential 2.3).**
- **Airspace disease** can be diffuse or focal but generally spares the lung periphery, where some interstitial processes are most prominent. In its earliest form, airspace disease can appear as ground-glass attenuation or small ill-defined nodules. These become confluent, resulting in lobular, subsegmental, or lobar **consolidation,** which is depicted as homogenous increased parenchymal attenuation that obscures vessels, producing air bronchograms **(Fig. 2.3).** The most common cause is bacterial pneumonia, but there are many etiologies **(Differential 2.4). Pulmonary hemorrhage** often presents as an airspace pattern **(Fig. 2.4).** The most common causes are bronchiectasis, pulmonary contusion, and vasculititis, particularly

2.1 LUNG DISEASE DISTRIBUTION

Peripheral—fibrosis, BOOP, eosinophilic pneumonia, septic emboli, metastases
Perihilar—pulmonary edema, bronchitis, viral pneumonia, PCP, sarcoidosis
Bronchovascular—sarcoidosis, Kaposi sarcoma
Upper lung—granulomatous disease, cystic fibrosis, sarcoidosis, eosinophilic granuloma, silicosis and coal worker's pneumoconiosis, *ankylosing spondylitis*
Lower lung—pneumonia, atelectasis, pulmonary fibrosis, bronchiectasis, metastases, *Kaposi sarcoma*

Key: BOOP, bronchiolitis obliterans with organizing pneumonia; PCP, *Pneumocystis carinii* pneumonia.

2.2 INTERSTITIAL LUNG DISEASE

Pulmonary edema
Pneumonia—PCP*; *Mycoplasma, H. influenzae;* granulomatous
Pulmonary fibrosis
Sarcoidosis
Tumor–lymphangitic carcinomatosis, leukemia, lymphoma
Hypersensitivity pneumonitis
Eosinophilic granuloma
Rare—lymphocytic interstitial pneumonia, lymphangiectasia, lymphangioleiomyomatosis, tuberous sclerosis, idiopathic pulmonary hemosiderosis, silicosis or coal worker's pneumoconiosis, amyloidosis

**Pneumocystis carinii* pneumonia.

2.3 GROUND-GLASS OPACITIES

Pulmonary edema
Infection—PCP, **bacterial** (alveolitis), **viral** (acute interstitial pneumonitis, CMV), mycobacterial
Fibrosing alveolitis
Connective tissue disease—particularly lupus
Hemorrhage
Hypersensitivity pneumonitis
Bronchiolitis obliterans
Eosinophilic pneumonia
Sarcoidosis
Alveolar proteinosis

Key: PCP, *Pneumocystis carinii* pneumonia; CMV, cytomegalovirus.

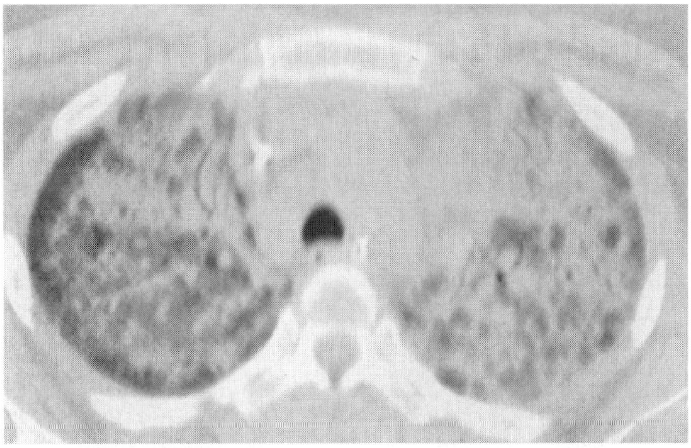

FIGURE 2.3 Acute respiratory distress syndrome. Chest CT shows severe pulmonary consolidation, which spares the lung periphery.

Wegener granulomatosis and Goodpasture disease. Hemorrhage can also result from impaired coagulation, metastases, and, uncommonly, arteriovenous malformations (AVMs), bronchogenic carcinoma, and pulmonary embolism.

- A **nodular pattern** suggests sarcoidosis, aspiration, granulomatous disease, extrinsic allergic alveolitis, bronchoalveolar cell carcinoma (BAC), or lymphoma **(Fig. 2.5). Chronic consolidation** represents recurrent or persistent pneumonia due to bronchial narrowing or obstruction, bronchiectasis, repeated aspiration, cystic fibrosis, or lipoid pneumonia **(Fig. 2.6).** Fungal, mycobacterial, and eosinophilic pneumonias are often chronic. Malignancies, such as BAC or lymphoma, can mimic persistent pneumonia, as can pulmonary sequestration.
- **Decreased pulmonary attenuation** can be seen in emphysema, compensatory hyperinflation, pulmonary artery hypertension (PAH), a right-to-left shunt, bronchiolitis obliterans **(Fig. 2.7)**, endobronchial obstruction, thromboembolism, pulmonary artery hypoplasia, congenital lobar emphysema, and congenital bronchial atresia.
- **Air trapping** is due to fixed bronchial narrowing or reactive airway disease from bronchial spasms in asthma or chronic obstructive

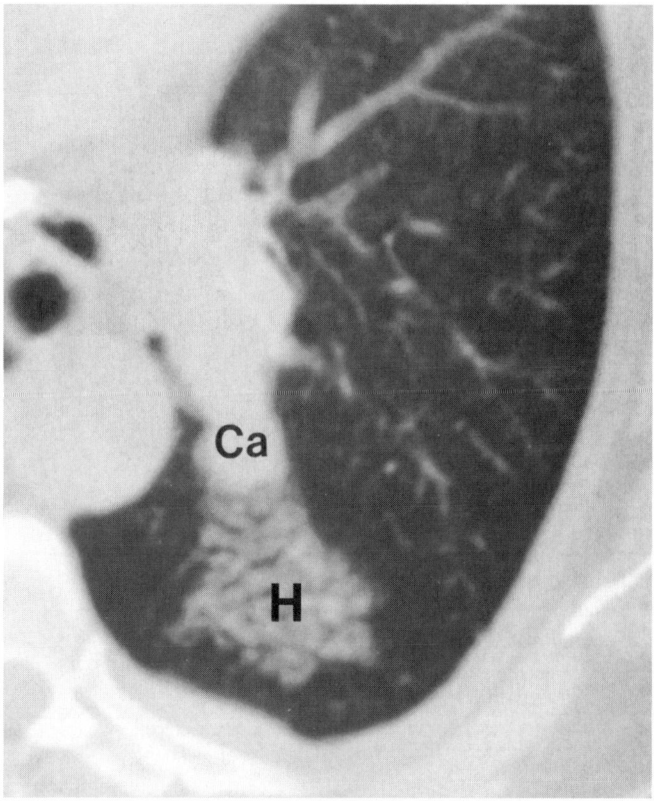

FIGURE 2.4 Pulmonary hemorrhage. Chest CT obtained immediately following CT-guided biopsy of a left lower lobe cancer (Ca) shows a classic pattern of focal airspace disease (H) as a result of bleeding.

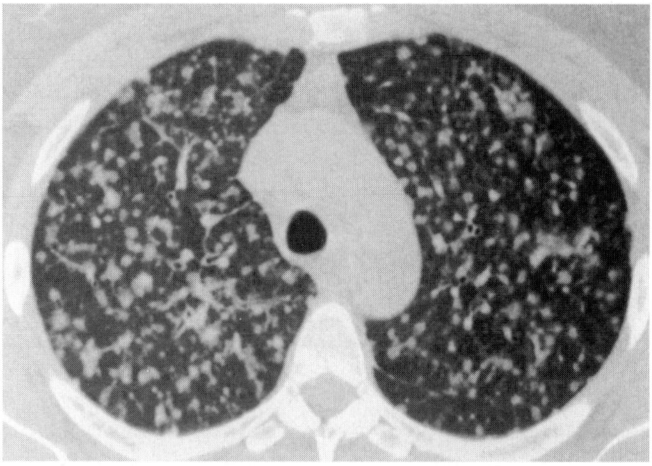

FIGURE 2.5 Bronchoalveolar cell carcinoma (BAC). HRCT in a 48-year-old woman shows innumerable small pulmonary nodules proven to be widespread BAC. (From Slone RM, Gutierrez FR, Fisher, AJ. *Thoracic Imaging: A Practical Approach*. New York: McGraw-Hill; 1999. With permission.)

2.4 PULMONARY CONSOLIDATION

Pneumonia—bacterial, aspiration, postobstructive; mycoplasma; mycobacterial—tuberculosis, BOOP; fungal; lipoid
Pulmonary hemorrhage
Pulmonary edema and ARDS
Pulmonary infarct
Tumor—BAC and lymphoma
Eosinophilic pneumonia
Sarcoidosis
Hypersensitivity pneumonitis
Radiation pneumonitis
Alveolar proteinosis
Pulmonary sequestration

Key: BOOP, bronchiolitis obliterans with organizing pneumonia; ARDS, acute respiratory distress syndrome; BAC, bronchoalveolar cell carcinoma.

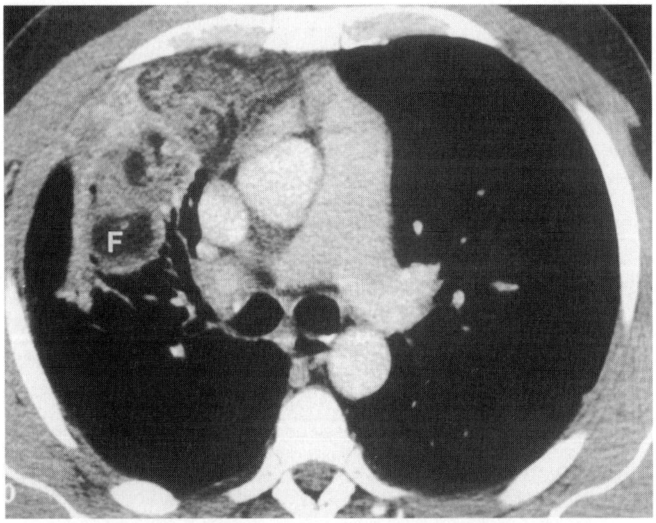

FIGURE 2.6 Lipoid pneumonia. A 36-year-old man with pneumonia. Although his symptoms improved with antibiotics, the radiographic abnormality persisted. Contrast-enhanced CT shows complex mass-like consolidation in the right upper lobe, with areas of fat attenuation (F) representing aspirated lipids.

pulmonary disease. It is also a characteristic finding in bronchiolitis obliterans. **Expiratory HRCT** is sensitive for demonstrating the differential attenuation between areas of air trapping and normal lung **(Fig. 2.8).**

- **Mosaic perfusion** is a lobular patchwork of varied attenuation due to regional differences in perfusion. The more lucent, oligemic lung has fewer and smaller pulmonary vessels compared with normal lung. Causes include thromboembolic disease, cystic fibrosis, and

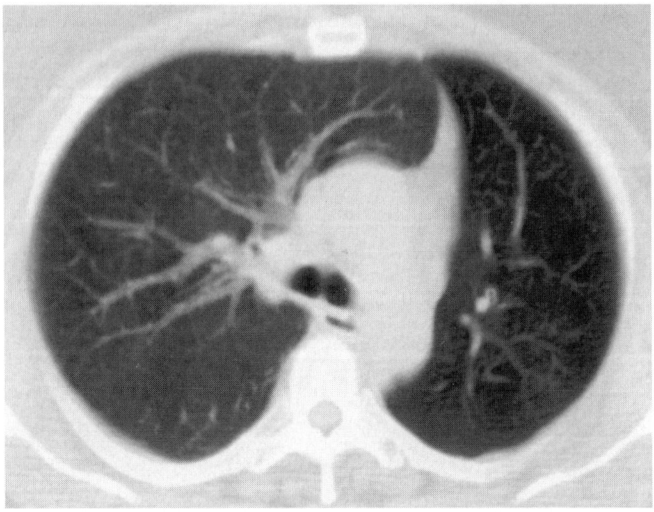

FIGURE 2.7 Swyer-James syndrome. Chest CT in a 54-year-old woman with a history of severe pneumonia as a child. A small, lucent left lung is seen, with decreased vessel size and number. (From Pickhardt PJ, Fisher KC. Unilateral hypoperfusion or absent perfusion on pulmonary scintigraphy; differential diagnosis. *AJR* 1998; 171:145–150. With permission.)

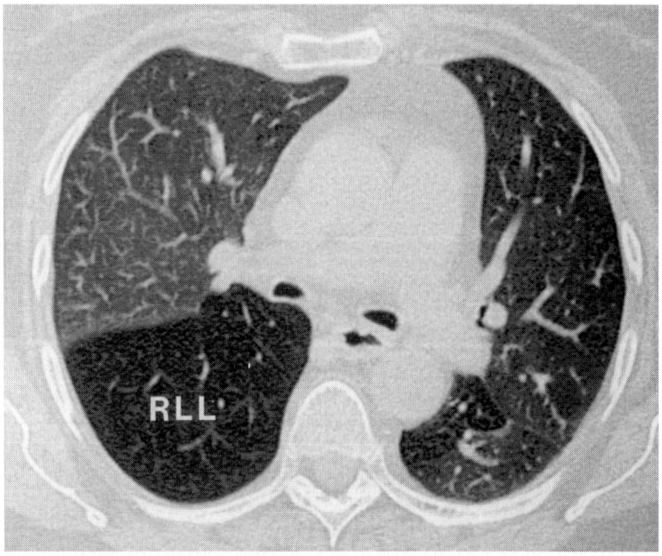

FIGURE 2.8 Air trapping from bronchial obstruction. HRCT in expiration shows a lucent right lower lobe (RLL) in contrast to normal lung that has increased attenuation and decreased in volume. This patient had an endobronchial foreign body. (From Sagel SS, Slone RM. The lung. In: Lee JKT, Sagel SS, Stanley RJ, Heiken JP (eds.): *Computed Body Tomography with MRI Correlation.* Philadelphia: Lippincott-Raven; 1998. With permission.)

bronchiolitis obliterans. **Mosaic attenuation** can be produced by infiltrative or inflammatory lung disease, with patchy areas of high attenuation, but there is no variation in vessel size. Patients with small airway disease, such as asthma or bronchiolitis obliterans, can have mosaic attenuation only on expiration, with lucent areas of air trapping adjacent to normal parenchyma.

- **Cystic lung disease** comprises abnormal pulmonary airspaces from inflammatory, congenital, idiopathic, or neoplastic conditions **(Differential 2.5). Bullae**, thin-walled airspaces larger than 1 cm, generally represent emphysema. **Blebs** are airspaces within the pleural layers. A **cyst** is a well-defined airspace lined by epithelium or fibrous tissue but without emphysema **(Fig. 2.9). Honeycomb cysts** are focal airspaces (less than 1 cm in size) formed by pulmonary fibrosis and retraction. Honeycomb cysts and bronchiolectasis become smaller on expiration, since they communicate freely with the airway, whereas bullae maintain their size on expiration.

2.5

LUCENT LESIONS OR CYSTS

Bullae and blebs
Pneumatoceles
Bronchiectasis
Fibrosis with honeycombing
Eosinophilic granuloma
Infection—abscess cavity, prior echinococcal cyst
Neoplasm—necrotic metastases, *tracheobronchial papillomatosis*
Congenital—cystic adenomatoid malformation, congenital lobar emphysema, sequestration
Lymphangioleiomyomatosis and tuberous sclerosis

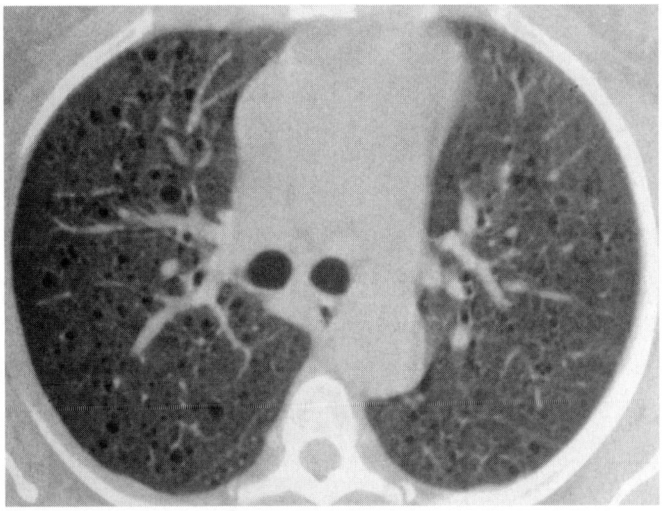

FIGURE 2.9 **Lymphangioleiomyomatosis.** CT in a young woman shows diffusely distributed pulmonary cysts with thin walls.

- **Pneumatoceles** are transient, thin-walled cysts, resulting from overdistention and contained rupture of small airways or alveoli. They are the sequelae of infection, most commonly *Staphylococcus* and less commonly *Klebsiella* and *Pneumococcus*. Pneumatoceles can also occur following trauma or as a complication of hydrocarbon aspiration.
- **Parenchymal high attenuation** can be caused by calcification, iodine, barium, Perflubron (for treatment of acute respiratory distress syndrome, or ARDS), or foreign bodies. Multiple pulmonary calcifications are usually the result of prior granulomatous infections (histoplasmosis or tuberculosis) but can occur with other infections and pneumoconioses. Metastases from osteogenic sarcoma, mucin-producing adenocarcinomas, and treated metastases can also calcify. Areas of **pulmonary ossification** are rare, occurring in chronic cardiopulmonary disease (mitral stenosis), but they can also be idiopathic or associated with hemorrhage or pulmonary fibrosis from chemotherapy, asbestos exposure, hemodialysis, hyperparathyroidism, or metastatic cancer.

2.3 ATELECTASIS AND PULMONARY COLLAPSE

- CT helps clarify the extent and potential etiology of **pulmonary atelectasis.** Collapse refers to a larger degree of atelectasis. The typical patterns of collapse are well known but can vary because of congenital variants or pleural adhesions.
- **Obstructive or resorptive atelectasis** is a result of endobronchial tumors, foreign bodies, mucous plugging, or occasionally benign strictures. Bronchoscopy can be required when CT is unrevealing. **Compressive atelectasis** results from a mass compressing normal lung, while **passive at electasis** is the result of decreased thoracic volume from pleural effusion **(see Fig. 3.6)** or pneumothorax. **Adhesive atelectasis** is seen in respiratory distress syndrome and pulmonary embolism. **Cicatrizing atelectasis** results from pulmonary fibrosis and is common following radiation therapy.
- The **right upper lobe collapses** superiorly and medially, producing a sharply defined triangular density adjacent to the superior vena cava and trachea, bordered by the minor fissure laterally and the major fissure posteriorly. The right hemidiaphragm and hilum will be elevated and the middle and lower lobes hyperexpanded. In **right-middle-lobe collapse,** the opacity contacts the right atrial border **(Fig. 2.10).** The **right lower lobe collapses** posteromedially, retracting the major and minor fissures inferoposteriorly, displacing the hilum inferiorly, and elevating the right hemidiaphragm.
- The **left upper lobe collapses** in an anterosuperior direction, creating a triangular density in the left paramediastinal region **(Fig. 2.11).** The hilum and left hemidiaphragm are elevated and the left lower lobe is hyperexpanded. **Left-lower-lobe collapse** causes downward displacement of the hilum and a triangular left paraspinal density behind the heart **(Fig. 2.12).** The oblique fissure is displaced posteriorly and the hyperexpanded left upper lobe will be lucent.
- **Rounded atelectasis** occurs after a previous exudative pleural effusion that forms adhesions, "trapping" the lung as the fluid reabsorbs. Asbestos exposure is the most common cause. Characteristic CT findings include a swirling of the pulmonary vessels and bronchi, producing a "comet tail" adjacent to the medial aspect of the atelectatic parenchyma **(Fig. 2.13).** The lesion may enlarge over time. Adjacent pleural thickening is always present.

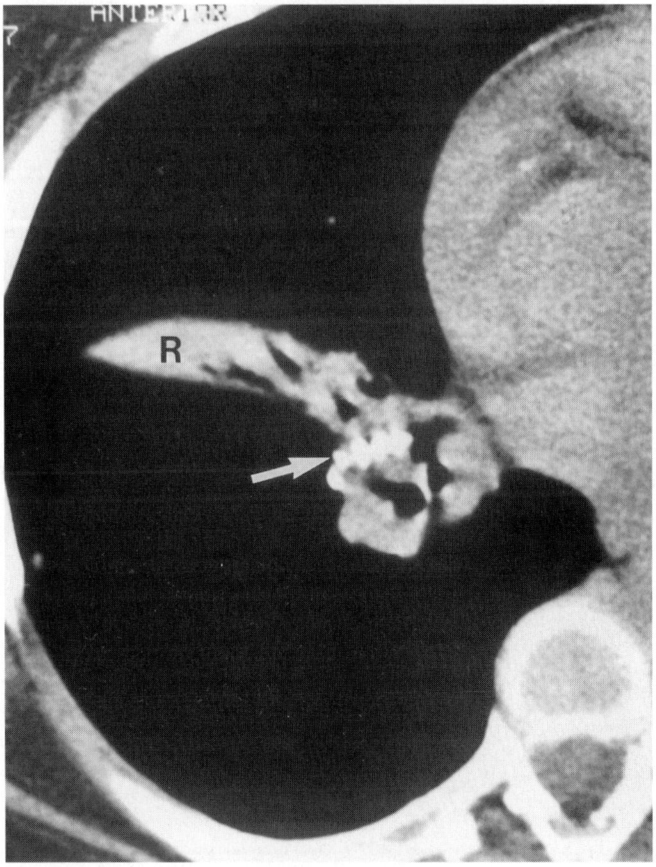

FIGURE 2.10 **Right-middle-lobe syndrome.** CT shows collapse of the lateral segment of the right middle lobe (R) due to obstruction of the segmental bronchus by calcified lymph nodes (broncholithiasis) *(arrow)*.

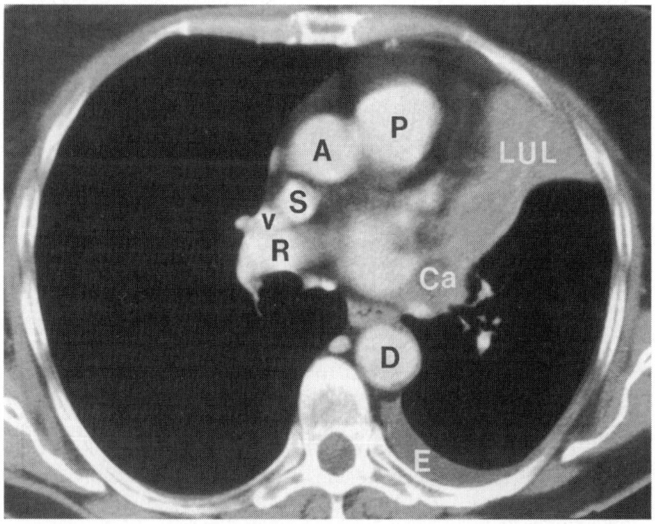

FIGURE 2.11 Left-upper-lobe collapse. Contrast-enhanced CT shows a central bronchogenic carcinoma (Ca) invading the left pulmonary artery and causing left-upper-lobe collapse (LUL). Note small pleural effusion (E). A, ascending aorta; P, pulmonary trunk; S, superior vena cava; R, right pulmonary artery; v, right superior pulmonary vein; D, descending thoracic aorta.

The findings are characteristic, but in atypical cases, close follow-up or biopsy may be necessary to exclude malignancy.

2.4 PULMONARY INFECTIONS

- **Pulmonary infections** result from a variety of organisms and the patterns of disease vary widely. In complex cases, CT can demonstrate features that narrow the differential diagnosis and detect complications such as abscess, empyema, and underlying obstructive lesions **(Fig. 2.14).** The patient's age, clinical symptoms, and predisposing conditions must be taken into account. Pneumonias are grouped as bronchopneumonias, lobar, rounded, or interstitial. **Cavitation,** representing necrosis, suggests a bacterial infection *(Staphylococcus aureus,* gram-negative, anaerobic, mycobacterial).

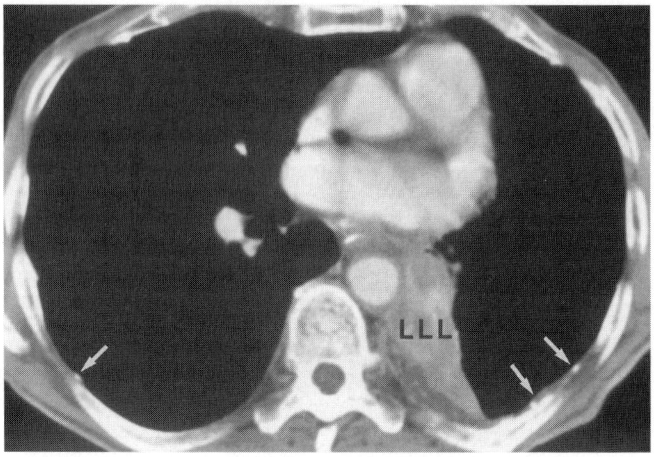

FIGURE 2.12 Left-lower-lobe collapse. A 71-year-old man with bronchogenic carcinoma invading the mediastinum and causing left-lower-lobe collapse (LLL). Note ipsilateral mediastinal shift due to volume loss and calcified pleural plaques *(arrows),* characteristic of prior asbestos exposure.

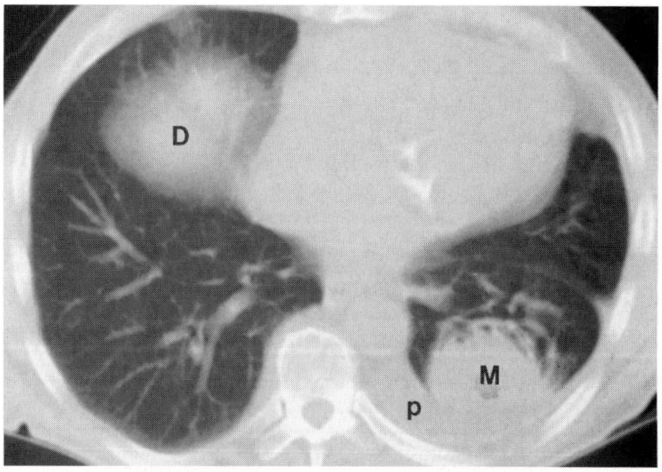

FIGURE 2.13 Rounded atelectasis. Chest CT in a 48-year-old man with a left-lower-lobe mass (M) that developed several years following coronary artery bypass surgery. Note the ill-defined margins, "swirling" of adjacent bronchovascular markings, and adjacent pleural thickening (p). D, dome of the right hemidiaphragm.

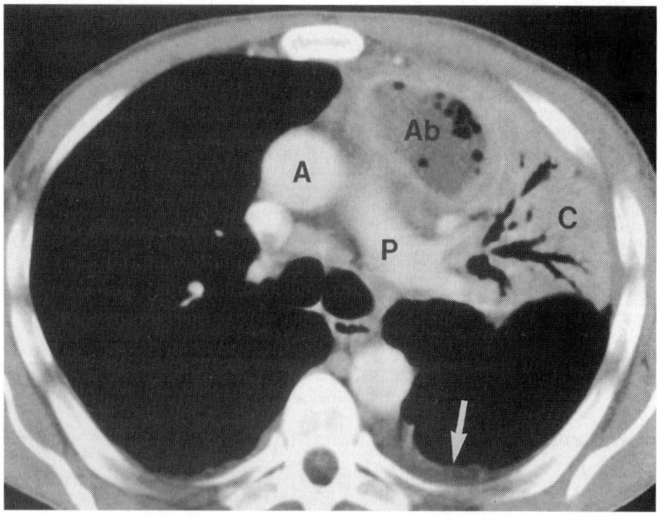

FIGURE 2.14 Pneumonia with lung abscess. Contrast-enhanced CT in a 46-year-old man shows left-upper-lobe consolidation (C) and lung destruction with abscess (Ab) formation. Note small peripneumonic pleural effusion *(arrow).* P, pulmonary trunk; A, ascending aorta.

- **Bronchopneumonia,** characterized by a patchy distribution and volume loss, is common. **Lobar pneumonia** with partial or complete lobar consolidation can be multifocal. Air bronchograms are present, and lung volumes are usually preserved. *Streptococcus, Klebsiella,* tuberculosis, and postobstructive infections are common. **Round pneumonia** is mass-like consolidation that does not follow lobar boundaries. It is much more common in children, typically occurring in the superior segments of the lower lobes.
- **Interstitial pneumonia** (infiltrate) is a pattern of septal or peribronchial inflammation, often with associated atelectasis. This pattern can be seen with viral, mycoplasmal, and *Pneumocystis carinii* infections and can be difficult to differentiate from other causes of interstitial lung disease. A **miliary pattern** of 2- to 4-mm nodules is an unusual presentation that can be seen with tuberculosis, histoplasmosis, and varicella.
- **Mycoplasmal pneumonia** is a common community-acquired infection with variable symptoms and does not respond to usual antibiotic regimens. Skin rash, gastroenteritis, and myalgias are frequent. Reticular interstitial infiltrates can progress to patchy or focal consolidation. Small pleural effusions develop in 20 percent. The diagnosis can be determined serologically.

Bacterial Pneumonia

- Bacterial pneumonias can occur de novo or complicate viral infections as a result of impaired mucociliary action. Pleural effusions are common and, when present, argue against a purely viral infection. Bacterial infections are either community-acquired or nosocomial.
- **Streptococcal** (pneumococcal) pneumonia is the most common community-acquired bacterial pneumonia. Lobar consolidation with air bronchograms is classic, but the infection can also form patchy interstitial infiltrates and spread across segmental boundaries. Pleural effusions are common and can become infected, creating an empyema. **Staphylococcal** pneumonia is a frequent cause of bronchopneumonia in old or debilitated patients, sometimes complicating viral influenza. It begins as bilateral patchy infiltrates that spread to involve several lobes. Volume loss, concomitant pleural effusions, abscess formation, and pneumatoceles are common.
- **Gram-negative pneumonias** (due to *Klebsiella, Enterobacter, Escherichia coli,* and *Haemophilus influenzae)* are frequently hospital-acquired, occurring in patients with predisposing or debilitating conditions. Patchy consolidation, segmental or lobar involvement, and ill-defined nodules can be seen. Pleural effusions, cavitation, and empyema formation are common.
- **Legionnaire disease** is due to *Legionella pneumophila,* an organism found in water towers and humidifiers. Systemic symptoms are frequently associated with rapidly developing peripheral consolidation, which is often bilateral and resolves slowly. Pleural effusions and empyema are common. The diagnosis is confirmed serologically.
- **Actinomycosis** is due to a gram-positive anaerobe *(Actinomyces israeli),* formerly classified as a fungus, that is part of the normal oral flora and can proliferate in immunocompromised patients or injured tissues. Pulmonary infection usually results from aspiration in patients with poor oral hygiene. Fever, chills, chest pain, and weight loss are typical. CT usually shows focal consolidation which can extend across fissures **(Fig. 2.15)** or into the chest wall. Pleural thickening, empyema, as well as destruction of ribs and spine can occur adjacent to the pulmonary consolidation. Cavitation, pleural effusions, empyema, and adenopathy are common. Penicillin is the treatment of choice, and drainage is often required.

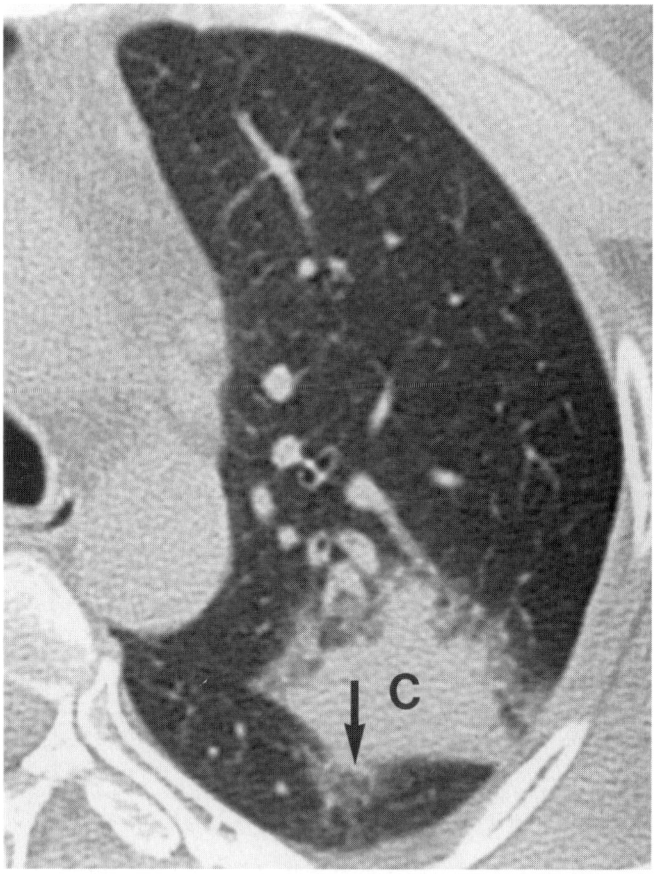

FIGURE 2.15 Actinomycosis. HRCT shows a focal area of consolidation (C), which is spreading through the major fissure *(arrow)*—a sign of an aggressive process. Lower images revealed cavitation.

- **Aspiration pneumonia** is most common in the posterior segment of the right upper lobe **(Fig. 2.16)** and superior segments of the lower lobes. Chemical pneumonitis can be followed by bacterial superinfection. Anaerobic bacteria and polymicrobial infections are common. Necrotizing pneumonia and abscess are frequent. Chronic aspiration leads to scarring and bronchiectasis.
- A **lung abscess** is the result of parenchymal destruction by a necrotizing pneumonia due to such organisms as *Staphylococcus, Klebsiella,* or *Pseudomonas* following aspiration or hematogenous seeding. A central lung abscess can be difficult to distinguish from a cavitary neoplasm, and a peripheral abscess can be difficult to distinguish from an empyema. Differentiation is crucial because an empyema requires thoracostomy tube drainage, whereas a lung abscess is managed with antibiotics and postural or bronchoscopic drainage.

  An **abscess** is spherical and lung destruction results in abrupt termination of bronchi and vessels at its margin **(Fig. 2.14).** An **empyema** is oval or crescentic, forming an obtuse angle with the

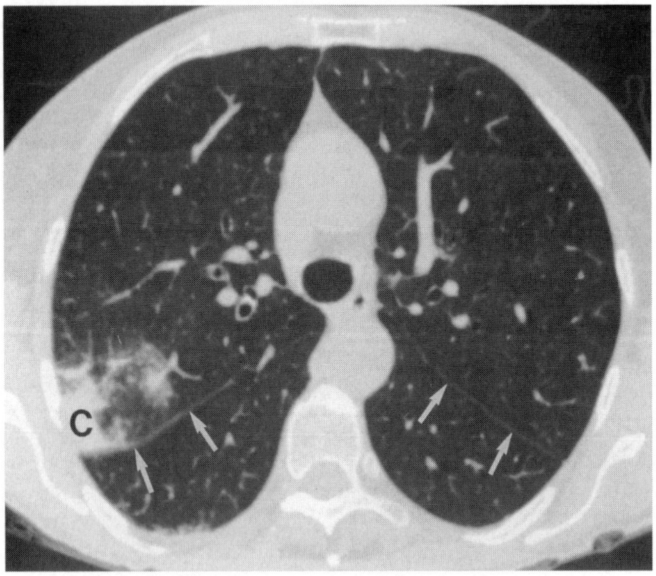

FIGURE 2.16 Aspiration pneumonia. HRCT in a 75-year-old woman shows a focal area of consolidation in the posterior segment of the right upper lobe (C). Note the major fissures *(small arrows)* separating the superior segment of the lower lobe from the upper lobe. [From Sagel SS, Slone RM. The lung. In: Lee JKT, Sagel SS, Stanley RJ, Heiken JP (eds.): *Computed Body Tomography with MRI Correlation.* Philadelphia: Lippincott-Raven; 1998. With permission.]

pleura. There is displacement of adjacent lung and atelectasis **(see Fig. 3.10).** An air-fluid level can be seen in a lung abscess due to communication with the bronchial tree or in an empyema as a result of a bronchopleural fistula. Consolidated lung, pleural fluid, and septate collections can be associated with either an empyema or lung abscess. Some patients have both an abscess and empyema **(see Fig. 3.11).**

Viral Pneumonia

- Most **viral pneumonias** begin as bronchitis and bronchiolitis, with patchy multifocal interstitial infiltrates, and may evolve to more confluent opacities that are difficult to differentiate from superimposed bacterial infection. Pleural effusions and cavitation are uncommon.

  Influenza is a common cause of respiratory infections and associated bacterial infection is common. **Adenovirus** infections in children and young adults produce air trapping and lobar collapse due to bronchial and peribronchial inflammation with bronchiolitis obliterans. Bronchiectasis and Swyer-James syndrome **(see Fig. 2.7)** are sequelae of adenovirus infection.

  Respiratory infections also occur by dissemination of a virus that primarily affects the skin. Disseminated **varicella zoster** causes severe pneumonia in immunocompromised adults afflicted with chickenpox. The skin rash invariably precedes the pneumonia by several days. Mortality approaches 10 percent. CT demonstrates innumerable tiny pulmonary nodules, which can become confluent. The nodular densities can disappear within a few days, persist for months, or calcify. Hilar adenopathy and small effusions can occur. Measles **(rubeola)** causes pneumonia with widespread reticular infiltrates, lobar atelectasis, and hilar adenopathy. CT findings clear slowly.

Fungal Infections

- Pulmonary fungal infections are usually the result of inhaled yeasts or molds, although normal flora, such as *Candida,* can infect immunocompromised patients. Fungi in the lungs can remain localized or disseminate via bronchial, hematogenous, or lymphatic routes, producing severe and potentially fatal infection. Disease extent depends on pathogen virulence, infecting dose, and host immune status.

- **Pulmonary aspergillosis,** due to *Aspergillus fumigatus,* is common in patients with bronchial asthma and chronic pulmonary disease. It produces a spectrum of disease ranging from simple colonization to life-threatening invasive infection in immunocompromised patients. Nodules of aspergillosis infection are often associated with surrounding increased parenchymal density from hemorrhage or edema, a nonspecific pattern called the **"CT halo sign" (Fig. 2.17).** A **fungus ball** (mycetoma or aspergilloma) results from colonization of a preexisting cavity by mycelial hyphae. The upper lobes are most common. CT demonstrates a crescent of air between the mass and the cavity wall. Repositioning the patient can show mobility of the fungus ball **(Fig. 2.18).**

  Allergic bronchopulmonary aspergillosis (ABPA) from colonization of the proximal bronchi is seen in asthmatics who develop sensitivity to the fungus. It presents as central, upper-lobe-predominant bronchiectasis with normal peripheral bronchi **(Fig. 2.19).** Mucous

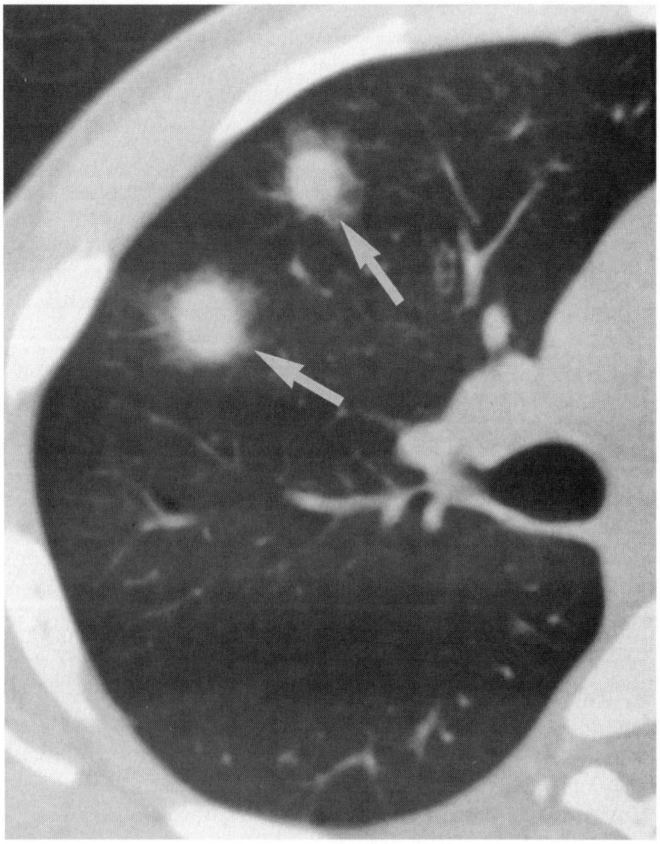

FIGURE 2.17 Aspergillus infection with CT halo sign. Chest CT shows nodules with surrounding ground-glass attenuation *(arrows)* representing hemorrhage from an *Aspergillus* infection.

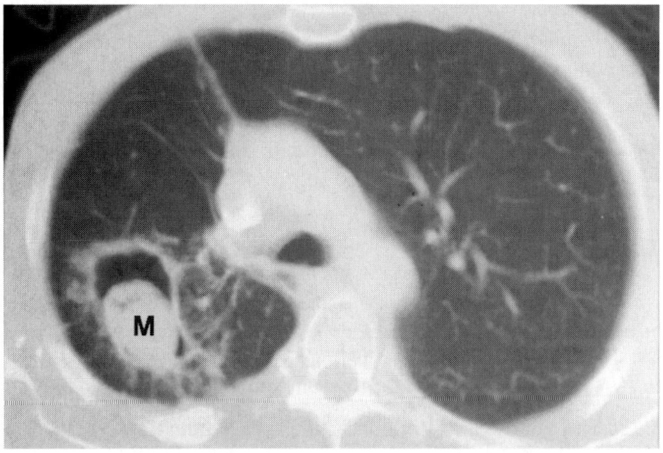

FIGURE 2.18 Aspergilloma. Chest CT in a 55-year-old man shows a mass (M), proven to be a mycetoma, within a thin-walled cavity, presumably the sequela of tuberculosis. There is surrounding fibrosis and associated volume loss. The mass was shown to be mobile when the patient was scanned in a prone position.

impaction in bronchi creates branching opacities described as "finger in glove." Atelectasis and transient pneumonitis can be seen and pulmonary fibrosis can develop. Patients have blood eosinophilia, a positive skin reaction, and elevated serum IgE.

- **Histoplasmosis** is due to *Histoplasma capsulatum,* an organism found in soil and the excrement of birds and bats. It is endemic in the central United States. Most infected individuals are asymptomatic. Severity is related to the quantity of exposure. A focal infiltrate eventually clears, commonly leaving a focus of calcification. Calcific hilar and mediastinal adenopathy is common **(Fig. 2.20).**

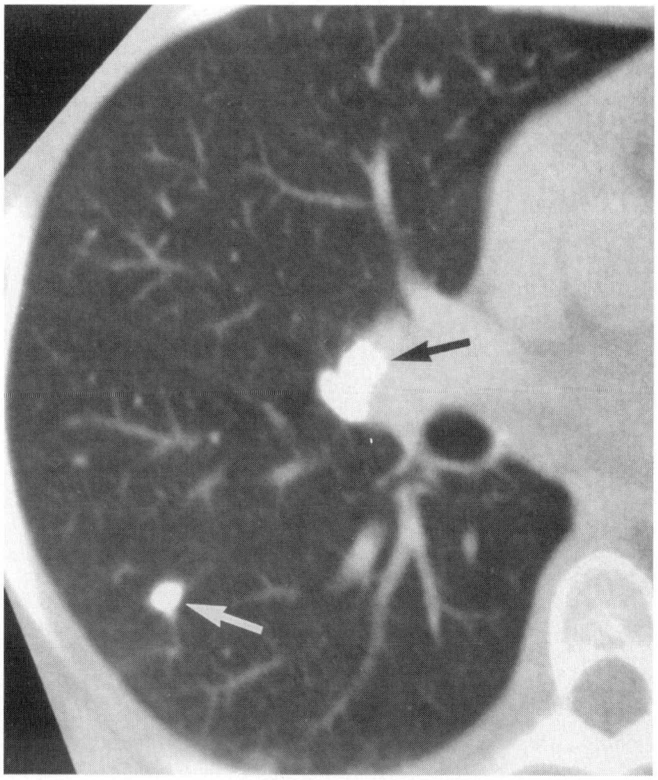

FIGURE 2.20 Old healed granulomatous disease. Chest CT shows a calcified pulmonary nodule *(white arrow)* and calcified hilar adenopathy *(black arrow).*

A disseminated pneumonia with miliary infiltrates can be seen with massive exposure (cave exploration) or in immunocompromised patients. High fever, respiratory failure, and hepatosplenomegaly can be present. **Complications** of histoplasmosis include fibrosing mediastinitis, pericarditis, and broncholithiasis **(see Fig. 2.10),** with erosion of calcified granulomas into the airways. A **histoplasmoma** is a well-defined necrotic focus of infection surrounded by an inflammatory reaction. It frequently calcifies, but slow growth may simulate bronchogenic carcinoma.

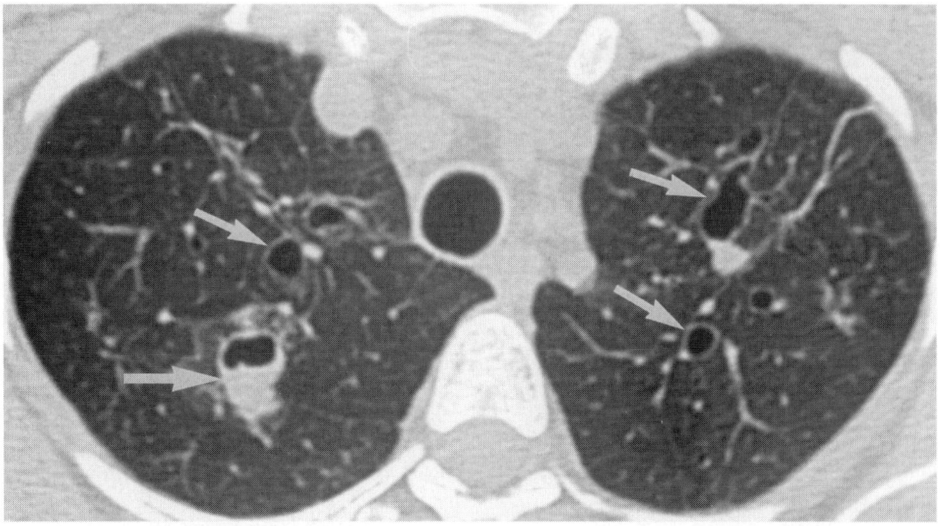

FIGURE 2.19 Allergic bronchopulmonary aspergillosis. CT shows central cylindrical bronchiectasis *(small arrows),* some with mucus plugging *(large arrow).* (From Slone RM, Gutierrez FR, Fisher, AJ. *Thoracic Imaging: A Practical Approach.* New York: McGraw-Hill; 1999. With permission.)

- **North American blastomycosis** is caused by *Blastomyces dermatitidis,* which is present in soil and can spread hematogenously to the gastrointestinal tract, skin, or skeleton following pulmonary infection. Small nodular lesions or consolidation with cavitation can mimic tuberculosis or cancer **(Fig. 2.21).** Pleural effusions and thickening are common, and blastomycosis can invade the chest wall, simulating an aggressive neoplasm. Adenopathy is uncommon.

- **Cryptococcosis** is caused by *Cryptococcus neoformans,* found in

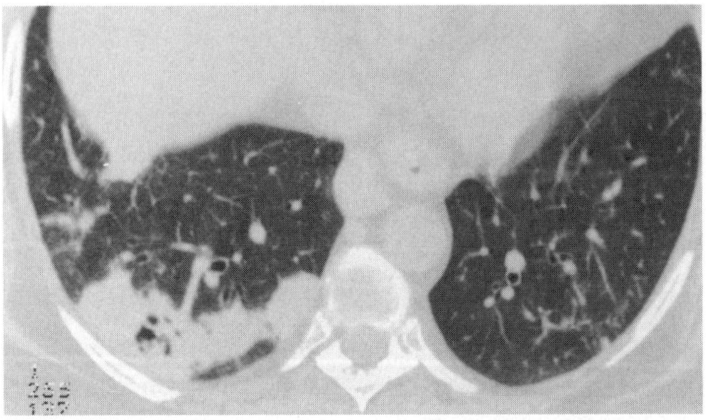

FIGURE 2.21 Blastomycosis. HRCT in a 53-year-old woman shows multifocal confluent nodular opacities with cavitation in the right lower lobe.

pigeon droppings; it is a facultative intracellular yeast infecting immunocompromised patients or individuals with chronic lung disease. Pulmonary patterns vary from patchy interstitial infiltrates to nodules or mass-like areas of consolidation, which can cavitate and simulate lung cancer. Pleural effusions and adenopathy occur, particularly in immunocompromised individuals. Pulmonary infection can lead to systemic dissemination, causing meningitis and encephalitis.

- **Coccidioidomycosis,** caused by *Coccidioides immitis,* is endemic in southwestern North America and Latin America. Patients can develop flu-like symptoms after a short incubation period, but most are asymptomatic. A few patients have persistent symptoms or infiltrates. Pulmonary findings depend on the severity of infection. Early patchy infiltrates can be accompanied by adenopathy and, less frequently, by pleural effusions. There is an upper-lobe and peripheral predominance, and cavitation similar to that in tuberculosis is common. The infiltrates can become nodular, multiple, or miliary in cases of hematogenous spread. In immunocompromised patients, dissemination to the skin, bone, lymph nodes, and urinary tract may occur.

Mycobacterial Infections

- **Tuberculosis (TB),** due to *Mycobacterium tuberculosis,* is the most common pulmonary mycobacterial infection. Acquired by inhalation of aerosolized bacilli from infected individuals, TB is widespread in underdeveloped countries, areas with poor sanitation, and the AIDS population. Pulmonary features include lymphadenopathy, parenchymal consolidation, collapse, cavitation, and pleural effusion or thickening. Multidrug therapy is necessary, and resistant organisms are increasingly common.

  In **primary tuberculosis,** phagocytized organisms are carried to regional lymph nodes and patients can be asymptomatic or present with flu-like symptoms. In most cases, a focal peripheral infiltrate and ipsilateral adenopathy can be identified **(Gohn complex),** but patients occasionally present with adenopathy alone. Pleural effusions are common but cavitation is uncommon. In most cases, the immune response inhibits disease progression and later fibrosis—often with calcification—eventually develops. In malnourished or immunodeficient patients, the disease can rapidly progress to caseation, bronchopneumonia, or miliary tuberculosis **(Fig. 2.22).**

  A **tuberculoma** is a well-defined chronic granulomatous lesion that can mimic a neoplasm if calcification is absent. Chronic infection also leads to pulmonary scarring and distortion with traction bronchiectasis and bronchial stenosis. Calcified tuberculous nodes can erode into the bronchus, producing broncholithiasis, or extrinsic bronchial compression that can cause recurrent lobar or segmental collapse. The right middle lobe is frequently affected.

  Secondary tuberculosis is the result of **reinfection** or **reactivation** of "dormant" bacilli due to immunity breakdown. Symptoms include fever, night sweats, and cough. The lung apex and superior segments of the lower lobes are most commonly affected, since the higher oxygen concentration allows aerobic bacilli to proliferate. As the organisms multiply, granulomatous inflammation and consolidation develop. CT can reveal bilateral or multilobar disease with cavitation, which facilitates endobronchial spread **(Fig. 2.23).** Thick-walled cavities with air-fluid levels form and are often multiple. **Miliary tuberculosis** is the result of hematogenous dissemination and is more common in children and immunocompromised adults.

- Less common **"atypical" mycobacterial infections**—due to *Mycobacterium kansasii* and *M. avium-intracellulare* (MAI)—become pathologic in patients with chronic lung disease, debilitation, or altered immune systems. Their disease course can be protracted, extending over several years. Cavitation and reticulonodular infiltrates are common, usually with associated fibrotic changes (fibrocavitary) and focal bronchiectasis **(Fig. 2.24).** It can be difficult to distinguish atypical mycobacterial infections from tuberculosis.

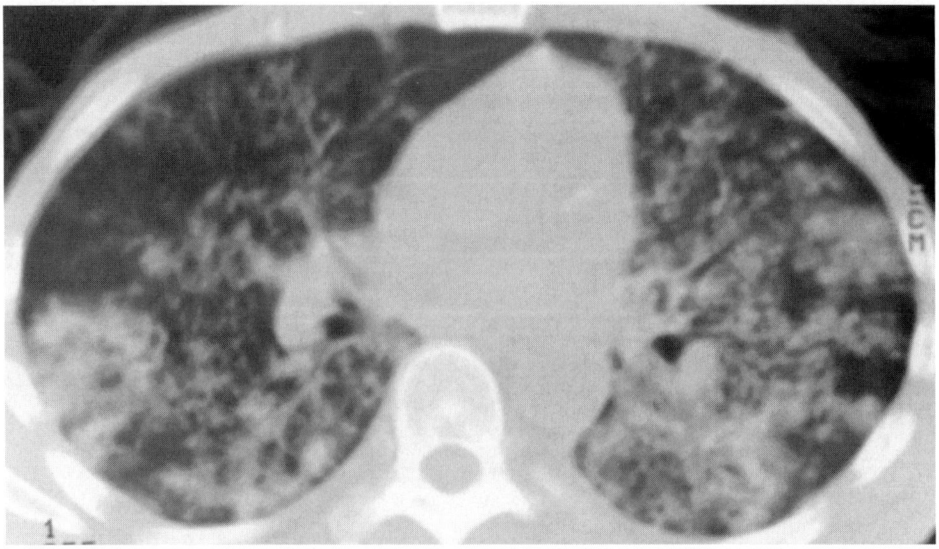

FIGURE 2.22 Tuberculosis. Diffuse nodular infiltrates and multifocal consolidation representing widespread tuberculosis in this 51-year-old man.

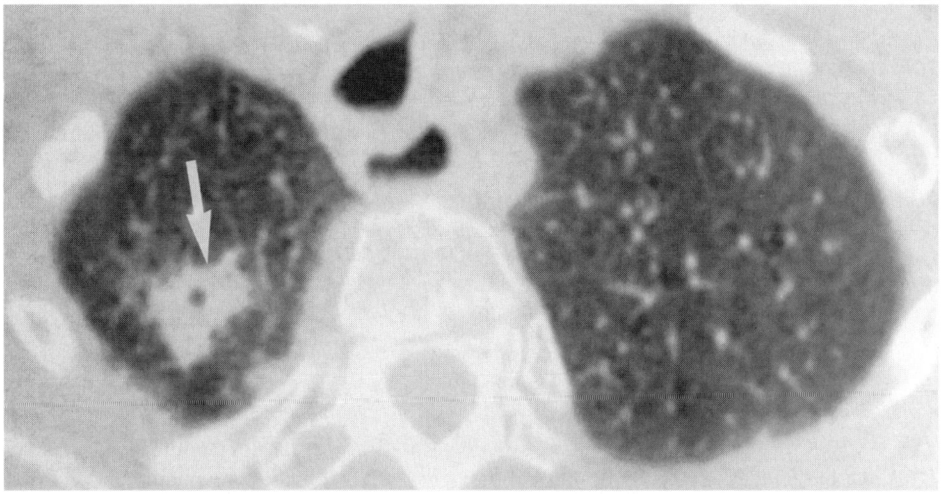

FIGURE 2.23 Tuberculosis. Chest CT through the lung apex shows a focal area of consolidation with central necrosis *(arrow)*. Bronchogenic carcinoma was the leading diagnosis. Transthoracic fine-needle biopsy revealed tuberculosis.

Pleural effusions and adenopathy are uncommon, and there is a poor response to traditional therapy.

Opportunistic Infections

- There has been a dramatic increase in the number of opportunistic infections over the past two decades as a result of AIDS, broad-spectrum antibiotic therapy, immunosuppressive treatment following transplantation, and chemotherapy for cancer. Immune status determines susceptibility, type, and severity of infection.

- The most common **bacterial** infections in immunocompromised patients are due to *S. aureus, Pseudomonas, Legionella,* and *Nocardia*. ***Nocardia*** is especially common in patients with lymphoma, alveolar proteinosis, and leukemia. The findings are similar to those of tuberculosis **(Fig. 2.25).** Nodules can cavitate, and infiltrates and pleural effusions can be present. **Tuberculosis** is a common opportunistic infection. Patterns include primary, reactivation, and miliary infection, depending on the severity of immunosuppression. MAI is also common. **Cytomegalovirus** (CMV) is the most common opportunistic **viral** infection and is common in transplant patients. The most common pattern is diffuse lower-lobe-predominant nodular interstitial infiltrates. Varicella zoster and herpes also occur.

- The most common opportunistic **fungal** infection is caused by *Aspergillus*. **Invasive pulmonary aspergillosis** can produce

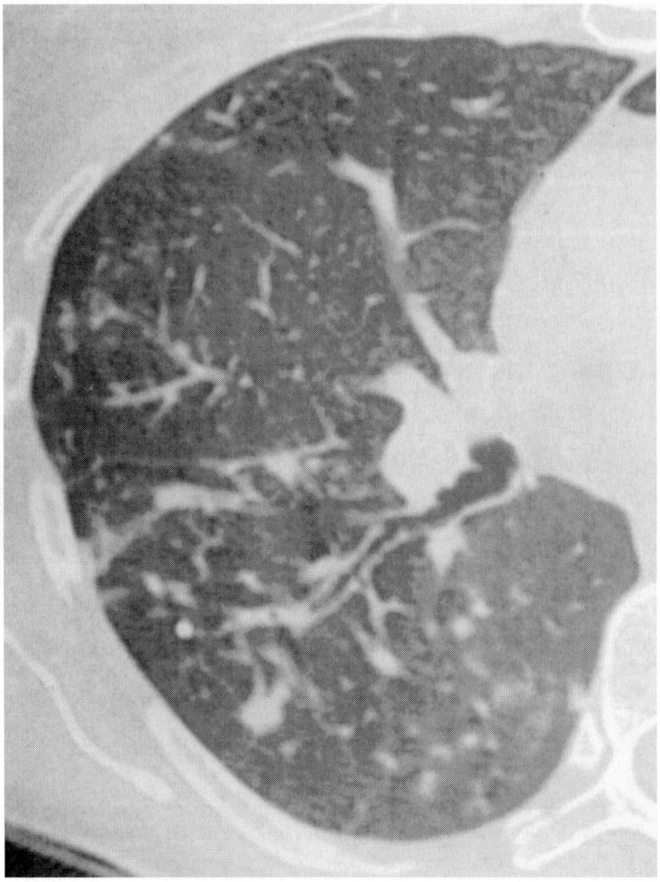

FIGURE 2.24 *Mycobacterium avium intracellulare* (MAI). Chest CT in a middle-aged woman shows a nodular infiltrate and focal bronchiectasis typical of MAI.

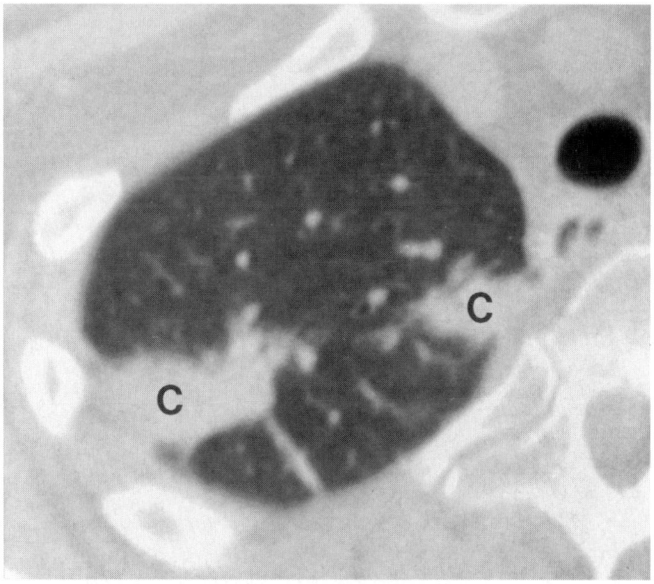

FIGURE 2.25 *Nocardia.* Chest CT in a 61-year-old woman shows two focal areas of "mass-like" consolidation (C) in the right lung apex, shown by fine-needle biopsy to be *Nocardia*.

nonspecific infiltrates and consolidation. This aggressive infection can invade the chest wall and be fatal. Amphotericin B is the treatment of choice, but fewer than 30 percent of patients survive. **Disseminated histoplasmosis** is a rare disease that occurs in patients with AIDS or lymphoma. The most common pattern takes the form of bilateral pulmonary infiltrates or diffuse nodules, similar to miliary tuberculosis.

- **Mucormycosis** is a fungal infection that occurs in patients with diabetes, leukemia, or lymphoma; it is rarely seen in healthy individuals. Mucormycosis is characterized by large, sometimes multiple consolidative masses, which grow insidiously up to but not across pleural boundaries. These organisms erode through bronchial walls and invade vessels, particularly arteries, causing infarction. Infarcted areas tend to be round centrally and wedge-shaped peripherally. Cavitation is common. Diagnosis is difficult and mortality is high even with aggressive treatment.
- Pulmonary infections and tumors in the **AIDS population** have a variable presentation. The CD4 T-lymphocyte count can narrow the differential. The major consideration in patients with consolidation and a CD4 cell count above 200/mm^3 is bacterial pneumonia *(Streptococcus pneumoniae, H. influenzae, Legionella, Mycoplasma,* and *M. tuberculosis).* The most likely diagnosis in patients with CD4 cell counts below 200/mm^3 is *Pneumocystis carinii* pneumonia (PCP), although disseminated fungal infections and Kaposi sarcoma are also prevalent. At CD4 cell counts below 50/mm^3, a reticular or nodular pattern suggests AIDS-related lymphoma, CMV, or MAI infections.
- ***Pneumocystis carinii* pneumonia (PCP)** is the most common opportunistic pulmonary infection in HIV disease. Chest radiographs may be minimally abnormal despite severe respiratory symptoms. A fine, bilateral interstitial or ground-glass appearance, sometimes with patchy consolidation, is the most common CT pattern **(Fig. 2.26).** Lobar consolidation, pleural effusion, and adenopathy are uncommon. Calcified lymph nodes are rare. Pneumatoceles can occur after treatment, and spontaneous pneumothorax can occur. *P. carinii* can be diagnosed by bronchoalveolar lavage.

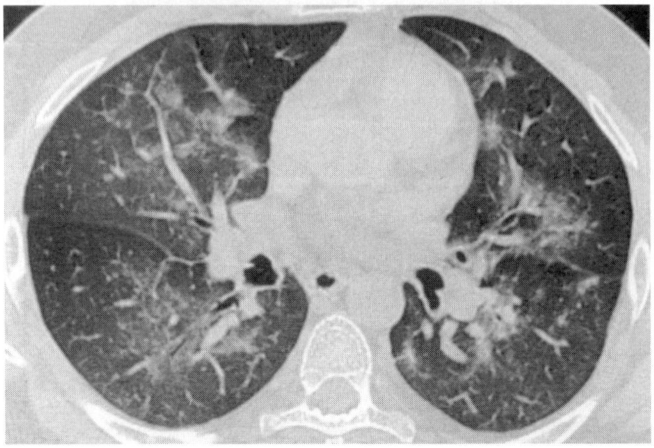

FIGURE 2.26 *Pneumocystis carinii* pneumonia. HRCT in a 40-year-old man shows bilateral perihilar ground-glass attenuation.

2.5 INTERSTITIAL LUNG DISEASE

- **HRCT** is well suited for evaluating interstitial lung disease. The most common and earliest signs are indistinct bronchovascular margins and thickening of the visceral pleura. Fluid or cellular infiltrates in interlobular septa appear as peripheral 1- to 2-cm linear opacities, although visualization of a few peripheral interlobular septa is normal. Most interstitial lung disease results in reduced **lung volumes** and restrictive pulmonary function; normal or increased lung volumes, however, can be seen in eosinophilic granuloma (EG), lymphangioleiomyomatosis (LAM), cystic fibrosis, and coexisting emphysema.
- **Smooth septal thickening** is the result of fluid or cellular infiltrates within the interlobular septa, most commonly from pulmonary edema **(Fig. 2.27)**. There is often a dependent distribution, cardiac enlargement, and pleural effusions. **Irregular or nodular septal thickening** without architectural distortion ***(beaded-septum sign)*** is common in patients with lymphangitic carcinomatosis **(Fig. 2.28)**, sarcoidosis, coal worker's pneumoconiosis, lymphoma, hypersensitivity pneumonitis, EG, and infections (particularly histoplasmosis, mycoplasma, and PCP). **Peribronchovascular** interstitial thickening, distinct from bronchial thickening (bronchi-

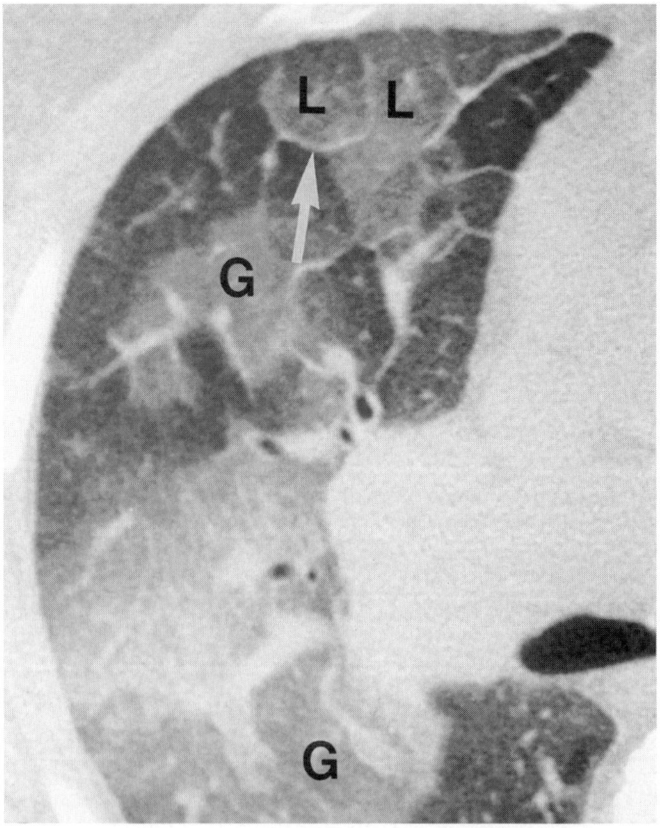

FIGURE 2.27 Smooth septal thickening and ground-glass attenuation. The thickened interlobular septa *(arrow)* outline several secondary pulmonary lobules (L). Note the areas of ground-glass attenuation (G), which increase opacity but do not obscure vessels. [From Sagel SS, Slone RM. The lung. In: Lee JKT, Sagel SS, Stanley RJ, Heiken JP (eds.): *Computed Body Tomography with MRI Correlation.* Philadelphia: Lippincott-Raven; 1998. With permission.]

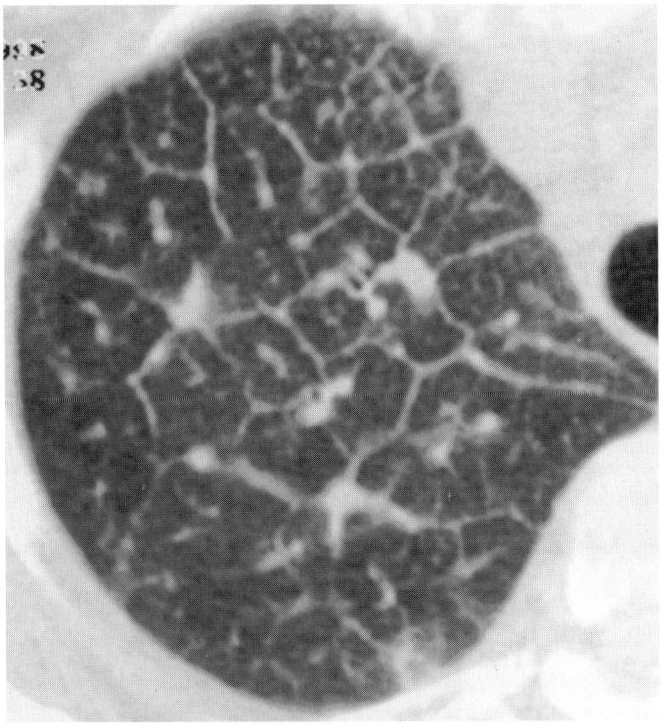

FIGURE 2.28 Lymphangitic spread. HRCT in a 74-year-old woman shows nodular septal thickening in the right lung apex, proven to be interstitial spread of adenocarcinoma.

tis), is common with pulmonary edema, sarcoidosis **(Fig. 2.29)**, lymphangitic carcinomatosis, Kaposi sarcoma, and lymphoma. **Septal thickening** with architectural distortion is the result of pulmonary fibrosis.

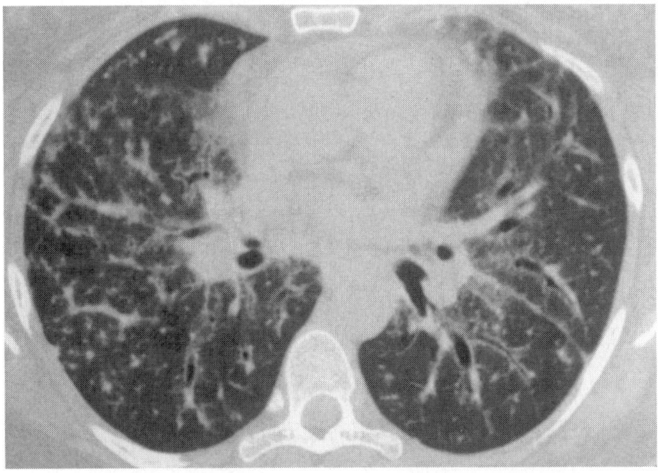

FIGURE 2.29 Sarcoidosis. HRCT in a 42-year-old woman shows nodular peribronchial thickening and ill-defined pulmonary opacities. [From Sagel SS, Slone RM. The lung. In: Lee JKT, Sagel SS, Stanley RJ, Heiken JP (eds.): *Computed Body Tomography with MRI Correlation*. Philadelphia: Lippincott-Raven; 1998. With permission.]

- Associated findings can help narrow the differential diagnosis in patients with interstitial lung disease. **Pleural effusions** can be seen with pulmonary edema, pneumonia, collagen vascular disease, lymphangitic carcinomatosis, lymphoma, leukemia, or LAM. **Adenopathy** is common with sarcoidosis, lymphoma or leukemia, silicosis, infections (particularly fungal and tubercular), and lymphangitic carcinomatosis.
- **Small interstitial nodules** can be seen with inflammatory, occupational, or neoplastic conditions. Close proximity to blood vessels suggests metastases. **Centrilobular nodules** can be seen on HRCT as a result of inflammation of the terminal bronchioles. The ***"tree-in-bud" sign*** is nodular dilatation of the centrilobular branching structures. **(See Sec. 2.6 for more information on small nodules.)**

Pulmonary Fibrosis

- **Pulmonary fibrosis** is irreversible pulmonary scarring caused by infection, chemotherapy, radiation, occupational lung disease, or collagen vascular disease. CT shows irregular septal thickening with architectural distortion **(Fig. 2.30)**. Depending on severity, patients can have dyspnea, dry cough, reduced lung volumes, and eventually pulmonary artery hypertension. A **honeycomb pattern** results from small cystic airspaces and traction bronchiolectasis. **Parenchymal bands** are elongated fibrotic opacities that extend to the pleura. **Subpleural lines** are parallel curvilinear opacities a few millimeters in thickness and less than 1 cm from the pleura that result from fibrosis, atelectasis, edema, or inflammation. CT scans obtained with the patient supine often have an area of gravity-induced ***dependent atelectasis*** adjacent to the posterior chest wall, simulating fibrosis. Prone positioning can be used to reverse the distribution of this microatelectasis and thus can exclude fibrosis **(Fig. 2.31)**.

  Although it is often impossible to determine the etiology of pulmonary fibrosis, its distribution can suggest a specific diagnosis. Idiopathic pulmonary fibrosis (IPF) is subpleural- and lower-lung-predominant. Asbestosis appears similar to IPF but includes pleural plaques or thickening **(Fig. 2.32)**. Connective tissue disease can lead to fibrosis in the lung bases. Chronic hypersensitivity pneumonitis is diffuse, with random areas of ground-glass appearance

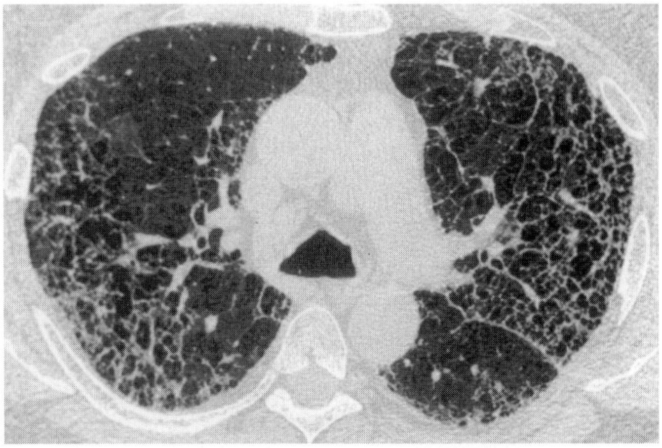

FIGURE 2.30 Idiopathic pulmonary fibrosis. HRCT in a 57-year-old man shows coarse peripheral interstitial septal thickening with associated architectural distortion characteristic of pulmonary fibrosis.

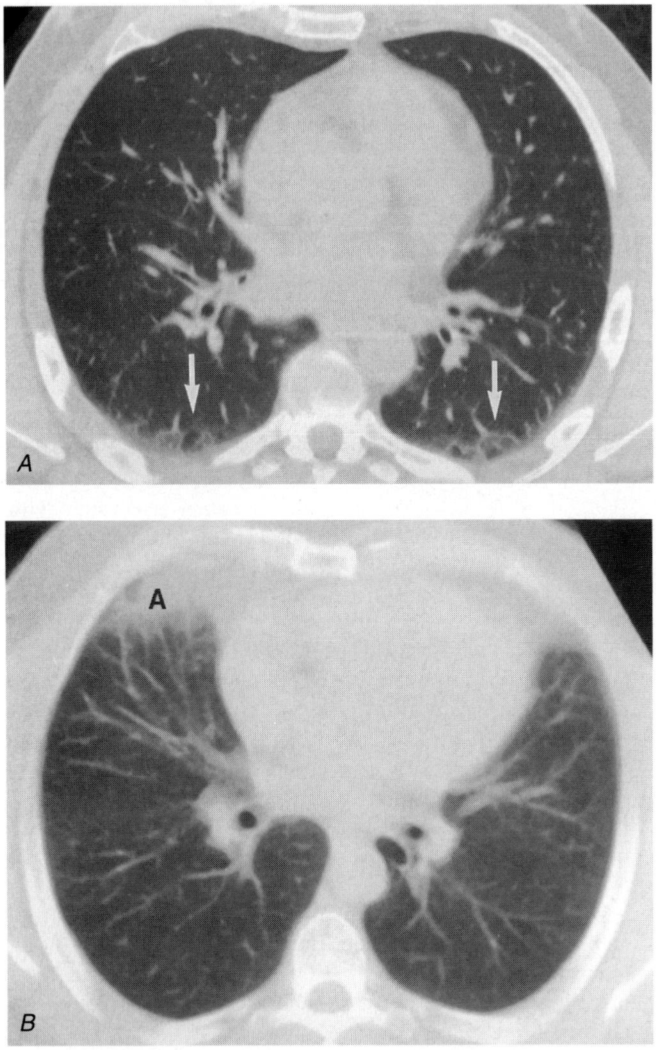

FIGURE 2.31 Dependent atelectasis simulating interstitial disease. *A*. Supine HRCT performed in a 51-year-old man shows increased linear parenchymal densities in both posterior lung bases *(arrows)*. The pattern is highly suggestive of pulmonary fibrosis. *B*. Subsequent chest CT performed in the prone position demonstrates complete reversal of the abnormality. Note that atelectasis (A) is now seen anteriorly adjacent to pericardial fat.

and subpleural fibrosis. Sarcoidosis is diffuse or upper-lobe-predominant and can have an irregular distribution **(Fig. 2.33).** Silicosis presents with upper-lobe nodules, and conglomerate fibrotic masses can develop. EG has upper-lung-predominant cystic spaces.

- **Idiopathic pulmonary fibrosis (IPF)** or fibrosing alveolitis is the cryptogenic form of the disease. Desquamative interstitial pneumonia (DIP) is the early inflammatory phase, and usual interstitial pneumonia (UIP) is nonspecific interstitial pneumonitis and fibrosis. Hamman-Rich syndrome is the rapidly progressive form. Early on, HRCT can demonstrate areas of ground-glass opacity representing active inflammation, which generally responds to treatment. These areas eventually progress to fibrosis. Adenopathy can be present due to the inflammation. Pleural effusions are rare.

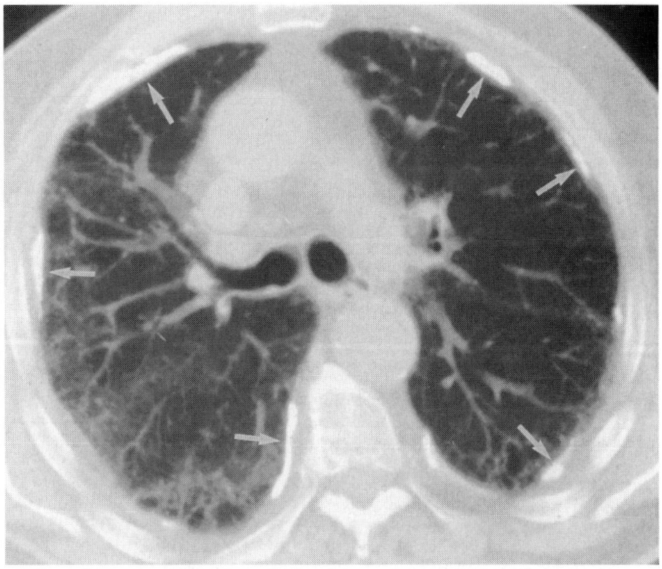

FIGURE 2.32 Asbestosis. HRCT shows peripheral pulmonary fibrosis consistent with asbestosis. Asbestos-related pleural disease is also present *(arrows)*.

- **Drugs** that can cause pulmonary fibrosis include bleomycin, amiodarone, nitrofurantoin, BCNU, methysergide, procainamide, busulfan, and cyclophosphamide.

Autoimmune and Connective Tissue Disease

- **Collagen vascular diseases** are chronic inflammatory autoimmune conditions that frequently produce interstitial pneumonitis and occasionally fibrosis. CT findings correlate well with the duration of

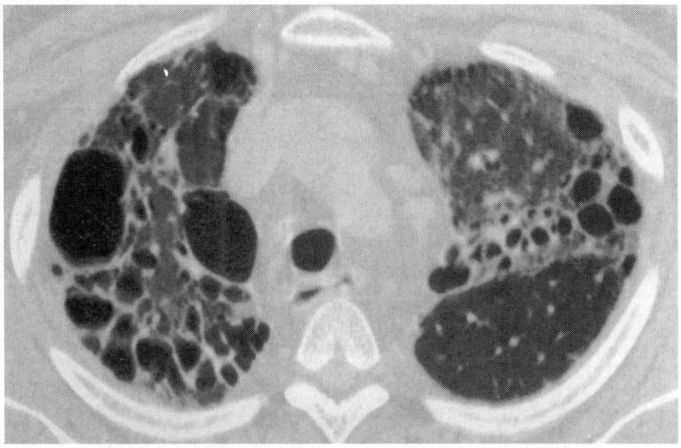

FIGURE 2.33 Pulmonary fibrosis from sarcoidosis. HRCT in a 48-year-old woman with advanced pulmonary sarcoidosis shows honeycombing with cystic airspaces adjacent to normal lung. This juxtaposition of normal and abnormal lung is typical of end-stage sarcoidosis. [From Sagel SS, Slone RM. The lung. In: Lee JKT, Sagel SS, Stanley RJ, Heiken JP (eds.): *Computed Body Tomography with MRI Correlation*. Philadelphia: Lippincott-Raven; 1998. With permission.]

symptoms and pulmonary function measurements, but HRCT can detect subtle abnormalities in patients with normal chest radiographs and no clinical symptoms. Findings include basilar interstitial infiltrates or fibrosis, pleural effusions, and pulmonary nodules in some disorders.

- **Systemic lupus erythematosus** affects young women primarily and has a predilection for African Americans. Lower-lobe-predominant septal thickening and ground-glass opacities representing pneumonitis are the most common findings. Small pericardial and chronic exudative pleural effusions are common and often lead to pleural fibrosis. Pulmonary fibrosis is uncommon. Patients can develop cardiomyopathy, glomerulonephritis, polyarteritis, or PAH.
- **Scleroderma,** most common in young women, affects the skin and gastrointestinal tract, often producing a dilated esophagus. Pulmonary involvement usually takes the form of basilar fibrosis, probably a manifestation of the systemic disease rather than aspiration from esophageal dysmotility. **CREST syndrome** is a combination of **c**alcification in soft tissues, **R**aynaud phenomenon, **e**sophageal dysmotility, **s**clerodactyly, and **t**elangectasias in patients with systemic sclerosis. One-third develop pulmonary fibrosis **(see Fig. 14.8)**. **Dermatomyositis** is a rare cause of interstitial pneumonitis and fibrosis.
- **Rheumatoid arthritis** is more common in women, but pulmonary manifestations are more common in men. Exudative pleural effusions, alveolitis, and basilar fibrosis are the most frequent findings and are usually preceded by joint involvement. Fibrosis is typically peripheral and lower-lobe in distribution, indistinguishable from IPF. Patients can have peripheral **"necrobiotic nodules,"** which are usually smaller than 1 cm but can be larger and may cavitate. Necrobiotic nodules are temporally related to subcutaneous nodules and can recede and recur. Arteritis, PAH, and bronchiolitis obliterans can occur. **Caplan syndrome** involves fibrotic nodules that occur in coal miners with rheumatoid arthritis.
- **Sjögren syndrome** is an autoimmune collagen vascular disorder characterized by dry mouth and eyes, chronic bronchitis, recurrent pneumonia, and an increased incidence of chronic active hepatitis, cirrhosis, thyroiditis, bronchiectasis, and lymphoproliferative disorders. Secondary Sjögren syndrome is seen in association with other connective tissue disorders. Patients can develop pleural effusions, lipoid interstitial pneumonia, or pulmonary fibrosis.
- **Ankylosing spondylitis,** seen mostly in young men, involves the lungs only after bone abnormalities are obvious. CT can show apical fibrosis as well as cavities and bronchiectasis. **Vasculitides** occasionally affecting the lung and leading to fibrosis include polyarteritis nodosa, Churg-Strauss disease, allergic angiitis, and lymphomatoid granulomatosis.

Malignancy

- **Lymphangitic carcinomatosis** is the interstitial spread of carcinoma. Hematogenous metastases penetrate the interstitium and lymphatic vessels, spreading along septa, the subpleural space, and connective tissue lining the bronchovascular bundles. The metastases usually arise from primary adenocarcinomas of the breast, lung, stomach, colon, or pancreas. The carcinomatosis can be focal or diffuse, involving both the central and peripheral lung. It is more common in the lower lung zones; associated adenopathy or pleural effusion is common. HRCT demonstrates irregular septal, subpleural, and bronchovascular thickening, which becomes nodular as the disease progresses **(see Fig. 2.28)**. Direct local lymphangitic spread can sometimes be seen around bronchogenic carcinomas.

Pulmonary Edema and ARDS

- **Pulmonary edema** is the most common cause of pulmonary infiltrates and a common finding in intensive care unit (ICU) patients. Edema results from increased pulmonary vascular pressure (congestive heart failure, volume overload, or renal failure), reduced intravascular oncotic pressure, lymphatic obstruction, or increased vascular permeability (noncardiogenic edema). CT findings of hydrostatic edema can precede clinical manifestations of dyspnea, peripheral edema, or hypoxemia and can persist after clinical recovery.
- **Hydrostatic edema** is associated with vascular enlargement and cardiomegaly except in cases of acute myocardial infarction or valve dysfunction. Redistribution of pulmonary blood flow appears as relative enlargement of the anterior pulmonary vessels in the supine position. As pulmonary venous pressures increase, fluid leaks into the interstitium and smooth septal, peribronchial, and fissural thickening develops, as do pleural effusions. Diffuse, patchy, and occasionally asymmetrical airspace disease develops with increasing pulmonary capillary wedge pressure **(see Fig. 2.27)**. Marked asymmetry can be the consequence of lateral decubitus positioning, thromboembolism, tumor invasion of the pulmonary vessels, or underlying lung disease. Emphysema and fibrosis alter the normal pattern of edema, leading to atypical patterns that may mimic pneumonia. Pulmonary edema can make the diagnosis of concomitant disease such as pneumonia difficult.
- **Noncardiogenic pulmonary edema** is the result of increased capillary permeability or reduced oncotic pressure with leakage of fluid into the alveoli **(see Fig. 2.2)**. Pulmonary vessel size and pressures are normal, and pleural effusions and cardiomegaly are absent. **Acute upper airway obstruction** from strangulation or laryngospasm can occasionally cause pulmonary edema. **Neurogenic edema** is the result of systemic vasoconstriction and increased capillary permeability associated with brain trauma, hemorrhage, or tumor. Near-drowning produces a similar appearance. **High-altitude edema** can occur following ascents over 9000 ft. Patchy edema develops over 1 to 2 days and clears with oxygen therapy and return to normal altitude. **Reexpansion pulmonary edema** occurs after rapid drainage of a large pneumothorax or pleural effusion. It develops within a few hours, can progress over 1 to 2 days, and usually resolves within a week.
- **Acute respiratory distress syndrome (ARDS)** is a clinical constellation consisting of severe respiratory distress, dyspnea, hypoxemia, and diffuse airspace disease from severe pulmonary or systemic injury. Causes include septic or hemorrhagic shock, massive trauma, burns, pancreatitis, aspiration, drug or transfusion reactions, severe pneumonia, fat or amniotic fluid embolism, inhalation injury, neurologic insult, and anaphylaxis. ARDS can develop rapidly, but radiologic abnormalities can be delayed up to 12 h after onset of clinical symptoms. Diffuse, patchy, ill-defined opacities initially develop, progressing to diffuse consolidation with hemorrhagic edema and microatelectasis by 48 h **(see Fig. 2.3)**. Cardiomegaly and pleural effusions are absent. Lung volumes are decreased from reduced compliance. Treatment is supportive to maintain cerebral and renal perfusion, prevent infection, and minimize barotrauma. Pneumothoraces, pneumomediastinum, and pneumonia are frequent complications. Death, usually from multisystem failure, is common.

2.6 PULMONARY NODULES

Solitary Pulmonary Nodule

- A **pulmonary nodule** is a well-circumscribed opacity measuring <3 cm. In three-quarters of cases, the final diagnosis is either granuloma or bronchogenic carcinoma. A distinction between these common entities is crucial **(Differential 2.6).** CT evaluation must include contiguous imaging of the entire chest with 5- to 8-mm collimation to identify associated mediastinal adenopathy, effusion, or other lung disease that may have been overlooked on radiography. Sections 2 to 3 mm thick targeted to the region of interest improve spatial resolution for lesion characterization. Several centers are evaluating the degree of enhancement following intravenous contrast administration as a differential point. Occasionally, CT can demonstrate a bone island, healing rib fracture, osteophyte, nipple shadow, or other benign extrapulmonary density mimicking an intrapulmonary lesion as the explanation for a radiographic abnormality. Lesions larger than 3 cm are a "mass" and typically malignant, so unless clearly benign they should be biopsied or resected.

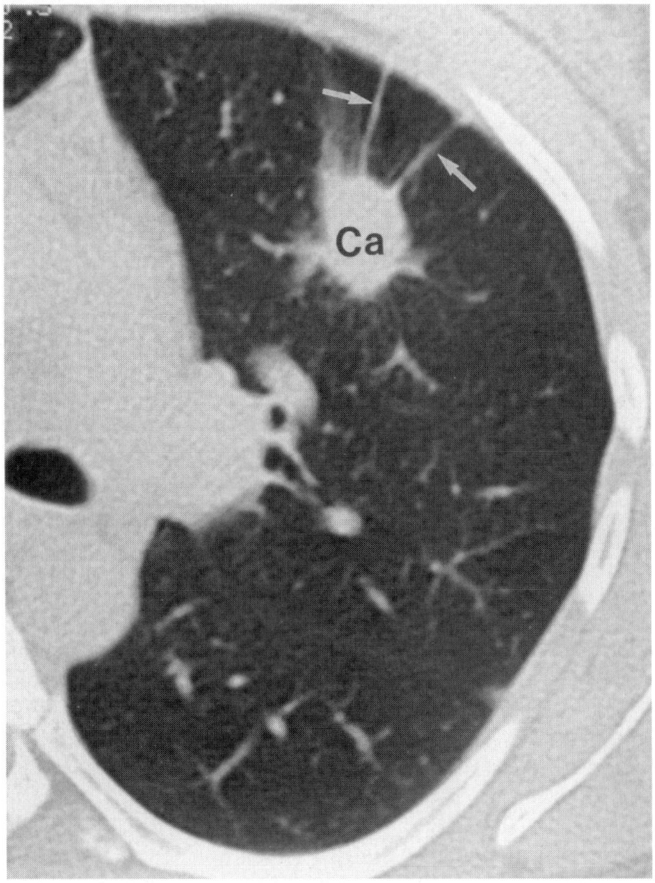

FIGURE 2.34 Adenocarcinoma with pleural tags. A 43-year-old woman with a spiculated mass in the left upper lobe. Percutaneous biopsy revealed adenocarcinoma. Pleural tags *(arrows)* are a nonspecific finding that can be seen in both benign and malignant processes.

2.6 SOLITARY PULMONARY NODULE OR MASS

Inflammatory—granuloma, scar, round pneumonia, fungus, organizing pneumonia, lung abscess, *lipoid pneumonia, rheumatoid, echinococcal cyst*

Neoplasm—bronchogenic carcinoma, solitary metastasis, carcinoid, hamartoma, pseudotumor, *pleural tumor, lymphoma*

Vascular—Wegener granulomatosis, pulmonary infarct, arteriovenous malformation, hematoma, *pulmonary sequestration, pulmonary artery pseudoaneurysm, pulmonary vein varix*

Rounded atelectasis

Progressive massive fibrosis

Bronchocele—mucoid impaction

Bronchogenic cyst

Amyloidosis

- Nodules with spiculated or ill-defined **margins** are more likely malignant than nodules with round, well-defined margins **(Fig. 2.34).** Lobulation implies differential growth rates and is also a common finding in malignant lesions. The **"halo sign,"** originally described in association with invasive pulmonary aspergillosis, refers to a rim of ground-glass attenuation due to surrounding edema or hemorrhage **(see Fig. 2.17).**
- **Calcification** is particularly helpful in distinguishing benign from malignant nodules. **Central** or **complete calcification** excludes malignancy. The calcification pattern must be symmetrical (diffuse, central, laminated, or ring-like); common causes include old healed granulomatous disease (OGD), particularly histoplasmosis, coccidiomycosis, or tuberculosis. Coarse, irregular **"popcorn"** calcifications can be seen in hamartomas **(Fig. 2.35). Eccentric calcifications** require further investigation, and although **diffuse, stippled calcifications** can be seen in hamartomas, this pattern is occasionally related to dystrophic calcification or necrosis in a malignant

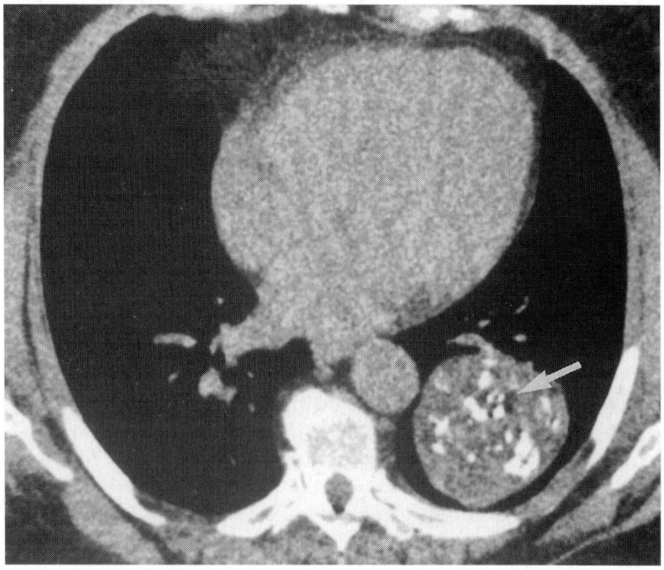

FIGURE 2.35 Hamartoma. Thin-section CT through a large soft tissue mass in the left lower lobe shows areas of fat *(arrow)* and coarse calcification.

2.7

CAVITARY LUNG LESION

Inflammatory—lung abscess, necrotizing pneumonia, mycobacterial cavity, *rheumatoid, echinococcal cyst*
Tumor—bronchogenic carcinoma, metastasis
Vascular—Wegener granulomatosis, septic embolus, pulmonary infarct, hematoma
Congenital—bronchogenic cyst, *cystic adenomatoid malformation, intrapulmonary sequestration*
Progressive massive fibrosis

tumor. In investigating multiple pulmonary nodules, the presence of calcification in one is not helpful in determining the likelihood of malignancy in the others.

- **Cavitation** indicates an active disease process and can be seen in benign and malignant nodules **(Differential 2.7). Air bronchograms** within the nodule suggest an infectious etiology, although BAC and lymphoma frequently have air bronchograms. **Pleural tags** are a nonspecific finding and can be seen in both benign and malignant lesions **(see Fig. 2.34).**
- The **rate of growth** is helpful in evaluating indeterminate lesions, and serial studies are invaluable for establishing the time course. Rapid development suggests infection. A 25 percent increase in diameter is equivalent to a doubling of volume. Most bronchogenic carcinomas double their volume in 1 to 18 months. Granulomas and hamartomas can enlarge slowly, as can low-grade adenocarcinomas and some metastases, such as renal cell carcinoma. If suspicion for malignancy is low, follow-up can establish the benign nature of a lesion. Protocols vary, but an initial 3-month follow-up that shows no change can be extended to 6 months and subsequently 1 year. Two-year stability is widely accepted as indicative of a benign lesion.
- **Other factors** to consider include the patient's age and immune status, history of smoking, prior infections, or known malignancy; however, even in patients with a known extrathoracic primary, a solitary pulmonary nodule is more likely to represent a primary lung cancer than a metastasis. The most likely cause of a **solitary metastasis** is colon, renal cell, testicular, or breast cancer, sarcoma, or melanoma.

Multiple Pulmonary Nodules

- As with solitary pulmonary nodules, there are many causes of multiple pulmonary nodules **(Differential 2.8).** CT can provide accurate assessment of size, number, and location as well as identify calcifications or cavitation and characterize lesion margins. **Multiple cavitary nodules** can be seen as a result of septic emboli, pulmonary metastases, BAC, Wegener granulomatosis, eosinophilic granuloma, and some pneumonias. Lymphoma, tracheobronchial papillomatosis, and rheumatoid arthritis are rare causes. When **adenopathy** is seen in association with multiple pulmonary nodules, it suggests sarcoidosis, metastatic disease, and granulomatous infections. Lymphoma, silicosis, and coal worker's pneumoconiosis can also present with nodules and adenopathy.
- **Pulmonary metastases** are a common clinical concern. They tend to be round, well-defined, and more numerous in the lower lobes **(Fig. 2.36).** CT can demonstrate their typical proximity to pulmonary arterial branches. The tumors **most likely to metastasize** to the lung are sarcomas, melanomas, choriocarcinomas, and renal cell, breast, testicular, and thyroid carcinomas; however, because many of these primary sites occur with low frequency, the most common primary tumors to produce pulmonary metastases are breast, renal, and colon cancer and squamous cancer of the head and neck.
- **Large metastases** are common with sarcomas and with testicular, colon, and renal cell carcinoma. Central necrosis and **cavitation** is most common with squamous cell cancers but can be seen with sarcomas, colon cancer, adenocarcinoma, and melanoma **(Fig. 2.37).** Hemorrhagic pulmonary metastases typically have **ill-defined margins** and are most often due to choriocarcinoma, melanoma,

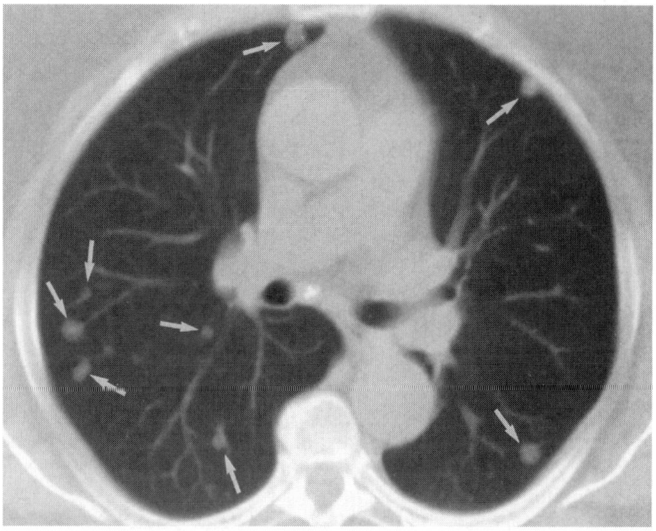

FIGURE 2.36 Metastatic breast cancer. Chest CT shows multiple pulmonary nodules *(arrows)*. Note the peripheral distribution and variation in size. The margins are smooth and there are no calcifications.

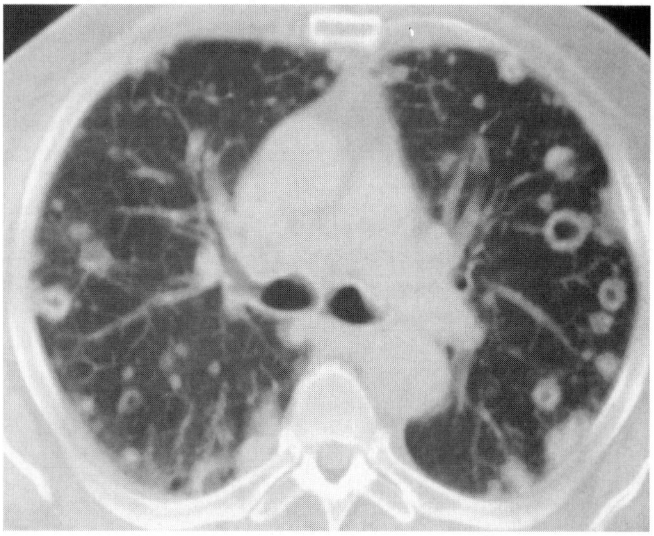

FIGURE 2.37 Metastatic squamous cell carcinoma. Chest CT in a 71-year-old man with head and neck cancer shows multiple solid and cavitary nodules, predominantly peripheral in location.

2.8

MULTIPLE PULMONARY NODULES

Granulomatous disease
Tumors—metastases, BAC,* Kaposi sarcoma,* *papillomas, lymphoma*
Infection*
Granulomatous disease
Bacterial—organizing bronchopneumonia, *Nocardia, Actinomyces, Legionella*
Vascular—Wegener granulomatosis, septic emboli,* arteriovenous malformations, pulmonary infarcts
Silicosis and coal worker's pneumoconiosis
Eosinophilic granuloma*
Mucoid impaction
Hypersensitivity pneumonitis*
*Sarcoidosis**
Amyloidosis
Rheumatoid

*Can be ill defined.

and renal cell, colon, and thyroid cancer. **Endobronchial metastases** can be seen with lung, renal cell, breast, and colon cancers and with lymphoma.

- Innumerable tiny **(miliary)** nodules are usually the sequelae of granulomatous disease but can also be seen with metastases, particularly thyroid carcinoma and melanoma **(Differential 2.9).**

- The most common cause for multiple calcified pulmonary nodules is **old healed granulomatous disease.** Other causes include silicosis, coal worker's pneumoconiosis, and healed varicella pneumonia. Alveolar microlithiasis, hypercalcemia, and mitral stenosis are rare causes. **Calcification** occurs in less than 1 percent of pulmonary metastases, typically osteosarcoma, chondrosarcoma, mucinous breast or colon adenocarcinomas, papillary adenocarcinoma from ovary or thyroid, and in others following radiation or chemotherapy.

2.7 PULMONARY NEOPLASMS

- CT is well suited for evaluating pulmonary neoplasms. Specific characteristics help determine the etiology, and the exact size and location are established. Adenopathy and associated findings such as effusion or occult lung disease can be detected. Pulmonary neoplasms can be divided into benign, primary malignant, and metastatic **(Sec. 2.6)** categories.

- A **hamartoma,** the most common benign pulmonary neoplasm, is slow-growing and typically circumscribed, round, or lobulated. A hamartoma arises within peripheral bronchi and is usually discovered incidentally in middle age. If present, symptoms are related to bronchial obstruction with atelectasis or hemoptysis. Fat within the tumor is a specific finding and is seen in about half of the cases on thin-section CT. One-third contain cartilage, depicted as coarse calcification on CT **(Fig. 2.35).**

- **Bronchial carcinoids** are very slow-growing vascular tumors that arise from neuroendocrine cells (Kulchitsky cells) of the bronchial mucosa. Some 5 percent occur in the lung, typically in central bronchi **(Fig. 2.38). Typical carcinoid** (low-grade neuroendocrine tumor) is a form that rarely metastasizes and is usually centrally located. They have a 90 percent 10-year survival. **Atypical carcinoids** (intermediate-grade neuroendocrine tumors) are more aggressive and have cytologic features resembling small cell carcinoma. They arise peripherally and often have metastases. They have a 60 percent 5-year survival. **Carcinoid syndrome** (flushing, tachycardia) is seen in patients with liver metastases. Carcinoid tumors can secrete adrenocorticotrophic hormone (ACTH), causing **Cushing syndrome.**

CT shows smooth, round soft tissue nodules. Calcification is common, sometimes involving large portions of the tumor. **Octreotide nuclear scintigraphy** has been used with some success in diagnosing carcinoid tumors because of their somatostatin receptors, but specificity is low. Percutaneous biopsy is usually diagnostic, although bronchoscopy is frequently more appropriate.

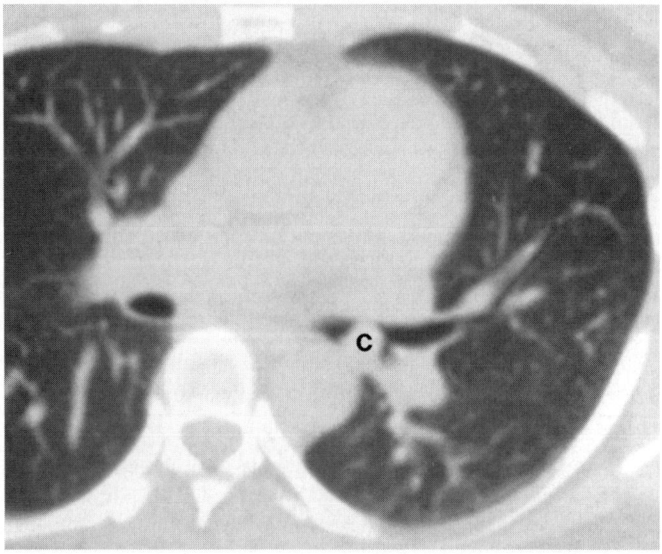

FIGURE 2.38 Endobronchial carcinoid. A 34-year-old woman who presented with wheezing unresponsive to bronchodilators. Chest CT reveals a nodule representing a well-differentiated neuroendocrine tumor (c) within the left main bronchus. There was neither postobstruction collapse nor infection.

2.9

TINY NODULES (<5 mm; MICRONODULAR; MILIARY)

Inflammatory—bronchopneumonia, granulomatous disease (miliary TB), bronchiolitis obliterans, hypersensitivity pneumonitis, viral pneumonia (particularly varicella), Asian panbronchiolitis, lymphocytic interstitial pneumonia
Malignancy—metastases (thyroid, melanoma), BAC*, lymphangitic carcinomatosis, *lymphoma*
Sarcoidosis
Silicosis and coal worker's pneumoconiosis
Eosinophilic granuloma
Alveolar microlithiasis
Amyloidosis
Idiopathic pulmonary hemosiderosis

*Bronchoalveolar cell carcinoma.

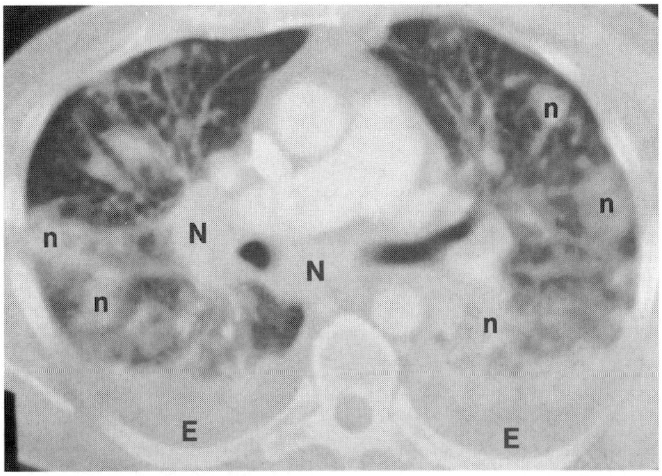

FIGURE 2.39 **Pulmonary lymphoma.** Chest CT in a 60-year-old man with widespread adenopathy shows bilateral pleural effusions (E), subcarinal and hilar adenopathy (N), and multifocal nodules (n) and consolidation, proven to be anaplastic large T-cell lymphoma.

- **Pulmonary lymphoma** is rare. It is more common with Hodgkin disease and is almost always accompanied by intrathoracic adenopathy. Isolated parenchymal involvement can be seen in non-Hodgkin lymphoma. Pulmonary patterns include patchy consolidation and ill-defined nodules or masses, often with air bronchograms or cavitation **(Fig. 2.39).** Less commonly, a nonspecific diffuse reticulonodular form can occur. Associated pleural and pericardial effusions can occur from mesothelial spread and lymphatic obstruction.

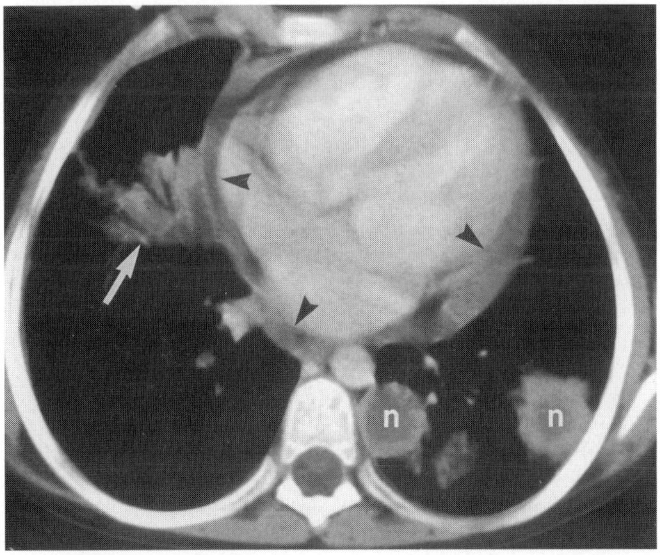

FIGURE 2.40 Posttransplant lymphoproliferative disorder (PTLD). Contrast-enhanced CT shows two nodules in the left lower lobe *(n)*, an area of consolidation on the right *(arrow)*, and a small pericardial effusion *(arrowheads)*, all representing PTLD. (Pickhardt PJ, Seigel MJ, Hayashi RJ, DeBaun MR. Chest radiography as a predictor of outcome in posttransplantation lymphoproliferative disorder in lung allograft recipients. *AJR* 1998; 171:375–385. With permission.)

- **MALT** (mucosa-associated lymphoid tissue) and **BALT** (bronchus-associated lymphoid tissue) refer to forms of non-Hodgkin lymphoma that involve the pulmonary parenchyma in the form of multiple nodules or masses. **Pseudolymphoma** is histologically identical to well-differentiated small lymphocytic lymphoma but can be differentiated using immunofluorescence techniques. It has a better prognosis than lymphoma. CT demonstrates nodules or consolidation with air bronchograms.
- **Posttransplantation lymphoproliferative disease (PTLD)** refers to a spectrum of disorders ranging from polyclonal lymphoid hyperplasia to aggressive lymphoma. PTLD occurs in 2 to 5 percent of organ-transplant recipients and is related to immunosuppression and Epstein-Barr virus infection. Treatment requires a delicate balance of reduced immunosuppression and efforts to prevent graft rejection. Chemotherapy or radiation may be considered when the disease is advanced. The most common presentation is solitary or multiple pulmonary nodules or patchy infiltrates. Adenopathy and pleural effusions are less frequent **(Fig. 2.40).**
- **Kaposi sarcoma** occurs in patients with AIDS and is usually present on the skin when pulmonary involvement is present. Focal parenchymal infiltrates with a bronchovascular distribution are most common. Concomitant infections can be present.

2.8 BRONCHOGENIC CARCINOMA

- **Bronchogenic carcinoma** is the leading cause of cancer death in the United States, accounting for 140,000 deaths annually. The male:female ratio is 2:1. Presenting symptoms include cough, hemoptysis, wheezing, and paraneoplastic syndromes. One-fourth of patients are asymptomatic at diagnosis. Heavy cigarette smoking (>40 pack years) increases the risk of bronchogenic carcinoma 20-fold. Approximately 10 percent of heavy smokers develop lung cancer. Relative risk falls to that of a nonsmoker after 10 years of abstinence from smoking. Cigarette smoking is associated with squamous cell, small cell, and, to a lesser degree, adenocarcinoma. Other carcinogens include radon gas, asbestos, heavy metals, radiation, and urban pollutants. Although controversial, chest radiography is frequently used for screening high-risk patients. Investigations using CT for screening show promising results. A spiculated peripheral nodule is the most common manifestation of bronchogenic carcinoma **(Fig. 2.41)**, particularly with adenocarcinoma and large cell tumors and less commonly squamous and small cell types.
- Lung cancer is classified into four major histologic types and subdivided into well, moderate, and poorly differentiated forms. **Squamous cell (epidermoid) carcinoma** arises in metaplastic squamous epithelium of the central bronchi and frequently remains localized. There is a strong male predominance among heavy smokers. Its incidence is decreasing (presently about one-third of lung cancers). A common manifestation is collapse and consolidation beyond the central bronchial obstruction. Squamous cell carcinoma can attain a large size and is the most common cell type to cavitate **(Fig. 2.42).**
- **Adenocarcinoma** accounts for about one-third of primary lung cancers and the incidence is rising, particularly in women. **Bronchoalveolar cell carcinoma (BAC)** is a form of well-differentiated adenocarcinoma that proliferates along preexist-

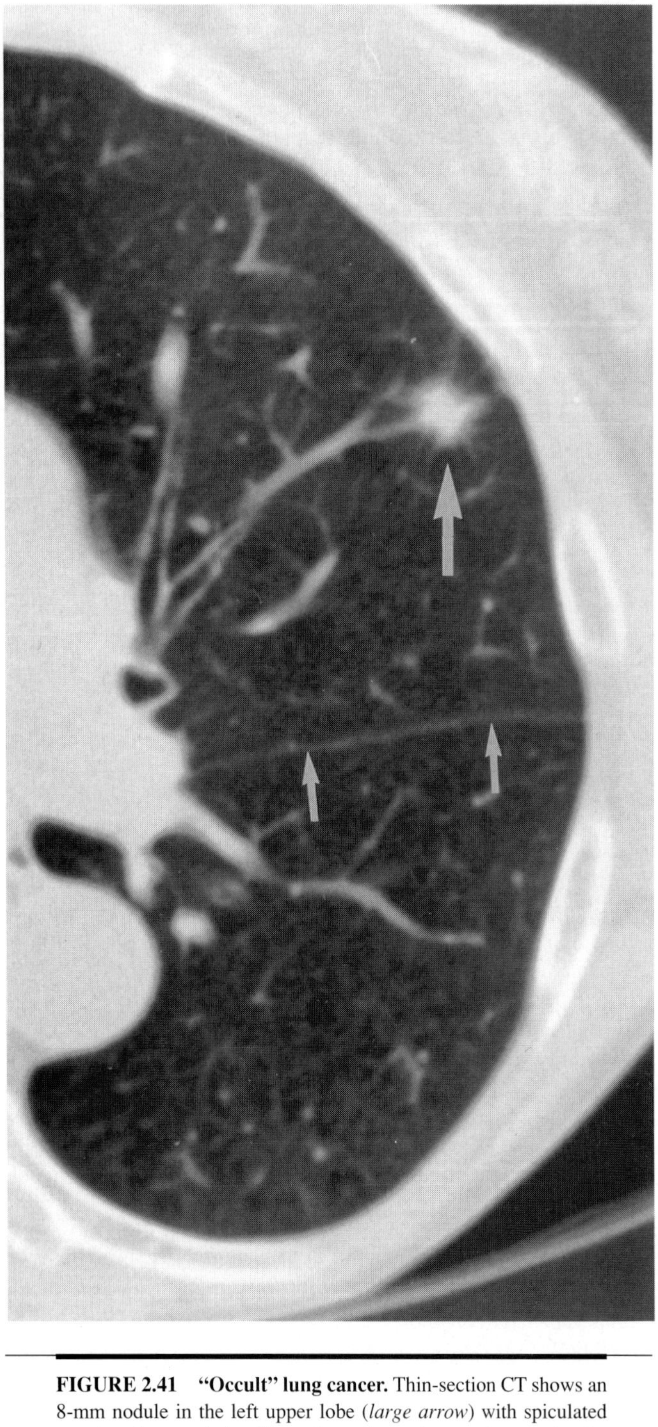

FIGURE 2.41 "Occult" lung cancer. Thin-section CT shows an 8-mm nodule in the left upper lobe (*large arrow*) with spiculated margins characteristic of bronchogenic carcinoma. Note major fissure (*small arrows*).

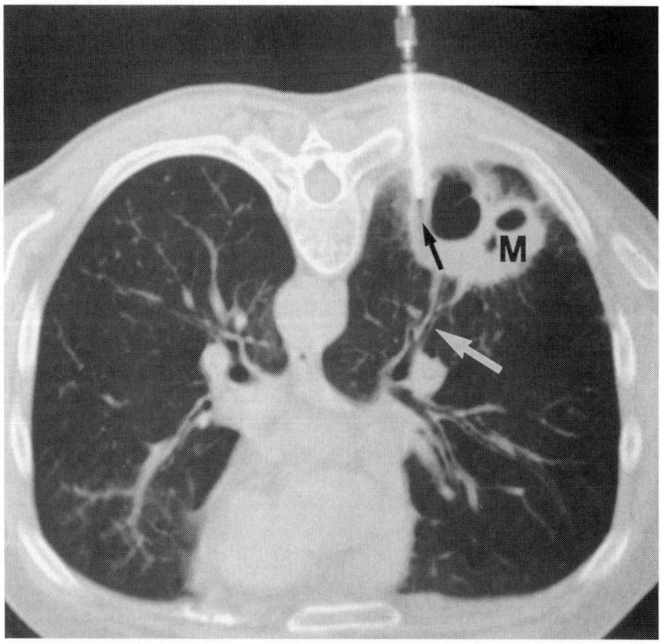

FIGURE 2.42 CT-guided percutaneous lung biopsy. Cavitary mass (M) with spiculated margins. Note superior segment bronchus *(white arrow)*, leading directly to the mass. CT facilitated placement of the biopsy needle into the wall of the lesion, where viable tissue could be aspirated. Note the characteristic needle-tip artifact *(black arrow)*. The lesion was a primary squamous cell carcinoma. (Figure courtesy of Christopher Gordon, MD.)

ing alveolar structures without invasive growth. It is a frequent component of bronchogenic carcinomas but is uncommon in pure form. BAC has a variable appearance, including a solitary nodule (best prognosis), mass, focal consolidation simulating pneumonia **(Fig. 2.43)**, or multifocal solid or cavitary nodules (poor prognosis). Mucinous BAC can present as low-attenuation nodules and in some cases mimics alveolar proteinosis. An HRCT pattern of ground-glass opacity with superimposed smooth septal thickening and a patchy geographic distribution ("crazy paving") suggests alveolar proteinosis or BAC.

- **Large cell undifferentiated carcinoma** accounts for about 10 percent of lung cancers. It is composed of large cells without clear squamous or glandular differentiation. **Mixed tumor types,** such as adenosquamous carcinoma, probably arise from pleuripotent cells.
- **Small cell carcinoma,** classified as a high grade neuroendocrine tumor and historically referred to as "oat cell," arises from neuroendocrine cells of the bronchial mucosa. It accounts for 20 percent of lung cancers and is more common in men. Two-thirds of patients have metastases at presentation. The primary tumor is typically small and often difficult to identify. The predominant feature at diagnosis is mediastinal and hilar adenopathy **(Fig. 2.44).** Five-year survival is only 10 percent.
- **Mucoepidermoid carcinoma** and **adenoid cystic carcinoma** can arise from bronchial mucous glands in the trachea and central bronchi **(see Fig. 4.27).** They infiltrate locally, grow slowly, and have a very low incidence of metastasis. Other primary lung malignancies are rare and include carcinosarcoma, pulmonary blastoma **(Fig. 2.45)**, and pleomorphic carcinomas with spindle or giant cells. These aggressive malignancies are typically large and peripheral; they often invade the chest wall. All have a poor prognosis.
- Lung carcinoma can **spread** in several ways. **Local invasion** of the adjacent pleura, chest wall, and mediastinal structures is common. BAC can spread along the airways. **Local lymph node metastasis** can occur in all types but tends to occur early with small cell carci-

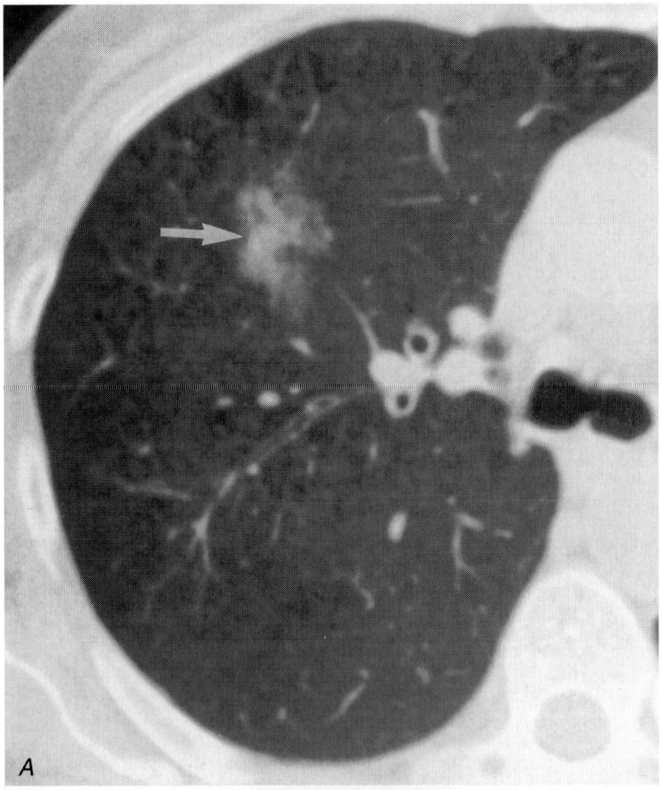

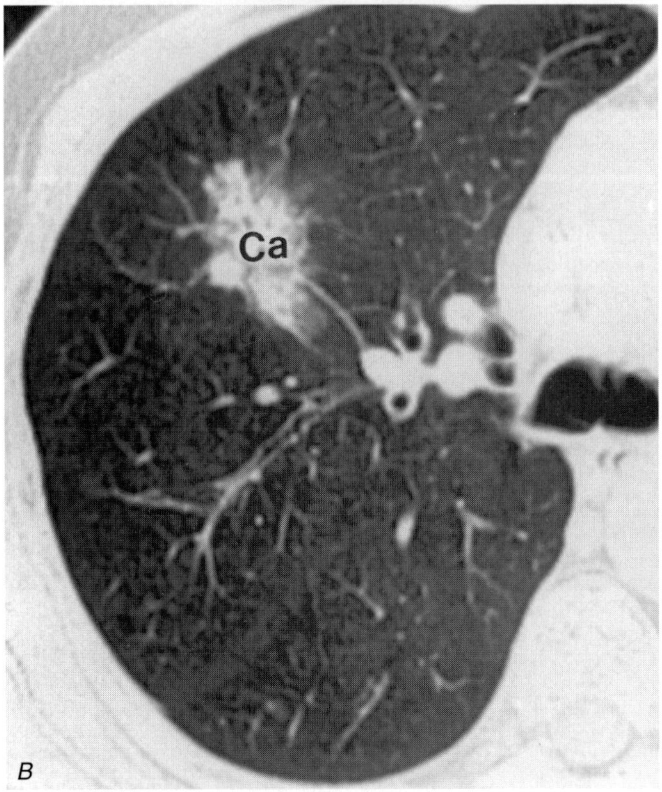

FIGURE 2.43 Bronchoalveolar cell carcinoma (BAC) simulating pneumonia. *A*. Chest CT shows a nonspecific focal area of consolidation *(arrow)*. *B*. Chest CT obtained 4 years later shows progressive "consolidation" in the same location, proven to be BAC (Ca) by transthoracic fine-needle aspiration.

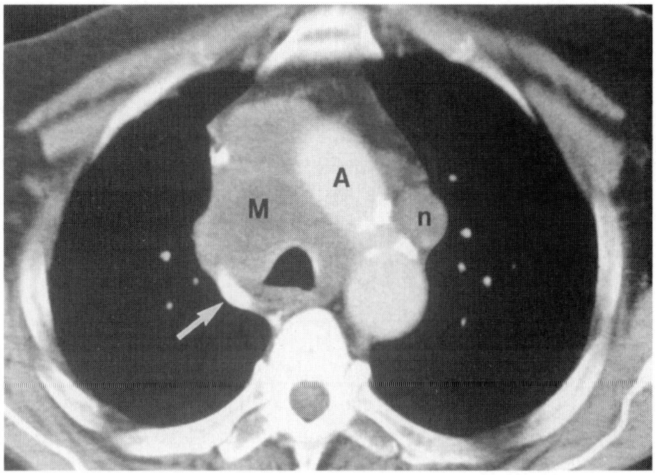

FIGURE 2.44 Small cell carcinoma. Contrast-enhanced CT shows a mediastinal mass (M) and adenopathy (n). Mediastinal invasion was causing obstruction of the superior vena cava. Note collateral flow through the azygos vein *(arrow)*. A, aortic arch.

noma. Hematogenous metastases to the adrenal glands, liver, bone, and brain are most common. Late in the disease, interstitial **lymphangitic spread** can also be seen **(Fig 2.46).**

CT has a low accuracy for **assessing chest wall invasion.** Pleural thickening is sensitive but nonspecific, since there is a high prevalence of benign pleural thickening. In general, the thicker the pleura and larger the contact area, the greater the risk of parietal pleural invasion. An extrapleural soft tissue component or increase in the extrapleural fat density can be the result of inflammation, fibrosis, or hemorrhage rather than tumor extension. It is also possible to have microscopic tumor invasion while the extrapleural fat appears normal. Bone destruction is a definitive finding and often accompanied by evidence of soft tissue extension **(Fig. 2.47).** Although not as sensitive, chest pain is more specific than CT and can be the best indicator of parietal pleural invasion. **Magnetic resonance imaging (MRI)** is better than CT for assessing invasion through the lung apex or diaphragm, or into the spinal canal.

- **Superior sulcus (Pancoast) tumor** is an apical, pleural-based bronchogenic carcinoma with a propensity for chest wall invasion. Tumors that invade the parietal pleura can lead to Pancoast syndrome, with arm pain and muscle wasting due to C8 and T1 nerve root involvement and Horner syndrome (enophthalmos, ptosis, myosis, and anhidrosis) due to invasion of the sympathetic chain. Superior sulcus tumors can also invade the subclavian vessels and spine. Low-grade squamous cell is the most common cell type. Breast cancer, multiple myeloma, metastases, lymphoma, and mesothelioma can produce the same syndrome. Coronal or sagittal reformatting are helpful in assessing the superior extent of tumor, but MRI is preferred. Surgery is contraindicated in patients with extensive involvement of the subclavian artery, spine, or brachial plexus.

Paraneoplastic Syndromes

Bronchogenic carcinoma can be associated with a number of paraneoplastic syndromes, including migratory thrombophlebitis, Trousseau syndrome, and **hypertrophic osteoarthropathy,** a syndrome of

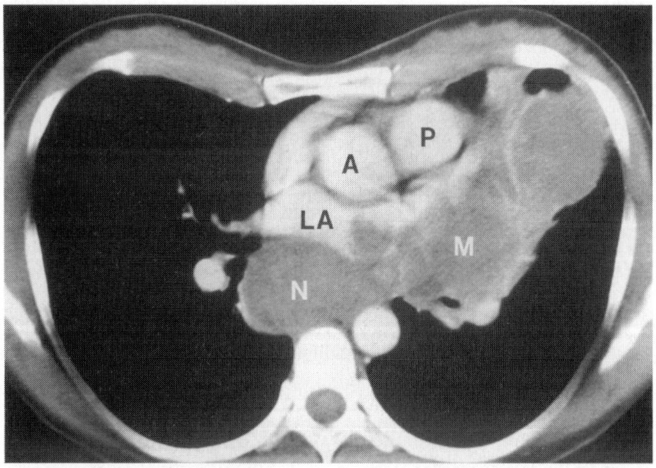

FIGURE 2.45 Pulmonary blastoma invading heart. Contrast-enhanced chest CT in a 43-year-old woman shows a large left hilar mass (M) invading the mediastinum, including the left atrium (LA). There is massive subcarinal adenopathy (N). A, ascending aorta; P, pulmonary trunk.

arthralgias, swelling, and stiffness of the joints. Although hypertrophic osteoarthropathy is most common in patients with an intrathoracic malignancy, benign tumors—particularly fibrous tumor of the pleura, infections, and other thoracic conditions—can be the cause. Endocrine manifestations of bronchogenic carcinoma can include Cushing syndrome and inappropriate secretion of antidiuretic hormone.

Staging

- Staging of **small cell carcinoma** is confined to two categories. **Limited disease** is local involvement of one hemithorax with regional hilar and mediastinal adenopathy amenable to a single radiation therapy portal. **Extensive disease** involves spread beyond the boundaries of a single radiation therapy portal.

- **Non–small cell carcinoma** is staged using the **TNM system,** which divides patients by prognosis. T (tumor location and size), N (lymph node involvement), and M (distant metastases) are determined with CT, bronchoscopy, and often mediastinoscopy, as CT lacks specificity in determining nodal involvement. Mediastinal lymph node involvement should be classified using the American Thoracic Society System **(see Fig. 4.3).**

  T1 refers to tumors <3 cm in diameter that are surrounded by lung or pleura and do not invade a lobar bronchus. **T2** denotes lesions ≥ 3 cm in diameter but >2 cm from the carina or tumors with visceral pleural invasion, atelectasis, or consolidation extending to the hilum. **T3** refers to tumors ≤ 2 cm from the carina; tumors producing total lung collapse or consolidation; or tumors that invade the parietal pleura, chest wall, diaphragm, or pericardium. **T4** denotes tumor invading the heart, great vessels, trachea, carina, esophagus, or spine or that give rise to a malignant effusion.

  Stage I includes T1 and T2 lesions without positive lymph nodes (N0) or metastases (M0). They are usually resectable, and 5-year survival is 65 percent.

  Stage II includes T1 or T2 lesions with ipsilateral hilar or peribronchial lymph node involvement (N1) but no distant metastases (M0). Most are resectable, with an average survival of 45 percent at 5 years.

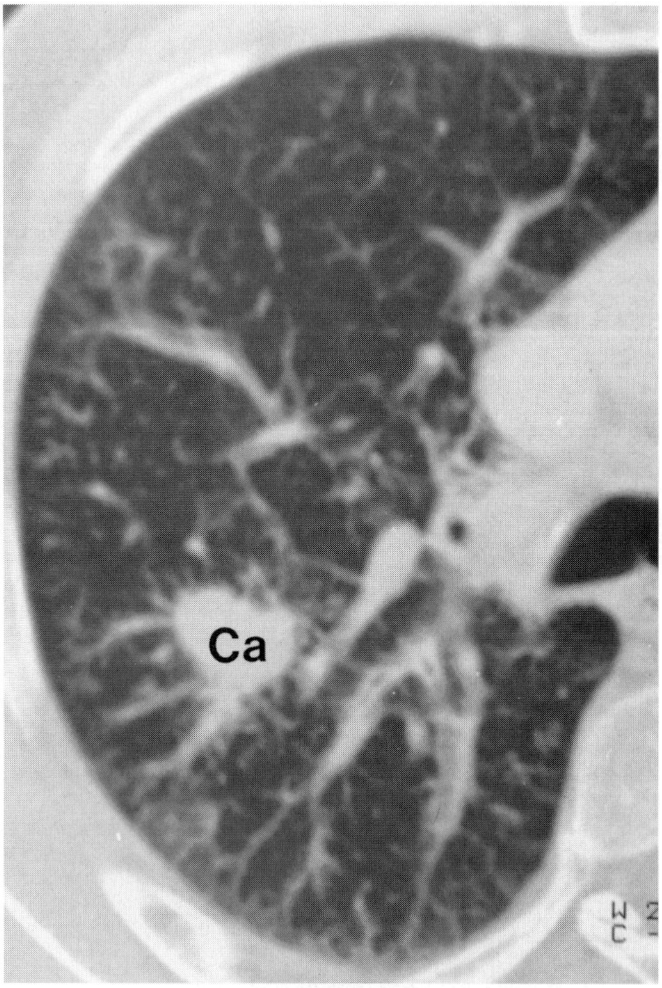

FIGURE 2.46 Local lymphangitic spread of lung cancer. Chest CT shows a spiculated nodule proven to be bronchogenic carcinoma (Ca). Note the nodular bronchovascular and septal thickening in the surrounding lung.

  Stage IIIA has limited and potentially resectable invasion of the chest wall or adjacent organs (T3) or metastases to subcarinal **(Fig. 2.48)** or ipsilateral peribronchial, hilar, or mediastinal lymph nodes (N2). Five-year survival is 25 percent.

  Stage IIIB are nonresectable tumors that invade vital organs, have supraclavicular, scalene, or contralateral hilar lymph node involvement (N3), or have a malignant effusion (T4) but no distant metastases (M0) **(Figs. 2.49 and 2.50).** They are treated with radiation therapy.

  Stage IV includes tumors with distant metastases (M1).

Treatment

- Untreated, small cell carcinoma is rapidly fatal, but most cases are very sensitive to chemotherapy. Radiation therapy further increases survival. A peripheral small cell cancer without mediastinal involvement is the only presentation in which resection is indicated, but this only occurs in a small fraction of patients.

- A **lobectomy** is the treatment of choice for patients with non–small cell bronchogenic carcinoma. Unfortunately, over two-thirds of lung cancers are unresectable due to advanced disease or inopera-

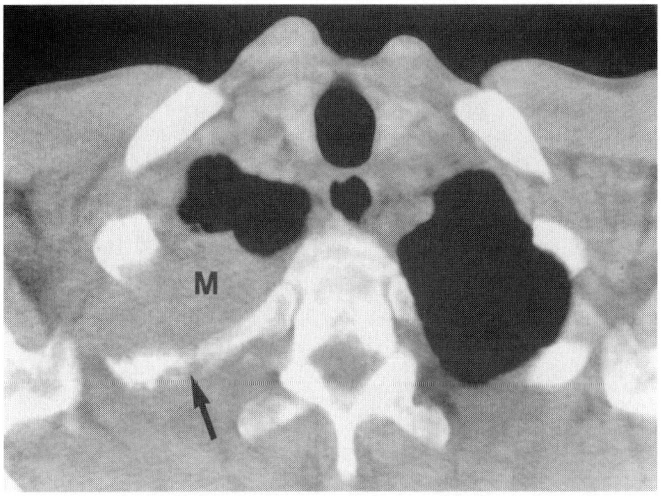

FIGURE 2.47 Chest wall invasion by lung cancer. CT through the lung apex shows a large right-upper-lobe mass (M) invading the chest wall, as evidenced by rib destruction *(arrow)*.

ble because of the patient's poor pulmonary function or significant cardiac disease. A segmentectomy can be considered in patients with limited pulmonary reserve, but it has a higher incidence of recurrence. Large tumors crossing the fissures or involving the main bronchus require pneumonectomy. Some patients with chest wall invasion can be successfully managed with a lobectomy and full-thickness chest wall resection. Five-year survival is 30 percent when regional nodes are negative.

- CT is valuable in assessing postoperative complications and recurrence **(Fig. 2.51).** In general, the **risk of recurrence** increases with the number and level of involved lymph nodes. Few patients with **stage IV** lung cancer live beyond 1 year (median survival <6 months). Treatment is palliative.

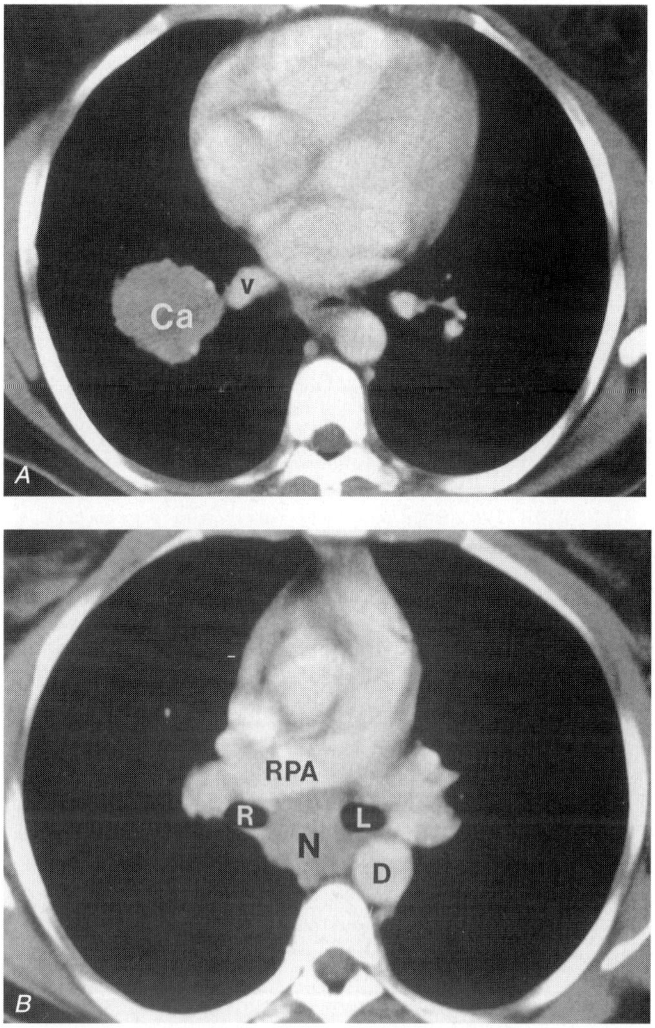

FIGURE 2.48 Stage IIIA lung cancer. *A*. Contrast-enhanced CT in a 42-year-old woman shows a 3-cm mass in the right lower lobe proven to be bronchogenic carcinoma (Ca). v, inferior pulmonary vein. *B*. Image at a higher level shows extensive subcarinal adenopathy (N) interposed between the right (R) and left (L) main bronchi, right pulmonary artery (RPA), and descending thoracic aorta (D).

2.9 CONGENITAL AND VASCULAR PULMONARY LESIONS

- **Pulmonary agenesis** results in complete absence of the pulmonary artery and lung with ipsilateral shift of the heart and mediastinum. Half of these patients have congenital heart disease. In **pulmonary aplasia,** the pulmonary artery and parenchyma are absent, but a blind-ending bronchial stump persists, predisposing patients to recurrent infections. Pulmonary agenesis and aplasia most commonly involve the right lung.

- **Pulmonary hypoplasia** associated with partial anomalous pulmonary venous return is the **pulmonary venolobar, hypogenetic lung,** or **scimitar syndrome.** There is right lung hypoplasia with a small pulmonary artery and partial anomalous pulmonary venous drainage to the inferior vena cava (IVC) or the hepatic or portal veins via a scimitar vein. There is volume loss of the right chest with mediastinal shift and frequent blunting of the right cardiophrenic angle.

- **Acquired pulmonary hypoplasia,** typically unilateral, is most often the result of postviral bronchiolitis obliterans in childhood **(Swyer-James syndrome).** The lung is small and hyperlucent with underdeveloped pulmonary vascularity **(see Fig. 2.7).** There is typically cylindrical bronchiectasis and early termination of the bronchial tree. Although it usually affects an entire lung, the process can be limited to a lobe or segment, simulating congenital lobar emphysema.

- **Congenital lobar emphysema** is progressive hyperinflation of one or more lobes, probably due to bronchial cartilage deficiency, bronchial compression, or endobronchial obstruction. Most patients present in the first year of life with respiratory distress. The middle and left upper lobes are the most common locations. Treatment is surgical resection.

- **Congenital cystic adenomatoid malformations** (CCAMs) comprise a spectrum of cystic and solid lesions resulting from anomalous development and proliferation of terminal respiratory structures. Patients typically present by the first year of life with respiratory symptoms. CCAMs usually involve a single lobe and

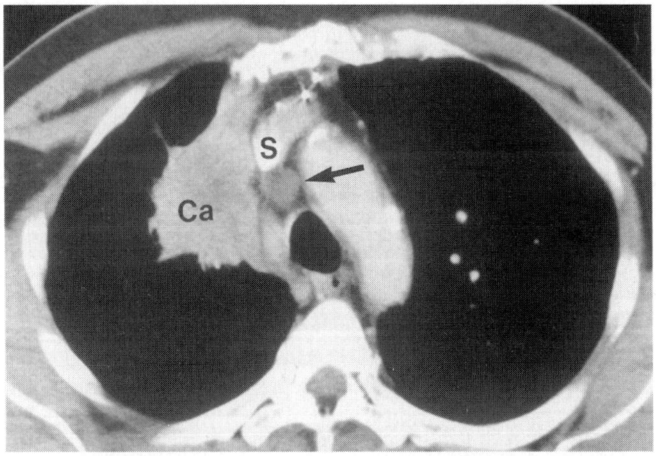

FIGURE 2.49 Right-upper-lobe cancer with paratracheal adenopathy. CT in a 55-year-old man shows a large soft tissue mass in the right upper lobe (Ca). There is a large interface with the mediastinum and suggestion of invasion. There is an enlarged low-density high right paratracheal lymph node *(arrow)*. Mediastinoscopy revealed malignancy, rendering this an unresectable cancer. S, superior vena cava.

appear as a parenchymal mass with a variable cystic component, depending on the degree of communication with the tracheobronchial tree **(Fig. 2.52).** Type I consist of one or more large (>2-cm) air-filled cysts; these are the most common and have the best prognosis. Surgical lobectomy is usually curative. Type II are composed of small cysts (<2 cm) mixed with a solid mass, and type III are solid, without cysts.

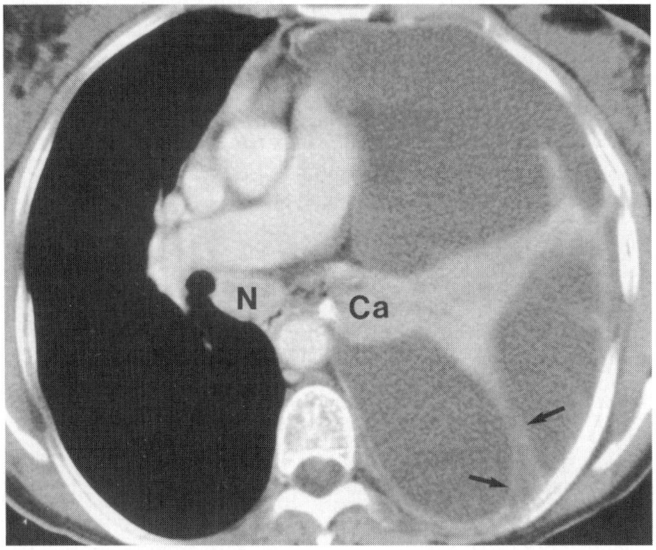

FIGURE 2.50 Advanced bronchogenic carcinoma. A 62-year-old woman with a central lung cancer (Ca) obstructing the left main bronchus and causing postobstructive collapse. Pleural adhesions *(arrows)* are seen attaching the visceral and parietal pleura. There is subcarinal adenopathy (N) and a malignant pleural effusion with thickened enhancing pleura. Note contralateral shift of the mediastinum.

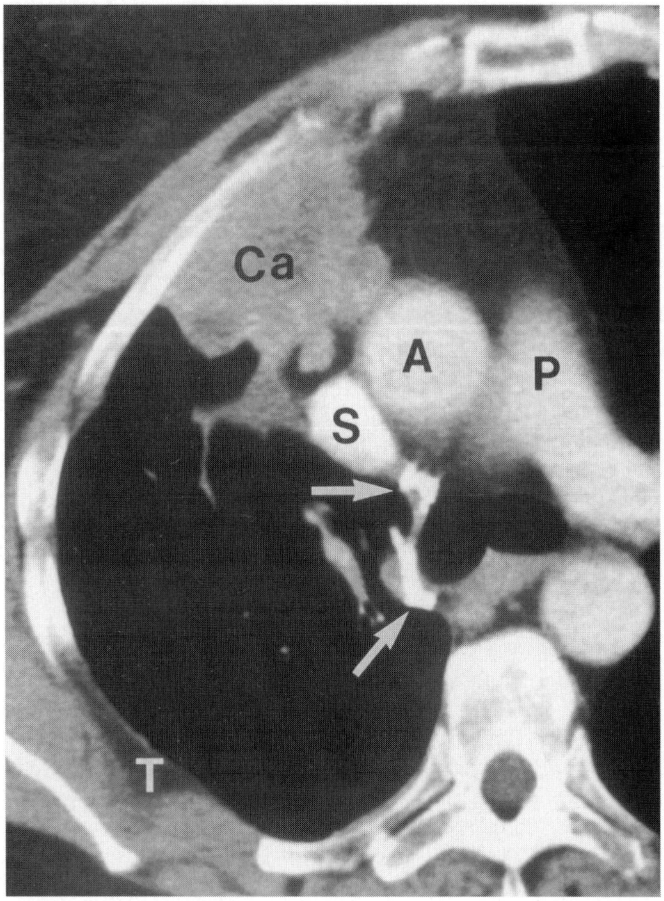

FIGURE 2.51 Recurrent lung cancer. Contrast-enhanced CT shows a mass (Ca) adjacent to the chest wall and ascending aorta (A), proven to be bronchogenic carcinoma by CT-guided biopsy. The patient had a prior right upper lobectomy for cancer, as evidenced by the staples *(arrows)*, ipsilateral mediastinal shift, and prior thoracotomy (T). S, superior vena cava; P, pulmonary trunk.

- **Pulmonary sequestration** is a congenital portion of lung tissue that lacks normal communication with the tracheobronchial tree **(Fig. 2.53).** Sequestrations have a systemic, usually aortic arterial supply. Patients often present with recurrent or persistent infection. Treatment is surgical resection. **Extralobar sequestration** is separated from surrounding normal lung by visceral pleura. It is located in the posterior lung base, most often on the left (90 percent). Venous return is via systemic vessels, usually the IVC or azygos system. **Intralobar sequestration** resides within normal lung parenchyma and has no separate pleural covering. It occurs in the lower lobes. Venous return is usually via the pulmonary veins or occasionally directly into the left atrium.

Vascular Disease

- **Arteriovenous malformations (AVMs)** are abnormal collections of vessels allowing direct communication between the pulmonary arterial and venous systems, resulting in a right-to-left shunt. CT demonstrates the feeding artery and draining vein associated with an enhancing lobulated lesion **(Fig. 2.54).** Dyspnea and hemoptysis are common presentations. Transcatheter coil embolization is therapeutic. The vast majority of AVMs are congenital. **Osler-Weber-**

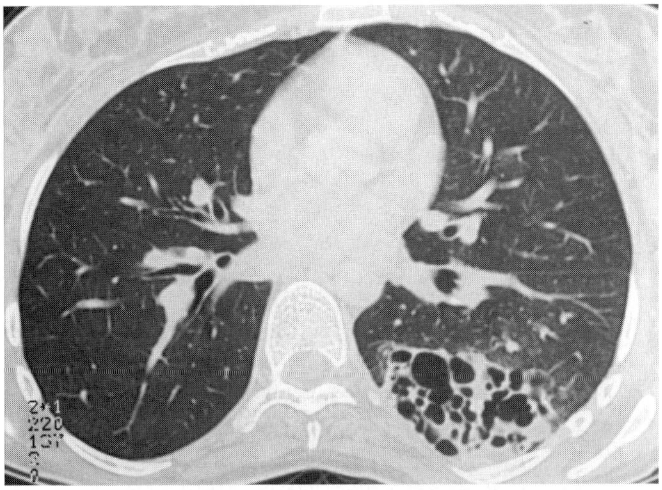

FIGURE 2.52 Cystic adenomatoid malformation. HRCT in a 24-year-old woman with chronic left-lower-lobe "consolidation" shows a multilocular cystic mass. There were no associated vessels to suggest pulmonary sequestration. The cyst size is characteristic of a type I lesion. [Sagel SS, Slone RM. The lung. In: Lee JKT, Sagel SS, Stanley RJ, Heiken JP (eds.): *Computed Body Tomography with MRI Correlation*. Philadelphia: Lippincott-Raven; 1998. With permission.]

Rendu syndrome *(hereditary hemorrhagic telangiectasis)* accounts for half of patients with pulmonary AVMs and is characterized by epistaxis, telangiectasias of the skin and mucous membranes, gastrointestinal bleeding, and multiple pulmonary arteriovenous malformations, which occur in about 15 percent of patients.

- **Pulmonary infarction** is seen in about 15 percent of patients surviving thromboembolism. Peripheral areas of consolidation (Hampton's hump) and pleural effusions are characteristic findings. Spiral CT for diagnosis of pulmonary embolism is discussed in **Section 5.3. Septic emboli** are usually the result of bacterial endocarditis, intravenous drug usage, or infected vascular grafts. Nodules with cavitation are frequently present. **Fat embolism** is usually the result of traumatic long bone fractures with fat droplets gaining access to the central circulation. In the lung parenchyma, fat acts as a chemical irritant. The usual presentation is airspace disease occurring 24 to 48 h after trauma.

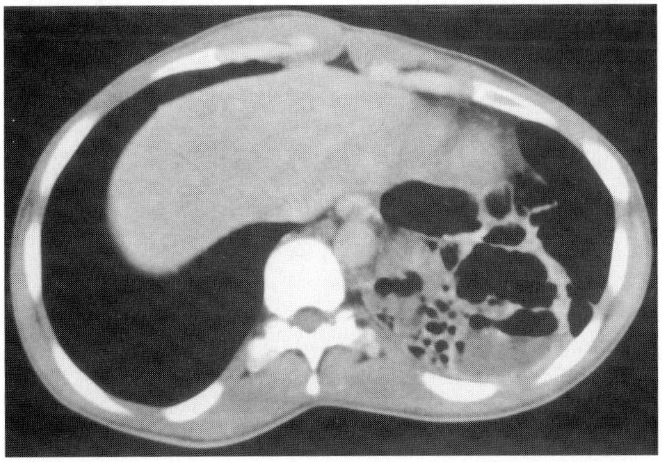

FIGURE 2.53 Bronchopulmonary sequestration. Contrast-enhanced chest CT in a 26-year-old man shows a complex cystic mass in the left lower lobe.

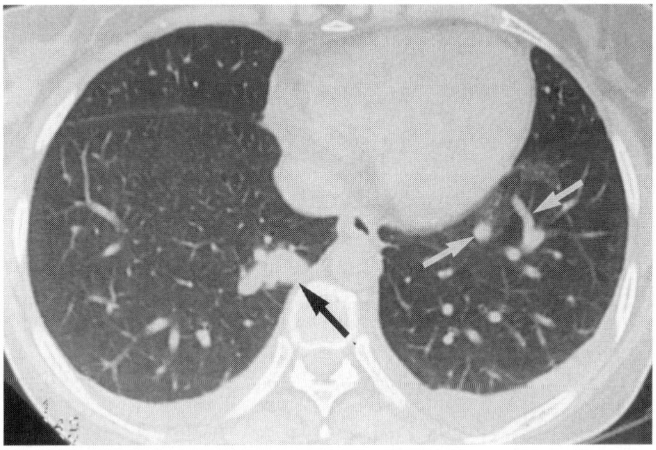

FIGURE 2.54 Arteriovenous malformations. Chest CT shows a lobulated nodule in the right lower lobe *(black arrow)* and enlarged vessels in the left lower lobe *(white arrows)*, which were supplying another lesion.

- **Sickle cell disease** produces cardiomegaly and congestive heart failure (CHF) due to chronic anemia and high cardiac output. The spleen becomes small, fibrotic, and sometimes calcifies. **Acute chest syndrome** ("sickle cell lung") comprises chest pain, fever, and pulmonary infiltrates; sometimes effusions and pericarditis occur during acute crises. No infectious organisms are recovered. HRCT can demonstrate septal thickening during the acute phase and fibrosis after recurrent episodes.

- **Goodpasture syndrome** is an autoimmune disease primarily affecting young men. Antibodies against glomerular and alveolar basement membranes produce cough, dyspnea, and pulmonary hemorrhage, leading to fibrosis. Patients also have glomerulonephritis, hypertension, and hematuria. Renal biopsy shows glomerulonephritis with characteristic IgG deposits. Death usually occurs from renal failure. CT shows patchy perihilar and lower-lobe-predominant consolidation similar to pulmonary edema. Adenopathy and hepatosplenomegaly can be present.

- **Wegener granulomatosis** is a necrotizing autoimmune vasculitis of middle-aged adults characterized by granulomatous involvement of small- and medium-sized vessels, upper respiratory ulcerations, and glomerulonephritis. Isolated thoracic involvement is uncommon. The most common CT finding is solitary or multiple peripheral nodules that cavititate **(Fig. 2.55).** Thrombosed vessels can be seen adjacent to the nodules. The nodules often resolve and new nodules develop. Endobronchial granulomas can cause obstruction and pulmonary hemorrhage can occur. Tracheal involvement can cause thickening and narrowing.

2.10 LARGE AIRWAY DISEASE AND BRONCHIECTASIS

- Disorders of the trachea are covered in **Section 4.6.**
- **Congenital airway disorders** include primary tracheal stenosis,

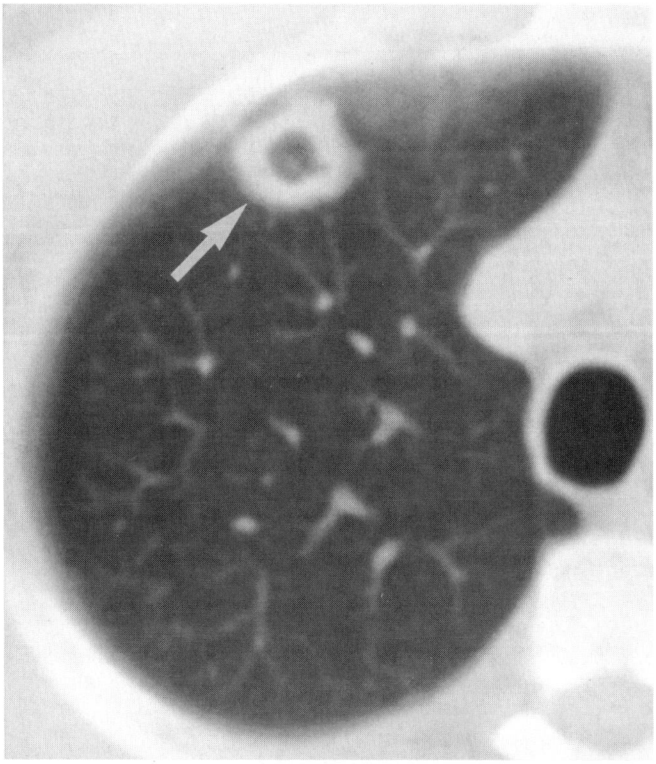

FIGURE 2.55 Wegener granulomatosis. CT in a 50-year-old man shows a cavitary nodule *(arrow)* in the right upper lobe. There were several other nodules at other levels.

bronchial atresia, and bronchial stenosis. In **bronchial atresia,** a normal bronchus ends blindly within the lung parenchyma, resulting in a focal area of emphysema. The airway proximal to the atresia fills with secretions, creating a **bronchocele,** often seen as a smooth opacity **(Fig. 2.56).** Surgical resection is necessary to prevent recurrent infections.

- **Bronchial wall thickening** or stenosis without dilatation is most commonly the result of bronchitis but can be seen with sarcoidosis, Wegener granulomatosis, amyloid deposition, and other inflammatory conditions. Normally, the thickness of the bronchial wall is no more than 10 percent of the bronchial diameter. **Chronic bronchitis** is a clinical diagnosis based on excessive sputum production. CT is usually normal.
- **Bronchiectasis** is irreversible bronchial dilatation with bronchial wall thickening. It is the result of inflammation and can result from pneumonia, obstruction, or congenital abnormalities such as cystic fibrosis, dysmotile cilia (Kartagener) syndrome, allergic bronchopulmonary aspergillosis (ABPA), impaired mucociliary clearance, hypogammaglobulinemia, or other immunodeficiencies. The specific cause is often unknown. Symptoms include chronic cough; frequent, recurrent infections; and hemoptysis. Medical management with antibiotics and respiratory therapy are the mainstays, but surgical resection of advanced localized disease can be warranted. Life-threatening bronchial artery hemorrhage can require embolization.
- **HRCT** is the method of choice for evaluating bronchiectasis; mild bronchiectasis can be overlooked on conventional CT. Abnormal findings include lack of bronchial tapering, bronchial dilatation, wall thickening, and mucoid filling. The most striking abnormality is visualization of bronchi further into the lung periphery than typically seen. The presence of bronchi in the peripheral third of the lung on conventional CT or within a few centimeters of the pleura on HRCT suggests bronchiectasis. Bronchi in cross section appear as thickened rings, and bronchi in the plane of section look like parallel, thickened "tram lines." In general, bronchi should be no larger than 1.2 times the diameter of the accompanying pulmonary artery. The "signet ring" sign is relative enlargement of the bronchi compared with the pulmonary artery, resulting in the artery forming the stone and the ectatic bronchi the band of the ring **(Fig. 2.57).**

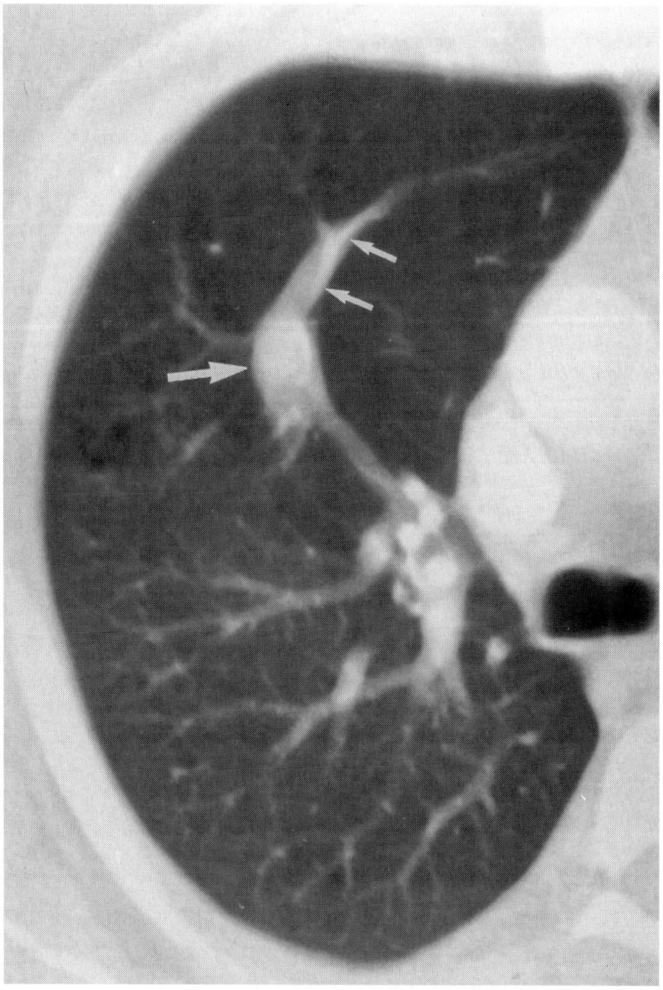

FIGURE 2.56 Bronchial atresia with bronchocele and regional hyperinflation. CT at the level of the carina shows regional emphysema surrounding a dilated mucus-filled bronchus *(large arrow).* Note the adjacent enhancing pulmonary artery branch *(small arrows).*

- **Mucoid impaction** in dilated bronchi is common. It can be isolated or seen in association with cystic fibrosis, ABPA, bronchial atresia, pulmonary sequestration, or bronchial obstruction **(Fig. 2.58).** The branching tubular opacities do not enhance following intravenous contrast, allowing distinction from vascular structures.
- The **distribution and morphology** of bronchiectasis varies according to the cause, but there is considerable overlap. Idiopathic bronchiectasis is often focal and is common in the lower lobes.

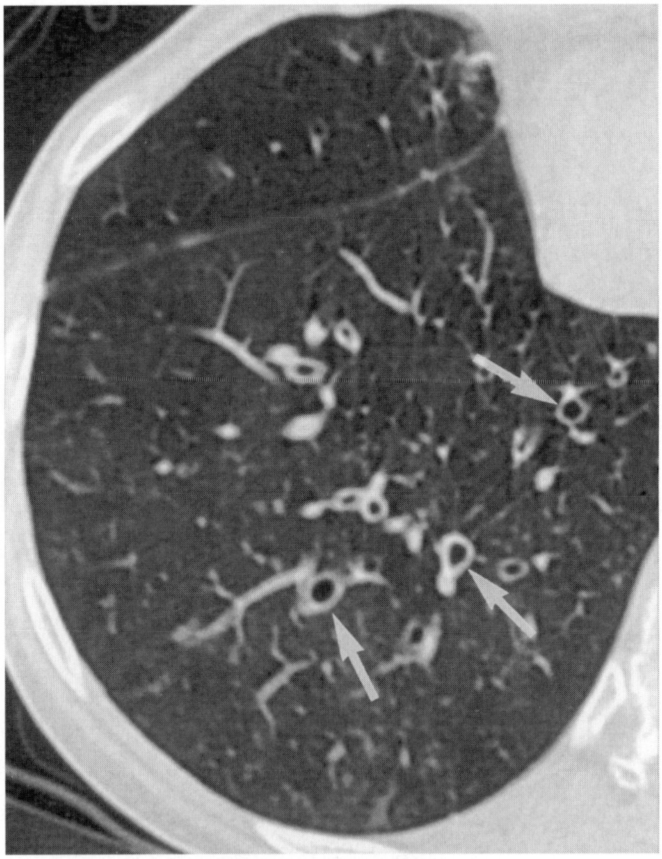

FIGURE 2.57 **Mild cylindrical bronchiectasis.** Note subtle thickening and enlargement of bronchi *(arrows)* as compared with their accompanying pulmonary artery branch.

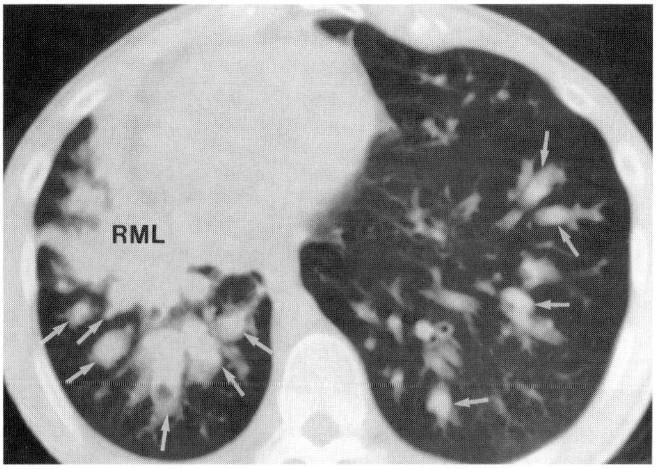

FIGURE 2.58 **Mucous plugging.** A 26-year-old man with cystic fibrosis and hypoxemia. CT revealed advanced mucoid impaction of dilated bronchi *(arrows)* and right-sided volume loss, with ipsilateral shift of the mediastinum and middle-lobe collapse (RML).

Focal bronchiectasis can also result from bronchial stenosis or endobronchial lesions with resultant mucoid impaction. Impaired mucociliary clearance and hypogammaglobulinemia have a lower-lobe predominance; cystic fibrosis has an upper-lobe predominance. APBA is often central **(see Fig. 2.19).**

Bronchiectasis is **classified morphologically** as cylindrical, varicose, or saccular (cystic), although mixed patterns are common and distinction has little clinical impact. **Cylindrical** (tubular) bronchiectasis involves fusiform dilatation with loss of normal tapering and abrupt termination. When confined to the central lung in asthmatics, ABPA is often the cause. **Varicose** bronchiectasis has a beaded appearance and is common with cystic fibrosis. **Cystic** (saccular) bronchiectasis causes marked bronchial dilatation, with peripheral ballooning producing cystic cavities, often with thick walls and air-fluid levels due to retained secretions **(Fig. 2.59).** It is often associated with bronchial stenosis.

Traction bronchiectasis is caused by fibrotic distortion of the lung parenchyma from infection, radiation therapy, or end-stage lung disease and is not due to intrinsic bronchial inflammation. Traction bronchiolectasis is common in the lung periphery of patients with fibrosis and contributes to the appearance of honeycombing.

- **Bronchiectasis** can be mimicked by respiratory or cardiac motion, causing blurring of the fissures and vessels simulating dilated bronchi in longitudinal section. Inspection of adjacent images almost always confirms the true nature of this finding. Inappropriate window settings can also produce a misleading appearance.
- **"Reversible or pseudobronchiectasis"** is a transient, cylindrical bronchial dilatation seen as a result of bronchial inflammation from bacterial pneumonia. The bronchial dilatation can persist for several months, but eventually there is a return to the normal diameter.
- **Immotile** or **dysmotile cilia syndrome** is an autosomal recessive deficiency resulting in sinusitis, deafness, and infertility. Pulmonary findings include atelectasis, infection, and bronchiectasis from chronic mucoid impaction. When associated with situs inversus, the disorder is known as **Kartagener syndrome. Congenital bronchiectasis** (Williams-Campbell syndrome) is a rare disorder of bronchial cartilage deficiency producing bronchiectasis and distal

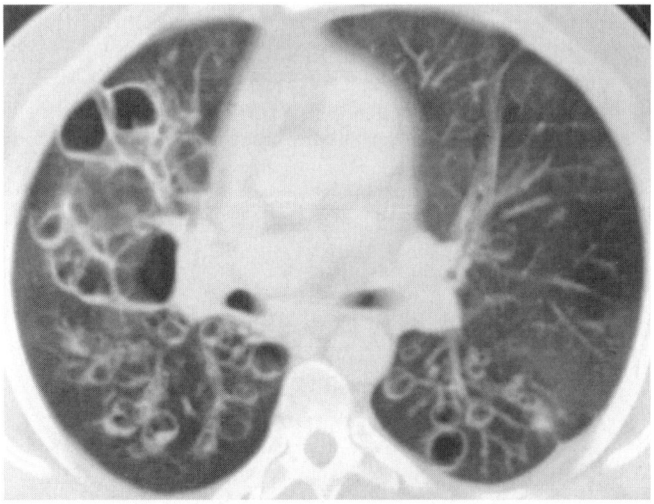

FIGURE 2.59 **Cystic bronchiectasis.** CT shows advanced cystic bronchiectasis in the right lung and superior segment of the left lower lobe. The most likely etiology was prior bacterial infections. (Slone RM, Gutierrez FR, Fisher AJ. *Thoracic Imaging: A Practical Approach*. New York: McGraw-Hill; 1999. With permission.)

emphysema. Unlike immotile cilia syndrome, there is no association with sinus disease, otitis, or abnormal situs. **Mounier-Kuhn syndrome *(tracheobronchomegaly)*** is a rare disorder presenting as tracheal and central bronchial enlargement, often with bronchiectasis **(see Fig. 4.25).** Patients have recurrent pulmonary infections, increased sputum production, and dyspnea.

- **Cystic fibrosis** (CF) is an autosomal recessive metabolic disorder characterized by abnormal exocrine gland function. Pancreatic insufficiency, biliary cirrhosis, and fertility problems are seen. Upper respiratory involvement includes sinusitis, nasal polyps, and recurrent otitis. Recurrent bronchitis and pneumonia lead to purulent cough, hemoptysis, dypsnea, and hypoxemia due to mucoid impaction. CT shows increased lung volumes with upper-lobe interstitial infiltrates, and bronchiectasis with peribronchial thickening, atelectasis, mucoid impaction, and air-fluid levels within bronchiectatic airways **(Fig. 2.60).**

  Complications include lung abscesses, empyemas, and pneumothorax due to rupture of emphysematous blebs. A delayed presentation and mild course are seen in some patients who present as adults with cylindrical bronchiectasis, as opposed to younger patients, who have cystic or varicose patterns. Pulmonary arterial and right heart enlargement as well as hilar adenopathy from chronic infection can be seen. *Pseudomonas* is the most common pathogen, and antibiotic resistance is problematic. Patients with CF are predisposed to invasive infections, including aspergillus and other fungi. Death results from respiratory failure, massive hemoptysis, or cor pulmonale. Improved medical management and lung transplantation have improved survival.

2.11 SMALL AIRWAY AND OBSTRUCTIVE LUNG DISEASE

- Chest radiographs and conventional CT can sometimes appear normal in patients with small airway disease. Detection of subtle disease is best accomplished using expiratory HRCT, which can demonstrate the structural and functional abnormalities to better advantage.
- **Asthma** is a hypersensitivity reaction producing reversible bronchoconstriction with dyspnea, cough, and wheezing. Findings can include hyperinflation, bronchial wall thickening, atelectasis, ABPA, and localized air trapping due to mucoid plugging. Patients are predisposed to bacterial and mycoplasma pneumonias. Chronic changes include bronchiectasis and scarring from recurring infections. Complications include pneumomediastinum and pneumothorax.
- **Bronchiolitis** is an inflammation of the small airways, sometimes with fibrosis, resulting from damage to the bronchiolar epithelium. Causes include pulmonary infections, smoke inhalation, toxic fumes, dust exposure, drug toxicity, graft-versus-host disease, autoimmune disease, lung transplantation, and connective tissue disorders. However, bronchiolitis is often idiopathic. Patients present with nonproductive cough, dyspnea, fever, or nonspecific symptoms that do not respond to antibiotics. HRCT can show patchy air trapping on expiration, centrilobular branching structures and nodules **(Fig. 2.61)**, and mosaic perfusion with areas of hypoventilation, and decreased blood flow due to vessel constriction.
- **Bronchiolitis obliterans** is characterized by granulomatous inflammation within bronchioles and alveolar ducts, producing small

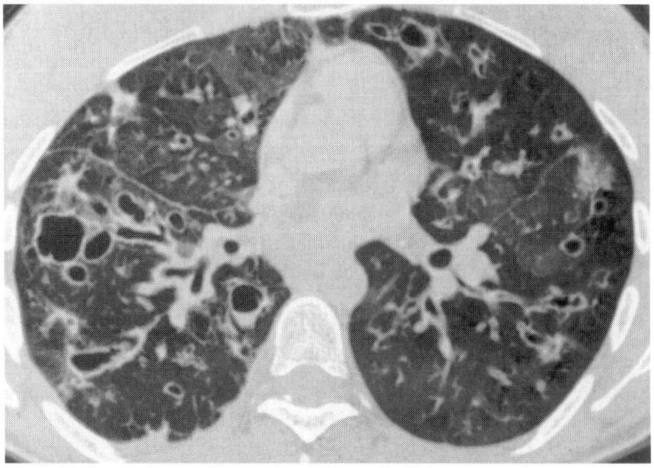

FIGURE 2.60 Cystic fibrosis. HRCT in a 26-year-old woman shows severe cylindrical and saccular bronchiectasis.

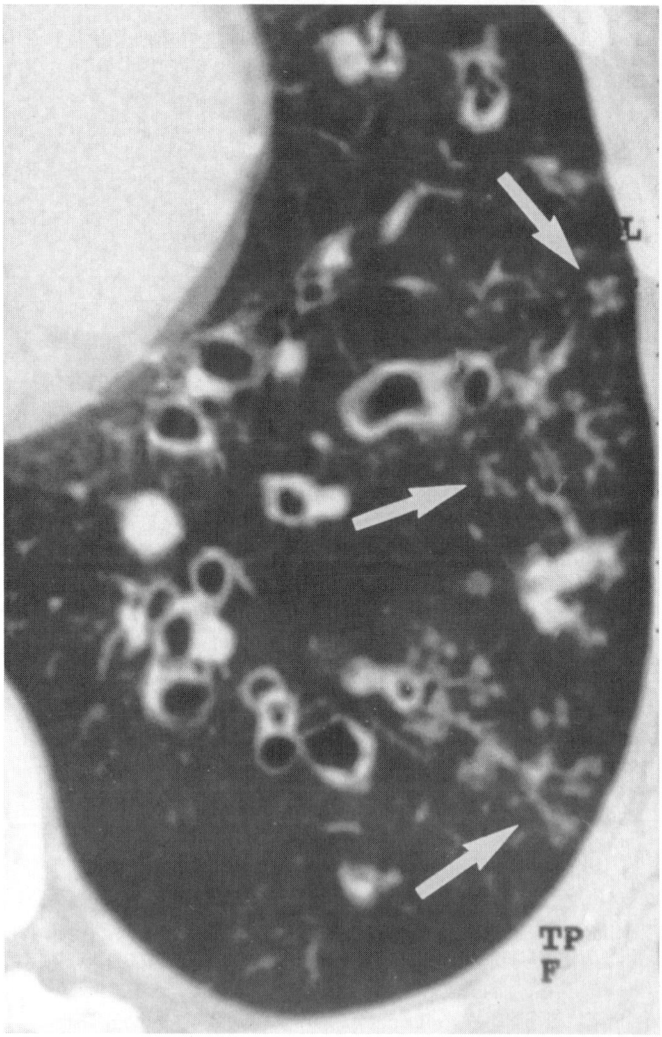

FIGURE 2.61 Bronchiectasis and bronchiolitis. HRCT in the left lower lobe shows bronchiectasis as well as multiple "tree-in-bud" opacities in the lung periphery *(arrows)*, representing terminal airway inflammation.

airway obstruction. Cough, wheezing, chest pain, and dyspnea are out of proportion to radiographic abnormalities; in fact, radiographs are often normal. **Diffuse panbronchiolitis,** characterized by diffuse airway inflammation, affects primarily people of Asian origin. Patients present with bronchiectasis and bronchiolectasis and peripheral nodular opacities representing dilated opacified bronchioles.

- **Bronchiolitis obliterans with organizing pneumonia (BOOP)**, also referred to as cryptogenic organizing pneumonia (COP), is the most common cause of proliferative bronchiolitis. It is the result of granulation tissue obstructing bronchioles and alveolar ducts, with organizing pneumonia and inflammatory cells infiltrating the airspace and interstitium. Patients typically present with upper respiratory symptoms and nonproductive cough. CT findings include bilateral patchy ground-glass infiltrates and areas of peripheral consolidation, presumably representing postobstructive pneumonitis, sometimes with pulmonary nodules, bronchial wall thickening, and dilation. The appearance often simulates bronchopneumonia, but steroid therapy reduces the inflammation and is the treatment of choice **(Fig. 2.62).**

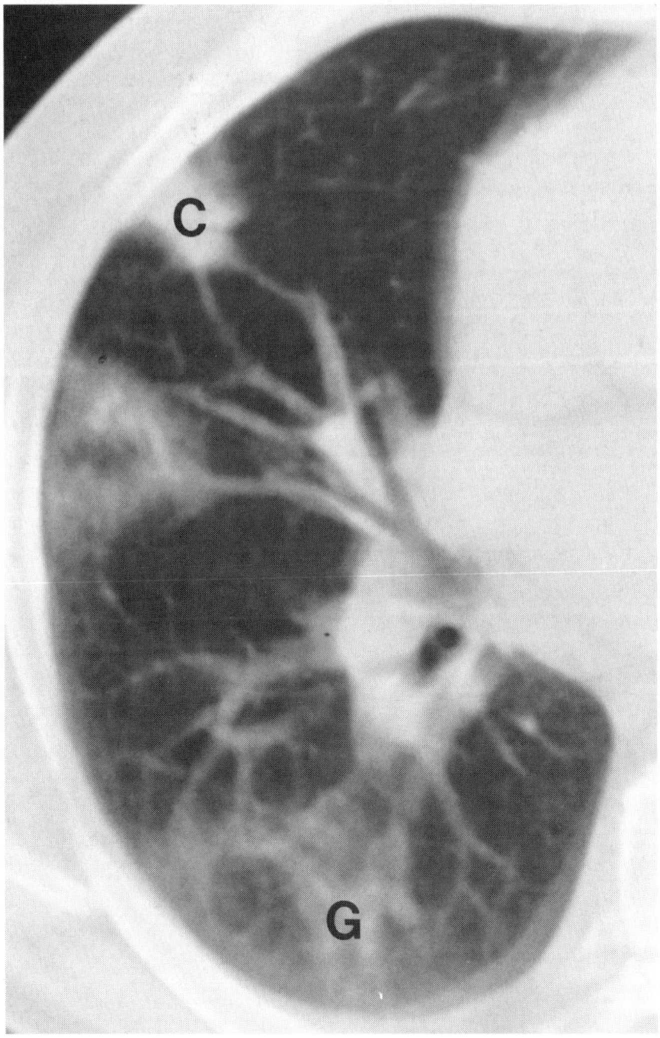

FIGURE 2.62 Bronchiolitis obliterans with organizing pneumonia (BOOP). Focal peripheral areas of consolidation (C) and ground-glass attenuation (G) shown to be BOOP on transbronchial biopsy. The infiltrates resolved with steroid therapy.

Pulmonary Emphysema

- **Pulmonary emphysema** is irreversible enlargement of airspaces distal to the terminal bronchiole, with destruction of the alveolar walls and no obvious fibrosis. This results in loss of pulmonary elastic recoil, causing airflow obstruction, hyperinflation, hypoxemia, and hypercapnea. Pulmonary function testing demonstrates an obstructive pattern with increased lung volumes. The term *chronic obstructive pulmonary disease* refers to a specific clinical presentation and should not be used to described the CT abnormalities.

  CT, particularly HRCT, permits identification of destroyed lung parenchyma that correlates well with direct pathologic examination. CT characteristics of emphysema include areas of decreased attenuation without visible walls and pulmonary vessel distortion and pruning. HRCT can reliably depict even mild emphysema that escapes detection by pulmonary function testing. Expiratory CT accentuates areas of lung destruction and air trapping. Blebs and bullae are frequently associated with emphysema but can be seen as a localized process in otherwise normal lungs. Although pulmonary artery enlargement and mild pulmonary hypertension are common in patients with advanced emphysema, pulmonary artery size is a poor indicator of pressure and, despite enlargement and advanced emphysema, significant pulmonary arterial hypertension is uncommon. Pulmonary emphysema is often seen in combination with other pulmonary disease processes and can alter the appearance of diffuse and focal lung diseases. Pulmonary edema, for example, can take on a more focal, patchy appearance, simulating pneumonia. This is because the edema primarily involves the areas of normal, better-perfused lung and spares the severely emphysematous, oligemic regions.

- **Four principal types** of emphysema have been described pathologically, although it is common for them to coexist. **Centrilobular** emphysema is the most common form and is the result of destruction at the center of the pulmonary lobule. It is found predominantly in cigarette smokers and is thought to be due to an imbalance between lung proteases and antiproteases. CT shows well-defined lucencies surrounded by normal lung parenchyma **(Fig. 2.63).** These holes become confluent and the vessels become peripherally attenuated as the destruction progresses. The apical and posterior segments of the upper lobes and superior segments of the lower lobes are most severely affected.

- **Panlobular** emphysema affects the entire secondary pulmonary lobule. It occurs in smokers and in alpha$_1$-antitrypsin deficiency as a result of unchecked proteolytic digestion of lung parenchyma. **Alpha$_1$-antitrypsin,** a glycoprotein synthesized in the liver, is a proteolytic inhibitor of trypsin, bacterial proteases, and proteolytic enzymes. Deficiency of this protein is a rare autosomal recessive disorder resulting in panacinar pulmonary emphysema. There is a lower-lobe predominance, presumably due to greater blood flow.

- **Paraseptal** emphysema is often an isolated phenomenon. Localized destruction and airspace enlargement are seen within otherwise normal lung, primarily in the lung periphery, characteristically adjacent to the visceral pleura. "Vanishing lung" describes massive bullae **(Fig. 2.64).**

- **Paracicatricial** ("scar") emphysema is airspace enlargement and lung destruction from adjacent pulmonary fibrosis. There is often associated traction bronchiectasis and "honeycomb lung." **Compensatory emphysema** involves hyperinflation in normal lung adjacent to an area of volume loss. It is not true emphysema, since there is no actual lung destruction.

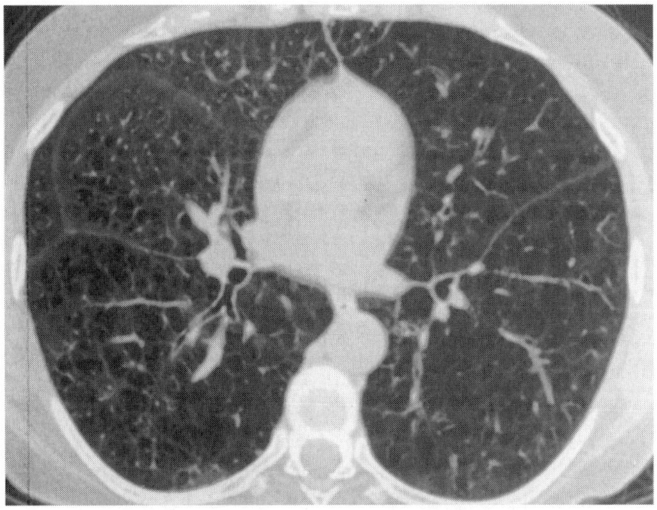

FIGURE 2.63 Severe diffuse centrilobular emphysema. HRCT in a 59-year-old man with severe dyspnea shows evidence of advanced pulmonary emphysema with hyperinflation and multiple small, circular areas of lung destruction. There was no evidence of interstitial lung disease or bronchiectasis.

- Medical management options for emphysema are palliative and include bronchodilators, steroids, supplemental oxygen, antibiotics, and smoking cessation. Surgical management options include lung volume reduction and transplantation.

2.12 ENVIRONMENTAL, OCCUPATIONAL, AND IATROGENIC LUNG DISEASE

- **The pneumoconioses** are lung diseases resulting from exposure to inorganic environmental materials. Foreign-body and inflammatory reactions lead to interstitial nodules or fibrosis. CT, particularly HRCT, is significantly more sensitive and specific than chest radiography for detecting and assessing disease.

- **Silicosis** is the result of inhaling silicon dioxide dust, typically affecting sandblasters, stone grinders, and foundry workers. Pulmonary nodules develop from phagocytized dust and fibroblasts. The disease progresses slowly. **Acute silicoses** (silicoproteinosis) can develop after massive exposure, in which pulmonary consolidation caused by abundant surfactant, similar to alveolar proteinosis, predominates.

  Simple silicosis takes the form of multiple discrete pulmonary nodules, typically only a few millimeters in diameter, with an upper-lobe predominance; some calcify. Mediastinal adenopathy is common, classically with eggshell calcification **(see Fig. 4.7). Complicated silicosis** (progressive massive fibrosis) involves ***conglomerate masses*** formed by coalescence of smaller silicotic nodules. They are usually symmetrical and located in the upper lobes; they sometimes cavitate. The fibrosis produces upper-lobe volume loss, paracicatricial emphysema, and progressive functional impairment **(Fig. 2.65).** Tuberculosis occurs with an increased incidence in these patients, a condition called ***silicotuberculosis.***

- **Coal worker's pneumoconiosis** is the result of incomplete clearing of inhaled inert coal dust containing fibrinogenic silica dioxide dust. The appearance is nearly indistinguishable from that of silicosis, although the distinction can be made pathologically. Simple coal worker's pneumoconiosis involves aggregates of "coal dust macules" measuring a few millimeters in diameter, found predominantly in the upper lobes. As with complicated silicosis, fibrosis and progressive massive fibrosis can develop.

- **Asbestosis** is asbestos-induced pulmonary fibrosis, in distinction from ***asbestos-related pleural disease,*** which refers to pleural plaques indicating prior asbestos exposure. Fibrosis can take 10 to 20 years to develop. Shortness of breath is the primary symptom. The earliest abnormality is septal thickening, parenchymal bands, subpleural curvilinear lines, nodules, and honeycombing in the lung bases **(see Figs. 2.1 and 2.32).** Traction bronchiectasis and pericicatricial emphysema occur with advanced asbestosis. Definitive diagnosis usually requires biopsy, revealing phagocytized asbestos fibers termed ***ferruginous bodies.*** Asbestos exposure increases the risk of mesothelioma and bronchogenic carcinoma.

- **Extrinsic allergic alveolitis** (hypersensitivity pneumonitis) is an immunologically mediated response to organic dust, producing inflammation, shortness of breath, and hypoxemia. The precipitating

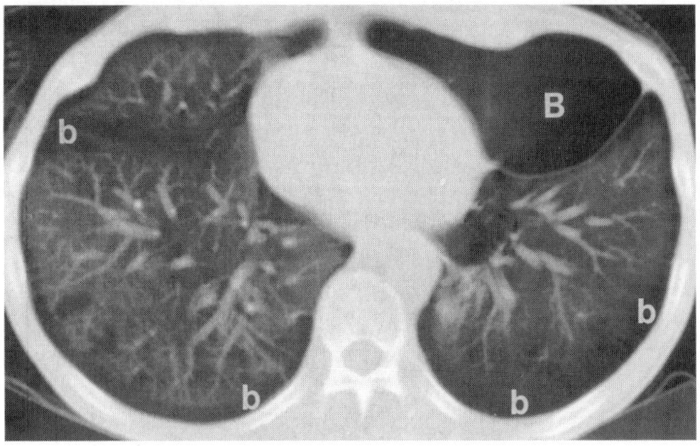

FIGURE 2.64 Advanced paraseptal emphysema. Chest CT in a 48-year-old man shows a large left upper lobe bulla (B) and characteristic subpleural lung destruction (b). The central lung tissue is normal.

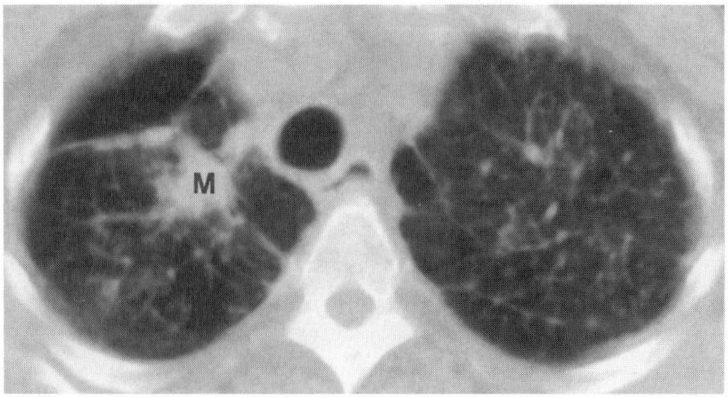

FIGURE 2.65 Silicosis with progressive massive fibrosis. Chest CT shows nodular interstitial disease in both lung apices. There is a conglomerate mass (M) in the right lung with surrounding fibrosis, architectural distortion of the lung parenchyma, and pericicatricial emphysema.

agent is primarily fungal antigens, in contrast to pneumoconioses caused by inorganic dust. Common eponyms include ***farmer's lung*** (moldy hay) and ***bird-fancier's*** or ***pigeon breeder's lung*** (excrement or feathers). CT demonstrates patchy ground-glass attenuation and ill-defined centrilobular opacities **(Fig. 2.66).**

- **Noxious gas inhalation** can produce bronchial irritation and inflammation, causing cough and dyspnea. It is usually a result of occupational accidents. Potential causative substances include chlorine, phosgene, ammonia, sulfur dioxide, toluene, and nitrous oxide ***(silo filler's disease).*** CT can reveal mild bronchitis and noncardiogenic edema. Recovery can take weeks. Bronchiolitis obliterans can develop as a complication.

Chemotherapy

- **Drug-induced lung disease** is a potential complication of several therapeutic agents. Toxic effects are often dose-related and cumulative. Pulmonary manifestations include interstitial infiltrates, effusions, nodules, and fibrosis. Narcotic overdose often leads to edema. Methotrexate, aspirin, penicillin, and nitrofurantoin can cause eosinophilia and pulmonary infiltrates. Procainamide, isoniazid, and penicillin can cause pneumonitis and pleural effusions. Busulfan, amiodarone, azathioprine, bleomycin, and cyclophosphamide are associated with fibrosis, primarily within the posterior lung. **Amiodarone,** used to treat refractory arrhythmias, accumulates in the liver and lung and can cause progressive pneumonitis. Ground-glass opacities on HRCT suggest reversible infiltrative lung disease. Advanced disease is associated with fibrosis. Increased liver attenuation can be seen due to iodine deposition **(see Fig. 7.4).** Rarely, bleomycin can cause pulmonary nodules indistinguishable from metastases. HRCT is sensitive in evaluating these complications and allows early detection of active inflammatory disease, making it possible to discontinue the drug before substantial fibrosis occurs.

Radiation Therapy

- **Complications** of thoracic radiation therapy include pneumonitis, esophagitis, pericarditis, esophageal stricture, and rarely myelopathy. **Radiation pneumonitis** does not always develop following radiation therapy, but when it does, it usually occurs 1 to 3 months following therapy and is self-limited. Symptoms include dyspnea, nonproductive cough, hypoxemia, a low-grade fever, and mild leukocytosis. Individual susceptibility varies. Risk factors include a high dose, less fractionation, greater volume of lung, and concomitant administration of chemotherapy. Radiologic evidence of injury is rare below 20 Gy (2000 rads).

  Typically there is gradual evolution from a homogeneous increase in density to discrete areas of consolidation. Small, nodular abnormalities can be confused with pulmonary metastases. Positron emission tomography (PET) can be useful in differentiating radiation fibrosis from recurrent tumor. The pneumonitis gradually transforms to radiation fibrosis, which usually stabilizes 9 to 12 months following treatment **(Fig. 2.67).** Bronchiolectasis and volume loss also occur, producing honeycombing. The findings cross anatomic boundaries and conform to the shape of the radiation port.

2.13 IDIOPATHIC LUNG DISEASE

- **Alveolar proteinosis** is the result of abnormal accumulation of surfactant in alveoli. The exact etiology is unknown. Men are affected more often than women. Symptoms include dyspnea, cough, weight loss, weakness, and hemoptysis. CT shows predominantly perihilar and lower-lobe ground-glass attenuation and consolidation. HRCT can show a pattern of "crazy paving" with smooth, linear opacities. There is no adenopathy, cardiomegaly, or pleural effusion. There is slow progression with a variable course of clinical and radiologic improvement and exacerbation. Superimposed pneumonia with *Nocardia,* mycobacteria, or CMV is common. Treatment is large-volume bronchopulmonary lavage.

- **Alveolar microlithiasis** is a rare disease of unknown etiology affecting middle-aged patients. CT features are disproportionately worse than clinical symptoms and include diffuse fine, sand-like microcalcifications, measuring <1 mm. The microliths can

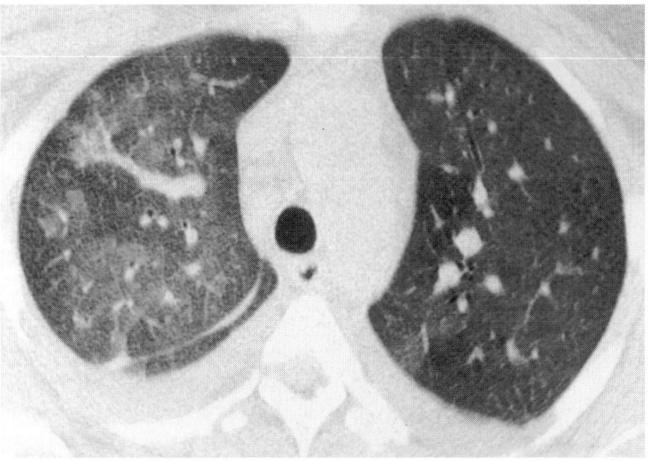

FIGURE 2.66 Hypersensitivity pneumonitis. HRCT through the upper lobes in a 32-year-old woman shows patchy ground-glass attenuation, primarily in the right lung. (Slone RM, Gutierrez FR, Fisher AJ. *Thoracic Imaging: A Practical Approach.* New York: McGraw-Hill, 1999. With permission.)

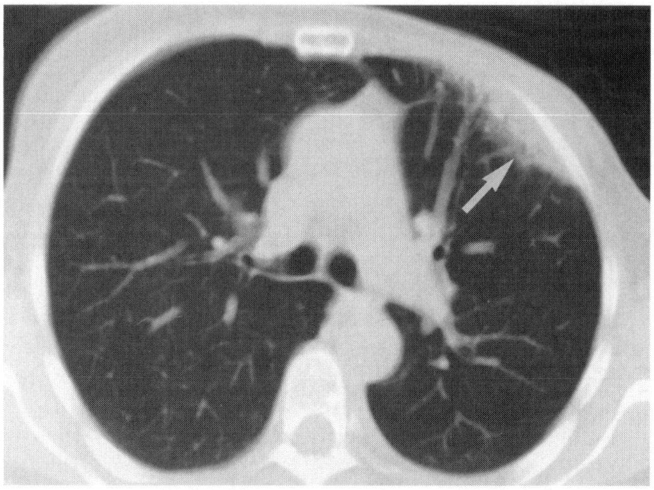

FIGURE 2.67 Radiation fibrosis. Chest CT in 52-year-old woman who had undergone a left mastectomy and radiation therapy for treatment of breast cancer. The geographic peripheral consolidation *(arrow)* and volume loss is a result of radiation pneumonitis and fibrosis. The radiation port passed tangential to the anterolateral chest wall.

continue to enlarge, progress to pulmonary fibrosis, or become arrested.

- **Lymphangioleiomyomatosis (LAM)** is a rare disease of unknown etiology that affects young women of reproductive age. The disease is characterized by smooth muscle proliferation in the airway, causing pulmonary cysts and pneumothoraces; in lymphatics, leading to chylothoraces and adenopathy; and in arterioles and venules to a lesser degree. It is exacerbated during pregnancy.

  HRCT shows well-defined, thin-walled cysts ranging from a few millimeters to several centimeters distributed uniformly throughout the lung **(see Fig. 2.9).** Septal thickening can result from lymphatic engorgement, smooth muscle proliferation, and fibrosis. The lung volumes are typically normal or increased. Pulmonary artery pressure increases as the disease progresses, leading to cor pulmonale and hemoptysis. Medical therapy includes progesterone or oophorectomy. LAM is uniformly fatal, typically within 10 years of diagnosis. Lung transplantation is an option for some patients. **Tuberous sclerosis** is an autosomal dominant neurocutaneous syndrome that rarely involves the lungs (1 percent); when it does, it can be indistinguishable from LAM, although small nodules can also be present.

- **Neurofibromatosis** (type I) is an autosomal dominant condition characterized by café au lait spots, mesenchymal dysplasia, and subcutaneous neurofibromas. Neurofibrosarcomas can develop and metastasize to the lung. About one-fifth of patients develop pulmonary fibrosis, typically with a basal predominance. Upper-lobe bullae are relatively common.

- **Acute eosinophilic pneumonia** (Loffler syndrome) consists of acute transient pulmonary infiltrates with blood eosinophilia that is either idiopathic or an allergic reaction to parasites such as *Strongyloides* or *Schistosoma*. CT shows migratory nonsegmental peripheral infiltrates, changing over days and clearing within a month. Pulmonary eosinophilia can also be caused by *Aspergillus* or medications. **Chronic eosinophilic pneumonia** is idiopathic and affects middle-aged women more than men. Patients have blood eosinophilia and sometimes cough, wheezing, fever, and malaise or dyspnea. CT demonstrates nonsegmental peripheral consolidation which changes slowly, lasting a month or more. Treatment is with steroids.

- **Pulmonary amyloidosis** is a rare disease characterized by extracellular protein accumulation; it can be primary or secondary to an underlying chronic disease. Chest involvement includes nodular tracheobronchial thickening, infiltrates, and parenchymal nodules that can cavitate or calcify. Fibrosis and adenopathy can develop but effusions are rare.

- **Langerhans cell histiocytosis** or eosinophilic granuloma (EG) is an idiopathic systemic disease with variable expression, ranging from solitary bone or skin disease to a multisystem process leading to organ failure and death. Pulmonary manifestations are present in half the patients, most of whom are female cigarette smokers. Symptoms include dry cough, dyspnea, and pneumothorax. The most common CT findings are upper-lobe-predominant interstitial nodules, pulmonary cysts, or combinations of both **(Fig. 2.68).** The nodules are usually less than 5 mm in diameter and are often distributed in the center of the pulmonary lobules and around small airways. The nodules likely progress to cavitary nodules, thick-walled cysts, and then thin-walled cysts. When both nodules and cysts are seen, it helps differentiate EG from the other diseases that can present with small nodules alone, including granulomatous infections, and silicosis. Interlobular septal thickening, ground-glass opacities, and fibrosis with paracicatricial emphysema can also be seen. Hyperinflation and spontaneous pneumothorax are also observed. There is no lymphadenopathy. Geographic lytic bone lesions can sometimes be seen in the ribs or spine.

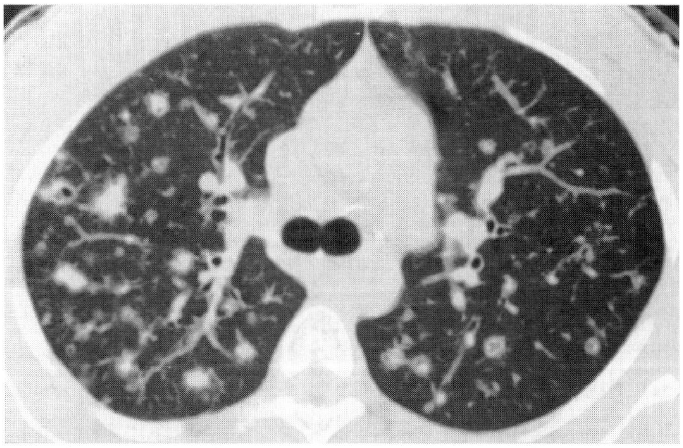

FIGURE 2.68 Eosinophilic granuloma. HRCT in a 33-year-old woman who is a heavy smoker. There are both smooth and ill-defined nodules, some with cavitation. There was an upper-lobe predominance of findings. [Sagel SS, Slone RM. The lung. In: Lee JKT, Sagel SS, Stanley RJ, Heiken JP (eds.): *Computed Body Tomography with MRI Correlation*. Philadelphia: Lippincott-Raven, 1998. With permission.]

- **Pulmonary hemosiderosis** is the result of recurrent alveolar hemorrhage with the deposition of iron and hemosiderin in alveolar macrophages. It is commonly idiopathic and probably autoimmune but can occur secondary to cardiac disease, such as mitral stenosis or vasculitis. CT findings include transient patchy bilateral airspace disease during acute episodes. With repeated hemorrhage, a reticular interstitial infiltrate can develop, progressing to fibrosis. Clubbing, pulmonary hypertension, iron deficiency anemia, and hepatosplenomegaly can develop. The prognosis is poorest for the idiopathic form.

- **Sarcoidosis** is a systemic disease characterized by noncaseating granulomas involving primarily mediastinal lymph nodes and the lung. The etiology is unknown, but it may be an immunologically mediated response to an unidentified agent. Women are more often affected than men. Uveal, cardiac, liver, spleen, skin, bone, and salivary involvement can also occur. Laboratory studies show an elevated sedimentation rate, hypercalcemia, and elevated levels of angiotensin-converting enzyme (ACE) in serum.

  Patients with adenopathy alone are usually asymptomatic, but patients with pulmonary involvement can experience weight loss, fatigue, fever, cough, or dyspnea. Hemoptysis is rare. Diagnosis is usually confirmed by transbronchial biopsy. Beryllliosis is indistinguishable radiologically and pathologically from sarcoidosis. Treatment of sarcoidosis is with steroids. Death is directly attributed to sarcoid in less than 5 percent of patients and is a result of cor pulmonale, hemorrhage, mycetoma, or respiratory failure. **Lofgren syndrome** is a constellation of fever, erythema nodosum, arthralgias, hilar adenopathy, and focal pulmonary infiltrates in patients with sarcoidosis. It portends a favorable prognosis.

  Staging is based on the radiographic appearance of adenopathy alone (stage I), adenopathy with pulmonary disease (stage II), pulmonary disease alone (stage III), or fibrosis (stage IV). Most patients present with stage I (50 percent) or stage II disease (30 percent). Less than one- third of patients with stage I progress to develop lung disease. The thoracic manifestations eventually resolve in over half of patients with stage I or II disease. **Mediastinal adenopathy** is usually depicted as symmetrical hilar and right paratracheal involvement **(see Figs. 2.69 and 4.4).** Subcarinal adenopathy is also common. Peripheral "eggshell" lymph node calcification is occasionally seen.

Pulmonary manifestations include 1- to 10-mm irregular interstitial and subpleural nodules and interstitial infiltrates resulting from noncaseating granulomas. Cavitation is rare. HRCT shows nodular, irregular bronchovascular and interlobular septal thickening similar to that seen in lymphangitic carcinomatosis **(see Fig. 2.29).** The middle and upper lung zones are most commonly involved and the periphery and bases of the lungs are generally spared. Adenopathy typically decreases as lung disease progresses. Pleural effusions are exceedingly rare. Pulmonary involvement usually resolves but progresses to fibrosis in about one-fifth of patients. The distribution is often patchy **(see Fig. 2.33)**, in contrast to the peripheral, lower-lobe distribution of IPF. Occasionally, pulmonary sarcoid can present as diffuse ground-glass opacities or consolidation, termed **alveolar sarcoid (Fig. 2.69).**

2.14 CT-GUIDED BIOPSY AND THORACIC SURGERY

- **CT-guided percutaneous lung biopsy** is an important tool for evaluating thoracic masses and fluid collections. CT facilitates accurate needle placement, allowing very small lesions to be interrogated. Tissue sampling techniques include fine-needle aspiration (FNA) for cytologic evaluation, and cutting needles and core biopsies for histology. If lymphoma is a diagnostic consideration, then core biopsy rather than FNA may be required to obtain adequate material. If infection is suspected, a sample should be sent for microbiologic evaluation. Commitment to biopsy a lesion should occur only after careful review of imaging studies, consideration of the differential diagnosis, and impact on clinical management.
- Important factors to consider in biopsy planning include patient positioning (prone, supine, or decubitus) and phase of respiration (end-expiration or inspiration). End-expiration is more reproducible, but inspiration may be required to facilitate approaching a lesion behind a rib. The patient should be as comfortable as possible and have a good understanding of the procedure to ensure cooperation. Breathing instruction should be rehearsed. Familiarity with the biopsy equipment and management plan for complications, particularly pneumothorax, is critical. Almost all biopsies can be performed as outpatient procedures. Conscious sedation is seldom necessary but can be used selectively for anxious or uncomfortable patients. Local anesthesia is typically adequate. A pulse oximeter for monitoring heart rate and oxygen saturation is useful.
- A needle path should be selected that avoids vessels, bullae, and pleural fissures. The needle should be positioned within the wall of necrotic lesions so as to obtain viable tissue **(see Fig. 2.42).** Care should be taken to avoid unnecessary contact of the needle tip with the pleura—i.e., the needle should always be well outside the pleura and within the chest wall or well through the pleura and into lung. It is critical that the patient suspend breathing while the needle is advanced through the pleura. Contact between the needle tip and moving visceral pleura will invariably lead to pneumothorax. A **coaxial technique** involves positioning an outer guiding needle (thin-walled 19-gauge) in or near the lesion and obtaining aspirates by deploying a smaller biopsy needle (20-gauge for biopsy, 22-gauge for FNA) through the guide needle **(Fig. 2.70).** Once positioned, the guiding needle facilitates successive biopsies and

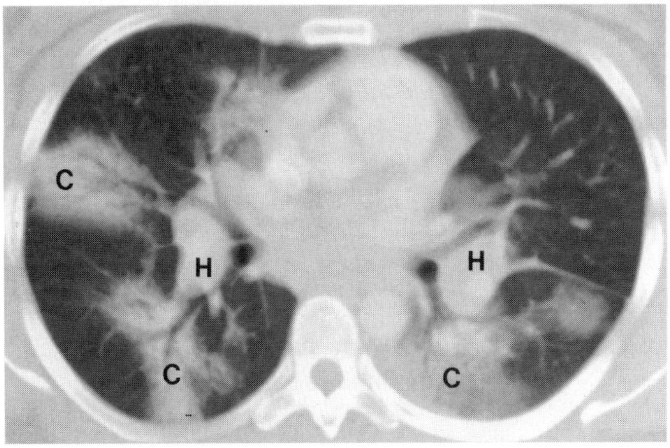

FIGURE 2.69 Alveolar sarcoidosis. CT in a 29-year-old woman with multifocal consolidation (C) and marked hilar adenopathy (H).

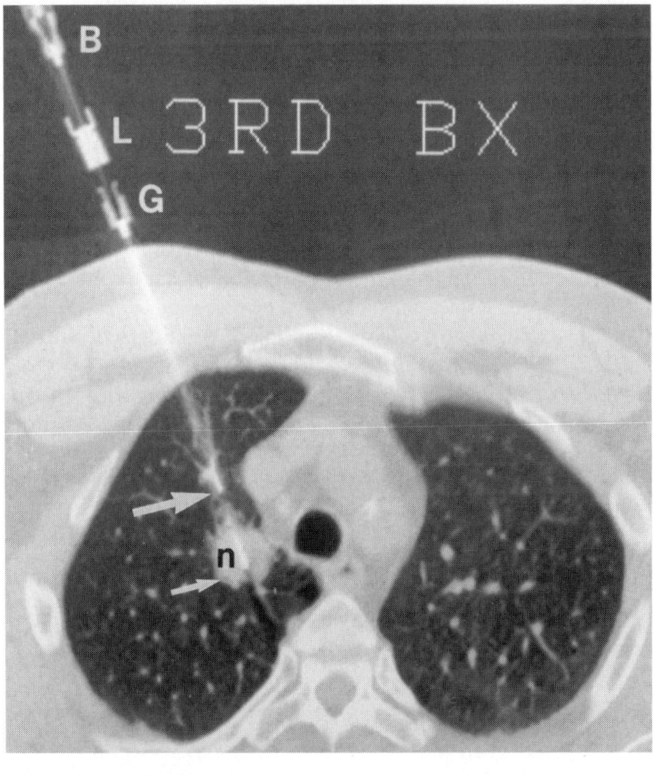

FIGURE 2.70 CT-guided percutaneous lung biopsy using coaxial technique. A thin-walled 19-gauge "guiding" needle was placed through the chest wall and within 1 cm of the nodule (n). Multiple biopsies were then performed by passing a 22-gauge Chiba needle through the guiding needle and into the nodule. A plastic lock device (L) was placed on the needle to mark the desired depth. G, hub of the guiding needle; B, hub of the biopsy needle; tip of the guide needle *(large arrow)*; tip of 22-gauge biopsy needle *(small arrow)*.

can be left in place while specimens are reviewed for adequacy by the cytotechnologist. This obviates repeated puncture of the visceral pleura, thus reducing the risk of pneumothorax and procedure time.

- The lesion is localized under CT guidance and the skin and subcutaneous tissues are anesthetized. The anesthesia needle can be left in place while a scan is performed to confirm needle orientation. Distance measurements are made from the skin surface to the pleura and to the edge of the lesion. A small skin nick is made and the guide needle with its stylet is placed into the chest wall, taking care to stop at least 1 cm short of the pleura. The needle's direction and depth are confirmed by CT. Then, during suspended respiration and with a single smooth but quick motion, the needle is advanced through the pleura and into lung. The location is confirmed by CT and the needle is repositioned during suspended respiration as necessary. FNA is performed by removing the stylet during suspended respiration and placing the aspirating needle into the guide needle. The patient can then breathe. Then, during suspended respiration, the aspiration needle is advanced into the lesion. The location can be confirmed by CT if indicated. Finally, during suspended respiration, with aspiration applied, the needle is moved in and out 5 to 10 mm within the lesion 6 to 10 times to obtain a sample. Suction is released and the patient can again breathe. During suspended respiration, the aspirating needle is removed and the stylet is placed in the guide needle. The procedure is repeated for subsequent aspirates. The needle should never be open to room air during inspiration, since air embolism can occur if the tip is in a pulmonary vein branch. Yield is generally optimized with three to four aspirates. If the result is nondiagnostic after five to six passes, core biopsy should be considered. A small amount of parenchymal **bleeding** can occur around the lesion **(see Fig. 2.4).** Mild **hemoptysis** is uncommon and usually self-limited.
- **Pneumothorax** occurs in about one-third of patients undergoing percutaneous lung biopsy, but chest tube drainage is required in less than half of these. In general, the risk of pneumothorax increases with needle size, number of visceral pleural punctures, duration of time the needle spans the pleura, depth of respiration, and presence of underlying lung disease, particularly emphysema. A small, asymptomatic pneumothorax can be observed, but when a pneumothorax is large or symptomatic, drainage is required. Several easy-to-use pneumothorax drainage sets are available, and these should be readily at hand. A delayed pneumothorax can occur spontaneously following biopsy or may be induced by coughing, laughing, or straining the thorax or abdomen. **Precautions** to reduce delayed pneumothorax include moving patients from the CT scanner to a stretcher rather than having them move themselves, positioning patients with the pleural puncture site in a dependent position (i.e., for a biopsy performed prone, patients should lie supine). Patients should remain relaxed on a stretcher for 1 h, after which radiographs can be obtained to assess the lung and pleura. If there is no evidence of pneumothorax, patients can be allowed to ambulate, use the rest room, and eat or drink. The idea is to engage patients in routine activities so that a delayed pneumothorax would occur under observation rather than at home. If patients remain asymptomatic and radiographs obtained 3 to 4 h after biopsy show no complications, patients can be discharged with instructions to seek immediate medical assistance if they develop chest pain, shortness of breath, or hemoptysis.
- **Fiberoptic bronchoscopy** allows direct visualization of the tracheobronchial tree for evaluation of hemoptysis, nodules, cough, unresolved pneumonia, diffuse lung disease, atelectasis, or infection. **Bronchoalveolar lavage** involves instillation and recovery of liquid aliquots into a bronchial segment to identify infection, alveolar proteinosis, and bronchoalveolar cell carcinoma. **Tissue sampling** techniques include bronchial washings, brush biopsies, and endobronchial, transbronchial, and transtracheal needle aspirates.
- **Mediastinoscopy** allows direct visualization and access to portions of the mediastinum for sampling mediastinal lymph nodes and occasionally to biopsy a mediastinal mass. **Cervical mediastinoscopy** is carried out through a suprasternal incision. Paratracheal, azygos, right tracheobronchial, and ***subcarinal*** lymph nodes are directly accessible. **Parasternal mediastinotomy *(Chamberlain procedure)*,** is an anterior mediastinal exploration through the second left ***intercostal*** space to access a mass or lymph nodes in the anterior mediastinum or aortopulmonary window.
- A **median sternotomy** is the incision of choice for cardiac operations, anterior mediastinal lesions, and some bilateral pulmonary procedures. Fluid and inflammatory changes are normally seen in the anterior mediastinum and adjacent soft tissues for several weeks. Air can remain for up to 1 week. **Wound dehiscence and mediastinitis** are uncommon but can carry a high mortality unless antibiotics, drainage, or surgical debridement are performed. CT can detect the location of fluid collections and extent of inflammation. Needle aspiration may be needed to determine whether collections are infected.
- **Pulmonary resections** range from wedge resection of small peripheral lesions to extrapleural pneumonectomy for mesothelioma. Excisions for malignancy may be extended to include portions of the chest wall, pericardium, diaphragm, or adjacent vascular structures if they contain tumor. A **segmentectomy** is most frequently performed for removal of the superior segment of the lower lobe or resection of the lingula. A **lobectomy** is performed through a posterolateral thoracotomy. With expansion of the remaining lung, elevation of the hemidiaphragm, and ipsilateral shift of the mediastinum, the lobectomy space, initially filled with fluid and air, is usually obliterated within a week. The CT findings of lobectomy are similar to those of lobar collapse.
- **Pneumonectomy** is most often performed for treatment of bronchogenic carcinoma. The pneumonectomy space slowly accumulates serosanguinous fluid and an air-fluid level may persist for months. Any increase in the air component signals bronchial dehiscence. Eventually the space fills completely with fluid and then decreases in size as fluid is resorbed. In most patients some fluid remains and becomes organized, but the transverse diameter of the collection is typically less than 5 cm. The hemithorax decreases in size with inward displacement of the chest wall. The remaining volume is filled by the shifted mediastinum and hyperinflated contralateral lung.
- A postoperative **bronchopleural fistula** is uncommon, usually occurring approximately 1 week following surgery. Delayed detection is often associated with empyema. This complication requires tube drainage followed by an open-window thoracostomy (Clagett window), allowing open drainage and irrigation **(see Fig. 3.5).** The Clagett window is eventually closed with a muscle flap or omentum.
- **Decortication of the lung** consists of removing a restrictive fibrous membrane from the pleural surface to treat fibrothorax resulting from an organized hemothorax or empyema.
- **Video-assisted thoracic surgery (VATS)** allows less invasive thoracic procedures to be performed, such as pleural biopsies,

small wedge resections, apical bleb resection, and pleural abrasion to induce fibrosis in patients with recurrent spontaneous pneumothoraces.

Bibliography

Akira M. Uncommon pneumoconioses: CT and pathologic findings. *Radiology* 1995;197:403–409.

Armstrong P, Wilson AG, Dee P, Hansell DM. *Imaging of Diseases of the Chest*, 2nd ed. St. Louis: Mosby-Year Book; 1995.

Austin JHM, Müller NL, Friedman PJ, Hansell DM, Naidich DP, Remy-Jardin M, Webb WR, Zerhouni EA. Glossary of terms for CT of the lungs: Recommendations of the Nomenclature Committee of the Fleischner Society. *Radiology* 1996;200:327–331.

Fishman AP, Elias JA, Fishman JA, Grippi MA, Kaiser LR, Senior RM. *Fishman's Pulmonary Diseases and Disorders*, 3rd ed. New York: McGraw-Hill; 1998.

Garg K, Lynch DA, Newell JD, King JTE. Proliferative and constrictive bronchiolitis: Classification and radiologic features. *AJR* 1994;162:803–808.

Gurney JW. The pathophysiology of airways disease. *J Thorac Imaging* 1995;10:227–235.

Haaga JR, Lanzieri CF, Sartoris DJ, Zerhouni EA, (eds.) *Computed Tomography and Magnetic Resonance Imaging of the Whole Body*, 3rd ed. St. Louis: Mosby; 1994.

Hartman TE, Primack SL, Lee KS, Swensen SJ, Müller NL. CT of bronchial and bronchiolar diseases. *Radiographics* 1994;14:991–1003.

McLoud T. Occupational lung disease. *Radiol Clin North Am* 1991;29:931–941.

Miller WT Jr. Spectrum of pulmonary nontuberculous mycobacterial infection. *Radiology* 1994;191:343–350.

Moss AA, Gamsu G, Genant HK (eds). *Computed Tomography of the Body with Magnetic Resonance Imaging*, 2nd ed. Philadelphia: WB Saunders; 1992.

Müller NL, Miller RR. Diseases of the bronchioles: CT and histopathologic findings. *Radiology* 1995;196:3–12.

Naidich DP, Zerhouni EA, Siegelman SS. *CT and MRI of Thorax*, 3rd ed. New York: Lippincott-Raven; 1999.

Sagel SS, Slone RM. The lung. In: Lee JKT, Sagel SS, Stanley RJ, Heiken JP (eds.) *Computed Body Tomography with MRI Correlation*. Philadelphia: Lippincott-Raven; 1998.

Sha RM, Kaji AV, Ostrum BJ, Friedman AC. Interpretation of chest radiographs in AIDS patients: Usefulness of CD4 lymphocyte counts. *Radiographics* 1997;17:47–58.

Slone RM, Fisher AJ. *Pocket Guide to Body CT Differential Diagnosis*. New York: McGraw-Hill; 1999.

Slone RM, Gutierrez FR, Fisher AJ. *Thoracic Imaging: A Practical Approach*. New York: McGraw-Hill; 1999.

Stern EJ, Swensen SJ. *High-Resolution CT of the Chest: Comprehensive Atlas*. Philadelphia: Lippincott-Raven; 1996.

Thurlbeck WM, Müller NL. Emphysema: definition, imaging and quantification. *AJR* 1994;163:1017–1025.

Webb WR, Müller NL, Naidich DP. *High-Resolution CT of the Lung*, 2nd ed. Philadelphia: Lippincott-Raven; 1996.

Chapter 3

PLEURA AND DIAPHRAGM

Richard M. Slone

3.1 Pleural Anatomy
3.2 Pneumothorax
3.3 Pleural Effusion
3.4 Pleural Infections
3.5 Pleural Plaques
3.6 Pleural Tumors
3.7 The Diaphragm

3.1 PLEURAL ANATOMY

Anatomy

- The **visceral pleura** covering the lung includes mesothelial cells lining the surface, underlying connective tissue, and a vascular layer. Blood is supplied by both pulmonary (98 percent) and bronchial (2 percent) arteries. The **parietal pleura** lines the thoracic cavity, mediastinum, and diaphragm. There is overlying connective tissue and extrapleural fat of variable thickness along the surface of the chest wall just beneath the endothoracic fascia. Only the parietal pleura is innervated with sensory nerves. Blood is supplied by systemic vessels. The pleural layers, in combination with the innermost intercostal muscle, are indistinguishable on CT and appear as a thin "intercostal stripe." The intercostal fat separates the intercostal stripe from the internal and external intercostal muscles.
- **Extrapleural fat,** located outside the parietal pleura yet within the endothoracic fascia, is present to a varying degree. It is typically smooth, symmetrical, thickest over the lung apex and midthorax, and associated with generalized fat deposition in the mediastinum and subcutaneous tissues. Abundant extrapleural fat can simulate pleural plaques on chest radiographs, but CT demonstrates the characteristic fat attenuation **(Fig. 3.1).** Chronic pleural processes can produce localized thickening of the adjacent extrapleural fat. This finding can be helpful in establishing the chronic nature of an otherwise indeterminate process **(Fig. 3.2).** Increased density within the fat suggests an active pleural process.
- **Pleural fissures** are clefts in the lung formed by the interface of visceral pleura covering the lobes. The **major fissure** separates the lower lobes from the rest of the lung. The upper portion is typically concave toward the anterior chest; the inferior portion is concave toward the posterior chest. Fat can enter the inferior margin of the fissure. The **minor fissure,** only present on the right, extends from the anterior chest wall to the major fissure posteriorly, is typically convex upward, and separates the middle and right upper lobes. Since it lies in the plane of transaxial images, its location can be noted as a hypovascular section. The major fissures are incomplete in over half of patients and the minor fissure is incomplete even more frequently. This allows air, infection, and neoplastic disease to spread between lobes.

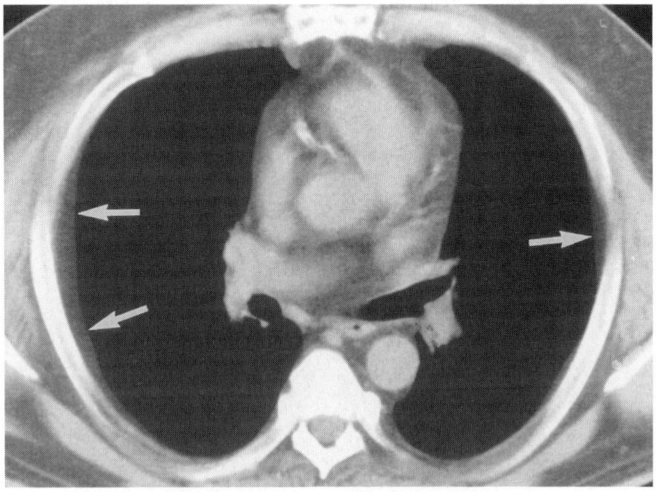

FIGURE 3.1 Abundant extrapleural fat. Noncontrast CT showing characteristic symmetric, smooth fat attenuation tissue *(arrows).*

- **Accessory fissures** represent invaginations of the visceral pleura between pulmonary segments, forming accessory "lobes." The **azygos fissure,** present in 1 percent of individuals, results when the right posterior cardinal vein fails to migrate over the pulmonary apex, trapping a portion of the right upper lobe. The pleural septum, comprising four pleural layers, is convex toward the chest wall and runs obliquely from the apex to the azygos vein **(Fig. 3.3).** The intrapulmonary course of the azygos vein is higher than that of the normal azygos and can mimic a pulmonary nodule. The azygos lobe varies in size and shares its bronchovascular supply with the right upper lobe.
- **The inferior pulmonary ligament** represents union of the mediastinal and visceral pleura at the hilum. It divides the medial pleural space into anterior and posterior compartments, demonstrated when pleural effusions are present. The ligament widens inferiorly and

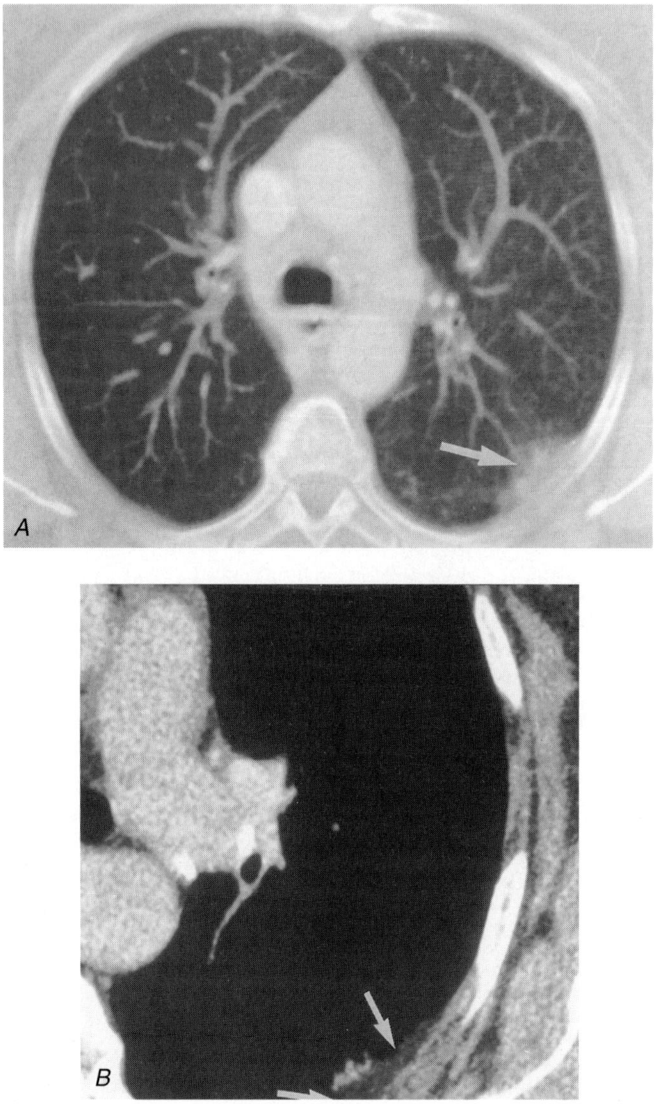

FIGURE 3.2 Focal extrapleural fat. *A.* Chest CT showing a focal pleural based parenchymal lesion *(arrow)*. *B.* Targeted image windowed for soft tissue detail shows abundant extrapleural fat below the parenchymal lesion *(arrows)* indicating a chronic process. The lesion was likely scarring from a prior pulmonary infarct.

can continue to the diaphragm, merging with the diaphragmatic pleura. A complete inferior pulmonary ligament tethers a collapsed lower lobe to the mediastinum. Paraesophageal varices and lymphadenopathy within the ligament can simulate parenchymal pathology.

- The **pleural space** normally contains a small amount of fluid (about 10 mL), primarily produced by the parietal pleura, which provides lubrication.

Imaging the Pleura

- **Computed tomography (CT)** can confirm the presence and determine the extent of a pleural lesion, characterize the abnormality, and distinguish between pleural and pulmonary processes. The fat in lipomas, calcification in asbestos-related plaques, and water density of loculated effusions can help distinguish benign from malignant lesions. CT can assess the amount of pleural fluid and characterize any associated lung disease. When a large effusion is present, performing CT after pleural drainage improves assessment of underlying lung. **Intravenous contrast** is generally not necessary, but it can help to differentiate atelectasis and consolidation from tumor, define areas of necrosis, and demonstrate peripheral enhancement in an abscess or empyema.
- **Magnetic resonance imaging (MRI)** plays a secondary role to CT in evaluating the pleura. The multiplanar imaging capability is useful in evaluating the extension of tumors into the chest wall, lung apex, or diaphragm. **Ultrasound** can be extremely helpful in corroborating pleural fluid and in guiding aspiration.

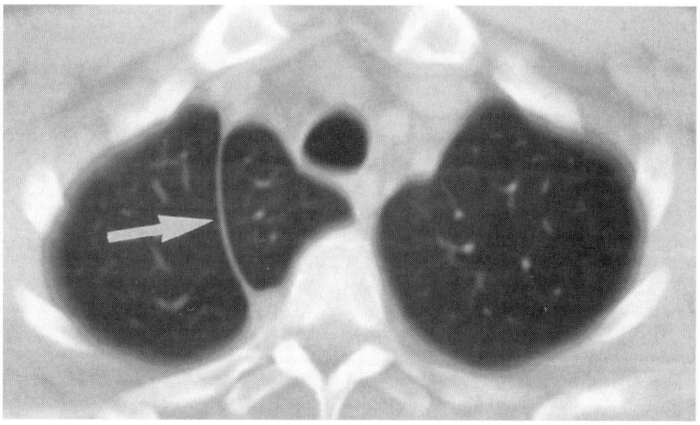

Figure 3.3 Azygos fissure. CT through the lung apex showing the azygos fissure *(arrow)*, created by entrapment of the azygos vein. The fissure comprises two layers of visceral and two layers of parietal pleura. (From Slone RM, Gutierrez FR, Fisher AJ. *Thoracic Imaging: A Practical Approach*. New York: McGraw-Hill; 1999. With permission.)

Evaluating Pleural Lesions

- The CT appearance of extrapleural, pleural, and peripheral lung lesions can overlap. A **pleural location** is suggested by a lenticular or crescent shape, tapering or obtuse angle at the chest wall interface, and well-defined margin with adjacent lung. Lesions forming an acute angle with the chest wall are typically **parenchymal** in origin. Exceptions include pedunculated pleural lesions, loculated pleural fluid collections that bulge into the lung, or a parenchymal lesion that infiltrates the pleura and creates an obtuse angle with the chest wall. An **extrapleural location** is confirmed by the presence of an associated extrapleural soft tissue mass, bone destruction, or displaced extrapleural fat **(Differential 3.1).**

3.1

EXTRAPLEURAL LESION

Lipoma
Hematoma—rib fracture, surgery, catheter placement
Rib metastasis or multiple myeloma—bone destruction with soft tissue extension
Chest wall infection—particularly tuberculosis, actinomycosis
Primary bone tumor—fibrous dysplasia, Ewing sarcoma, chondrosarcoma

3.2 PNEUMOTHORAX

- **Pneumothorax** refers to air in the pleural space, typically the result of a defect in the visceral pleura. Causes include penetrating trauma, iatrogenic puncture from central line placement, or biopsy, thoracentesis, rupture of a pulmonary cyst, or dissection from a pneumomediastinum or pneumoperitoneum **(Differential 3.2).** Symptoms include pleuritic chest pain and shortness of breath. **Conventional radiography** is the principal technique for evaluation. **CT** can be helpful in complex cases, such as differentiating a large bulla from a pneumothorax, assessing chest tube position, or when extensive subcutaneous air or artifact obscures radiographic findings **(Fig. 3.4).**
- A small pneumothorax can be asymptomatic and resolve spontaneously over a day, but larger pneumothoraces often produce hypoxemia, necessitating chest tube placement. Reexpansion can be delayed if there is underlying lung disease or pleural thickening or if the pneumothorax is chronic. Rapid reexpansion of a collapsed lung can cause **reexpansion pulmonary edema.**
- A primary **spontaneous pneumothorax** can occur in otherwise healthy individuals in the absence of a known traumatic event. These occur more frequently in tall, thin males in their third to fourth decades. Apical bullae or subpleural blebs may warrant resection to prevent recurrences. A **tension pneumothorax** occurs when air continues to enter the pleural space. There is ipsilateral hyperexpansion of the hemithorax, downward displacement of the diaphragm, and a contralateral shift of the mediastinum.
- **Bronchopleural fistula** is a communication between the airways and pleural space and can occur as an immediate or delayed complication of surgery, cancer, trauma, or infection. When it is present following pneumonectomy, air is seen in the postpneumonectomy space and fluid can be aspirated into the remaining lung. **Open-window thoractomy** (Clagett window) is an open pleural drainage for treatment of postpneumonectomy empyema or bronchopleural fistula that has failed thoracostomy tube management **(Fig. 3.5).** The opening is created by dissection through the chest wall and resection of several ribs. The skin is marsupialized into the wound to optimize drainage. The cavity is packed with dressing and, when fully healed, closed with soft tissue and a skin graft.

3.3 PLEURAL EFFUSION

- **Pleural effusions** are common and develop when fluid production is increased, as in heart failure, or when resorption is impaired, as in lymphatic obstruction by tumor. The most common causes are congestive heart failure, pneumonia, and tumor **(Differential 3.3).** CT can identify the cause of an effusion, particularly when it is parapneumonic or abdominal; however, the cause can be systemic (hypoalbuminemia). Patients with massive ascites can develop pleural effusions as a result of transdiaphragmatic flow of ascites through lymphatic channels or diaphragm defects. **Thoracentesis** is the mainstay for diagnosing the composition of pleural effusions and determining if the pleural space is infected or contains blood or malignant cells.

3.2 PNEUMOTHORAX

Trauma—iatrogenic, barotrauma, rib fracture, blunt or penetrating injury, esophageal rupture, dissection from pneumoperitoneum or pneumomediastinum

Focal lung disease—ruptured cystic airspace, bronchogenic carcinoma, necrotizing pneumonia or ruptured abscess, bronchopleural fistula, pulmonary metastases (osteosarcoma), catamenial

Diffuse lung disease—cystic fibrosis, PCP,* lymphangioleiomyomatosis, pulmonary fibrosis, eosinophilic granuloma, asthma

**Pneumocystis carinii* pneumonia.

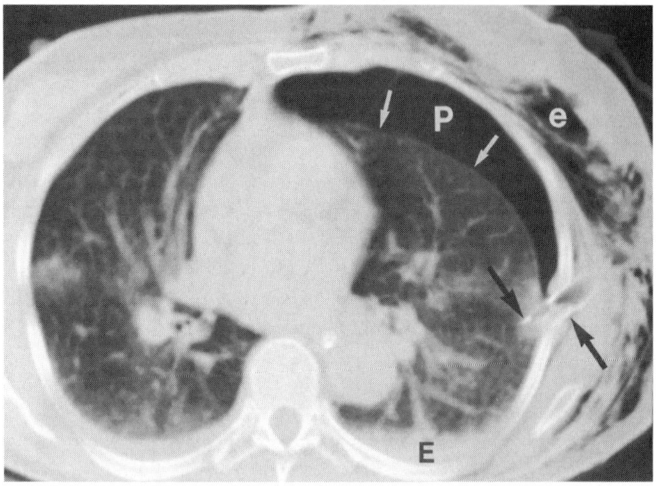

FIGURE 3.4 Pneumothorax and subcutaneous emphysema. Chest CT following emergent placement of a thoracostomy tube for treatment of a tension pneumothorax. The chest tube *(black arrow)* was aberrantly placed into the lung parenchyma. There is a persistent pneumothorax (P) and subcutaneous emphysema (e). Note sharp demarcation of the visceral pleural edge *(white arrows).* E, small pleural effusion.

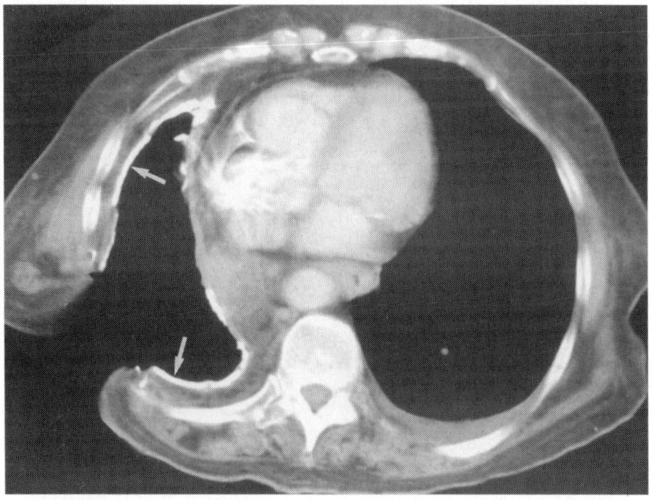

FIGURE 3.5 Clagett window. Contrast-enhanced CT showing a large defect in the chest wall. The dense calcification *(arrows)* is the result of an old tuberculous empyema. The pleural space became infected with *Aspergillus*, requiring open drainage.

3.3

PLEURAL EFFUSION

Cardiovascular—CHF,* pulmonary embolism, recent chest surgery, Dressler syndrome
Inflammatory—parapneumonic, pericarditis, pyelonephritis, pancreatitis, subphrenic abscess
Malignancy—pleural metastases (breast, lung, stomach, pancreas), bronchogenic carcinoma, mesothelioma, lymphoma, or leukemia
Collagen vascular—lupus, rheumatoid
Abdominal—renal failure, ascites, cirrhosis, nephrotic syndrome, *Meig syndrome*
Traumatic—vascular injury, pulmonary contusion or laceration, esophageal rupture or fistula, thoracic duct rupture
Uncommon—asbestos exposure, drugs, radiation therapy, Wegener granulomatosis

*Congestive heart failure.

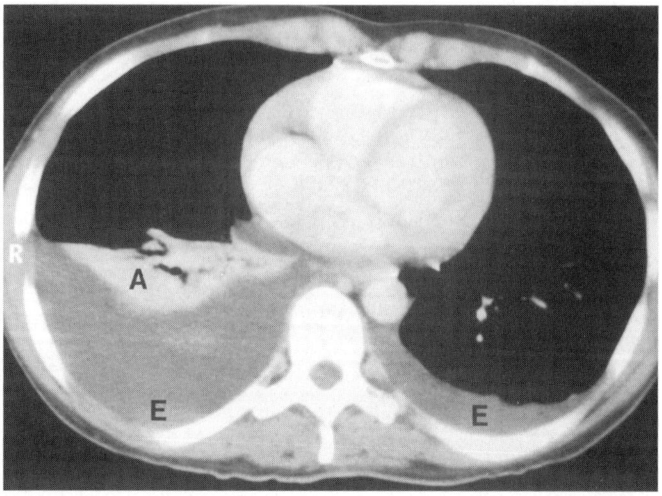

FIGURE 3.6 Pleural effusions with atelectasis. Contrast-enhanced CT in a 48-year-old woman showing a small left pleural effusion (E) and a large right effusion (E) with associated pulmonary atelectasis (A). Note the characteristic marked enhancement of the collapsed lung tissue.

- Pleural effusions usually cause some **atelectasis** of the underlying lung, and large pleural effusions can result in lower-lobe collapse. The adjacent atelectatic lung demonstrates marked enhancement, in contrast to infected, consolidated lung **(Figs. 3.6 and 3.7).**
- Effusions are classified clinically as transudates or exudates based on their composition. **Transudates** are the result of increased capillary hydrostatic pressure or decreased colloid osmotic pressure and result from systemic rather than pleural pathology. They typically have homogeneous water attenuation on CT and are bilateral. **Exudates** are the result of a local pathologic process involving the pleura, most commonly infection or tumor, disrupting the pleura or obstructing lymphatics. Other causes include collagen vascular disease and pulmonary thromboembolism. As compared with transudates, exudative effusions are more opaque, have increased protein content, higher specific gravity, and lactate dehydrogenase (LDH) concentration. Exudates also can have a high white blood cell (WBC) count (>15,000 cells per milliliter) and low glucose (<40 mg/dL); they may be bloody or chylous.
- **Bilateral** pleural effusions are usually transudates, although in some situations, such as congestive heart failure, they can be primarily right-sided due to cardiac motion, which stimulates lymphatic resorption. **Unilateral** effusions are often exudates. Left-sided effusions can be seen following rupture of the esophagus, dissecting aneurysms, and traumatic injury to the aorta. Pancreatitis typically leads to left-sided effusions but can cause isolated right-sided effusions and occasionally intrathoracic pseudocysts. A unilateral pleural effusion in an older patient without symptoms of infection or heart disease is often malignant.
- **Pleural thickening** or enhancement on CT usually indicates an exudate. However, it is not always seen with malignancy or parapneumonic effusion.
- **Hemothorax** is suggested by pleural fluid with a heterogeneous appearance, including fluid levels or attenuation higher than soft tissue **(Fig. 3.8).** The increased attenuation is due to a high protein content, which can be seen with other complex fluid collections. A hemothorax can lead to significant pleural fibrosis (fibrothorax) and calcification. Causes include trauma, malignancy, pleural endometriosis, anticoagulation, and pulmonary embolism. A torn pleural adhesion is the most common spontaneous cause.
- **Chylothorax** has a high triglyceride content and can result in a CT attenuation less than that of water. Chylous effusions are uncommon and can result from damage to the thoracic duct, slow leakage from pleural lymphatics, or communication of the pleural space with chylous ascites. About half of chylothoraces are related to tumors, mostly lymphoma. Surgery is the most common traumatic cause. Transection of the lower thoracic duct can produce an isolated left effusion, and transection of the upper duct, an isolated right effusion. Lymphangioleiomyomatosis, lymphangioma, and mediastinal fibrosis are uncommon causes.

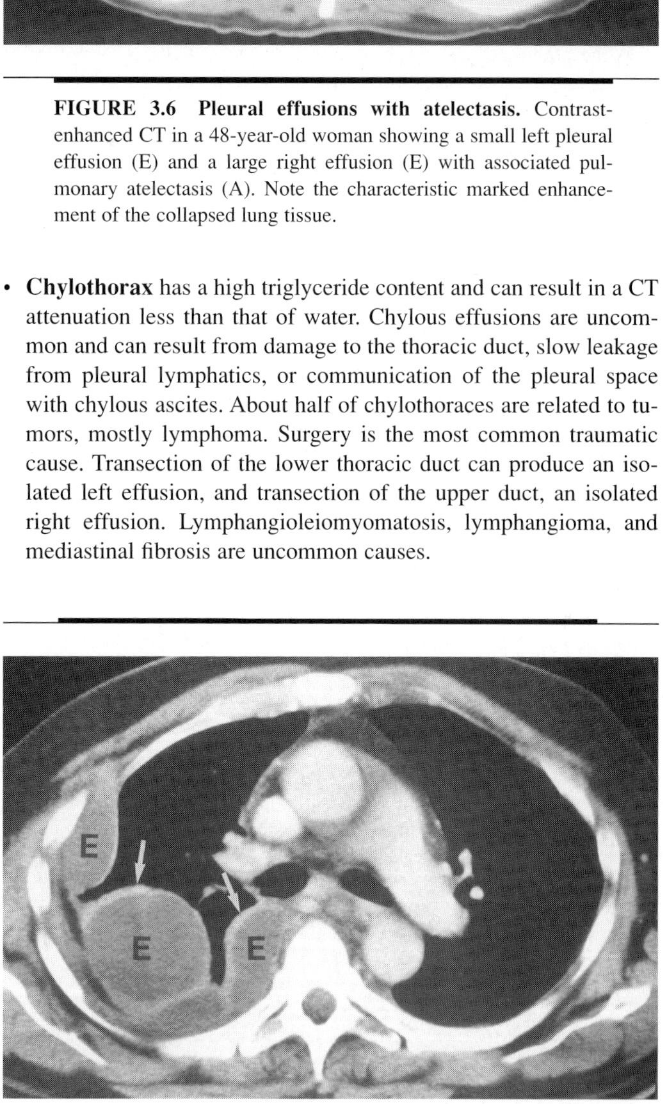

FIGURE 3.7 Loculated pleural effusion. Contrast-enhanced CT in a 59-year-old man showing loculated pleural fluid collections (E) in the right hemithorax. Note adjacent enhancing atelectatic lung *(arrows).* [From Slone RM, Gierada DS. Pleura, chest wall and diaphragm. In: Lee JKT, Sagel SS, Stanley RJ, Heiken JP (eds.): *Computed Body Tomography with MRI Correlation*, 3rd ed. Philadelphia: Lippincott-Raven, 1998. With permission.]

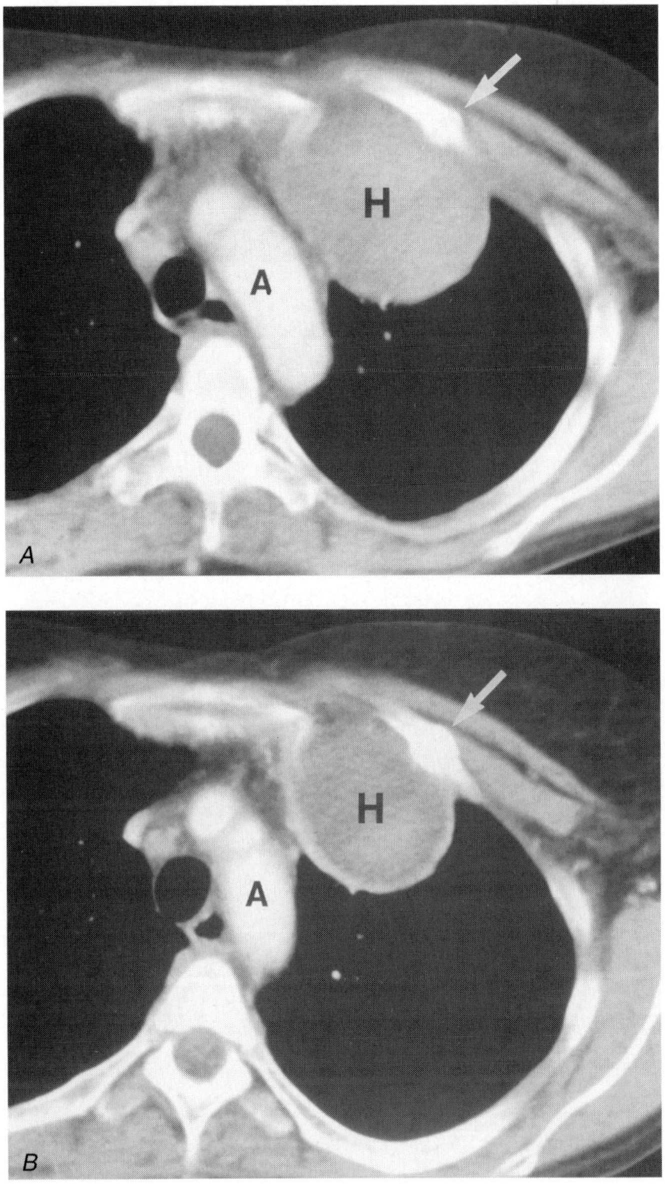

FIGURE 3.8 Extrapleural hematoma. A 47-year-old woman presenting with a left apical mass on radiography following trauma. *A*. Contrast-enhanced CT shows a high-attenuation mass (H). Note adjacent rib fracture *(arrow)*. *B*. CT 5 weeks later shows a decrease in size and attenuation of the hematoma. The callus around the rib fracture has increased *(arrow)*.

Fluid Location

- CT is sensitive for detecting small pleural effusions and frequently demonstrates fluid not appreciated on conventional radiographs. In the **supine position,** mobile pleural fluid collects in the posteromedial hemithorax. As an effusion increases in size, it conforms to the pleural space and can extend laterally, displacing lung away from the thoracic wall. The lateral aspect of the major fissure can become filled with fluid, noted as a superiorly marginated opacity pointing toward the hilum. Adhesions can lead to loculation of fluid, which can simulate a mass **(pseudotumor).** The sharp pleural margins and water density on CT are characteristic.

Several signs have been described to distinguish pleural fluid from ascites on CT. The **displaced crus sign** refers to pleural fluid lying posterior to the diaphragmatic crus, displacing the diaphragm away from the spine and decreasing inferiorly. Ascites is anterolateral to the crus, displaces the diaphragm toward the spine, and increases in volume inferiorly. The **diaphragm sign** is visualization of the diaphragm when both ascites and pleural fluid are present. Ascites is inside the diaphragm and effusions are peripheral. An exception occurs when large effusions invert the hemidiaphragm. A partially collapsed lower lobe within a pleural effusion can simulate the diaphragm.

The **bare-area sign** refers to the right coronary ligament, which restricts peritoneal fluid from moving posteromedially to the liver on the right, and the splenorenal ligament, which restricts fluid on the left **(Fig. 3.9).** Fluid adjacent to these areas is pleural, although massive ascites can extend medially beneath the hemidiaphragms above the bare area on either side. The **interface sign** refers to the sharp margin between ascites and the liver or spleen and the hazy interface between pleural fluid and the diaphragm.

3.4 PLEURAL INFECTIONS

- An **empyema** is an infected, exudative pleural effusion containing pus (WBC count >5000/mm^3); it most commonly occurs as a result of an infected parapneumonic effusion, particularly following bacterial pneumonia but also with tuberculosis or fungal infections. Infection can also occur as a complication of trauma, esophageal perforation, septic pulmonary infarction, or spread from osteomyelitis or abdominal abscess. Iatrogenic pleural infection can follow thoracic surgery, thoracentesis, or percutaneous biopsy.
- The incidence of **parapneumonic pleural effusions** is dependent upon the infecting organism, ranging from about 10 percent for pneumonias caused by *Pneumococcus* to over half of those caused

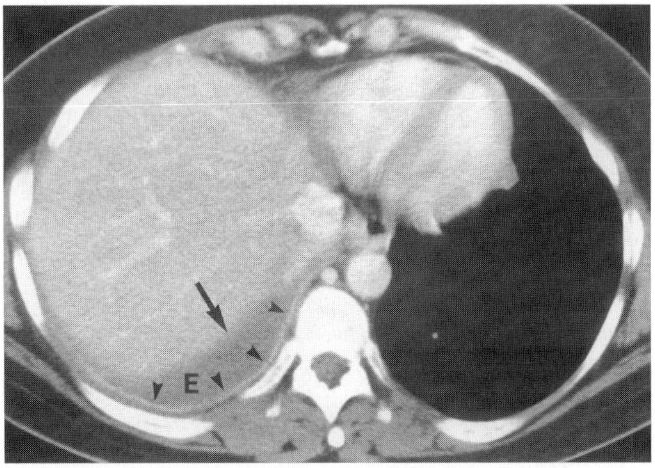

FIGURE 3.9 Pleural effusion behind liver. Contrast-enhanced CT in a 35-year-old woman with an exudative right pleural effusion (E). Note pleural enhancement *(arrowheads)*. Unlike ascites, the fluid is posteromedial in location and extends over the bare area of the liver *(arrow)*. Also note the indistinct interface with the diaphragm, which is in direct contact with the liver. Ascites would have a sharper interface.

by *Staphylococcus*. Most parapneumonic effusions are composed of sterile fluid from visceral pleura inflammation and resolve with antibiotics; however, some become infected and progress to an empyema, with fibrin deposited over the visceral and parietal pleura. Pleural thickening impairs fluid resorption and promotes loculation. Fluid can also accumulate in bullae due to adjacent pneumonitis, analogous to a parapneumonic pleural effusion.

- CT can reliably distinguish between an abscess and empyema. Differentiation is crucial because proper therapy of an empyema requires thoracostomy tube drainage, whereas a lung abscess is appropriately managed with antibiotics and postural or bronchoscopic drainage. **Empyemas** generally have smooth walls and a lenticular shape that conforms to the pleural space. They form a sharp border with the lung, which is frequently compressed, resulting in displacement of peripheral pulmonary vessels and bronchi **(Fig. 3.10). CT** can depict the thickened pleura which becomes organized with fibrosis and vascular ingrowth. **Intravenous contrast** can demonstrate enhancement of the pleural layers ***(split-pleura sign),*** seen in over two-thirds of empyemas. The extrapleural fat can be edematous, resulting in elevation of the parietal pleura away from the chest wall **(Fig. 3.11).**
- A **lung abscess** usually has thick, irregular walls and a spherical or oblong shape that forms an acute angle with the chest wall when peripheral. Lung destruction results in abrupt termination of bronchi and vessels at the margin of the abscess, and the lung around the abscess is often infected. An air-fluid level can be seen in a lung abscess because of communication with the bronchial tree or in an empyema as the result of a bronchopleural or esophageal fistula **(Fig. 3.12).** Consolidated lung, pleural fluid, and septated collections can be associated with either process; in some cases, an empyema and lung abscess coexist, typically the result of a necrotizing pneumonia.
- **Chest tube drainage** is the treatment of choice for management of empyemas. CT can be needed to clarify the exact site and extent of the empyema and its relation to the tube. An improperly drained empyema is much more commonly a consequence of tube malposition than of clogging of the tube with fibrin or debris. Improper treatment of an empyema usually results in progressive organization of the fibrous pleural lining surrounding the loculated pleural fluid. This thickened inelastic membrane traps the lung and contracts the hemithorax. The pleura can eventually calcify, particularly if the empyema was due to tuberculous infection. Effective therapy may require surgical pleural decortication.
- Infected pleural fluid can extend directly through the thoracic wall and present as a subcutaneous mass. Such an ***empyema necessitans*** is most commonly secondary to tuberculosis but can occur as a consequence of actinomycosis, blastomyocosis, tumor **(Fig. 3.13)**, or following thoracentesis of a pyogenic empyema.

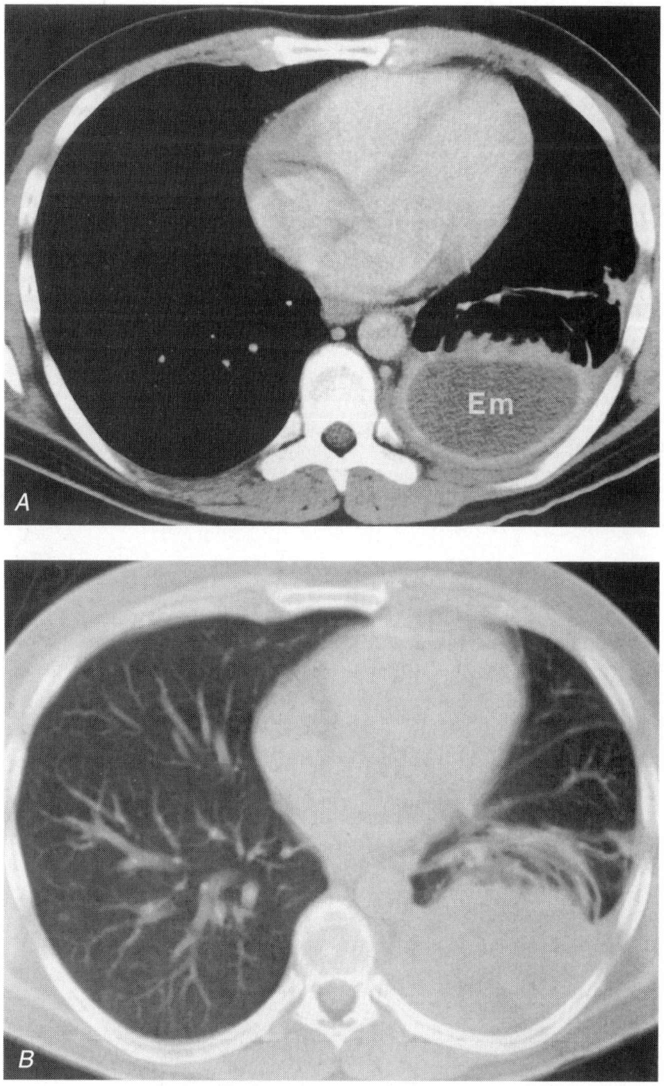

FIGURE 3.10 Classic empyema (Em) *A*. Contrast-enhanced CT showing a loculated pleural fluid collection with enhancing walls representing thickened pleura. Note extrapleural edema. *B*. Image windowed for lung detail showing displacement of lung with atelectasis, clearly distinguishing this process from a lung abscess. [From Slone RM, Gierada DS. Pleura, chest wall and diaphragm. In: Lee JKT, Sagel SS, Stanley RJ, Heiken JP (eds.): *Computed Body Tomography with MRI Correlation*, 3rd ed. Philadelphia: Lippincott-Raven, 1998. With permission.]

3.5 PLEURAL PLAQUES

- **Pleural thickening** can be focal or diffuse and is usually the result of a preceding inflammatory process, but it can be malignant **(Differential 3.4).** Normal anatomic structures such as the phrenic bundles or intercostal veins should not be mistaken for small pleural plaques. Peripheral pulmonary disease and occasionally a process involving the spine can extend into the paraspinal soft tissues and present as pleural disease. **Apical lung fibrosis** and adjacent pleural thickening are commonly seen as senescent changes, possibly related to relative ischemia or the result of prior granulomatous infections.
- **Localized pleural thickening** is often the result of a prior organized effusion, hemothorax, or empyema. Benign causes of **diffuse pleural thickening** include prior surgery, radiation therapy, asbestos exposure, drug reactions, and collagen vascular disease. Circumferential fibrous visceral pleural thickening, referred to as a ***fibrothorax,*** can restrict ventilatory excursion and reduce lung volumes. Calcification is common.
- **Malignant neoplasms**—including metastases, mesothelioma, and lymphoma—can also present as thickened pleura. When nodularity, a thickness over 1 cm, or mediastinal pleural involvement is seen, a malignant etiology should be suspected.

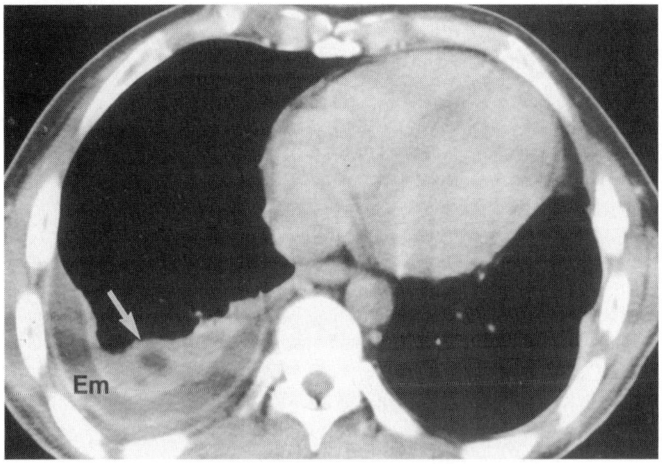

FIGURE 3.11 Occult empyema and small lung abscess. Contrast-enhanced CT in a 32-year-old man hospitalized for treatment of traumatic cervical spine fracture. There is a focal area of necrotic lung *(arrow)* and a pleural effusion with thickened enhancing pleura. Note extrapleural edema below enhancing parietal pleura.

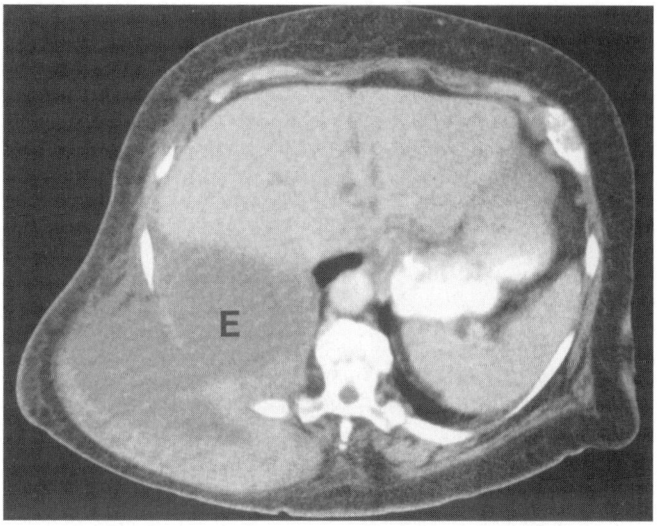

FIGURE 3.13 Empyema necessitans. Contrast-enhanced CT showing extension through the chest wall of a large pleural fluid collection (E), which began as a necrotic pleural metastasis.

- **Pleural calcification** is usually associated with pleural thickening and is most commonly the result of asbestos exposure, but it can be due to prior infection or hemorrhage, particularly if unilateral. A prior tuberculous empyema can cause dense unilateral pleural thickening with calcification and is often accompanied by substantial associated parenchymal disease and volume loss. Pleural calcification alone has no significant effect on lung volumes or pulmonary function, but extensive pleural thickening can result in impaired pulmonary function. Diffuse calcification can be seen as a consequence of a prior pleurodesis, with the apparent "calcifications" representing talc. Bilateral, symmetrical disease, particularly with calcified plaques on the diaphragm, is almost pathognomonic of asbestos-related pleural disease.

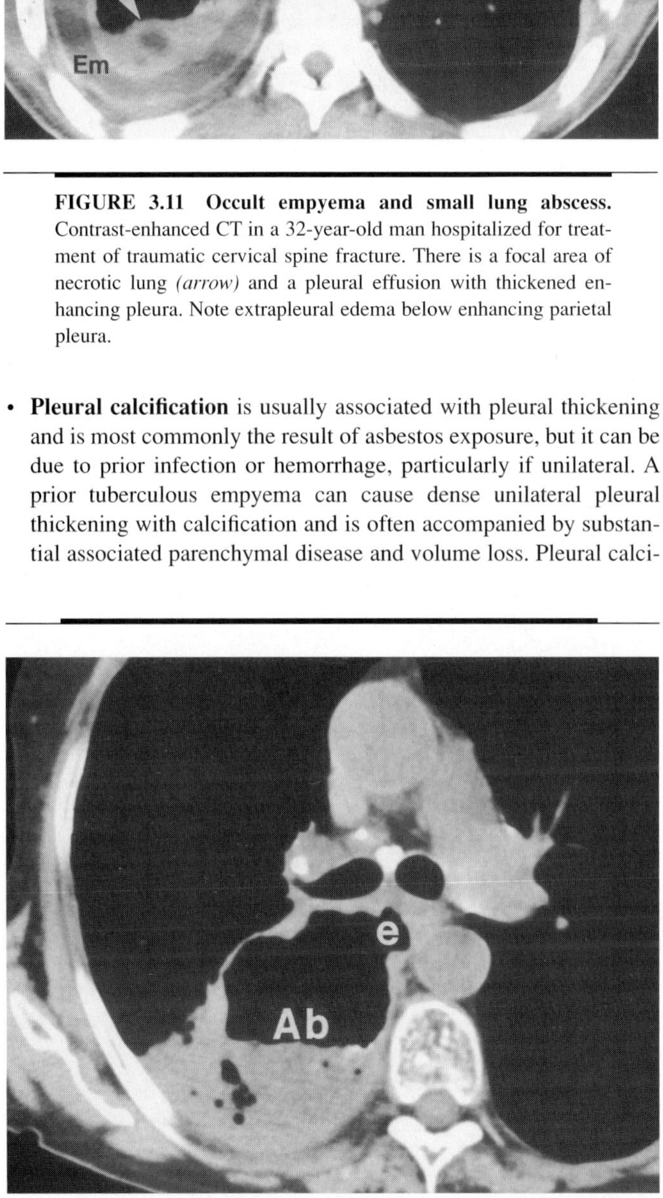

FIGURE 3.12 Esophagopleural fistula and empyema. Chest CT in a 64-year-old woman who sustained an esophageal perforation during endoscopic biopsy of an esophageal cancer. The enhancing abscess cavity (Ab) extends from the azygoesophageal recess to the posterior right chest cavity and contains air and fluid. e, esophagus. [From Slone RM, Gierada DS. Pleura, chest wall and diaphragm. In: Lee JKT, Sagel SS, Stanley RJ, Heiken JP (eds.): *Computed Body Tomography with MRI Correlation*, 3rd ed. Philadelphia: Lippincott-Raven, 1998. With permission.]

- **Asbestos dust exposure** causes pleural inflammation leading to effusions, thickening, plaque formation, pulmonary fibrosis, and malignant neoplasms of the lung, pleura, and abdomen. A chronic pleural effusion can be the first abnormality to develop after a latent period of 8 to 10 years. It is typically an exudate and can be hemorrhagic. Such an effusion can also be the first sign of mesothelioma or lung cancer. The term **asbestosis** refers to pulmonary fibrosis caused by asbestos exposure and should not be used to describe asbestos-related pleural abnormalities. Patients exposed to asbestos have an increased incidence of **bronchogenic carcinoma.** The risk is dose-related and there is a latency period of 20 years. Smoking combined with asbestos exposure greatly increases the risk. This synergistic effect leads to an over 50-fold risk of developing bronchogenic carcinoma.
- **Asbestos-related pleural plaques** are the most frequent manifestation of asbestos exposure. The latent period between exposure

3.4 PLEURAL THICKENING

Extrapleural fat deposition
Asbestos exposure
Prior empyema—particularly tuberculosis
Organized effusion—prior surgery, hemorrhage
Metastatic disease—adenocarcinoma; breast, lung, stomach, pancreas, ovary, renal
Pulmonary fibrosis—when advanced
Mesothelioma—focal or diffuse

and plaque formation is approximately 20 years. The plaques are composed of hyalinized collagen in the submesothelial layer of the parietal pleura. Visceral and mediastinal pleural involvement is rare and raises the suspicion of mesothelioma. These lesions have sharp margins, are typically bilateral, and are most common in the paravertebral and posterolateral midportion of the chest. **Plaque calcification** is common and can be punctate, linear, or cakelike, especially along the diaphragmatic surface, where they are almost pathognomonic of prior asbestos exposure **(Fig. 3.14).** They can occasionally be large, irregular, and up to 15 mm thick; they can also enlarge, thus resembling mesothelioma.

- **Rounded atelectasis** is a focal spiral infolding of lung seen exclusively adjacent to pleural thickening **(see Fig. 2.13).** It usually occurs in the posterior lower lobe and is most commonly associated with asbestos-related pleural disease. Patients usually are asymptomatic, and the finding is often incidental.

3.6 PLEURAL TUMORS

- The most common benign tumors involving the pleura are lipomas and fibrous tumors. Metastatic disease and direct tumor invasion of the pleura are more common than primary malignant tumors. Features suggesting malignancy include pleural thickening >1 cm, disseminated pleural nodules, extension into the fissures, mediastinal pleural involvement, and associated effusion, or volume loss. Definitive diagnosis usually requires biopsy **(Differential 3.6).**

Benign Tumors

- **Lipomas** are usually asymptomatic, incidental findings. Some can protrude through the chest wall into the pleural surface. CT allows definitive diagnosis based on homogeneous fat attenuation **(Fig. 3.15).** A capsule or small bands of fibrous soft tissue are sometimes identified.
- **Fibrous tumors** are the most common benign pleural tumors, but they are rare. They are slow-growing, found in patients of all ages, and are unrelated to asbestos exposure. Most are asymptomatic and discovered incidentally, but patients can present with cough, chest pain, dyspnea, hypertrophic osteoarthropathy, clubbing, or episodic hypoglycemia. The vast majority are benign, but some are histologically malignant and can invade the chest wall or mediastinum. They do not metastasize outside the thorax. Treatment is surgical excision, although local recurrence is common and can occur as late as 15 years after resection. Homogeneous contrast enhancement is depicted on CT. They appear as sharply defined, pleural-based, soft tissue masses without chest wall invasion **(Fig. 3.16).** Some are attached to the pleural surface by a pedicle, allowing mobility. Most arise from the visceral pleura and can occur within a fissure, simulating a pulmonary nodule. An effusion is rare, but calcification occurs in 10 percent. They can grow to be very large **(Fig. 3.17)**, displacing bronchi, producing atelectasis, and almost filling a hemithorax. Large tumors can have low-attenuation areas due to cystic necrosis or hemorrhage.
- **Thoracic splenosis** is the result of ectopic splenic tissue displaced into the thorax following a traumatic injury to the diaphragm. The splenic fragments become supplied by the pleural vessels and present as pleural masses **(Fig. 3.18).** CT is nonspecific, but splenic tissue can be diagnosed with nuclear medicine sulfur colloid or heat-labeled red blood cell scintigraphy.

Pleural Metastases

- **Pleural metastases** account for the majority of malignant pleural neoplasms. They involve both the visceral and parietal pleura and

3.6

PLEURAL MASS

Loculated effusion or empyema
Lipoma
Neoplasm—peripheral lung cancer, lymphoma, pleural metastases, extraosseous extension of a rib lesion, mesothelioma, invasive thymoma, fibrous tumor
Thoracic splenosis
Endometriosis

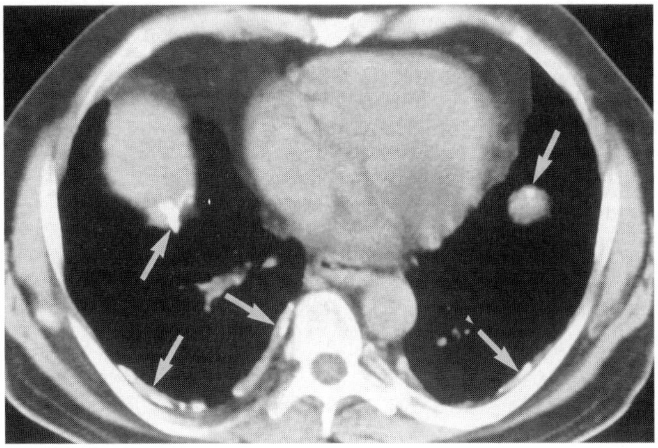

FIGURE 3.14 Calcified asbestos pleural plaques. Chest CT showing calcified pleural plaques characteristic of asbestos exposure along both chest walls and on the surface of the diaphragm.

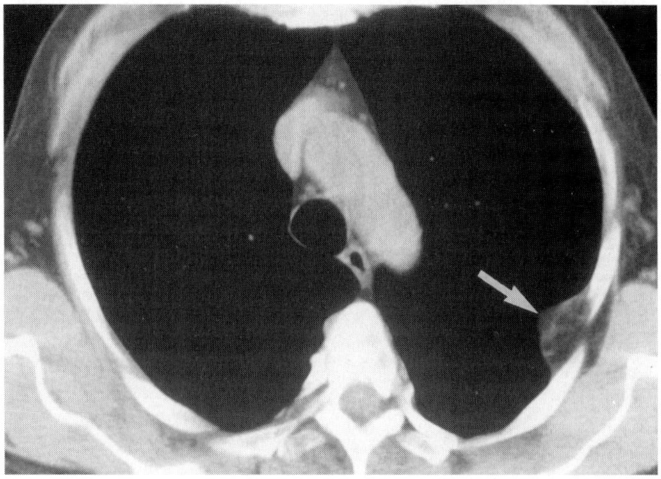

FIGURE 3.15 Extrapleural lipoma. Contrast-enhanced CT showing a fat-attenuation pleural-based mass *(arrow)* extending between the ribs and displacing the external intercostal muscle.

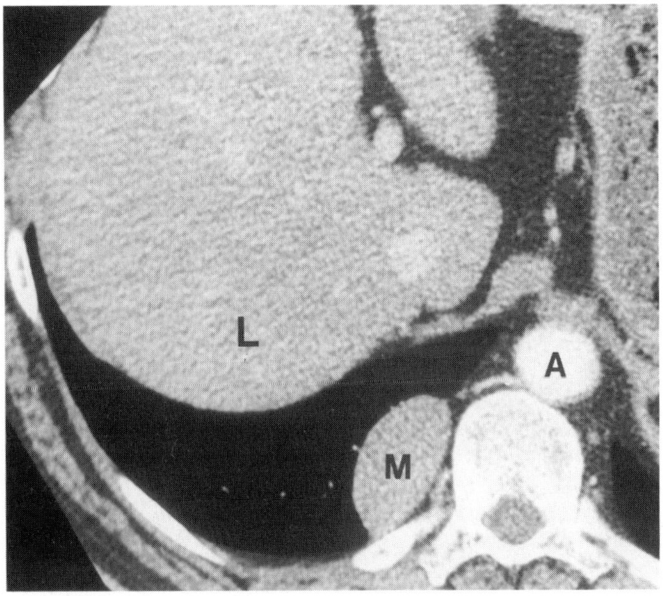

FIGURE 3.16 Localized fibrous tumor. Contrast-enhanced CT showing a smooth, soft tissue, pleural-based mass (M). L, liver: A, aorta.

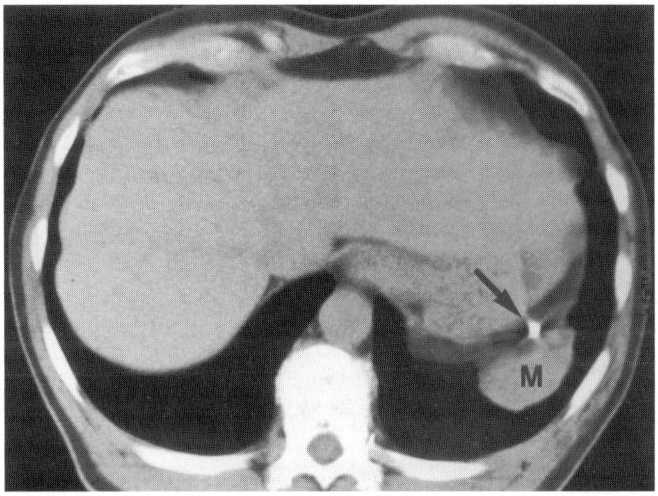

FIGURE 3.18 Splenosis. CT image through the upper abdomen showing a metallic density *(arrow)* adjacent to the left hemidiaphragm, representing a piece of shrapnel from a war injury. The pleural-based soft tissue mass (M) was confirmed on heat-damaged red blood cell scintigraphy to be ectopic splenic tissue.

almost always cause an effusion. Pleural metastases result from hematogenous spread of tumor emboli that lodge in distal branches of the pulmonary arteries. Adenocarcinoma is the most common cell type and most often the result of lung and breast carcinoma **(Figs. 3.19 and 3.20).** Lymphoma is another common cause. Invasive thymomas, lung cancer, and breast cancer can invade the pleura by direct spread. Pleural metastases usually appear as small, lenticular masses having obtuse margins with the chest wall. They enhance with contrast, allowing differentiation from fluid on CT. They can progress to encase the entire hemithorax and extend into the fissures, making differentiation from mesothelioma difficult.

Malignant Tumors

- **Liposarcomas** are exceedingly rare and typically more heterogeneous than lipomas, with substantial areas of soft tissue density and

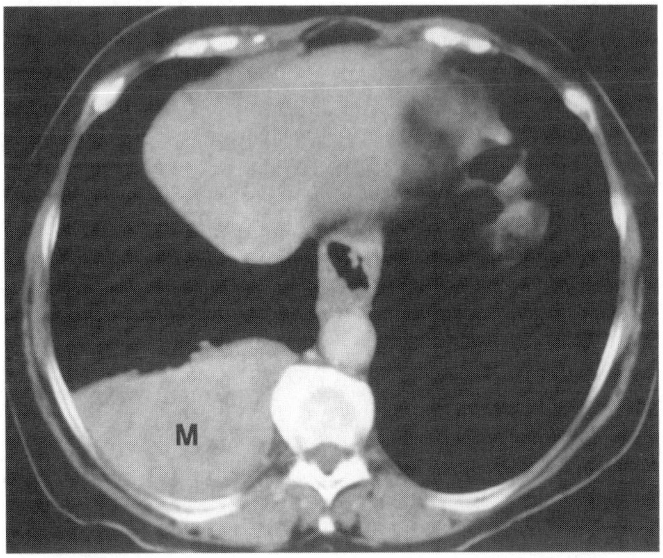

FIGURE 3.17
Large fibrous tumor. Contrast-enhanced CT showing large enhancing mass (M) proven to be a fibrous tumor.

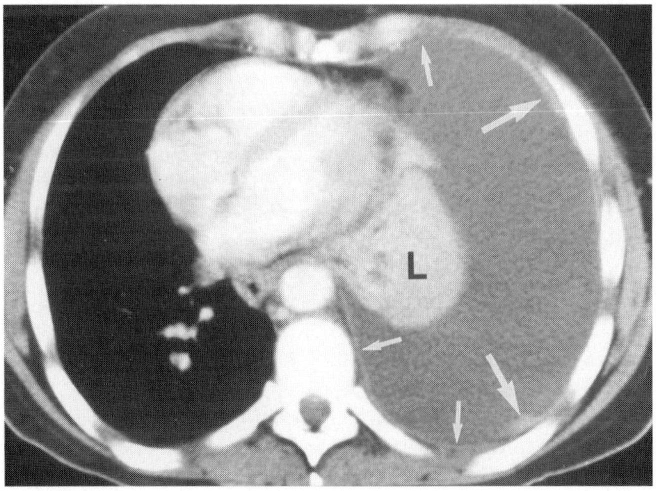

FIGURE 3.19 Malignant pleural effusion. Contrast-enhanced CT in a 45-year-old woman presenting with shortness of breath. There is a massive left pleural effusion causing contralateral mediastinal shift. The left lung (L) is collapsed and was found to contain adenocarcinoma. Note the thickened, enhancing pleura *(small arrows)* characteristic of an exudate. The enhancing nodules *(large arrows)* are characteristics of pleural metastases.

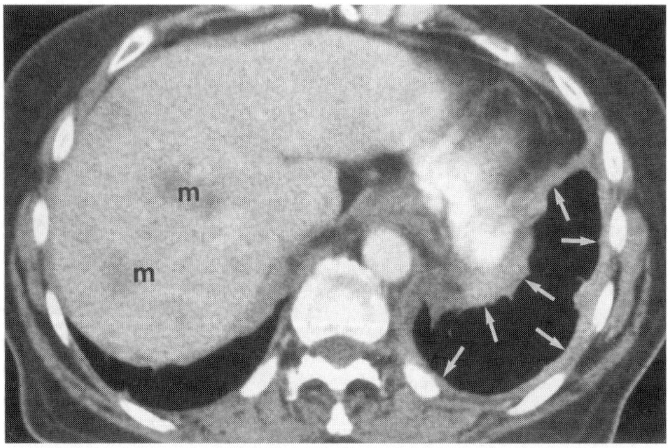

FIGURE 3.20 Pleural metastases. Contrast-enhanced CT in a 63-year-old woman with breast cancer showing liver metastases (m) and circumferential pleural thickening *(arrows)* proven to be adenocarcinoma.

infiltration of adjacent tissues. Inflammatory changes following infarction of a lipoma can produce a similar appearance.

- **Lymphoma,** including Hodgkin and non-Hodgkin disease, can involve the pleura but is rarely the initial manifestation of disease. It is more common with recurrence or in addition to thymic, mediastinal, or pulmonary disease by direct extension from the mediastinum or chest wall. A paraspinal location is common. Diffuse pleural involvement can occur.

  Lymphomatous involvement of the lymphatic channels and lymphoid aggregates found beneath the visceral pleura of the lung can present as subpleural nodules or plaques. Mediastinal adenopathy can cause lymphatic obstruction leading to a pleural effusion, which occurs in up to one-third of patients with Hodgkin disease at presentation. **Leukemia** can also cause pleural thickening.

- **Mesothelioma** is a rare, aggressive pleural tumor with an extremely poor prognosis. Mean survival following diagnosis is less than 1 year. It occurs more commonly in men. Chest pain, dyspnea, cough, weakness, and weight loss are late findings. Hypertrophic pulmonary osteoarthropathy is uncommon. The vast majority of patients have a history of occupational exposure to asbestos, but the risk is unrelated to the duration or degree of exposure. There is a 20- to 40-year latent period after initial exposure. Asbestos-related pleural disease is seen in the contralateral hemithorax in about half the patients. The pleural plaques themselves do not undergo malignant degeneration but are simply an indicator of prior asbestos exposure. Asbestosis (pulmonary fibrosis) is uncommon. Lung cancer is much more common than mesothelioma in patients exposed to asbestos. Mesothelioma is not smoking-related.

  Most patients present with a pleural effusion, which is usually exudative, often hemorrhagic, and can obscure the tumor **(Fig. 3.21).** The tumor is depicted on CT as a focal mass or diffuse nodular pleural thickening. Both the visceral and parietal pleura are involved, and extension into the fissures and along the mediastinal pleura is common. Disease is often advanced at diagnosis **(Fig. 3.22).** Calcification is extremely rare. As the tumor progresses, it can invade the lung, chest wall, pericardium, and mediastinum. It can penetrate the diaphragm and involve the peritoneal cavity or retroperitoneum. Surgery, radiation therapy, and chemotherapy have little impact on survival.

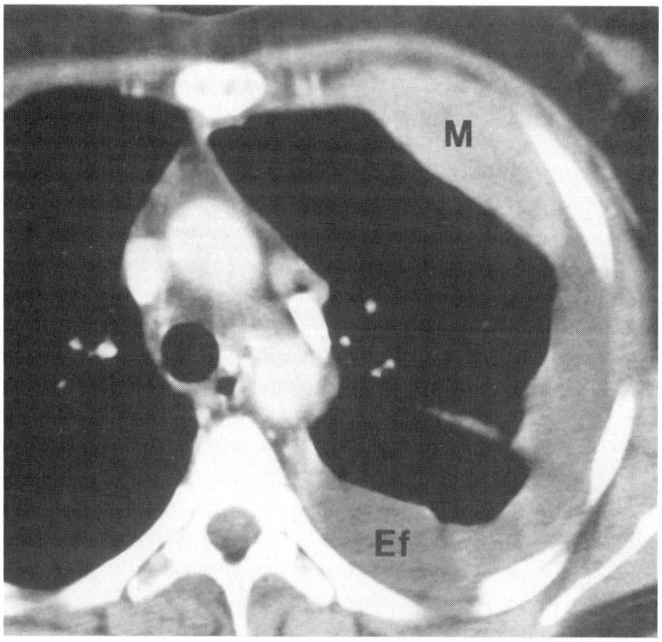

FIGURE 3.21 Occult mesothelioma. Contrast-enhanced CT in a 46-year-old man with a recurrent left pleural effusion (Ef). There is an enhancing soft tissue mass (M) anteriorly, proven to be mesothelioma.

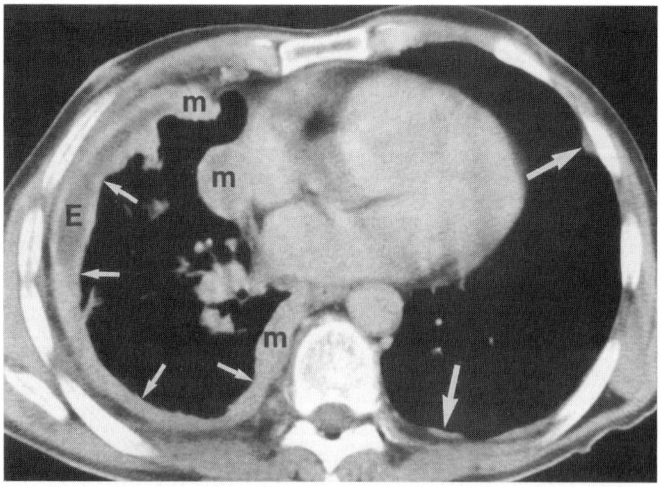

FIGURE 3.22 Advanced mesothelioma. Contrast-enhanced CT in a 65-year-old man showing circumferential pleural encasement *(small arrows)* with areas of nodular thickening (m) and a loculated effusion (E). Note contraction of the ipsilateral hemithorax and contralateral pleural plaques *(large arrows)* from prior asbestos exposure. [From Slone RM, Gierada DS. Pleura, chest wall and diaphragm. In: Lee JKT, Sagel SS, Stanley RJ, Heiken JP (eds.): *Computed Body Tomography with MRI Correlation*, 3rd ed. Philadelphia: Lippincott-Raven, 1998. With permission.]

3.7 THE DIAPHRAGM

- **The diaphragm** is a thin, domed, musculotendinous structure that separates the thorax from the abdomen, and is the primary muscle of respiration. The **muscular diaphragm** is made up of three groups, (1) the sternal portion of the diaphragm, arising from the xyphoid process; (2) the costal slips from the ribs; and (3) the crura from the upper three lumbar vertebrae. All three converge on the **central tendon.** There are three major openings for the inferior vena cava, esophagus, and aorta (along with the azygos and hemiazygos veins and thoracic duct). The **lateral arcuate ligaments** are thickened bands of fascia overlying the quadratus lumborum muscles and adjacent to the posterior pararenal space; they extend from the transverse process of L1 to the middle of the twelfth rib. A portion of the lumbar diaphragm is attached and can be mistaken for nodules or tumor implants.

- **CT** can be useful in assessing congenital or acquired defects in the structural integrity of the diaphragm. Peridiaphragmatic lesions can be localized and characterized. Primary diaphragmatic masses are rare. Spiral CT with multiplanar reconstructions improves depiction. The direct multiplanar imaging capability of **MRI** is advantageous in assessing the diaphragm and peridiaphragmatic processes.

- **Focal eventration** is a localized bulge in the diaphragm due to instrinsic thinning and weakness. It is most common in the anterior portion of the right hemidiaphragm. The exact etiology is unknown, but possibilities include congenital deficiency of muscle or acquired focal diaphragmatic dysfunction secondary to ischemia, infarction, or neuromuscular disease.

- **Anterior diaphragmatic lymph nodes** reside posterior to the xiphoid and behind the costal cartilages in the cardiophrenic angles. Up to two lymph nodes less than 5 mm in diameter can normally be seen on CT. Lymphadenopathy is often associated with lymphoma or lung, breast, or colon cancer. The diaphragm's attachment to the xiphoid can mimic adenopathy on CT.

- The **retrocrural space** contains the aorta, azygos vein, thoracic duct, nerves, and lymph nodes. **Lymphadenopathy** is suggested when discrete soft tissue masses larger than 6 mm are present on CT and is often accompanied by upper abdominal paraaortic lymphadenopathy. Lymphoma is the most common malignant process.

- **Vascular masses**, such as esophageal varices or aortic aneurysmal rupture, can also present as retrocrural masses and are easily confirmed with CT. Extension of disease from the adjacent spine—such as malignancy, infection, or fracture with hematoma—can also produce a retrocrural abnormality. **Azygos vein enlargement** can occur with congenital interruption, thrombosis, or obstruction of the inferior vena cava and should not be mistaken for retrocrural lymphadenopathy.

- Primary **tumors of the diaphragm** are rare and their appearance is generally nonspecific. Most are benign lipomas, neurofibromas, or mesothelial or teratoid cysts.

Hernias

- Diaphragmatic hernias are common, occur in a variety of forms, and can be congenital or acquired.

- The **Bochdalek hernia** is the most common congenital diaphragmatic hernia and results from incomplete closure of the embryonic pleuroperitoneal membrane. The defect is located posterolaterally and is most often left-sided. Small defects can contain only retroperitoneal fat **(Fig. 3.23).** Larger defects can contain the stomach, intestines, spleen, kidney, or liver. The majority of posterior diaphragmatic defects in adults are likely **acquired** rather than true Bochdalek hernias. The incidence increases with age, weight, and emphysema.

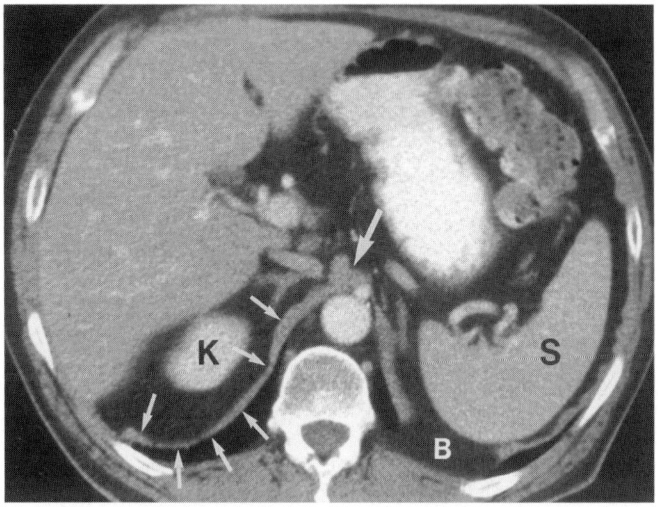

FIGURE 3.23 Bochdalek hernia. Contrast-enhanced CT showing a normal right hemidiaphragm *(small arrows).* There is a defect in the left hemidiaphragm, with herniation of retroperitoneal fat (B). Note the normal enlargement of the crux of the right diaphragm *(large arrow).* K, right kidney; S, spleen.

- **Morgagni hernias** are considerably less common than Bochdalek hernias. They occur more often on the right through an anterior defect in the sternocostal trigone. Associated with obesity, they usually contain omental fat, are covered by both peritoneum and parietal pleura, and present as asymptomatic right cardiophrenic an-

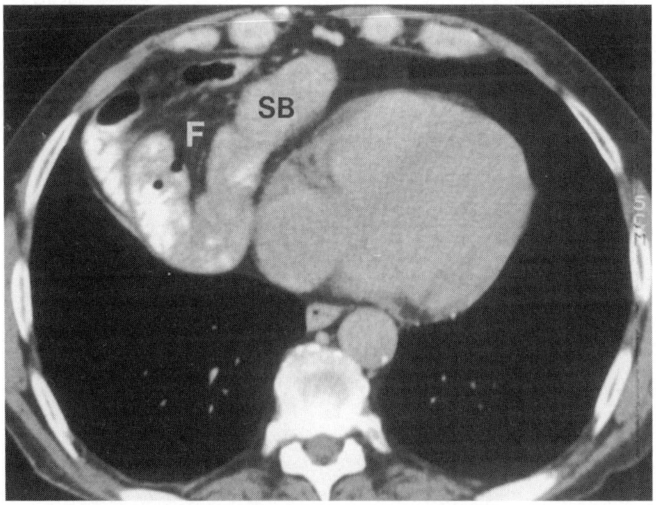

FIGURE 2.24 Morgagni hernia. Abdominal fat (F) and loops of small bowel (SB) presenting as a right cardiophrenic mass in this 70-year-old man.

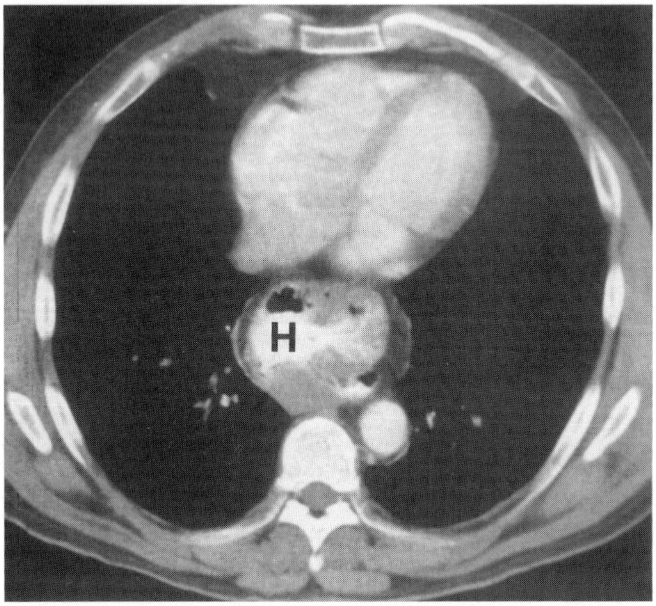

FIGURE 3.25 Hiatal hernia. Contrast-enhanced CT through the lower chest showing a large hiatal hernia (H) interposed between the spine and heart. The hernia contains air and oral contrast material.

gle masses **(Fig. 3.24).** The transverse colon is more frequently involved than the stomach, small bowel, or liver.

- **Hiatal hernias,** herniation of the stomach through the esophageal hiatus, are common in adults. The typical presentation is a retrocardiac mass with an air-fluid level **(Fig. 3.25).** This acquired abnormality is secondary to laxity and stretching of the phreno-esophageal ligament and widening of the esophageal hiatus. Obesity and increased intraabdominal pressure are contributing factors. The majority can be reduced or are reversible and are called ***sliding hiatal hernias.*** Some are ***paraesophageal,*** in which case the stomach herniates adjacent to the distal esophagus. A very large hernia or "intrathoracic stomach" can become incarcerated or undergo volvulus. When marked ascites occurs in a patient with a hiatal hernia, fluid can extend into the lower posterior mediastinum, mimicking a mediastinal abscess, necrotic tumor, or foregut cyst.
- **Traumatic disruption of the diaphragm** can result from penetrating or blunt trauma and often goes undetected initially. This lesion can enlarge over time and poses a high risk of eventual incarceration and strangulation. Herniation most often occurs on the left and involves the stomach but it can also involve the bowel, omentum, spleen, or liver. CT can show discontinuity of the diaphragm, abdominal organs, or peritoneal fat above the diaphragm, and focal constriction of the stomach or bowel at the site of herniation **(see Sec. 15.3).**

Bibliography

Armstrong P, Wilson AG, Dee P, Hansell DM. *Imaging of Diseases of the Chest*, 2nd ed. St. Louis: Mosby-Year Book; 1995.

Brink JA, Heiken JP, Semenkovich J, Teefey SA, McClennan BL, Sagel SS. Abnormalities of the diaphragm and adjacent structures: Findings on multiplanar spiral CT scans. *AJR* 1994;163:307–310.

Dynes MC, White EM, Fry WA, Ghahremani GG. Imaging manifestations of pleural tumors. *Radiographics* 1992;12:1191.

Freundlich IM, Bragg DG. *A Radiologic Approach to Diseases of the Chest*, 2nd ed. Baltimore: Williams & Wilkins; 1997.

Halvorsen RA, Fedyshin PJ, Korobkin M, Foster WLJ, Thompson WM. Ascites or pleural effusion? CT differentiation: Four useful criteria. *Radiographics* 1986;6:135–149.

Hanna JW, Reed JC, Choplin RH. Pleural infections: A clinical-radiologic review. *J Thorac Imaging* 1991;6:68.

Kawashima A, Libshitz HI. Malignant pleural mesothelioma: CT manifestations in 50 cases. *AJR* 1990;155:965.

Leung AN, Müller NL, Miller RR. CT in differential diagnosis of diffuse pleural disease. *AJR* 1990;154:487–492.

Light RW. *Pleural diseases*, 3rd ed. Baltimore: Williams & Wilkins; 1995.

Matthay RA, Coppage L, Shaw C, Filderman AE. Malignancies metastatic to the pleura. *Invest Radiol* 1990;25:601.

Müller NL. Imaging of the pleura. *Radiology* 1993;186:297–309.

Slone RM, Gierada DS. Pleura, chest wall and diaphragm. In: Lee JKT, Sagel SS, Stanley RJ, Heiken JP (eds): *Computed Body Tomography with MRI Correlation*, 3rd ed. Philadelphia: Lippincott-Raven, 1998.

Slone RM, Gutierrez FR, Fisher AJ. *Thoracic Imaging: A Practical Approach.* New York: McGraw-Hill, 1999.

Sofranik RM, Gross VH, Spizarny DL. Radiology of the pleural fissures. *Clin Imaging* 1992;16:221.

Tarver RD, Conces DJJ, Cory DA, Vix VA. Imaging the diaphragm and its disorders. *J Thorac Imaging* 1989;4:1–18.

Wechsler RJ, Steiner RM, Conant EF. Occupationally induced neoplasms of the lung and pleura. *Radiol Clin North Am* 1992;30:1245.

Chapter 4

MEDIASTINUM

Fernando R. Gutierrez and Sanjeev Bhalla

4.1 Anatomy and Technique
4.2 Thoracic Inlet
4.3 Lymphadenopathy and Inflammatory Changes
4.4 Pneumomediastinum and Low-Density Masses
4.5 Anterior Mediastinum
4.6 Middle Mediastinum
4.7 Posterior Mediastinum
4.8 Postoperative Mediastinum

4.1 ANATOMY AND TECHNIQUE

- Bordered by the lungs laterally, the chest wall anteriorly, and the spine posteriorly, the **mediastinum** is the space that contains the heart, great vessels, tracheobronchial tree, thymus, esophagus, lymph nodes, and lymphatics.
- Artificially dividing the mediastinum into four compartments can help in narrowing the differential diagnosis. The **thoracic inlet** or **superior mediastinum** marks the junction with the lower neck. The remainder of the mediastinum can be divided coronally into three spaces: the **anterior mediastinum, middle mediastinum,** and **posterior mediastinum.**
- The **anterior mediastinum** contains the thymus, lymph nodes, internal mammary veins and arteries, and fat. It is defined by the sternum anteriorly and the aorta, brachiocephalic vessels, and anterior pericardium posteriorly. The **middle mediastinum** contains the heart, ascending aorta, aortic arch, superior and inferior venae cavae, brachiocephalic vessels, trachea, right and left main bronchi, and central pulmonary arteries and veins. The **posterior mediastinum** contains the descending thoracic aorta, thoracic duct, esophagus, azygos and hemiazygos veins, autonomic nerves, and fat. It extends from the posterior portion of the pericardium to the paravertebral gutters posteriorly.

Technique

- Although chest radiographs are often used to screen for mediastinal pathology, computed tomography (CT) is usually necessary to characterize the location and nature of a lesion. CT can help to determine whether the abnormality is solid, cystic, or vascular. Scanning should be performed with the patient in suspended inspiration with a slice thickness of 5 to 8 mm and reconstruction interval of 5 to 10 mm. A slice thickness of 3 to 5 mm with overlapping reconstructions through selected regions of interest such as the trachea can be implemented if needed. Single or multiple breath-holds with a 10- to 15-s interscan delay should be utilized as indicated. The survey study should extend from the thoracic inlet to the level of the adrenal glands.
- Iodinated intravenous contrast can be very helpful and, in many cases, is essential in determining the relationship of abnormal structures to adjacent vasculature and in the detection of small lesions that could be mistaken for vessel on a noncontrast study. A total volume of 100 to 125 mL should be injected at a rate of 2 mL/s with a scan delay of about 25 s. Thoracic aorta and pulmonary thromboembolism protocols are discussed in Sec. 1.3. In cases of suspected esophageal pathology, the use of barium paste (Esophotrast) can be extremely useful for anatomic characterization.
- If a cystic mass is suspected, at least one noncontrast image should be made through the lesion. If it is water attenuation, the examination can be completed without intravenous contrast. If it is high in attenuation, the examination should be conducted with intravenous contrast. Some cystic masses have high attenuation due to proteinaceous contents but will not enhance after contrast.

4.2 THORACIC INLET

- A wide variety of lesions can be found in the thoracic inlet or superior mediastinal space **(Differential 4.1).**
- **Tumoral masses** arising from structures of the neck can extend along the fascial planes into the upper mediastinum **(Fig. 4.1).** Associated adenopathy may be necrotic, as in tonsillar and nasopharyngeal malignancies. Malignant adenopathy may also be secondary to lymphoma or to bronchogenic or breast cancer.

4.1

THORACIC INLET MASS

Thyroid mass—goiter, adenoma, carcinoma
Lymphoma or leukemia—particularly CLL* and Hodgkin disease
Adenopathy—reactive, metastases (head and neck, lung, breast)
Vascular—tortuous brachiocephalic vessels, cervical aorta
Thymic mass—thymoma, thymolipoma, thymic carcinoma, rebound hyperplasia, thymic cyst
Parathyroid mass—adenoma
Lymphangioma—cystic hygroma

*Chronic lymphocytic leukemia.

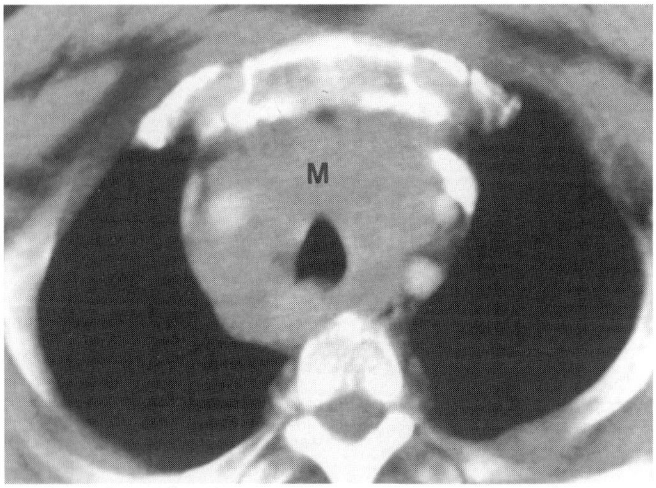

FIGURE 4.1 Nasopharyngeal tumor. Note tumoral mass (M) extending into superior mediastinum and displacing vessels.

- **Vascular masses** may be seen as manifestations of tortuous or aneurysmal brachiocephalic vessels, cervical aortic arch, posttraumatic pseudoaneurysm, asymmetrical jugular veins, and arteriovenous malformations, among others.
- **Thoracic goiters** (benign enlargement of the thyroid gland greater than 50 g) usually present as both superior and anterior mediastinal masses that have mass effect on the trachea. They are classified into simple and multinodular goiters. Although they usually extend anteriorly, in 20 percent of cases the goiter extends posterior to the trachea. In almost all cases, continuity with the cervical thyroid is seen. On CT, the goiter may have areas of low attenuation and calcification **(Fig. 4.2).** Contrast is rarely needed to make this diagnosis. If contrast is administered, the goiter enhances for a prolonged period.
- **Thyroid tumors** are usually thyroid adenomas and malignant neoplasms **(Differential 4.2). Adenomas** are usually solitary; they grow slowly and can be associated with hyperthyroidism. Although usually solid, they may undergo cystic degeneration. **Thyroid carcinoma** usually affects young adults and is mostly well differentiated. Papillary thyroid carcinoma represents about 70 percent of all thyroid cancers; it usually has a poorer prognosis in patients above 40 years of age, has a tendency to metastasize via the lymphatics, and can demonstrate cystic degeneration. Follicular carcinoma represents about 20 percent of the total, spreads hematogenously, and shows cystic degeneration less commonly. Medullary carcinoma is rare and can be associated with the multiple endocrine neoplasia syndromes. Anaplastic carcinomas of the thyroid represent about 5 percent of all thyroid malignancies; it is usually seen in elderly patients and is frequently associated with adjacent adenopathy.

4.2

THYROID LESION

Goiter
Adenoma
Thyroid carcinoma
Cystic lesion—colloid cyst, necrotic papillary cancer, adenoma or goiter
Inflammation—thyroiditis, abscess
Hemorrhage within an adenoma or colloid nodule
Lymphoma—particularly Hodgkin
Metastases—breast, lung, renal cell, melanoma

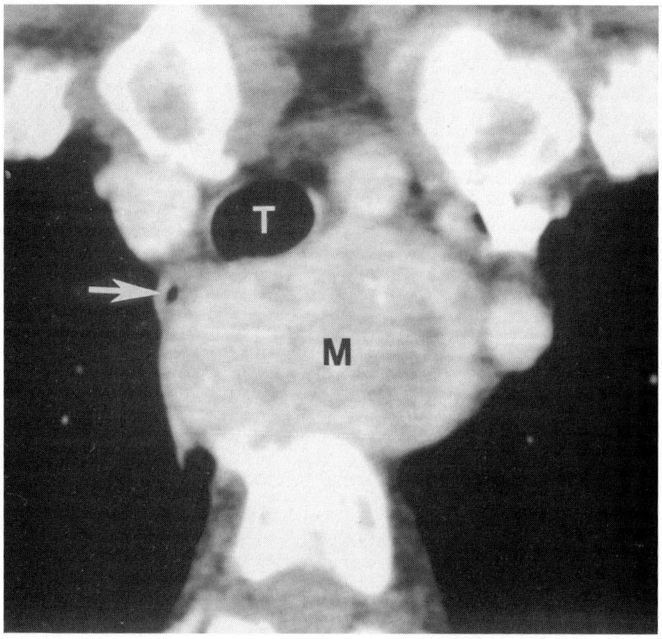

FIGURE 4.2 Ectopic goiter. CT of a 66-year-old woman shows a large heterogeneous enhancing mass (M) with areas of low attenuation and stippled calcifications posterior to the trachea (T). The mass was continuous with the left lobe of the thyroid gland. Note displacement of the esophagus to the right *(arrow)*.

- **Abscesses** originating in the neck can extend into the thoracic inlet and eventually involve lower mediastinal regions. They may start in the tonsils or parotid region or be a consequence of trauma. They usually show thick, enhancing walls with adjacent areas of inflammation and may contain gas.
- **Air-filled masses** may represent laryngoceles, Zenker diverticulae, or lateral pharyngeal diverticulae.

4.3 LYMPHADENOPATHY AND INFLAMMATORY CHANGES

- **Mediastinal lymphadenopathy,** pathologic involvement of lymph nodes, represents a common cause of mediastinal widening on chest radiographs. CT is more sensitive than conventional radiography for this process, which can be secondary to inflammation, infection, or neoplasm. Lymphadenopathy will have a similar CT appearance in all three conditions. Lymph nodes are present in the anterior, middle, and posterior mediastinum, so mediastinal lymphadenopathy can present as a mass in any one of these compartments.
- **CT criteria** for lymphadenopathy include abnormal size and number of lymph nodes. Specificity is increased when both criteria are used. CT, however, is not 100 percent sensitive. It cannot evaluate the internal architecture of the lymph nodes. Normal-sized lymph

nodes containing malignant deposits, therefore, can have the same CT appearance as uninvolved nodes. Intravenous contrast can be helpful in detecting adenopathy, particularly in the hila, where adjacent vessels may obscure or mimic lymph nodes. If a vascular etiology is suspected as the likely cause of the mediastinal abnormality, intravenous contrast material is necessary.

- **Normal sizes** for mediastinal lymph nodes vary by location and method of measurement. Though lymph nodes may be measured in the long or short axis, the latter has been advocated. Short-axis measurement of less than 1 cm has been used as the cutoff between normal and pathologic lymph nodes in most locations. Normal subcarinal lymph nodes may approach 12 mm; but hilar, cardiophrenic angle, and diaphragmatic lymph nodes should not exceed 5 mm. The American Thoracic Society's nomenclature for mediastinal lymph node locations is shown in **Fig. 4.3.**

- **Inflammatory or nonneoplastic** causes of mediastinal lymphadenopathy include sarcoidosis **(Fig. 4.4)** and pneumoconioses, such as silicosis. Fungal and mycobacterial infections may also result in mediastinal lymphadenopathy. Among patients with primary tuberculosis, mediastinal adenopathy is more common in children. **Neoplastic** adenopathy can result from lymphoma and bronchogenic carcinoma, which usually involves ipsilateral hilar nodes before involving mediastinal lymph nodes **(Fig. 4.5).** Small cell carcinoma is frequently associated with bulky mediastinal and hilar adenopathy **(Fig. 4.6).** Hilar and mediastinal lymphadenopathy may also be secondary to extrathoracic nodal metastases, most commonly renal, breast, testicular, and head and neck cancers as well as melanoma.

- **CT features** that may help in the evaluation of mediastinal lymphadenopathy include calcification, low attenuation, and enhancement. **Calcification** usually excludes malignancy. Frequently, it is secondary to healed granulomatous infection. Silicosis, sarcoidosis, and treated **Hodgkin disease** may also result in lymph node calcification in either a diffuse or eggshell pattern **(Fig. 4.7).** *Pneumocystis carinii* pneumonia can also result in calcified mediastinal lymph nodes from the granulomatous reaction. Rare causes of malignant calcification include metastatic osteosarcoma, mucinous adenocarcinoma of the colon or ovary, and bronchoalveolar carcinoma.

- **Low-attenuation lymph nodes** can result from infections that may incite a granulomatous response, particularly tuberculosis and fungal infections. Low-attenuation necrotic lymph nodes from aggressive malignancies can be seen with testicular, ovarian, or lung cancer metastases. They can also be seen in lymphoma prior to therapy or following radiation or chemotherapy. Fatty replacement of lymph nodes virtually excludes malignancy **(Fig. 4.8).** Rare causes of low-attenuation mediastinal lymph nodes include lymphangioleiomyomatosis and Whipple disease.

- **Enhancing lymph nodes** can be secondary to involvement from vascular tumors, such as renal cell cancer **(Fig. 4.9)**, thyroid cancer, Kaposi sarcoma, paraganglioma, melanoma, or carcinoid. Alternatively, enhancing lymph nodes may be secondary to angiofollicular lymph node hyperplasia (Castleman disease). Lymphoma can have moderate enhancement, as can nonspecific HIV-related adenopathy.

- **Castleman disease**—also known as giant lymph node hyperplasia, angiofollicular hyperplasia, lymphonodal hamartoma, and follicular lymphoreticuloma—is a benign condition of uncertain etiology that presents with enlarged lymph nodes in a variety of locations,

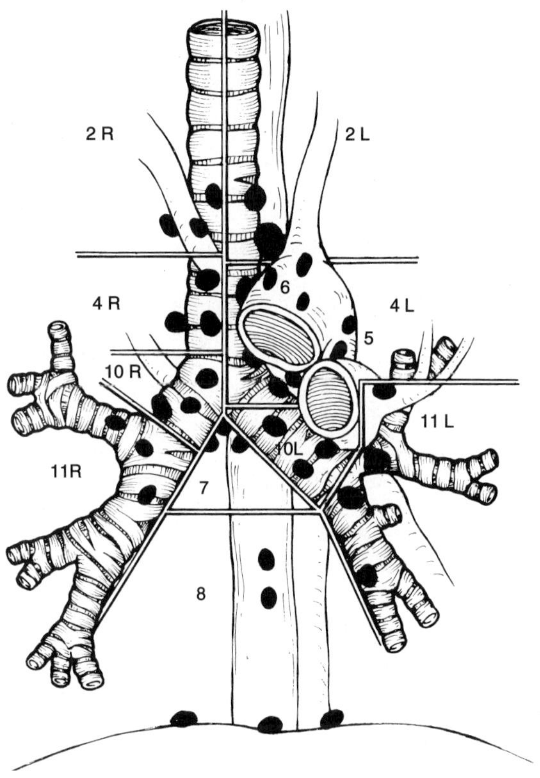

FIGURE 4.3 Modified American Thoracic Society classification of mediastinal lymph node stations. Right upper paratracheal nodes (2R). Nodes to the right of the midline of the trachea, above the level of the aortic arch. **Left upper paratracheal nodes (2L).** Nodes to the left of the midline of the trachea, between the top of the aortic arch and the apex of the lung. **Prevascular and retrotracheal nodes (3) (not shown). Right lower paratracheal nodes (4R).** Nodes to the right of the midline of the trachea, between the azygos vein and the top of the aortic arch. **Left lower paratracheal nodes (4L).** Nodes to the left of the midline of the trachea, between the top of the aortic arch and the level of the carina, medial to the ligamentum arteriosum. **Aortopulmonary nodes (5).** Subaortic and para-aortic nodes, lateral to the ligamentum arteriosum and proximal to the first branch of the left pulmonary artery. **Anterior mediastinal nodes (6).** Nodes anterior to the ascending aorta or the innominate artery. **Subcarinal nodes (7).** Nodes arising caudal to the carina. **Paraesophageal nodes (8).** Nodes dorsal to the posterior wall of the trachea and below the subcarinal region and around the descending aorta. **Pulmonary ligament nodes (9).** Nodes within the right or left inferior pulmonary ligament (not shown). **Right hilar nodes (10R).** Nodes to the right of the midline of the trachea, from the level of the azygos vein to the origin of the right-upper-lobe bronchus. **Left hilar nodes (10L).** Nodes to the left of the midline of the trachea, between the carina and the left-upper-lobe bronchus, medial to the ligamentum arteriosum. **Interlobar nodes (11).** Nodes removed in the right or left lung specimen, plus those distal to the main bronchi (includes interlobar, lobar, and segmental nodes). (From Slone RM, Gutierrez FR, Fisher AJ. *Thoracic Imaging: A Practical Approach.* New York: McGraw-Hill, 1999. With permission.)

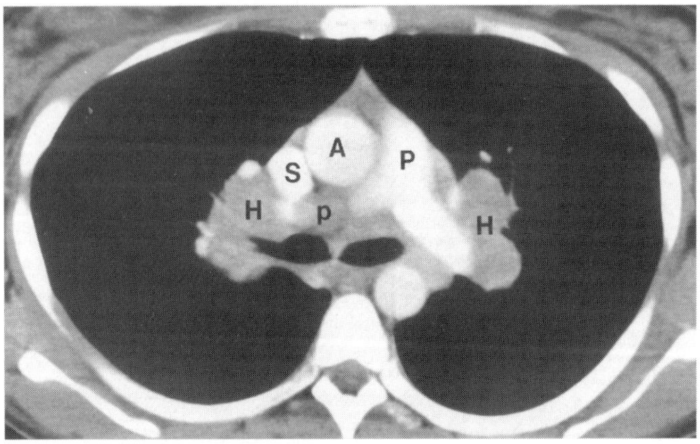

FIGURE 4.4 Sarcoidosis. Massive low-density bilateral hilar (H) and precarinal (p) adenopathy in a 32-year-old woman. Right paratracheal adenopathy was also present. A, ascending aorta; S, superior vena cava; P, pulmonary trunk.

predominantly in the mediastinum. There are two variants: plasma cell, an acute variant that can progress to malignant lymphoma, and an angiofollicular form, which tends to be more chronic and is not associated with an increased incidence of malignant lymphoma. It is unclear whether these two variants are two separate diseases or two ends of a spectrum.

Unlike lymphoma, Castleman disease has a predilection for the posterior mediastinum. It is most often found incidentally in young patients who are asymptomatic or have nonspecific constitutional symptoms, such as low-grade fevers and night sweats. Involved lymph nodes show diffuse enhancement and are highly vascular. Histologically, it can be difficult to differentiate involved nodes from thymoma or malignant lymphoma, making the imaging characteristics even more important in establishing a diagnosis. An association with Kaposi sarcoma has been reported.

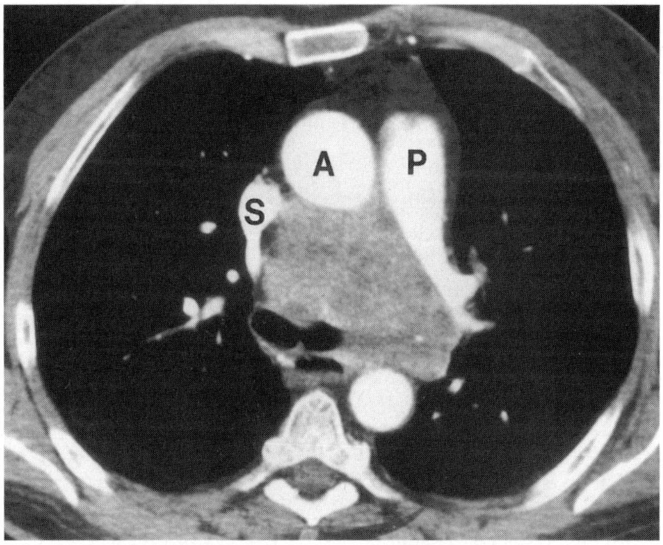

FIGURE 4.6 Bulky mediastinal lymphadenopathy. Encasement of the pulmonary arteries with virtual occlusion of the right branch in a patient with small cell carcinoma of the lung. A, ascending aorta; P, pulmonary trunk; S, superior vena cava.

- **Acute mediastinitis** may result from mediastinal surgery or esophageal perforation. Necrotic tumor may also cause the esophagus to rupture. Spread of infection from an adjacent structure, such as lung or sternum, may also result in acute mediastinitis. Early in the course of mediastinitis, streaky soft tissue infiltration of the fat can be seen. This may eventually result in a loculated fluid collection or abscess that may or may not contain gas **(Fig. 4.10).** The administration of intravenous contrast allows for visualization of the enhancing wall of the abscess. This can be helpful, particularly in the

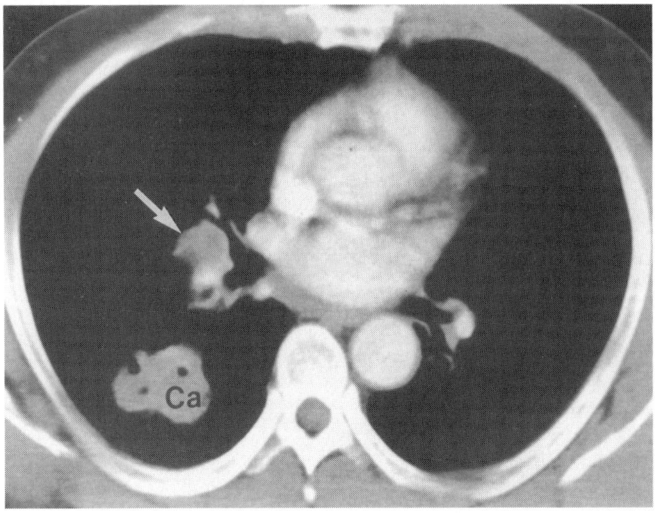

FIGURE 4.5 Bronchogenic carcinoma with hilar adenopathy. Contrast-enhanced CT in a 59-year-old man with a right-lower-lobe primary lung cancer (Ca) and ipsilateral hilar adenopathy *(arrow).*

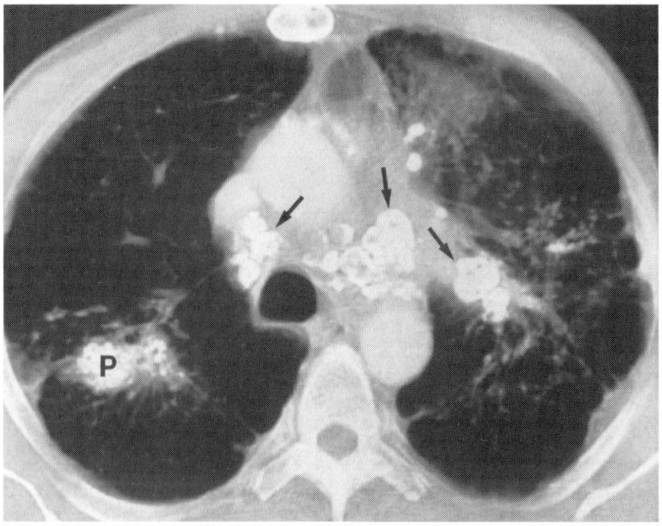

FIGURE 4.7 Silicosis with eggshell calcifications. Extensive calcification of mediastinal and hilar lymph nodes *(arrows)*, some with a peripheral pattern (eggshell calcification). Note also evidence of progressive massive fibrosis (P) in the right upper lobe with confluent calcified nodules and associated scarring.

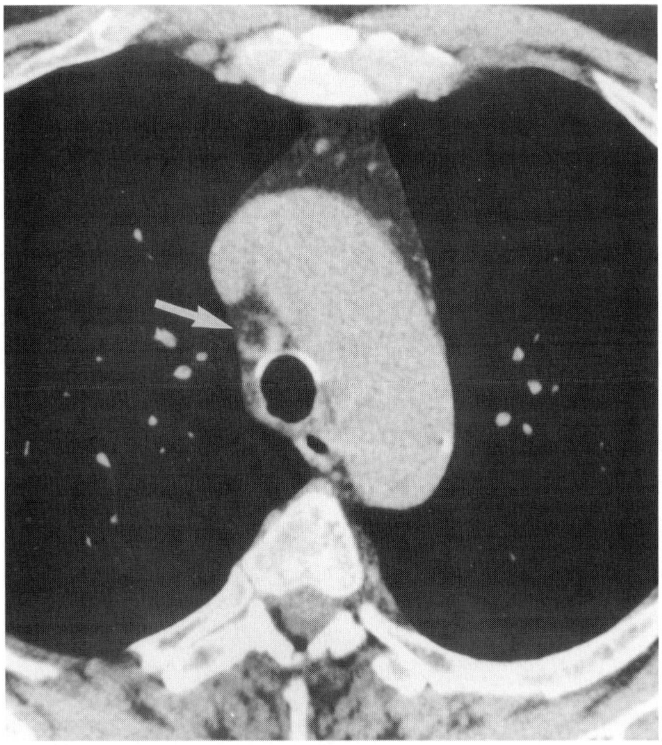

FIGURE 4.8 Normal lymph node. CT demonstrating fatty hilum of a precarinal lymph node *(arrow)*.

setting of a large pericardial or pleural effusion abutting the abscess, which might obscure it. If esophageal or gastroesophageal perforation is suspected, aqueous oral contrast should be administered.

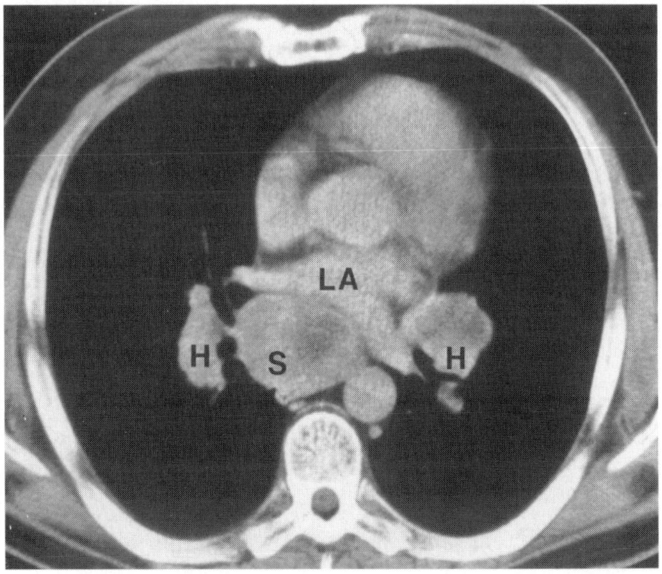

FIGURE 4.9 Metastatic renal cell carcinoma. CT 1 year following nephrectomy in a 51-year-old man showing bilateral hilar (H) and subcarinal adenopathy (S) displacing the left atrium (LA). Note the typical vascular enhancement of the adenopathy and central necrosis.

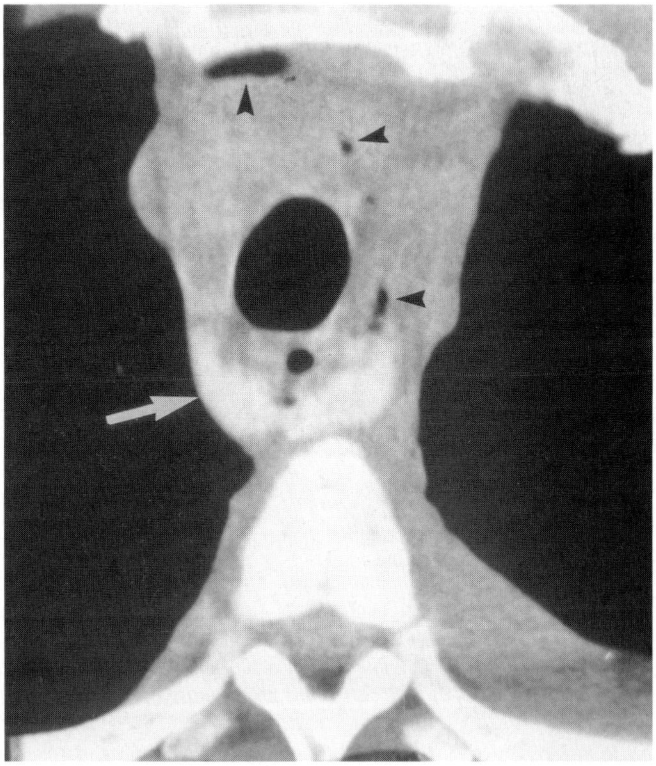

FIGURE 4.10 Esophageal perforation as a consequence of esophagoscopy. CT at the level of the manubrium demonstrates gas *(arrowheads)* and water-soluble oral contrast material *(arrow)* within the mediastinum.

- **Fibrosing mediastinitis** refers to exuberant fibrogenesis as a result of exposure to fungal infection, most commonly *Histoplasma capsulatum*. An immunologic host response has been postulated as the probable cause. The fibrosis can compress and occlude mediastinal structures. Symptoms depend on which structure is compressed. Involvement of veins, arteries, the tracheobronchial tree, and the pericardium may occur. Pulmonary infiltrates may result from arterial compression, resulting in infarct or edema from pulmonary venous obstruction.

  Compression of the superior vena cava (SVC) may result in SVC syndrome, with multiple venous collaterals seen throughout the chest wall. CT with intravenous contrast can readily show the vessels and the effect of the adjacent fibrosis **(Fig. 4.11).** Narrowing of the vessel lumen and complete occlusion can be seen. Coronal and sagittal reconstructions can sometimes be helpful in assessing the effect of the fibrosis on the pulmonary arteries and veins. Rarely, fibrosis of the mediastinum can occur simultaneously with retroperitoneal fibrosis (Ormond syndrome). This has been reported as a complication of methysergide therapy.

4.4 PNEUMOMEDIASTINUM AND LOW-DENSITY MASSES

Pneumomediastinum

- **Pneumomediastinum,** or air within the mediastinum but outside of the tracheobronchial tree or esophagus, can occur from a variety of causes **(Differential 4.3)**, among which alveolar rupture is the most

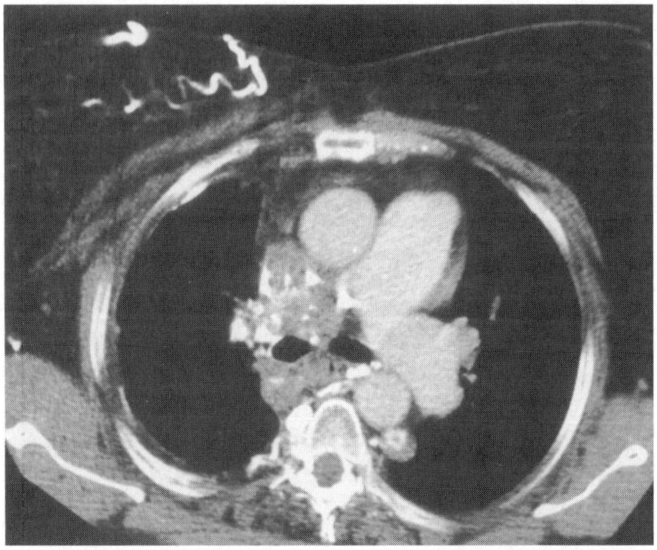

FIGURE 4.11 Fibrosing mediastinitis. A 68-year-old woman with extensive confluent calcified mediastinal adenopathy. There is obstruction of the superior vena cava with collateral flow through chest wall veins. There is also obstruction of the right pulmonary artery.

common. Volutrauma can occur in mechanically ventilated patients in whom air (under positive pressure) dissects along walls of the airway into the mediastinum. Perforation of the tracheobronchial tree or esophagus can also result in pneumomediastinum. Free air from the peritoneum or retroperitoneum can extend up through the esophageal hiatus and cause a pneumomediastinum.

- The diagnosis of a pneumomediastinum simply requires the visualization of air outside of the esophagus or tracheobronchial tree. Findings can vary from a single dot of air to extensive air collections surrounding the mediastinal structures. These findings are most easily seen on lung windows. Although pneumomediastinum may result in a pneumothorax, the opposite situation is less common. CT can be useful in distinguishing between a medial loculated pneumothorax and pneumomediastinum. It can also be useful in distinguishing pneumomediastinum from a **pneumopericardium,** a less common condition usually seen in cases of cardiac surgery or other interventions to the pericardium. The latter condition will not result in air in the superior mediastinum or around the aortic arch, as the pericardial reflections usually end just inferior to the arch. In addition, pneumomediastinum tends to contain streaky gas collections, as opposed to the broad band of gas (halo) seen around the heart in pneumopericardium, which can change in configuration with different patient positioning.

4.3

PNEUMOMEDIASTINUM

Recent surgery
Tracheobronchial trauma
Extension—pneumoperitoneum or subcutaneous emphysema
Esophageal tear—endoscopy, dilatation
Spontaneous—asthma, cough, vomiting, idiopathic
Tracheal or esophageal fistula—tumor, infection

Low-Attenuation Mediastinal Masses

- Low-attenuation mediastinal masses include cystic and fat-containing lesions **(Differential 4.4).**

Mediastinal Hemorrhage

- **Mediastinal hemorrhage** may be due to atherosclerotic disease (bleeding aneurysm, penetrating atherosclerotic ulcer, dissection) or secondary to trauma or surgery. Usually, patients present with chest pain and may have a history of prior trauma, severe atherosclerosis, or known thoracic aortic aneurysm. On noncontrast CT, high attenuation abutting the aorta is usually found. The appearance on magnetic resonance imaging (MRI) is more variable, depending on the age of the hematoma. It should be noted that not all high-attenuation collections abutting the aorta are due to arterial bleeding. In trauma cases, this high attenuation may be due to venous blood. The presence of this blood, however, is an indication that the mechanism of injury was severe enough to have potentially disrupted the aorta.

Cystic Mediastinal Masses

- **Bronchogenic cysts** are the most common congenital cysts of the mediastinum. Arising as a result of abnormal budding of the foregut, they are frequently in close proximity to the trachea, usually in the hilar, subcarinal, or right paratracheal regions. They may have a narrow stalk connecting them with the airway, although communication with the foregut is almost always lost. They occur within the mediastinum (85 percent) more frequently than within the pulmonary parenchyma (15 percent). These well-defined cysts are lined by columnar respiratory epithelium and may contain smooth muscle, cartilage, and mucous glands in their walls.

  Their contents can vary from water-like to viscous, proteinaceous fluid, but they do not enhance with intravenous contrast **(Fig. 4.12).** Because of the variability of the contents, the CT and MRI appearance can also be quite variable. Fluid-fluid levels may be seen within the cysts on cross-sectional imaging. When the connection with the airway is maintained or develops as a complication of infection, these cysts may contain an air-fluid level. Despite the variable attenuation or signal, the appearance of bronchogenic cysts usually allows for a confident diagnosis by CT. In equivocal or symptomatic cases, aspiration by CT guidance or surgery can be performed. Otherwise, conservative management is recommended.

- **Pericardial cysts** are usually asymptomatic and abut the parietal pericardium but have no communication with the pericardial space. If a persistent communication is found, these are referred to as **pericardial diverticula.** These cysts are most frequent in the right cardiophrenic angle and usually contain serous fluid. They may pre-

4.4

LOW-ATTENUATION MEDIASTINAL MASS

Fat—obesity, steroids, lipoma, thymolipoma, mature teratoma, *liposarcoma*
Cyst—bronchogenic or esophageal duplication; pericardial, thymic, pancreatic pseudocyst; *neuroenteric, lateral thoracic meningocele*
Fluid collection—seroma from trauma or surgery, perforated venous catheter, loculated pleural effusion, abscess
Gastrointestinal—hiatal, Morgagni, or Bochdalek hernia; gastric interposition; dilated esophagus; esophageal diverticulum
Lymphangioma—cystic hygroma

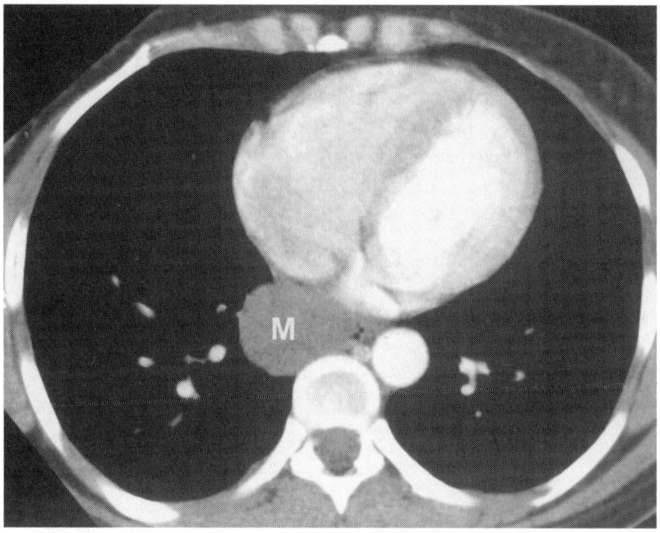

FIGURE 4.12 Duplication cyst. A 26-year-old woman with a mediastinal mass (M) noted on the chest radiograph. CT confirms the benign nature of the cystic lesion. The lesion measured 35 to 40 HU both before and after intravenous contrast.

sent anywhere along the pericardium and may extend to other parts of the mediastinum, making them hard to differentiate from bronchogenic cysts. On CT, they are often found abutting the right atrium and are near water attenuation unless the fluid is proteinaceous **(see Fig. 5.2).**

- **Esophageal duplication cysts** are a form of bronchopulmonary foregut malformation that may appear as cystic posterior mediastinal masses. On CT, they are well marginated, near water attenuation, and appose the esophagus. The differential diagnosis for these predominantly right-sided masses includes neurogenic tumors, abscess (in the appropriate clinical setting), and bronchogenic cyst. Duplication cysts may have a squamous or columnar epithelial lining as well as two muscular layers. These cysts may be intramural or paraesophageal and usually do not communicate with the esophageal lumen. Esophageal duplication cysts are most commonly seen arising from the distal esophagus and are more posterior than bronchogenic cysts.
- **Neuroenteric cysts** are foregut cysts of the posterior mediastinum that may be confused with esophageal duplication cysts. They develop as a result of failed separation of neuroectodermal and pulmonary elements in the third week of gestational development. Although they have a CT appearance similar to that of other mediastinal cysts (bronchogenic cysts, pericardial cysts, esophageal duplication cysts), they are found in conjunction with vertebral anomalies such as spina bifida or hemivertebrae. MRI may best show the relationship of the cyst to the thecal sac. They may be attached to the vertebrae by fibrous strands and do not necessarily arise at the level of the vertebral anomaly. They rarely communicate with the gastrointestinal tract.
- Rarely, **pancreatic pseudocysts** can dissect into the posterior mediastinum via the esophageal or aortic hiatus. Continuity with a pseudocyst arising inferior to the diaphragm and the appropriate clinical setting should be clues to the diagnosis.
- **Lymphangiomas** are benign multicystic tumors that are classified as capillary, cavernous, or **cystic** (hygromas). Often, individual tumors contain more than one type. These tumors arise from proliferating lymphatics and can develop around and eventually surround mediastinal structures. Mediastinal cystic hygromas may be seen as direct extensions of neck cystic hygromas. In less than 1 percent, the cystic hygroma is found exclusively in the mediastinum. These lesions present as multilocular cystic lesions with low attenuation on CT because of their chylous composition **(Fig. 4.13).** They may present anywhere in the mediastinum.

Fatty Masses

- **Mediastinal lipomatosis** represents an abundance of normal fat within the mediastinum. It does not exert mass effect on the mediastinal structures but may provide an explanation for mediastinal widening seen on a chest film **(Fig. 4.14).** This condition may be seen in obese patients or in patients exposed to excess endogenous or exogenous steroid. The fat is usually in the superior mediastinum but may extend into any mediastinal compartment.
- **Mediastinal lipomas** are rare. Unlike mediastinal lipomatosis, the fat of a lipoma is encapsulated but usually does not compress adjacent structures. These benign lesions may have thin septations on CT. Additional soft tissue attenuation is suggestive of other fatty tumors, such as liposarcoma, germ cell tumor, or myelolipoma.
- **Omental fat** or abdominal fat can herniate through the diaphragm via the foramen of Morgagni, esophageal hiatus, or foramen of Bochdalek **(see Sec. 3.7 and Figs. 3.23 and 3.24).** Soft tissue attenuation within the fat simply represents blood vessels. Continuity with the omentum establishes the diagnosis.

4.5 ANTERIOR MEDIASTINUM

- Mediastinal masses, which can be congenital or acquired, may be categorized based on the compartment in which they arise. This classification allows for the generation of a more specific differential diagnosis. The most common anterior mediastinal masses are lymphomas, thoracic goiters, and thymic lesions **(Differential 4.5).**

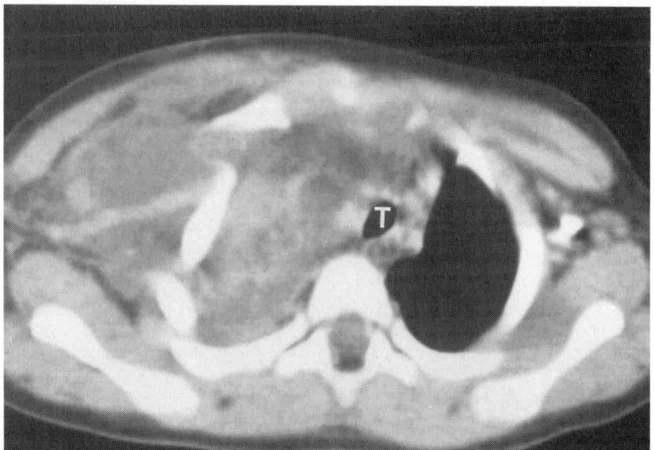

FIGURE 4.13 Lymphangioma. A 10-year-old with a large heterogeneous mass extending from the base of the neck and into the mediastinum. Note displacement of trachea (T) to the left.

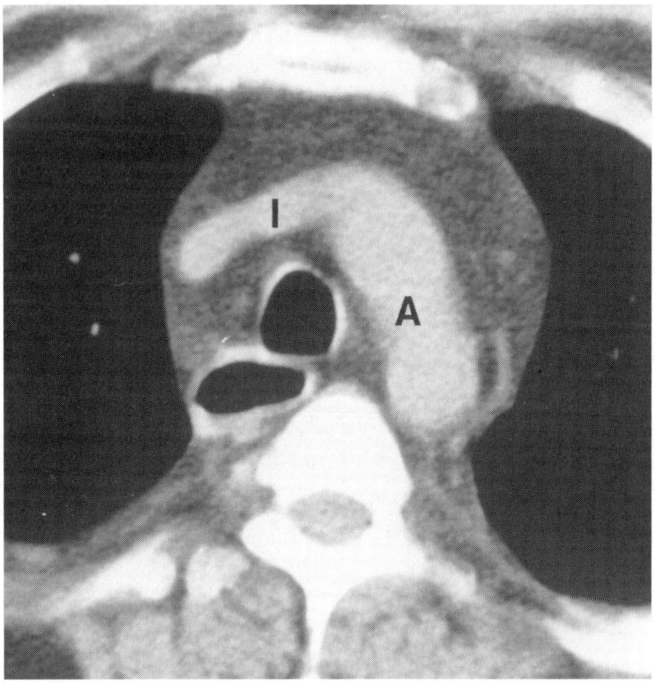

FIGURE 4.14 Fatty infiltration of the mediastinum. An asymptomatic patient with a widened mediastinum on routine chest radiograph. I, innominate vein; A, aortic arch.

Lymphoma

- **Malignant lymphomas** usually occur as solid tumors within lymph nodes, but they may involve extranodal sites. They are classified into **Hodgkin disease (HD) and non-Hodgkin lymphoma (NHL).** HD derives from an uncertain cell of origin. It has no sex predilection and has a bimodal age incidence (between 20 and 30 years or greater than 50 years). HD accounts for about 20 percent of all lymphomas. NHL derives from lymphocytes and is frequently seen in children after age 2, more commonly in males. While HD and NHL cannot be differentiated without tissue sampling, certain CT features may provide clues to the diagnosis. Involved lymph nodes are enlarged and show variable enhancement in both conditions.

4.5

ANTERIOR MEDIASTINAL MASS

Fat deposition—obesity, steroids, lipoma
Tumor
  Thyroid—goiter, adenoma, carcinoma
  Lymphoma—usually Hodgkin
  Thymic—thymoma, thymolipoma, thymic carcinoma, rebound hyperplasia, thymic cyst
  Germ cell neoplasm—teratoma, seminoma, choriocarcinoma
  Sternal metastasis or primary bone tumor
  Sarcoma
  Lymphangioma—cystic hygroma
Vascular—aortic aneurysm or pseudoaneurysm, tortuous vessels, coronary artery graft aneurysm
Fluid collection—hematoma, seroma, pericardial cyst, mediastinitis
Morgagni hernia

- **HD** involves the thorax in over 75 percent of patients, typically with anterior or superior mediastinal or hilar adenopathy. Cystic areas may be seen in newly diagnosed HD and calcifications may develop following treatment **(Fig. 4.15).** HD more commonly infiltrates the thymus and commonly involves multiple lymph node groups in the thorax. It spreads contiguously within the mediastinum and may be seen with pleural, pericardial, or chest wall invasion. Less than 10 percent of patients have lung involvement, but mediastinal adenopathy is invariably present.
- **NHL** involves the thorax in about 40 percent of patients and predominantly involves the middle mediastinum. Over 75 percent of cases of NHL have involvement outside of the mediastinum. A large posterior mediastinal or cardiophrenic lymph node may be the only site of NHL in the thorax. In children, NHL may involve the thymus. Pulmonary involvement is uncommon, and often occurs without mediastinal disease.

Thymus

- **The thymus** contains two lobes that are frequently asymmetrical (the left lobe is usually larger and extends more inferiorly). In younger patients, these triangular lobes may appear isointense to muscle on CT. With age, the thymus becomes replaced by fat, and only nodular or streaky densities can be seen in the anterior mediastinal fat in older individuals. In about 6 percent of patients, only one lobe is present. There are many anterior mediastinal masses that arise primarily from the thymus. CT is the method of choice in the evaluation of thymic abnormalities.
- **Thymic cysts** can be present anywhere along the developmental path of the thymus, from neck to mediastinum **(Fig. 4.16).** Congenital cysts represent persistence of the thymopharyngeal duct, whereas acquired cysts may be due to inflammation or neoplasia. Most patients with thymic cysts are asymptomatic. Simple cysts are primarily fluid-containing and do not have a sizable soft tissue component. This distinguishes them from cystic degeneration

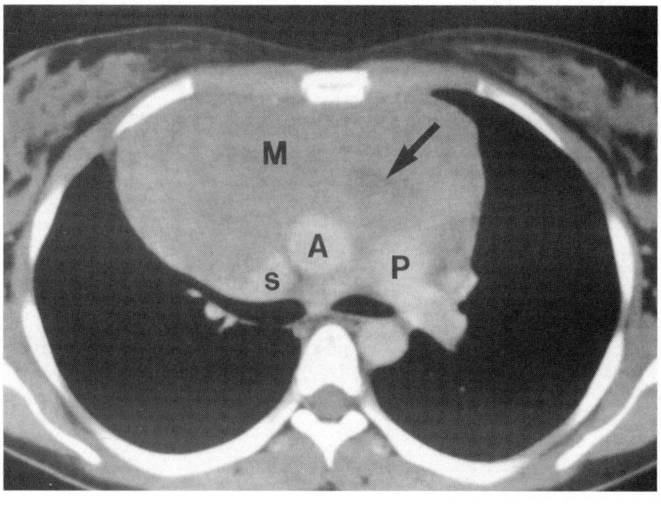

FIGURE 4.15 Hodgkin lymphoma. Very large anterior mediastinal mass (M) in a 23-year-old woman. Note the inhomogeneous enhancement and small area of necrosis *(arrow)*. s, superior vena cava; A, ascending aorta; P, pulmonary trunk.

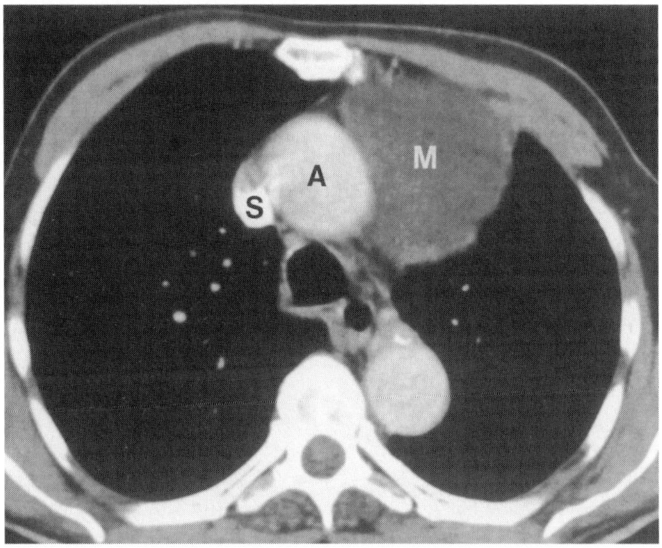

FIGURE 4.16 Thymic cyst. Large, low-attenuation anterior mediastinal mass (M) with no discernible wall or soft tissue component. A, ascending aorta; S, superior vena cava.

of a thymic malignancy, which usually has an associated soft tissue component. Thymic cysts may persist or enlarge after treatment for Hodgkin disease. Their presence does not reflect residual lymphoma. Hemorrhage into the cyst may increase the attenuation. Eventually, the hemorrhage may result in calcification of the thymic cyst wall.

- **Thymic hyperplasia** may be seen in up to 80 percent of patients with myasthenia gravis and may manifest on CT as simply a symmetrically enlarged thymus. Graves disease, Addison disease, and acromegaly are also associated with thymic hyperplasia.

- **Rebound thymic hyperplasia** refers to a period of thymic overgrowth that follows a period of thymic involution. After the period of stress, the thymus can enlarge, but it retains its arrowhead configuration. This condition is common in young patients after chemotherapy, particularly following treatment of Hodgkin disease. It may also be seen in the recovery period from severe illness or after treatment for Cushing disorder **(Fig. 4.17).** If history is supportive of prior chemotherapy, this condition may simply be followed. On occasion, gallium scintigraphy may be used to help differentiate atypical thymic rebound from recurrent lymphoma.

- **Thymomas** are traditionally thought of as anterior mediastinal masses, though they may occur anywhere in the mediastinum and occasionally in the neck. They represent the most common primary tumor of the anterior mediastinum and may be cystic, calcified, large, or small. The terms **invasive** and **noninvasive** are used to describe the behavior of the tumor (referring to whether the thymic capsule is invaded) as opposed to the histology, which is unrelated to prognosis. About 30 percent of thymomas are invasive. These spread by direct invasion, and distant metastases are very rare **(Fig. 4.18).** Gender incidence is equal for thymomas, and two-thirds present in the fifth and sixth decades of life. About half of these patients are asymptomatic, whereas others will present with symptoms of compression or invasion of mediastinal structures, including cough, chest pain, dysphagia, or dyspnea.

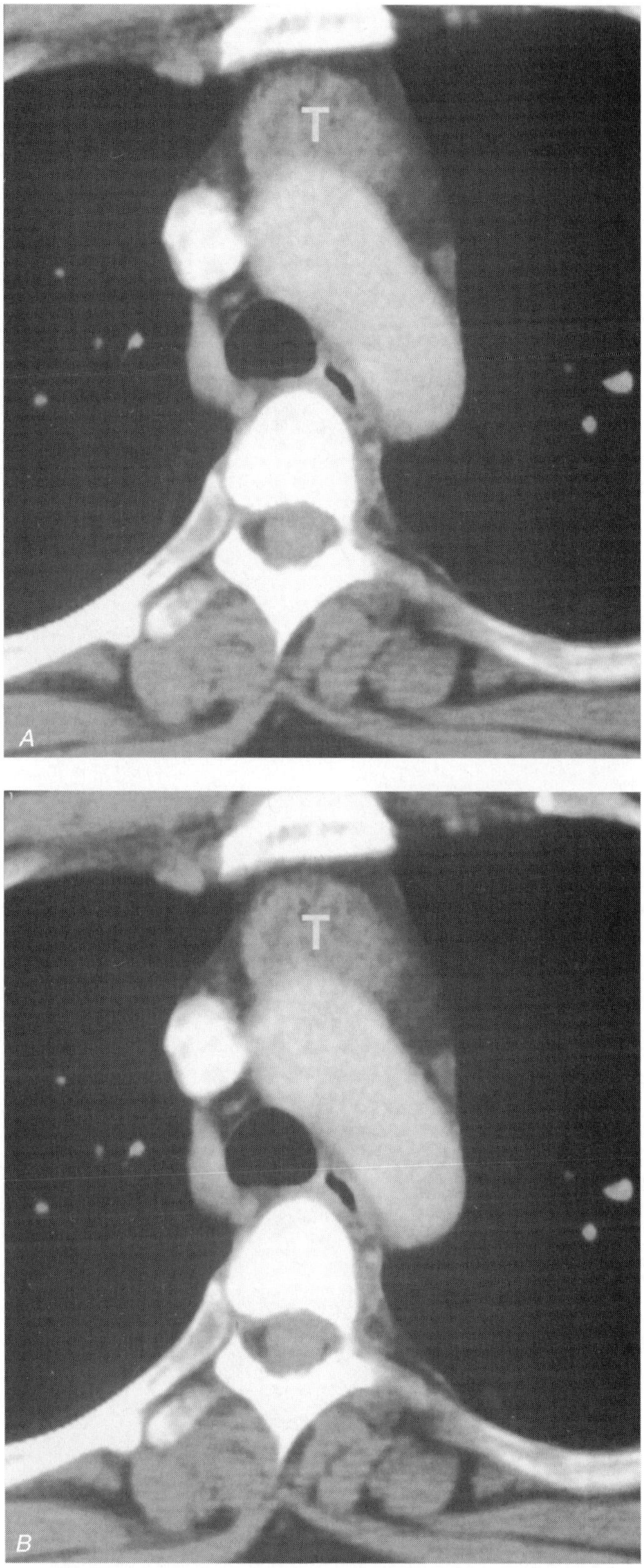

FIGURE 4.17 Rebound thymic hyperplasia. A 26-year-old with a prior history of sarcoma and leg amputation. *A*. CT immediately after chemotherapy treatment. Very small residual thymic tissue is present. *B*. CT performed 1 year later demonstrates interval enlargement of the thymus (T). Patient was disease-free at the time.

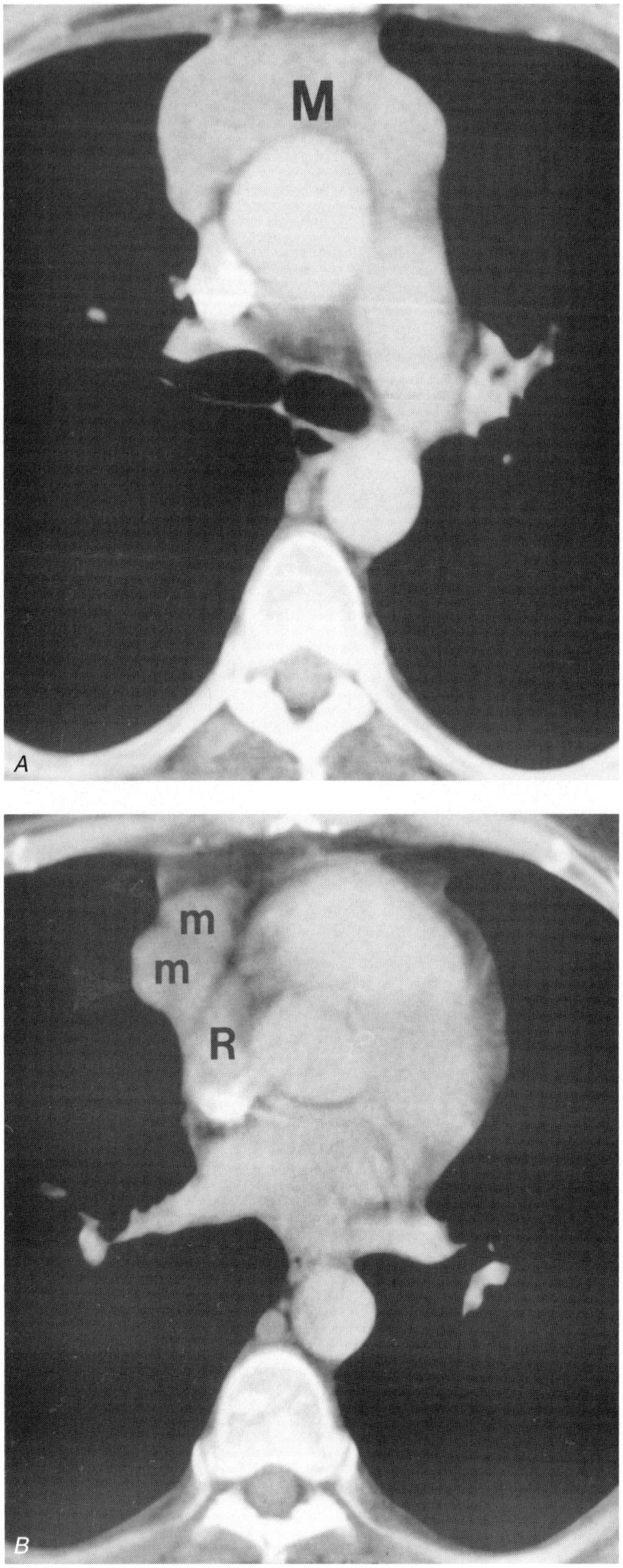

FIGURE 4.18 Invasive thymoma in a patient with myasthenia gravis. *A*. Bulging anterior mediastinal mass (M) occupying the thymic bed. *B*. CT scan at a lower level reveals tumoral mass (m) violating pericardium adjacent to the right atrial appendage (R).

In patients with myasthenia gravis, the size of the tumor is usually smaller, perhaps because a search for thymoma begins at an earlier age. Of all patients with thymomas, 40 percent have myasthenia gravis, while only 10 to 15 percent of patients with myasthenia gravis have thymomas. Even without a documented thymoma, thymectomy can bring some degree of symptomatic relief to the patient with myasthenia. The exact relationship of myasthenia gravis and these thymic tumors is not well understood.

Other conditions reported to have an association with thymoma include red cell aplasia, thyroid carcinoma, hypogammaglobulinemia (up to 10 percent may have thymomas), ulcerative colitis, and Crohn disease. The CT appearance of a noninvasive thymoma is that of a round, lobulated mass in the anterior mediastinum. No capsule is usually visualized. Mild, homogeneous enhancement is seen with noninvasive thymoma. Up to one-third of thymomas may have cyst formation or focal areas of hemorrhage. Invasive thymomas may present with heterogeneous enhancement. Pleural or pericardial implants may be seen. Absence of fat planes with the adjacent mediastinum does not necessarily indicate invasion.

- **Thymolipomas** are rare thymic masses that contain fat and septations made of involuting thymic tissue. Usually seen in young adults, they can be very large and are diagnosed by the presence of fat attenuation on CT and high signal on T1-weighted MRI. These masses are soft and may change shape when the patient changes position.

- **Thymic lymphoma** is common in patients with Hodgkin disease, especially the nodular sclerosing type. Enlargement can be asymmetrical and can include cystic components as well as calcification, which may develop after treatment **(Fig. 4.19).** Usually, they are seen in conjunction with lymphadenopathy elsewhere. In the younger patient, thymic lymphoma can look very similar to thymic rebound. Gallium scintigraphy may be helpful in this setting. Thymic lymphoma may be hard to differentiate from lymphocytic thymoma radiologically and histologically. Imaging features that favor lymphoma include invasion of the anterior chest wall and lymphadenopathy elsewhere. Pleural-based masses favor thymoma.

- **Thymic carcinoma** is a rare malignant neoplasm that arises from thymic epithelium. Unlike an invasive thymoma, the thymic carci-

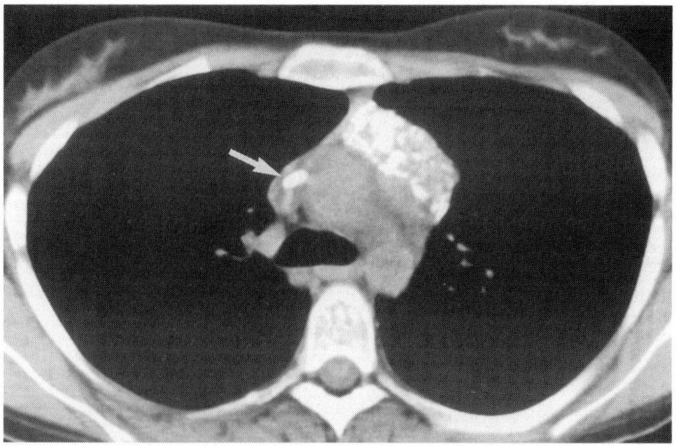

FIGURE 4.19 Calcified thymus following radiation therapy. Diffuse thymic calcification in a 19-year-old woman treated for Hodgkin lymphoma. Central venous catheter *(arrow)*.

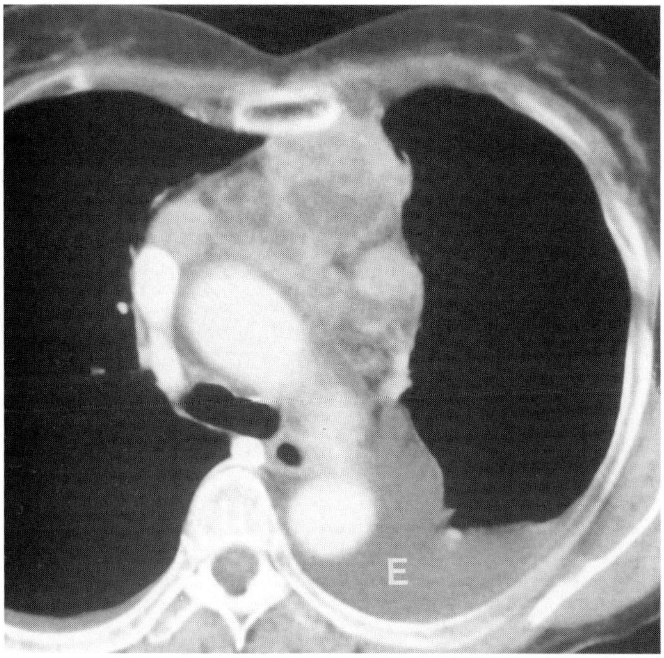

FIGURE 4.20 Mucoepidermoid thymic carcinoma. Contrast-enhanced CT in a 73-year-old patient demonstrating a large, heterogeneous mass in the anterior mediastinum. Note associated left pleural effusion (E).

noma is histologically more aggressive and more locally invasive. By CT, these two tumors may look very similar. Thymic carcinoma more often shows areas of calcification, cyst formation, or areas of necrosis **(Fig. 4.20).** Metastases may occur by hematogenous or lymphatic routes. Distant metastases and invasion of the adjacent mediastinum are indicative of a poor prognosis.

Other Anterior Mediastinal Masses

- **Germ-cell tumors** occur most often in the gonads; but when they are extragonadal, they occur most often in the midline. Usually found in the second through fourth decades, these are usually benign (mature teratoma) but can be malignant. They can arise from remnants of one or more primitive germ-cell layers (ectoderm, mesoderm, endoderm). Benign germ-cell tumors more commonly occur in women, while men usually present with malignant types. These are considered primary mediastinal germ-cell tumors if no gonadal or retroperitoneal mass is found.
- **Mature teratomas** are benign and do not invade the adjacent mediastinal structures. Found in young adults, the mature teratoma represents 75 percent of all mediastinal germ-cell tumors. They are usually multilocular and may contain areas of calcification, ossification, and soft tissue. Fat is found in about half of all cases **(Fig. 4.21).**
- **Seminomas** and **nonseminomatous germ-cell tumors** are malignant anterior mediastinal masses. Occurring more commonly in men than in women, these may metastasize to lung, pleura, or bone. On CT, these tend to be homogeneous and demonstrate uniform enhancement. They rarely calcify and low-attenuation areas are rare. Malignant germ-cell tumors may be indistinguishable on CT from invasive thymoma or lymphoma.

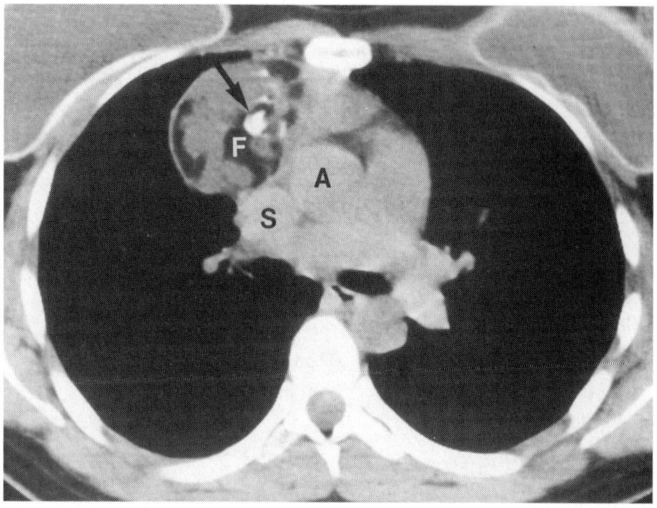

FIGURE 4.21 Mature teratoma. A 34-year-old woman with an anterior mediastinal mass detected on chest radiograph. CT shows a complex mass with characteristic fat (F), soft tissue, and calcified *(arrow)* components. S, superior vena cava; A, ascending aorta.

- **Ectopic parathyroid adenomas** can be seen in 20 percent of patients undergoing parathyroid resection surgery for hyperparathyroidism. Glands can frequently be located in the thymus and 80 percent occur within the anterior mediastinum. The size of the ectopic mass correlates with the degree of hypercalcemia. On CT, they are usually small, round masses that resemble lymph nodes.

4.6 MIDDLE MEDIASTINUM

- Most middle mediastinal processes, including masses, are associated with the trachea or lymph nodes **(Differential 4.6).**
- The **trachea** is a hollow, tubular structure that extends from the cricoid cartilage to the carina (located around T5) and is composed of 16 to 20 C-shaped cartilage rings with a posterior membrane. These rings may calcify with age, particularly in older females. Patients on warfarin therapy may show calcification at an earlier

4.6 MIDDLE MEDIASTINAL MASS

Vascular—aortic aneurysm, tortuous vessels, pulmonary artery enlargement, right-sided or double aortic arch, left superior vena cava, enlarged azygos vein, aberrant subclavian artery
Lymphadenopathy—lymphoma, bronchogenic carcinoma, leukemia, extrathoracic malignancy, reactive, silicosis, *Castleman disease*
Primary tumor—bronchogenic cancer, tracheal tumor, esophageal tumor, parathyroid adenoma, *angiosarcoma*
Cyst—bronchogenic or esophageal duplication, pericardial, pancreatic pseudocyst
Goiter
Fluid collection—hematoma, seroma, mediastinitis

4.7

TRACHEAL NARROWING

Extrinsic

- **Mediastinal mass—**thyroid mass (goiter), adenopathy (sarcoidosis, granulomatous disease), lymphoma, metastases (renal, lung, testicular), esophageal cancer, bronchogenic cyst
- Central bronchogenic cancer
- Fibrosis—radiation, fibrosing mediastinitis
- Saber-sheath trachea—advanced emphysema
- *Vascular ring*

Intrinsic

- **Trauma**—burn or chemical aspiration
- Cartilage deficiency—tracheomalacia, prior tracheostomy, trauma, radiation therapy, intubation injury, congenital
- Inflammation—croup, tuberculosis, fungus, epidermolysis bullosa
- Carcinoma—squamous cell, adenoid cystic, mucoepidermoid

With thickening

- Wegener granulomatosis
- Sarcoidosis
- *Infection*—tuberculosis, *Klebsiella rhinoscleromatis*
- *Relapsing polychondritis*
- *Tracheopathia osteochondroplastica*
- *Amyloidosis*

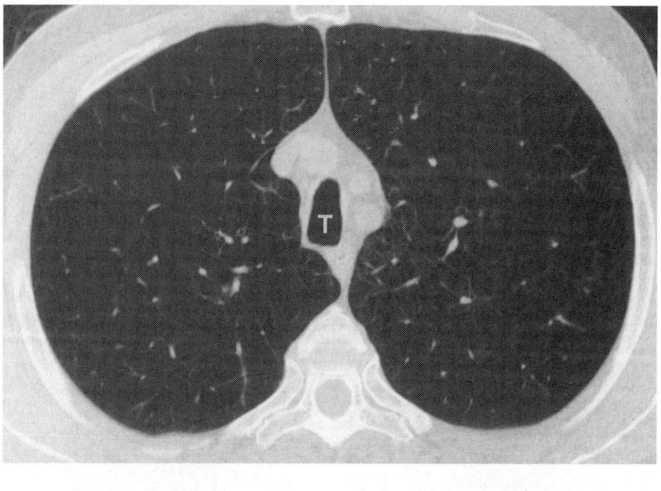

FIGURE 4.22 Saber-sheath trachea. Chest CT in a 69-year-old man with severe pulmonary emphysema shows advanced lung destruction and narrowed trachea (T) with an increased anteroposterior dimension.

age. **Tracheal narrowing** can be focal or diffuse, intrinsic or extrinsic; it may be associated with thickening of the wall **(Differential 4.7).**

- **Focal narrowing** can be iatrogenic, resulting from either prolonged intubation or tracheostomy insertion. Granulation tissue may narrow the airway near the insertion site of the tracheostomy. Complications from endotracheal tube insertion have decreased with the use of the high-volume, low-pressure cuffs. Extrinsic narrowing can be seen with goiters, adenopathy, esophageal cancer, or vascular compression.
- **Tracheomalacia** does not refer to tracheal narrowing; rather, there is increased compliance from cartilage destruction. Common causes include intrinsic and extrinsic tracheal compression that results in wall degeneration and collapse during expiration. The diagnosis can be made by fluoroscopy or CT. Imaging in inspiration and expiration may be necessary for better demonstration.
- **Diffuse narrowing** can result from a host of conditions. **Burn or chemical aspiration** can result in extensive tracheal narrowing secondary to inflammation and fibrosis. **Saber-sheath trachea** is usually seen in men with emphysema. It refers to the configuration of the trachea below the thoracic inlet. In this condition the trachea is normal in the neck but assumes a sheath-like configuration in the intrathoracic region, where it is narrower in the transverse dimension than in the anteroposterior dimension **(Fig. 4.22).**
- **Tracheopathia osteochondroplastica (TOP)** is a rare cause of tracheal narrowing seen in middle-aged patients presenting with cough and hemoptysis. The process primarily involves the trachea but can extend into the bronchi. Findings include thickening of tracheal cartilage with submucosal osteocartilaginous nodules **(Fig. 4.23).** Amyloidosis of the tracheobronchial tree involves the deposition of a protein-polysaccharide complex in the submucosa, which can narrow the lumen and cause wheezing or stridor. The CT appearance is similar to TOP **(Fig. 4.24).** Nodules of amyloid can be seen in the lung periphery and may calcify.

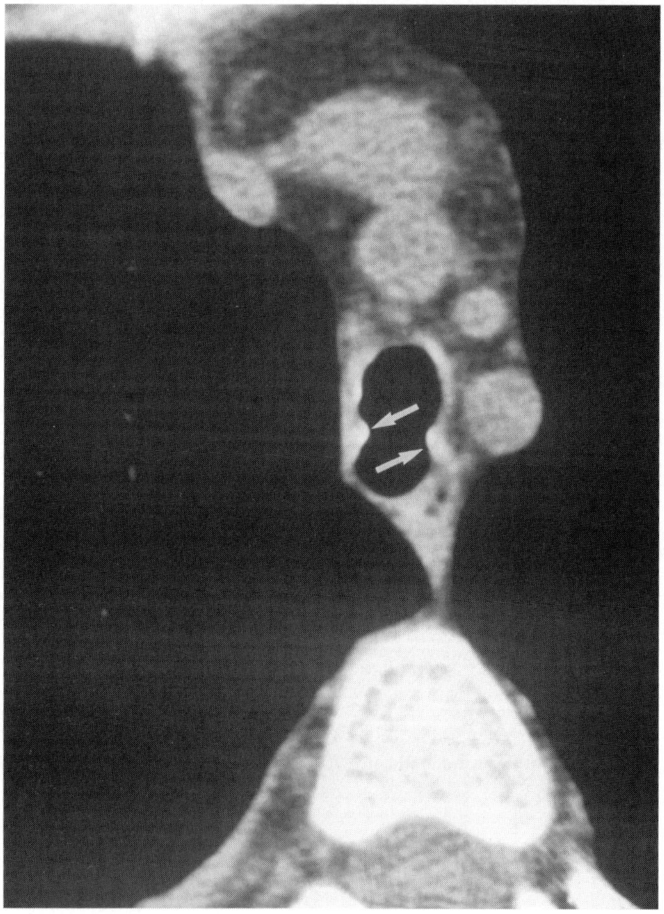

FIGURE 4.23 Tracheopathia osteochondroplastica (TOP). Chest CT shows nodular thickening and distortion of the trachea with submucosal calcifications *(arrows).*

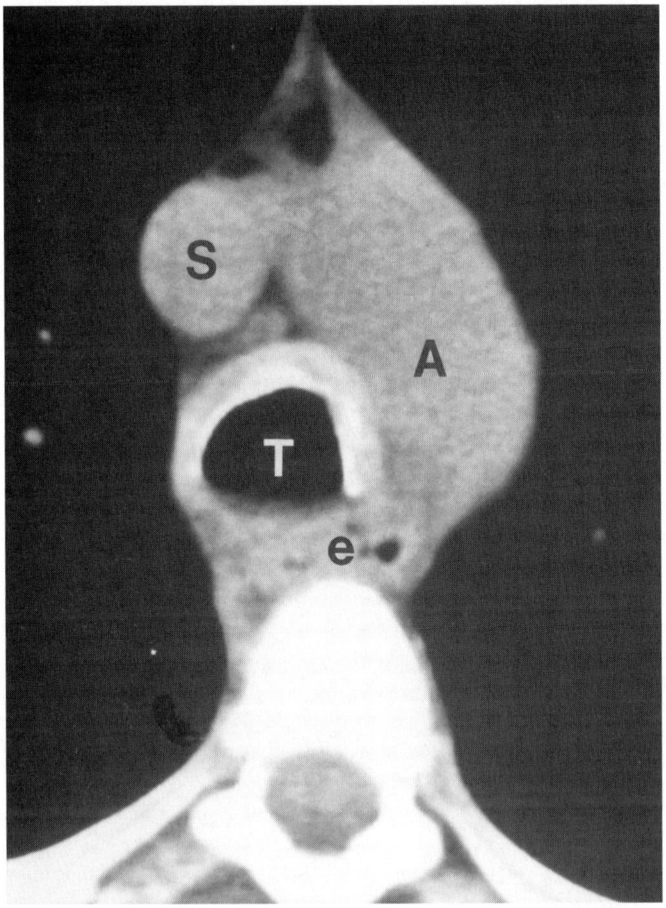

FIGURE 4.24 Amyloidosis. Note extensive thickening and calcification of the tracheal wall. T, trachea; A, aortic arch; S, superior vena cava; e, esophagus.

- **Relapsing polychondritis** narrows the airway in young and middle-aged adults by causing thickening and calcification of the tracheal cartilage. The lumen is usually quite deformed by the wall thickening and is prone to collapse. Although death associated with relapsing polychondritis is usually due to airway involvement, this condition may be associated with other findings, including aortitis and arthritis. Involvement of the ear and nose cartilage may result in floppy ears and a saddle-nose deformity.

- **Wegener granulomatosis** may demonstrate diffuse or focal tracheal narrowing with occasional cartilage distortion on CT. This condition is more commonly found in males and frequently involves the airway. It consists of acute necrotizing granulomas of the respiratory tract (both upper and lower), vasculitis, and glomerulonephritis.

- **Tracheomegaly** or tracheal widening may be acquired or congenital **(Differential 4.8).** The upper limit of normal for tracheal diameter is 26 mm in men and 23 mm in women. **Acquired tracheomegaly** may be due to chronic tracheal inflammation or adjacent pulmonary fibrosis with resultant traction on the trachea. Cystic fibrosis and idiopathic pulmonary fibrosis are two such conditions. They may result in acquired tracheomegaly that becomes more pronounced as the fibrosis progresses.

4.8

TRACHEAL ENLARGEMENT

Tracheomalacia
Adjacent pulmonary fibrosis
Cystic fibrosis
Tracheobronchomegaly—Mounier-Kuhn syndrome
Relapsing polychondritis
Uncommon—immunoglobulin deficiency, tracheocele

- **Congenital tracheobronchomegaly** or **Mounier-Kuhn syndrome** is a rare condition characterized by widening of the trachea and central bronchi **(Fig. 4.25).** It is associated with recurrent pulmonary infection and bronchiectasis. Patients may be asymptomatic or have chronic cough, hemoptysis, or dyspnea. The corrugated appearance seen on CT or conventional radiography represents atrophic mucosa prolapsing between the cartilage rings.

- **Tracheal tumors** are rare but may be seen on routine chest CT. In children, they are usually benign (hemangioma or papilloma) **(Fig. 4.26);** in adults, they are usually malignant (squamous cell or adenoid cystic carcinoma) **(Fig. 4.27).** Metastases to the trachea, either by direct invasion or by hematogenous spread from a distant primary, are more common than primary tracheal tumors **(Differential 4.9). Mucus** within the trachea may have a similar appearance to a tracheal tumor. If no tumor is suspected or if the patient has no symptoms of cough, stridor, or dyspnea, the patient can be asked to cough and be rescanned. On the rescan, the mucus will have changed configuration or will no longer be seen. Symptoms from tracheal tumors may have an insidious onset, since a large portion of the lumen must be compromised before symptoms become evident.

Hila

- The **pulmonary hila** are anatomic extensions of the middle mediastinum into the medial aspect of the lungs and are mainly composed of bronchi, pulmonary arteries, and veins as well as lymph nodes. The most common causes of bilateral hilar enlargement are

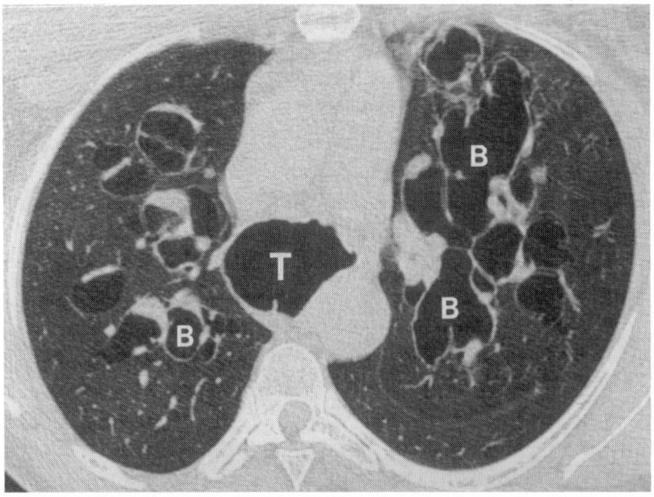

FIGURE 4.25 Mounier-Kuhn syndrome. CT at the level of the carina in a 50-year-old female demonstrating severe dilatation of the trachea (T) and central bronchi (B).

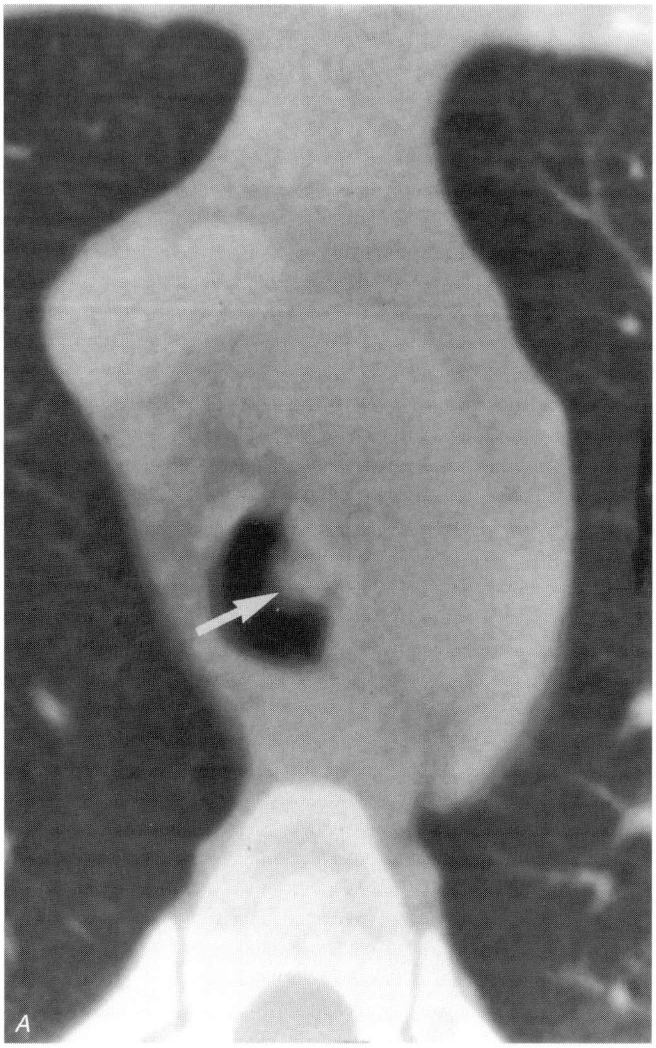

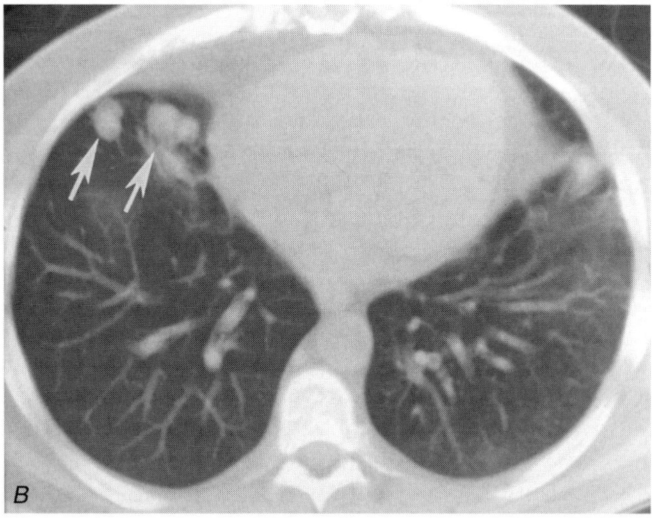

FIGURE 4.26 Tracheobronchial papillomatosis. A 35-year-old male with *(A)* a tracheal papilloma *(arrow)* as well as *(B)* multiple parenchymal papillomata in the right lung base *(arrows)*.

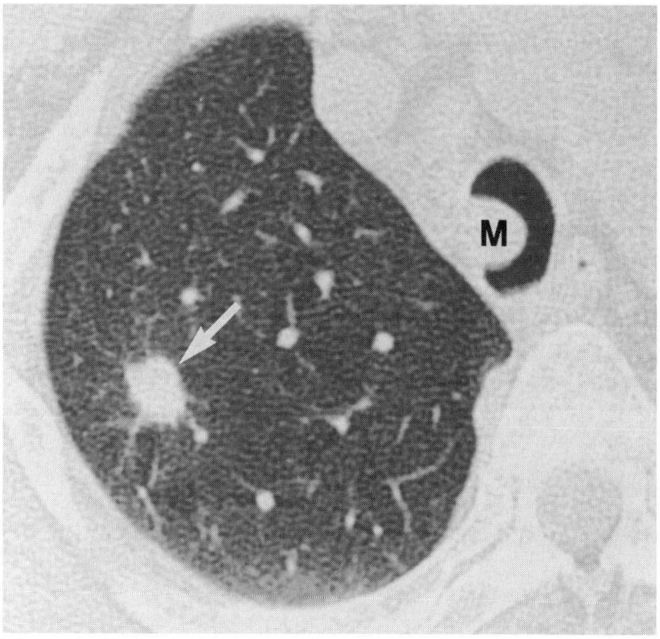

FIGURE 4.27 Mucoepidermoid carcinoma of the trachea. A 58-year-old man presenting with a tracheal soft tissue mass (M). Biopsy of the spiculated pulmonary nodule *(arrow)* revealed adenocarcinoma.

pulmonary artery hypertension and adenopathy **(Differential 4.10).** Unilateral hilar enlargement is most commonly due to tumor **(Differential 4.11).**

- **Vascular causes** of bilateral hilar enlargement include pulmonary arterial or venous hypertension, left-to-right shunts, and a normal variant in young patients. Unilateral vascular enlargement can be a result of pulmonary valvular stenosis (which results in preferential left hilar enlargement) **(see Fig. 5.15)** and surgical systemic-to–pulmonary artery shunts.
- **Hilar adenopathy** may result from inflammatory conditions such as tuberculosis, histoplasmosis, coccidiomycosis, and sarcoidosis **(see Fig. 4.4)** as well as bacterial or viral infections. Malignant diseases such as carcinomas; of the lung, head, and neck; renal and tes-

4.9

TRACHEAL OR ENDOBRONCHIAL MASS

Tumor
- **Bronchogenic carcinoma**
- **Adenoid cystic carcinoma**
- **Direct invasion**—esophageal, lung, thyroid cancer
- Carcinoid
- Mucoepidermoid carcinoma
- Endobronchial metastasis—renal cell, breast, melanoma, colon
- Benign tumor—pleomorphic adenoma, hemangioma, chondroma, fibroma
- Papilloma—most common laryngeal tumor in child
- Lymphoma

Mucus—asthma, allergic bronchopulmonary aspergillosis, congenital bronchial atresia

Foreign body

Broncholith

4.10

BILATERAL HILAR ENLARGEMENT

Pulmonary artery enlargement—pulmonary artery hypertension, normal variant, venous engorgement, left-to-right shunt, high-output heart disease
Adenopathy
- **Sarcoidosis**
- **Granulomatous—**tuberculosis, histoplasmosis, coccidiomycosis
- **Metastases—**lung, head and neck, renal, testicular
- Lymphoma or leukemia
- Reactive—bacterial, viral, AIDS
- *Cystic fibrosis*
- *Silicosis*
- *Castleman disease*

ticular carcinomas; and lymphoma and leukemia can frequently involve the hilar regions.

4.7 POSTERIOR MEDIASTINUM

- **Posterior mediastinal processes,** including masses, are frequently associated with the gastrointestinal or nervous system **(Differential 4.12).**
- The **esophagus** begins at the level of the cricopharyngeus muscle (usually about C4) and extends through the posterior mediastinum, exiting the thorax through its diaphragmatic hiatus, anterior to the aorta and to the left of midline. Unlike other portions of the gastrointestinal tract, the esophagus lacks a serosal covering and the proximal one-third is composed only of striated muscle.
- Sometimes the entire esophagus is dilated, occupying the majority of the posterior mediastinum **(Differential 4.13).** This is particularly true in **achalasia.** This condition results from decrease or absence of myenteric plexus ganglia in the distal esophagus, but the etiology is unknown. The lower esophageal sphincter fails to relax normally and food passage into the stomach is impaired. The esophagus dilates over time and can become quite massive. Patients usually present with dyspepsia, chest pain, dysphagia, frequent regurgitation, and aspiration pneumonia. The diagnosis of achalasia must be based on clinical history and other findings. An obstructing mass at the gastroesophageal junction or a stricture at this level may result in a dilated esophagus with a CT appearance similar to that of achalasia. In addition, patients with achalasia are predisposed to developing esophageal cancer.

4.11

UNILATERAL HILAR ENLARGEMENT

Primary tumor—bronchogenic, thymoma, germ cell, *lymphoma*
Adenopathy
- **Metastases—**lung, head and neck, renal, testicular
- **Granulomatous**
- Reactive
- *Sarcoidosis*
- *Castleman disease*

Pulmonary artery enlargement—pulmonary stenosis, surgical systemic-to-pulmonary shunt, *aneurysm*
Bronchogenic cyst

4.12

POSTERIOR MEDIASTINAL MASS

Hiatal hernia or gastric interposition
Neurogenic tumor—schwannoma, neurofibroma, neuroblastoma, ganglioneuroma, ganglioneuroblastoma, paraganglioma
Vascular—aortic aneurysm, enlarged azygos vein, paraesophageal varices
Paraspinal abscess
Primary tumor or metastasis involving spine or posterior ribs
Esophageal tumor, duplication cyst or diverticulum
Bochdalek hernia
Compression fracture—hematoma
Neuroenteric cyst
Extramedullary hematopoiesis
Pancreatic pseudocyst
Meningocele

- **Chagas disease,** which results from infection with *Trypanosoma cruzi,* may result in a condition similar to achalasia. In addition to the autonomic ganglia of the esophagus, Chagas disease may affect the ganglia of the duodenum, colon, and heart.
- **Hiatal hernias** may present as posterior or middle mediastinal masses **(see Fig. 3.25).** The diagnosis can frequently be made by plain film, especially when an air-fluid level is present. The vast majority of hiatal hernias are **sliding** hernias, in which the gastroesophageal junction is more cephalad than usual. A minority are **paraesophageal** hernias, in which the gastroesophageal junction retains its normal position below the diaphragm but the gastric cardia herniates through the hiatus. A very large hernia described as an **intrathoracic stomach** may require surgical repair due to the risk of volvulus.
- **Esophageal varices** may be seen by CT in the region of the gastroesophageal junction **(Fig. 4.28).** These may present as posterior mediastinal masses. Often, the patient is known to have a history of portal hypertension or superior vena cava thrombosis. These tubular structures enhance intensely with intravenous contrast on CT, allowing for the diagnosis to be readily made. Esophageal varices may be divided into uphill and downhill types. The former involve portosystemic collaterals that form in the setting of portal hypertension and are usually found near the gastroesophageal junction. The downhill varices usually appear more proximally and represent collaterals that form in the setting of superior vena cava occlusion.
- **Esophageal diverticulum** may be seen as a cystic structure on CT, similar to an esophageal duplication cyst. Unlike esophageal duplication cysts, esophageal diverticula do communicate with the esophageal lumen and are felt to be acquired. They may be classi-

4.13

DILATED ESOPHAGUS

Normal variant
Achalasia
Esophageal carcinoma
Scleroderma
Stricture—infection, inflammation, caustic ingestion
Gastric carcinoma—secondary achalasia
Vagotomy
Esophagitis
Amyloidosis
Chagas disease—Trypanosoma cruzi infection

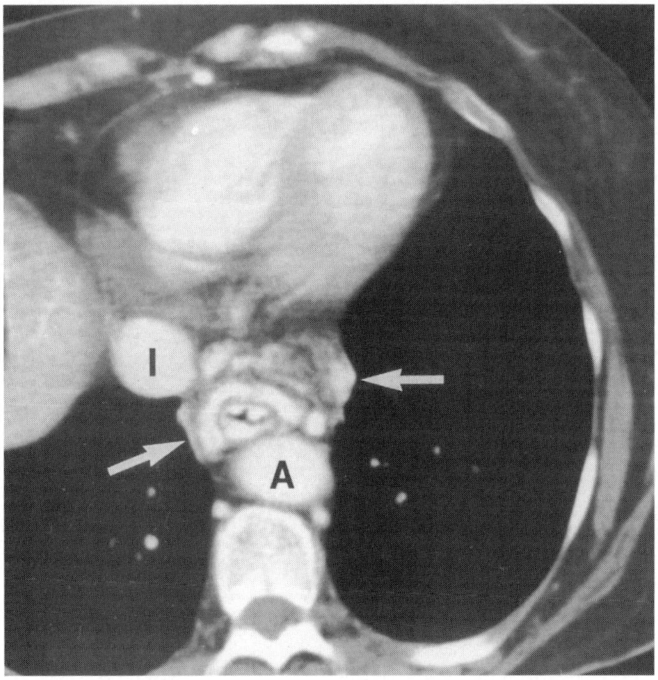

FIGURE 4.28 Esophageal varices. Note enlarged tortuous vessels *(arrow)* in a patient with cirrhotic liver disease. A, descending aorta; I, inferior vena cava.

fied into pulsion and traction types based on etiology of the diverticulum. **Zenker diverticulum** is a pharyngeal pulsion diverticulum at the level of the cricopharyngeus. The majority of esophageal diverticula are pulsion in nature and are most common in the middle and distal esophagus. Large distal (epiphrenic) diverticula are associated with symptomatic dysphagia due to dysmotility or mechanical obstruction from food trapping.

Esophageal Cancer

- **Esophageal carcinoma** can present as a posterior mediastinal mass and is often accompanied by lymphadenopathy or mediastinal spread. Esophageal carcinoma represents 1 percent of all gastrointestinal malignancies. It is a disease of older adults, more commonly affecting black males. Predisposing factors include lye strictures, Barrett esophagus, ethanol, smoking, tylosis, and tannins. The polypoid, ulcerated masses or annular, constricting masses seen on the esophagram usually manifest as areas of eccentric or circumferential thickening on CT **(Fig. 4.29).**

  Most esophageal carcinomas arise in the distal esophagus; they are adenocarcinomas arising in the columnar epithelium of a Barrett esophagus or represent direct extension of a gastric adenocarcinoma. Mid-esophageal cancers are more often squamous. Esophageal cancer may spread by direct extension to adjacent mediastinal structures; by lymphatic spread to mediastinal, cervical, or upper abdominal lymph nodes; or by hematogenous spread to lung or liver.

  CT is a sensitive indicator of metastatic disease to the liver and adjacent mediastinum. Visualization of an intact fat plane between the tumor and the aorta is necessary in order to exclude aortic invasion confidently. Routine staging of esophageal cancer (Table 4.1) by CT is not agreed to be useful, but its accuracy has been reported to be near 90 percent. There is a lower detection rate for tumors near the gastroesophageal junction. Sensitivity for the

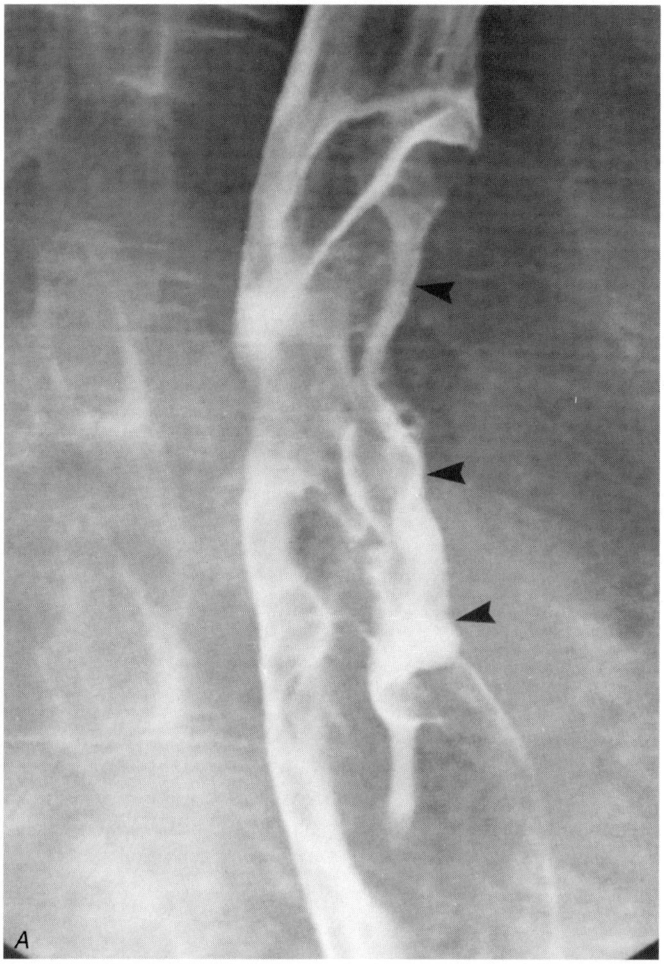

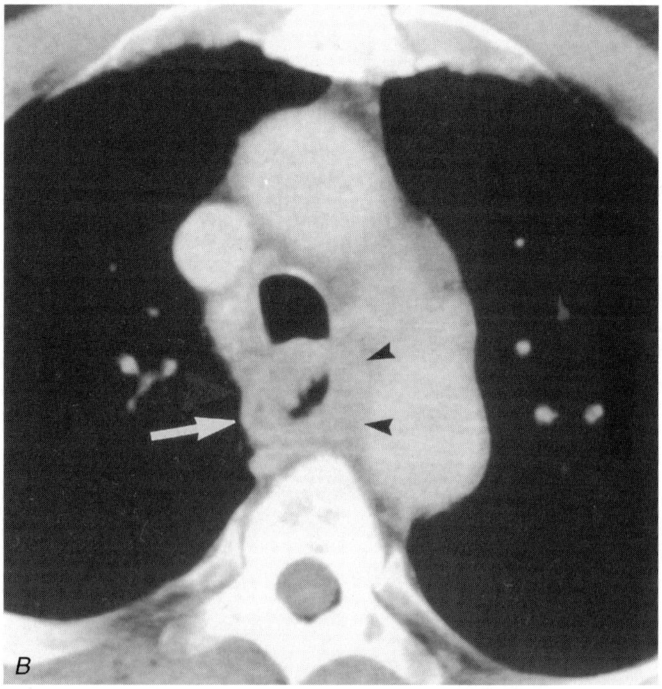

FIGURE 4.29 Esophageal cancer. Esophagram *(A)* and CT *(B)* from a 63-year-old with esophageal carcinoma showing a large fungating mass *(arrow, arrowheads).*

TABLE 4.1

CT STAGING OF ESOPHAGEAL CARCINOMA	
Stage I	Intraluminal mass or localized wall thickening (3–5 mm). No adenopathy.
Stage II	Greater than 5 mm of esophageal wall thickening. No adjacent or distant metastases.
Stage III	Wall thickening with direct extension into adjacent mediastinum. Lymphadenopathy may or may not be present.
Stage IV	Any stage with metastatic disease.

detection of lymph node involvement is reduced by the fact that normal-sized lymph nodes often contain tumor. Positron emission tomography (PET) is playing an increasing role in the detection of subtle metastases in liver and in normal-sized lymph nodes.

Benign esophageal tumors such as leiomyoma can have a similar CT appearance to esophageal carcinoma **(Fig. 4.30).**

Neurogenic Tumors

- Most posterior mediastinal masses are neurogenic **(Fig. 4.31).** They are divided into three groups based on tissue of origin: peripheral nerves, autonomic paraganglia, and sympathetic ganglia.
- **Schwannomas, neurofibromas,** and **malignant nerve-sheath tumors** arise from the peripheral nerves. Although the effect on adjacent structures can be helpful in their evaluation, differentiation of benign from malignant neurogenic tumors is not always possible on CT.
- **Schwannomas** or **neurilemmomas** are the most common peripheral nerve tumors. They are well encapsulated and do not involve the actual nerve fibers. Usually solitary and painless, they can go unnoticed unless they get large enough to have pressure effects. Schwannomas may enlarge intervertebral foramina if they involve the nerve roots. By CT, these well-defined masses can have areas of low attenuation and often enhance with iodinated contrast. Although present in other parts of the body, such as the head or neck, these tumors attain their largest size in the mediastinum. Once excised, schwannomas tend not to recur. Unlike neurofibromas (see below), they do not undergo malignant degeneration.

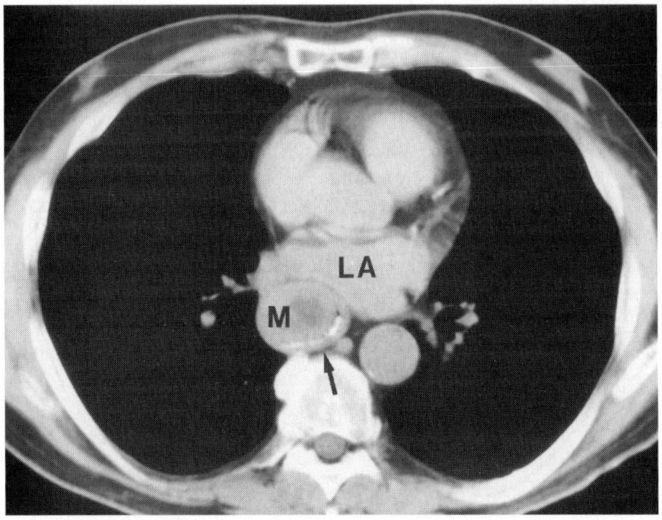

FIGURE 4.30 Leiomyoma. Contrast-enhanced CT showing a posterior mediastinal mass (M) indenting the posterior wall of the left atrium (LA). A small, eccentric crescent of oral contrast material is being displaced by the intramural mass.

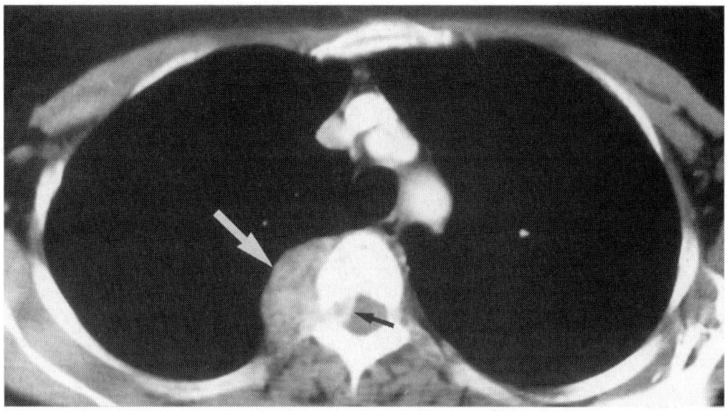

FIGURE 4.31 Neurogenic tumor. Contrast-enhanced CT at the level of the great vessels showing an enhancing paraspinal mass *(white arrow)* entering the spinal canal *(black arrow)* through the neural foramen.

- **Neurofibromas** as compared with schwannomas are usually seen in younger patients and can be single or multiple (neurofibromatosis). Unlike schwannomas, neurofibromas consist of masses composed of Schwann cells entangled with neurons and are unencapsulated. Dissection of the neurofibroma can be very difficult without damaging the accompanying nerve. Solitary neurofibromas have a similar prognostic significance to the solitary schwannoma. Multiple neurofibromas are more likely to undergo malignant degeneration and are more likely to recur. Approximately 30 percent of patients with neurofibromas have neurofibromatosis.
- **A malignant nerve-sheath tumor** is one of a variety of malignant tumors seen in the peripheral nerves of patients with and without neurofibromatosis. The earlier a neurofibroma appears, the more likely it is to undergo malignant degeneration. Patients with neurofibromatosis type I (von Recklinghausen disease) have a higher incidence of malignant nerve-sheath tumors. These tumors are highly aggressive and have a high recurrence rate. They have a similar appearance to their benign counterparts but can show destruction of adjacent tissues.
- **Paragangliomas** arise from the autonomic paraganglia cells, which normally function as chemoreceptors. When functional, these tumors may cause flushing or systemic hypertension. They are usually found in the adrenal gland (pheochromocytomas) or adjacent to the abdominal aorta. When they are in the thorax, functional paragangliomas are most frequently found in the posterior mediastinum or adjacent to the heart. They tend to enhance intensely on CT and are quite bright on T2-weighted MRI. Nonfunctional paragangliomas are known as **chemodectomas** and may be found near the aortic arch, in the aortopulmonary window, or near the right pulmonary artery.
- **Ganglioneuromas, ganglioneuroblastomas,** and **neuroblastomas** arise from the sympathetic ganglia. These ganglion-cell tumors are typically oriented more vertically, in the direction of the sympathetic chain, and frequently have a lenticular appearance.

- **Neuroblastomas** are highly malignant, undifferentiated tumors that arise from sympathetic ganglia in young children. Although Wilms tumor is more common than neuroblastoma in the abdomen, the high incidence of thoracic neuroblastoma explains why neuroblastoma is more common overall. **Ganglioneuroblastomas** are also considered malignant, but these have a better prognosis than neuroblastomas. They may have speckled calcifications on CT and are also seen in children. **Ganglioneuromas** are benign tumors of the sympathetic ganglia usually seen in teenagers and young adults.
- **Primitive neuroectodermal tumors (PNET)** are undifferentiated small round-cell sarcomas that mimic Ewing sarcoma radiologically, pathologically, and clinically. They may present anywhere in the soft tissues of the body, including the posterior mediastinum and chest wall (Askin tumor). Symptoms on presentation include dyspnea, cough, fever, and weight loss. Associated pleural effusions and rib destruction may be seen. Prognosis is poor and metastases are frequent.

Other Masses

- Not all posterior mediastinal masses arise from the nervous or gastrointestinal systems. **Extramedullary hematopoiesis** is a rare cause of a posterior mediastinal mass. It may be seen in patients with severe anemia and represents expansion of the erythropoietic tissue. In the thorax, it presents as lobulated paraspinal masses **(see Fig. 14.27)**.
- **Mediastinal abscess** may present in any mediastinal compartment. **Infection of the disk** (infectious spondylitis or **diskitis**) may present as a posterior mediastinal mass. Staphylococcal species are usually the offending organisms, though tuberculosis has classically been associated with this process. This disk-centered process is characterized by a paraspinal mass associated with vertebral endplate erosion and disk-space narrowing.

4.8 POSTOPERATIVE MEDIASTINUM

- The mediastinum may be affected by many different types of surgery. Coronary artery bypass grafting (CABG) has become well known by the configuration of mediastinal wires and surgical clips. Valvular surgeries also leave easily discernible metallic devices that have become well known and can easily be deduced from location.
- Surgical management for **gastroesophageal reflux** is indicated when medical management has failed or when esophagitis or pulmonary complications continue to progress in the setting of medical treatment. Antireflux procedures include open and laparoscopic techniques. A **Nissen fundoplication** is the most common and entails a 360-degree wrap of the gastric fundus around the distal esophagus. It has a 90 percent success rate in long-term control of reflux symptoms. **Minimally invasive antireflux surgery** refers to laparoscopic Nissen fundoplication. Potential complications include esophageal, gastric, or bowel perforation and distal esophageal ischemia. Potential side effects of fundoplication include dysphagia, bloating, and inability to belch.
- A **Belsey fundoplication** (Belsey Mark IV) is performed through a left thoracotomy and involves a 240- to 270-degree fundoplication. The procedure is a **Toupet** fundoplication if performed through the abdomen. Over 85 percent of patients have reduced symptoms with this procedure.
- The modified **Heller esophagomyotomy** for treatment of achalasia is performed through a left posterolateral thoracotomy. Complications include empyema, atelectasis, pneumonia, wound infection, and phlebitis. Gastroesophageal reflux develops in 5 percent of patients.
- **Esophagectomy** is the treatment of choice for esophageal cancer. Tumors that are unresectable or patients who are medically inoperable can be treated palliatively with stents, chemotherapy, or radiation. Postoperative radiation decreases local recurrence but does not improve survival. Five-year survival following complete resection is approximately 90 percent for stage I, 50 percent for stage II, and 20 percent for stage III disease.
- The technique for esophageal resection and replacement depends on tumor size and location and surgeon preference. Transhiatal esophagectomy and gastric replacement with a cervical anastomosis provides the best functional results for tumors in the distal third of the esophagus, small mobile tumors in the midesophagus, and Barrett esophagus with severe dysplasia or carcinoma in situ. It also works well for esophageal replacement in benign disease, such as chronic lye stricture, and motor disorders such as diffuse spasm, achalasia, and scleroderma.

  Complications include anastomotic leak, stricture, and recurrent laryngeal nerve palsy. One-quarter of patients have anastomotic leaks following transhiatal esophagectomy, although few of these are of clinical significance.

  Although the stomach is the preferred organ for esophageal replacement, the colon or jejunum can also be used. The left colon is preferred owing to its smaller diameter, more constant and reliable blood supply, and more adequate length for total esophageal replacement.
- An **Ivor-Lewis esophagectomy** is a partial esophagectomy and gastric interposition. In contrast to a transhiatal approach, in which the stomach is contained in the mediastinum, an Ivor-Lewis is performed via a right thoracotomy and leads to displacement of the stomach into the right chest.

Bibliography

Boiselle PM, Patz EF, Vining DJ, Weissleder R, Shepard J, McLoud T. Imaging of mediastinal lymph nodes: CT, MR, and FDG PET. *Radiographics* 1998;18:1061–1069.

Chandrasoma P, Taylor C. *Concise Pathology*, 2nd ed. Norwalk, CT: Appleton & Lange; 1995.

Lee JKT, Sagel SS, Stanley RJ, Heiken JP (eds.): *Computed Body Tomography with MRI Correlation*, 3rd ed. Philadelphia and New York: Lippincott-Raven; 1998.

Noh M, Fishman EK, Forastiere AA, Bliss DF, Calhoun PS. CT of the esophagus: Spectrum of disease with emphasis on esophageal carcinoma. *Radiographics* 1995;15:1113–1134.

Remy-Jardin M, Duyck P, Remy R, Petyt L, Wurtz A, Mensier E, Copin M, Riquet M. Hilar lymph nodes: Identification with spiral CT and histologic correlation. *Radiology* 1995;196:387–394.

Slone RM, Fisher AJ. *Pocket Guide to Body CT Differential Diagnosis*. New York: McGraw-Hill; 1999.

Slone RM, Gutierrez FR, Fisher AJ. *Thoracic Imaging: A Practical Approach*. New York: McGraw-Hill, 1999.

Tecce PM, Fishman EK, Kuhlman JE. CT evaluation of the anterior mediastinum: Spectrum of disease. *Radiographics* 1994;14:973–990.

Chapter 5

CARDIOVASCULAR CT

Fernando R. Gutierrez

5.1 Pericardium
5.2 Heart
5.3 Pulmonary Vessels
5.4 Aorta
5.5 Caval System
5.6 Cardiovascular Intervention and Surgery

5.1 PERICARDIUM

Anatomy and Function

- The **pericardium** is a two-layered sac enclosing the heart and proximal great vessels within the middle mediastinum. It is composed of an outer **fibrous pericardium** made of dense connective tissue that attaches to the diaphragm, sternum, and adventitial layer of the great arteries and an inner **serous pericardium.** The serous layer secretes pericardial fluid, an ultrafiltrate of plasma that allows the heart to move freely within the pericardium. The pericardial cavity is a completely collapsed sac lined by mesothelial cells. The monocellular serosa directly covering the heart is the visceral pericardium or epicardium.
- **Pericardial sinuses or recesses** are formed by pericardial reflections. The oblique sinus is the superior recess created around the pulmonary trunk and aorta posterior to the venae cavae and pulmonary veins. The transverse sinus is dorsal to the pulmonary trunk and aortic root. Variable amounts of fluid normally collect within these sinuses.
- The **arterial supply** to the pericardium is via small branches from the descending aorta and internal thoracic artery. The phrenic bundle—which includes the nerve, artery, and vein—courses through the anterior portion of the pericardium and is often visible on CT as a small enhancing dot. The phrenic and vagus nerves supply most of the pericardium. In many people, the left superior and inferior pulmonary veins join together to form a common trunk within the pericardium.
- Large amounts of **fat** can accumulate between the surface of the heart and the pericardial mesothelium, thus improving pericardial visualization on CT **(Fig. 5.1).** Epicardial fat is not necessarily related to total body fat but is increased in patients with coronary disease and those on corticosteroid therapy.
- The flexible pericardium, in combination with the normal serous fluid (15 to 35 mL), distributes the hydrostatic forces of cardiac contraction, gravity, and inertial forces. Intrapericardial pressure varies with pleural pressure during respiration and is usually slightly negative. The elasticity of the pericardium prevents intrapericardial pressure from rising with modest amounts of excess fluid **(pericardial reserve).** Chronic increases in pericardial fluid are therefore tolerated; however, acute increases can cause pressure elevation and tamponade.

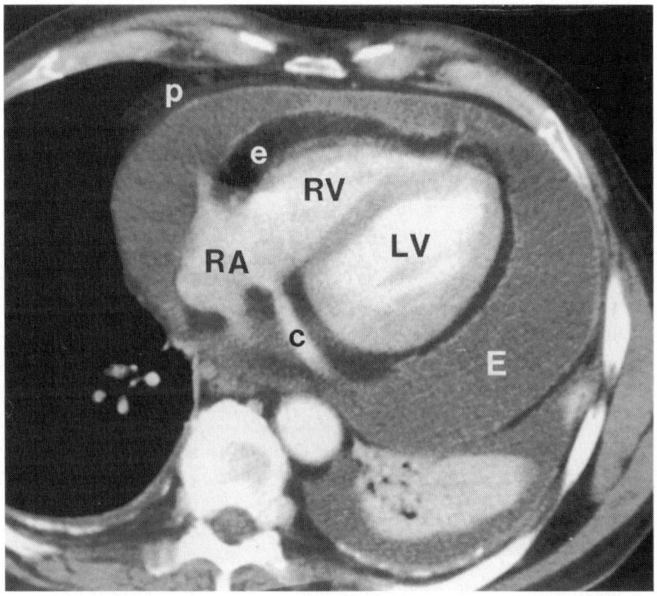

FIGURE 5.1 Large pericardial effusion (E). Note abundant epicardial fat (e), clearly delineating myocardial edge. Small pleural effusion and calcified pleural plaques are also present. p, pericardial fat; RV, right ventricle; LV, left ventricle; RA, right atrium; c, coronary sinus.

CT of the Pericardium

- **Echocardiography** is the noninvasive modality of choice for evaluating the pericardium, but it frequently becomes necessary to use other methods when sonography is limited by emphysema, thoracic deformities, or postoperative scarring. Computed tomography (CT), with its excellent spatial resolution and ability to differentiate fluid, soft tissue, and calcification, is well suited to assessing the integrity, thickness, and fluid content associated with pericardial disease. **Magnetic resonance imaging (MRI)** is preferred for assessing congenital anomalies, the myocardium, and flow dynamics.

- **Pericardial CT** should be performed with 3- to 5-mm collimation using spiral technique in suspended inspiration from the top of the aortic arch to just below the diaphragm. Intravenous contrast is not necessary but can be helpful in cases of pericarditis and for assessing the relationship of the great vessels and heart.
- The normal pericardium is depicted on CT as a thin (1 to 2 mm) curvilinear density best seen in front of the right ventricle and apex. While the cephalad extension of the pericardium is not readily observed except when distended by fluid, the caudal insertion of the normal pericardium is usually seen. Fat, coronary vessels, and myocardium are normally found beneath the visceral pericardium. The surrounding subpericardial fat serves to identify important anatomic landmarks, such as atrioventricular and interventricular grooves and coronary arteries.

Congenital Anomalies of the Pericardium

- Congenital anomalies are rare but more common than once thought. They include absence of the pericardium, pericardial cyst, diverticulum, and benign teratoma.
- **Congenital absence of the pericardium** can be total or partial (almost always left-sided), and can be associated with other congenital anomalies. Men are affected more often than women (3:1). Symptoms can include chest pain and, rarely, dyspnea. Herniation or entrapment of the heart is rare and occurs only with partial absence. On CT, absence of all or a portion of the fibrous layer of the parietal pericardium allows direct contact between the heart and lung. Lung can insinuate itself between the aorta and pulmonary artery. Absence of the preaortic pericardial recess, a structure normally seen in adults, is a specific finding.
- **Pericardial cysts** occur as a result of isolation of part of the pericardium during development. They appear as smooth, low-attenuation, unilocular cysts **(Fig. 5.2),** usually located in the right cardiophrenic angle. They do not communicate with the pericardial cavity. They can be of lymphangiomatous, bronchial, or teratomatous origin. They are usually asymptomatic but can rarely cause chest pain and arrhythmia, probably as a result of compression of adjacent structures. **Pericardial diverticula** are extremely rare. They contain all of the pericardial layers and communicate with the pericardial sac.

Acquired Pericardial Disease

- **Pericardial disease** can be primary but is more often secondary to a systemic process or prior therapy. Pericardial disease may be asymptomatic, present with gradual or sudden onset of symptoms, and can masquerade as cardiac disease, making clinical diagnosis difficult. The normal pericardium reacts to injury in three ways: fluid exudation, fibrin production, and cellular deposition. As a result, various degrees of effusion, thickening, adhesion, and calcification can be present.
- **Pericardial effusion** is an excess in the amount of pericardial fluid. Causes include inflammation, systemic fluid retention, bleeding, and infection. The fluid arises mainly from the visceral pericardium. Attenuation characteristics of the pericardial fluid can give an idea of the composition of the fluid (serous versus hemorrhagic). The fluid may be evenly distributed or loculated. Despite fluid sampling, one-third of pericardial effusions remain idiopathic in nature **(Differential 5.1).**

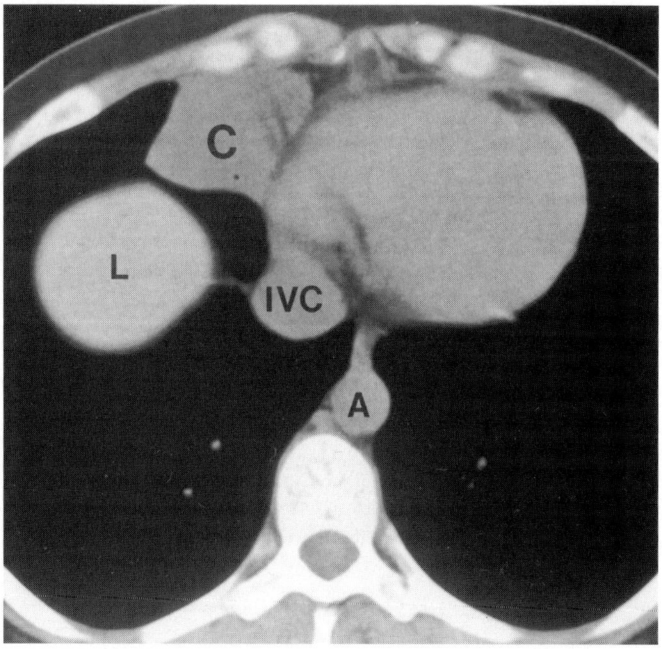

FIGURE 5.2 Pericardial cyst. Nonenhanced CT scan of an asymptomatic patient with a right cardiophrenic angle mass discovered on a chest radiograph. Note smooth, water-attenuation cyst (C). L, liver; IVC, inferior vena cava; A, descending aorta.

- **Pericardial thickening,** whether focal or diffuse, is evidence of inflammation. **Acute pericarditis** can result from a variety of causes and is usually not associated with a significant amount of fluid. Common causes include infections (viral, bacterial, tuberculous), systemic disorders (lupus), trauma, and malignancy. Pain, tachypnea, cough, dyspnea, and hiccups are common symptoms. A pericardial rub heard on auscultation is virtually pathognomonic of acute pericarditis. With intravenous contrast, enhancement of the pericardium can be appreciated on occasion **(Fig. 5.3).**
- **Constrictive pericarditis** results from scarring of the pericardium, which becomes thick and unyielding, thus restricting cardiac filling. Most cases are "idiopathic" in nature. Although constriction can occur on the heels of an acute process, the majority are subacute or chronic. Both CT and MRI are more specific than echocardiography in diagnosing constrictive pericarditis. The venae cavae—particularly the inferior vena cava (IVC)—are dilated compared with

5.1

PERICARDIAL EFFUSION

Idiopathic
Infectious pericarditis—tuberculosis, viral
Collagen vascular disease—lupus
Recent cardiac surgery—coronary bypass or valve replacement
Dressler syndrome
Uremia
Congestive heart failure
Tumor—metastases (lymphoma, breast, melanoma, carcinoid) or direct invasion (lung, cardiac tumors, thymoma)
Radiation therapy
Hemopericardium—aortic dissection, trauma, coagulopathy

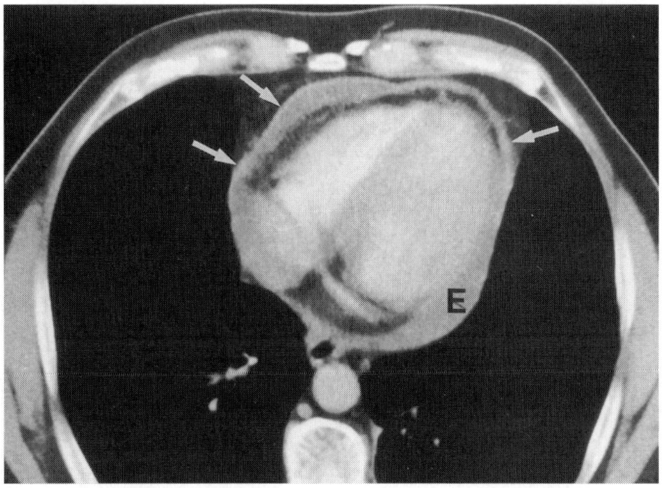

FIGURE 5.3 Acute pericarditis. Note contrast enhancement of the parietal pericardium *(arrows)* and small pericardial effusion (E).

the aorta and the ventricles are deformed and tube-like, whereas the atria enlarge **(Fig. 5.4).** The right ventricular wall and the interventricular septum can be deviated. The degree of pericardial thickening can vary greatly and be focal or generalized. Subtle degrees of pericardial thickening are frequent. Pericardial fibrosis can surround the caval orifices and atrioventricular grooves, thus producing a "tourniquet" effect by hampering diastolic filling. **Pericardial calcification** is a common finding but is not pathognomonic of pericardial constriction. Calcification establishes the presence of pericardial disease but not its hemodynamic significance. Pericardial thickening in association with IVC enlargement is a more reliable sign of constrictive physiology **(Fig. 5.5).** Other causes of cardiac calcification seen on CT are listed in **Differential 5.2**.

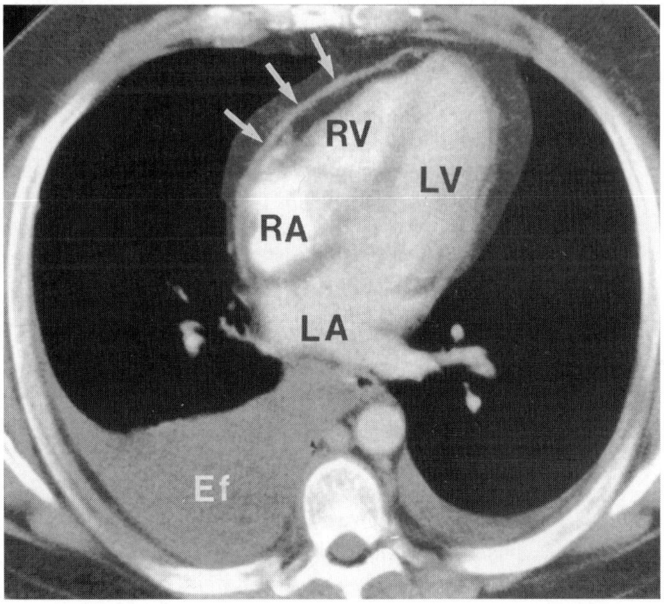

FIGURE 5.4 Constrictive pericarditis. A 42-year-old patient with clinical symptoms suggesting constrictive physiology. Thickened, enhancing pericardium is seen *(arrows)* associated with tube-like deformity of the ventricles. At a lower level, the inferior vena cava was enlarged. Note bilateral pleural effusions (Ef). RV, right ventricle; LV, left ventricle; RA, right atrium; LA, left atrium.

- It is important to differentiate constrictive pericarditis from **restrictive cardiomyopathy,** which is usually a result of amyloidosis; the pericardium is normal in such cases. Normal pericardium on CT in patients with symptoms, signs, and hemodynamic changes suggestive of constrictive pericarditis virtually excludes the presence of constrictive pericarditis. Restrictive cardiomyopathy can be diagnosed with endomyocardial biopsy. In rare cases, constrictive pericarditis can be so thin that it cannot be recognized as abnormal and requires open inspection for diagnosis.
- **Dressler syndrome** is a postcardiac injury syndrome, specifically following myocardial infarction. It is characterized by fever, chest pain, pneumonitis, high sedimentation rate, and pleural and pericardial inflammation. It can occur anywhere from weeks to months after the myocardial event. It occurs more commonly in patients with pericardial bleeding. The etiology is likely autoimmune, with development of cardiac antibodies during the latent period. The **postpericardiotomy syndrome** following surgery has similar characteristics and represents a form of the same entity. Pericardial and pleural effusions associated with focal pericardial thickening are the most frequent CT findings.
- **Radiation pericarditis** can be seen several months after therapy for lymphoma or breast, lung, or thyroid cancer. Any radiation port involving over 50 percent of the heart and over 25 Gy produces a definite risk. Echocardiography, CT, and MRI are frequently used in the diagnosis, usually demonstrating pericardial effusions, thickening, or constriction. Associated radiation-induced myocardial and mediastinal changes can complicate therapy.
- The pericardium is the most common site of **metastatic disease to the heart.** Noncardiac tumors can invade the pericardium directly or by hematogenous or retrograde lymphatic spread. Neoplastic in-

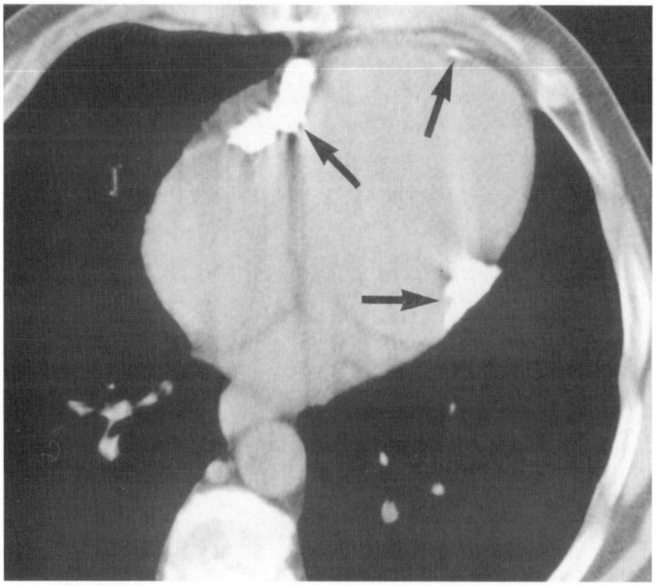

FIGURE 5.5 Calcific pericarditis. Note dense pericardial calcification *(arrows).*

5.2

CARDIAC CALCIFICATIONS

Coronary arteries
Aortic valve—bicuspid, rheumatic, endocarditis, atherosclerosis
Pericardium—prior viral or tuberculous pericarditis (often spares apex), rheumatic, syphilitic, asbestos
Mitral annulus
Mitral valve—rheumatic heart disease
Left atrium—mitral valve disease
Myocardium—aneurysm, old myocardial infarction (commonly involves cardiac apex) syphilis, trauma.
Ascending aorta—hyperlipoproteinemia, diabetes, syphilis, atherosclerotic
Left ventricular thrombus
Postoperative—right ventricular or septal patches
Ductus arteriosus—aortopulmonary window location
Left atrial myxoma

volvement of the pericardium is seen in up to one-fifth of patients on autopsy series, with breast and lung primarics accounting for about half the cases **(Fig. 5.6).** Pericardial involvement by leukemia, lymphoma, or melanoma is also relatively common. Pericardial effusion with or without pericardial thickening is the most common finding on CT. **Primary pericardial malignancies** are rare, with pericardial mesothelioma being the most common. This tumor often presents as a persistent pericardial effusion.

5.2 HEART

Anatomy

- The normal mediolateral dimension of the **left ventricle** (LV) is about 4.7 cm, while the right ventricle (RV) measures about 3.5 cm.

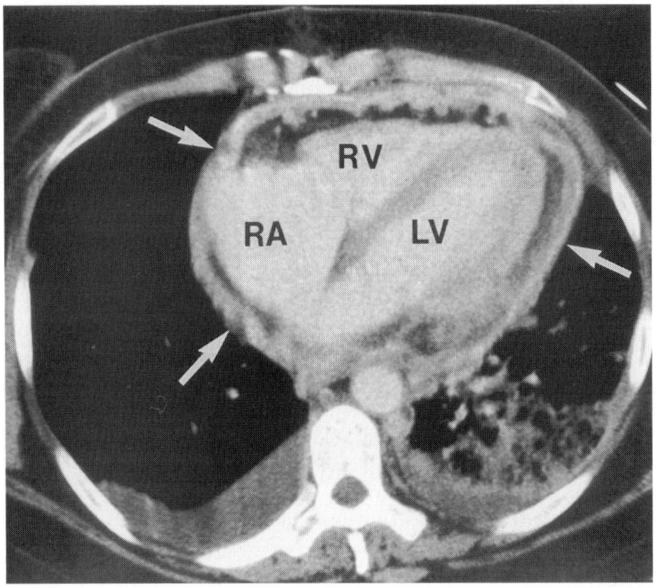

FIGURE 5.6 Pericardial metastases. Contrast-enhanced CT shows nodular, thickened, enhancing pericardium *(arrows).* RA, right atrium; RV, right ventricle; LV, left ventricle.

The tip of the LV forms most of the cardiac apex, and the RV, which is located behind the sternum, provides most of the anterior wall. Blood enters the LV from the left atrium via the mitral valve, which has two leaflets that prevent regurgitation into the left atrium during ventricular systole. The chordae tendineae extend from the papillary muscles inside the ventricle to the tips of the valve leaflets. The posterolateral papillary muscle can appear as a filling defect within the ventricular cavity on CT. Calcification can be seen in the papillary muscles or subchordal mitral valve area in patients with coronary atherosclerosis. The **RV** has a three-cusp atrioventricular valve (tricuspid valve) guarding the opening with the right atrium. The chordae tendineae attach the leaflets to the papillary muscles and **moderator band.**

CT Technique

- Even the fastest spiral CT scanners are too slow to properly assess ventricular dynamics; therefore, CT is limited to assessing cardiac anatomy rather than function. **Ultrafast,** cine, or electron-beam CT, however, can acquire an image in as little as 50 ms. Triggering image acquisition to the electrocardiogram can effectively freeze cardiac motion. This technique has been utilized to evaluate coronary bypass graft patency, left ventricular function, and coronary artery calcification.

Ischemic Heart Disease

- Ischemic heart disease is the most common cause of cardiac enlargement **(Differential 5.3),** but many potential etiologies exist. Ischemic heart disease remains the most common cause of death in the Western world. New methods of diagnosis and treatment are constantly being investigated. CT evaluation of ischemic heart disease has been rather limited, for the reasons noted above, but also because echocardiography and nuclear medicine studies have proven to be very effective.
- **Coronary artery calcification** has been utilized as a predictor of coronary disease based on the postmortem observation that the presence and quantity of calcium in the wall is related to the degree of coronary atherosclerosis. Substantial coronary calcification, calcification in the left main coronary artery, or the presence of calcium in younger patients has more importance than small amounts of calcium in the proximal left anterior descending or other branches in elderly patients **(Fig. 5.7).** Conventional CT is limited because of relatively slow scan times, motion artifacts, volume averaging, respiratory misregistration, and inability to accurately quantify the extent of calcification.

5.3

CARDIAC ENLARGEMENT

Cardiomyopathy—ischemic, viral, idiopathic, postpartum
Left ventricle—congestive heart failure, ischemic heart disease, high-output heart disease (anemia, sickle cell, fluid overload, AV fistula, polycythemia vera, pregnancy, thyrotoxicosis), valvular heart disease, coarctation, hypertension, congenital heart disease
Left atrium—mitral insufficiency, left-to-right shunts
Right ventricle—cor pulmonale, atrial septal defect, pulmonary or tricuspid insufficiency
Right atrium—RV failure, atrial septal defect, tricuspid insufficiency or stenosis, *congenital heart disease*

Key: AV; arteriovenous; RV, right ventricle.

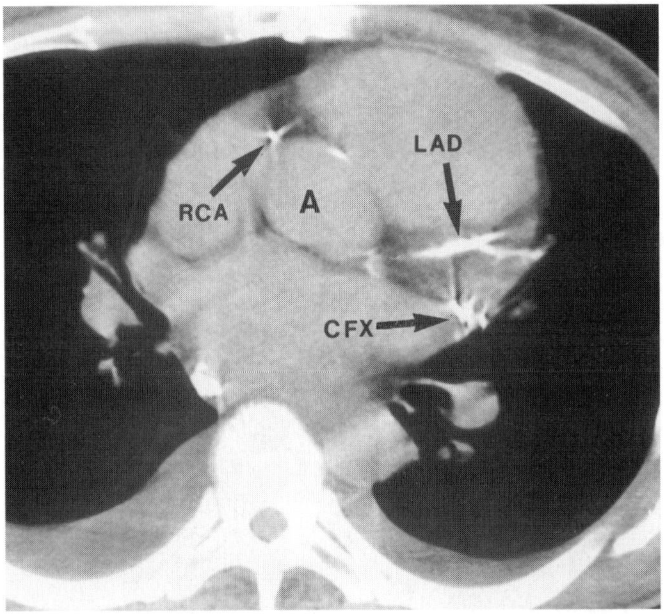

FIGURE 5.7 Three-vessel coronary artery calcification. Nonenhanced exam showing extensive intimal calcification in the left anterior descending (LAD), circumflex (CFX), and right coronary arteries (RCA) in this patient with history of angina pectoris. A, ascending aorta.

- Narrow collimation and rapid image acquisition are required to adequately determine the presence and extent of calcification. Ultrafast CT is very sensitive in detecting and quantifying coronary calcium. Spiral CT allows for faster acquisition of volumetric data than conventional CT, thus providing good sensitivity, although probably not to the same degree as ultrafast CT. New multirow detector CT, which effectively increases the scan volume and resolution, has a high sensitivity (90 to 100 percent) and specificity (about 70 percent). Because of the high prevalence of disease and occasional presence of calcification without an angiographic correlate, care must be taken in using calcium scoring for diagnosis or exclusion of disease until further studies are available.
- CT has been used to determine the **patency of coronary artery bypass grafts,** with varying success. Grafts to the left anterior descending and right coronary artery are better visualized than grafts to the circumflex artery **(Fig. 5.8).** Sequential scans obtained during opacification and clearance of intravenous contrast have been utilized to evaluate flow. Other abnormalities of coronary grafts can also be evaluated.
- **Coronary artery aneurysms** often calcify. Most are related to atherosclerosis, although they can rarely be congenital or a sequela of **Kawasaki disease.** In addition, coronary artery bypass grafts, particularly saphenous vein grafts, can, with time, become progressively ectatic and aneurysmal **(Fig. 5.9).**
- Sites of old myocardial infarction are demonstrated on CT as regions of wall thinning, making it possible to determine the extent of myocardial injury. Calcification may be seen. **Ventricular aneurysms** are depicted as areas of thinning and outpouching of the ventricular wall and represent a complication of myocardial infarction that is seen in about 10 percent of cases. Mural thrombus can be present within the aneurysm **(Fig. 5.10).** After myocardial infarction and open-heart surgery, mural thrombi develop within the LV cavity in up to one-third of patients.

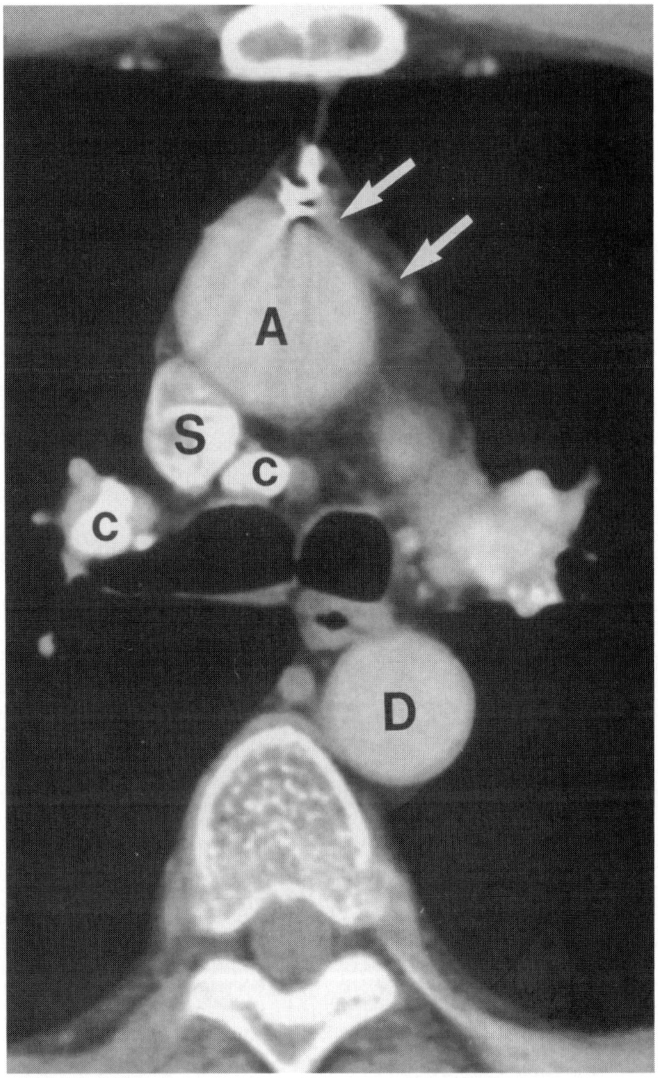

FIGURE 5.8 Coronary artery bypass surgery. Contrast-enhanced CT showing metallic artifact from several hemoclips and a patent saphenous vein graft *(arrows)* arising from the anterior surface of the aorta (A). Lower images demonstrated the anastomosis with the left anterior descending coronary artery. Note several calcified mediastinal lymph nodes (c) characteristic of old healed granulomatous disease. D, descending thoracic aorta; S, superior vena cava.

- CT can also help differentiate between true and false LV aneurysms. **False aneurysms**, which are contained myocardial ruptures, are usually located posteriorly or posterolaterally, have a narrow neck or ostium connecting the aneurysmal cavity with the ventricle, and tend to project beyond the ventricular contour. Ultrafast CT has been utilized to determine and quantify areas of regional contraction abnormalities. The presence and the site of regional contraction abnormalities defined by ultrafast CT had a greater than 90 percent correlation with wall motion abnormalities (demonstrated by left ventriculography) and critical coronary artery stenoses (shown by coronary arteriography).

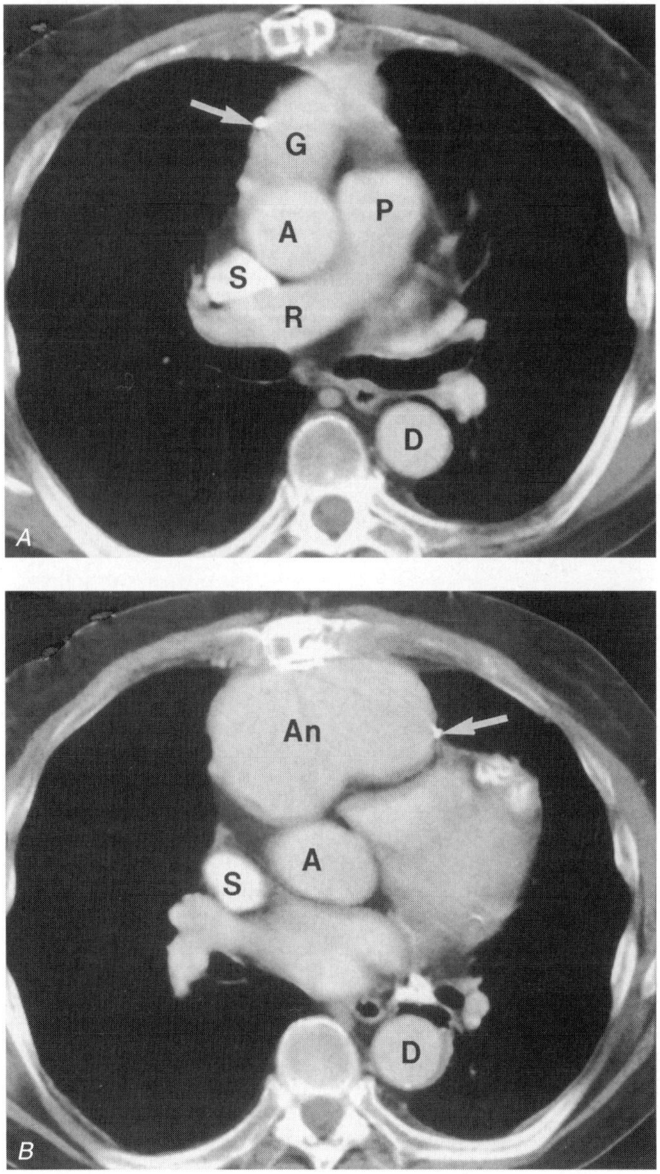

FIGURE 5.9 **Saphenous vein coronary graft aneurysm.** *A*. A large fusiform aneurysm of a right coronary artery graft (G) is seen as it arises from the anterior portion of the ascending aorta (A). *B*. The aneurysm (An) becomes very large at a lower level. Note displacement of the surgical clips *(arrow)*. P, pulmonary trunk; R, right pulmonary artery; S, superior vena cava; D, descending aorta.

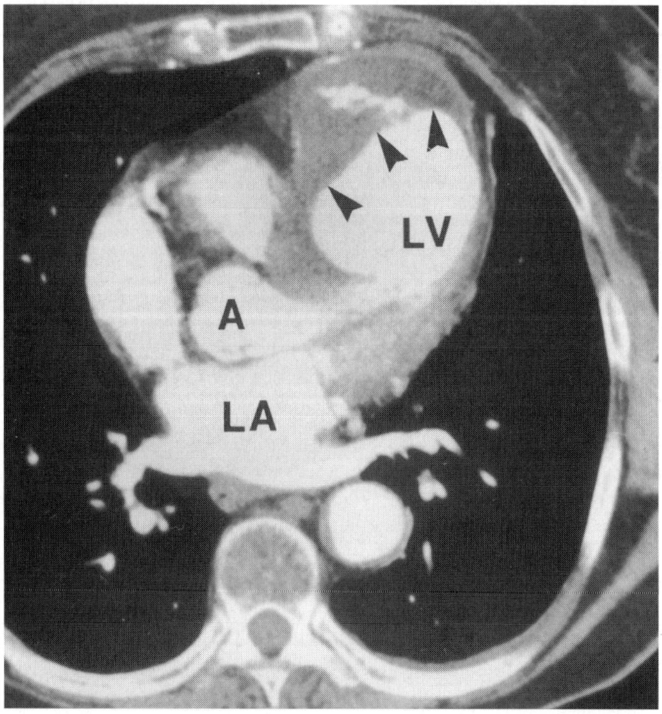

FIGURE 5.10 **Left ventricular aneurysm.** Large anteroseptal aneurysm demonstrating extensive mural thrombus *(arrowheads)* and calcification. A, aorta; LA, left atrium; LV, left ventricle.

Cardiac Neoplasms

- The most common cause for an intracardiac filling defect on CT, other than flow artifact or normal papillary muscle, is thrombus **(Differential 5.4).** Primary cardiac neoplasms are rare and most are benign. **Myxomas** account for about 50 percent of the total. They are generally located in the left atrium **(Fig. 5.11),** although the right atrium or right ventricle can be affected less frequently. They are usually seen as pedunculated intra-atrial masses attached to the atrial septum. **Lipomatous hypertrophy of the interatrial septum** represents nonencapsulated fatty tumefaction of the atrial septum **(Fig. 5.12).** This is usually a benign condition with no clinical consequences. In children, **rhabdomyoma** is the most common cardiac tumor, usually located in the RV or right atrium and generally associated with tuberous sclerosis. The most common primary malignant tumor of the heart is **angiosarcoma,** usually arising from the right atrial wall and rapidly extending into the adjacent pericardium **(Fig. 5.13). Metastatic tumors** of the heart are 40 times more common than primary malignant tumors; they frequently affect the pericardium first. Melanoma, lung cancer, breast carcinoma, and lymphoma are the most common. Intraluminal metastases, usually to the right side of the heart, can be seen with carcinoid tumor, hepatoma, and renal cell carcinoma.

Valvular Heart Disease

- **Aortic stenosis** is usually a consequence of degeneration of a bicuspid aortic valve, a condition seen in 2 percent of the population. Calcification of a bicuspid aortic valve is a common finding. In addition, because of systolic jetting across the valve, the proximal ascending aorta may show aneurysmal dilatation. Aortic valve

5.4

CARDIAC MASS

Bland thrombus—left atrium with atrial fibrillation or mitral valve disease; left ventricle within an aneurysm
Primary benign tumor—myxoma, lipomatous hypertrophy of the interatrial septa, rhabdomyoma, fibroma and fibromyxoma, hamartoma
Tumor emboli—renal cell carcinoma, hepatocellular carcinoma
Direct invasion—lymphoma, lung, esophagus, thymoma
Metastases—carcinoid, breast, melanoma, lymphoma, lung, osteosarcoma, chondrosarcoma
Primary malignant tumor—angiosarcoma

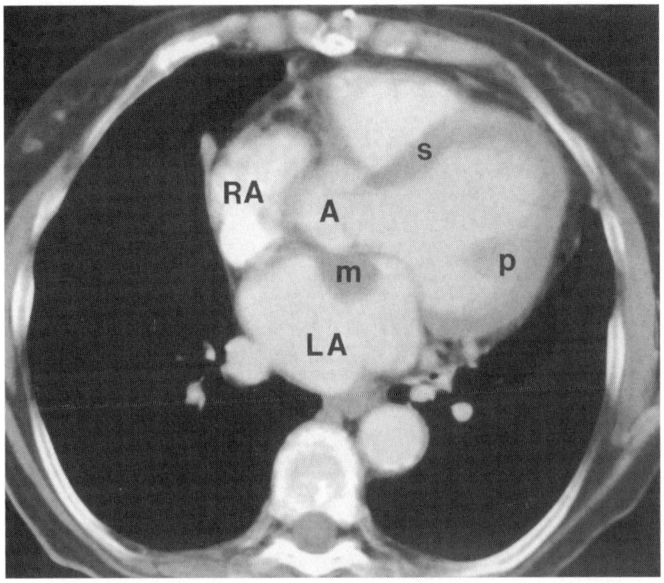

FIGURE 5.11 Left atrial myxoma. The tumor (m) in the left atrium (LA) was successfully resected several days later in this 76-year-old patient. Note the left ventricular filling defect created by a normal papillary muscle (p). A, aortic root; RA, right atrium; s, septum.

replacements show the characteristic metallic artifact in the location of the aortic valve.

- **Mitral valve disease** has become less common with the significant decrease in rheumatic fever in developed countries. Affected patients are usually elderly, with left atrial and RV enlargement. Small amounts of calcium may be seen in the mitral valve **(Fig. 5.14).** Calcification may also be present, within mural thrombus in the left atrium, particularly the appendage. Calcification of the mitral valve annulus is common but rarely clinically significant.
- **Pulmonary stenosis** is a congenital condition that results from commissural fusion. CT shows enlargement of the main and left pulmonary arteries as a result of poststenotic jetting across the valve **(Fig. 5.15).**
- **Tricuspid valve disease** is an uncommon and seldom significant entity that can be congenital or acquired. Most cases of tricuspid valve regurgitation are the result of elevated right-sided pressures from congestive heart failure. Early opacification of the inferior vena cava (IVC) and hepatic veins during the contrast bolus is indicative of tricuspid regurgitation. Another acquired cause of triscuspid valve disease is **carcinoid syndrome.** Carcinoid tumors secrete serotonin (5-hydroxytryptamine), which leads to fibrosis of the endocardium and right-sided valves. Since serotonin is rapidly metabolized in the lung, left-sided valves are rarely affected. CT can demonstrate hepatic lesions in association with evidence of tricuspid regurgitation **(Fig. 5-16).**

5.3 PULMONARY VESSELS

Anatomy

- The **pulmonary trunk** is a continuation of the RV outflow tract. It extends intrapericardially about 5 to 6 cm above the pulmonary valve before bifurcating into the right and left pulmonary arteries.

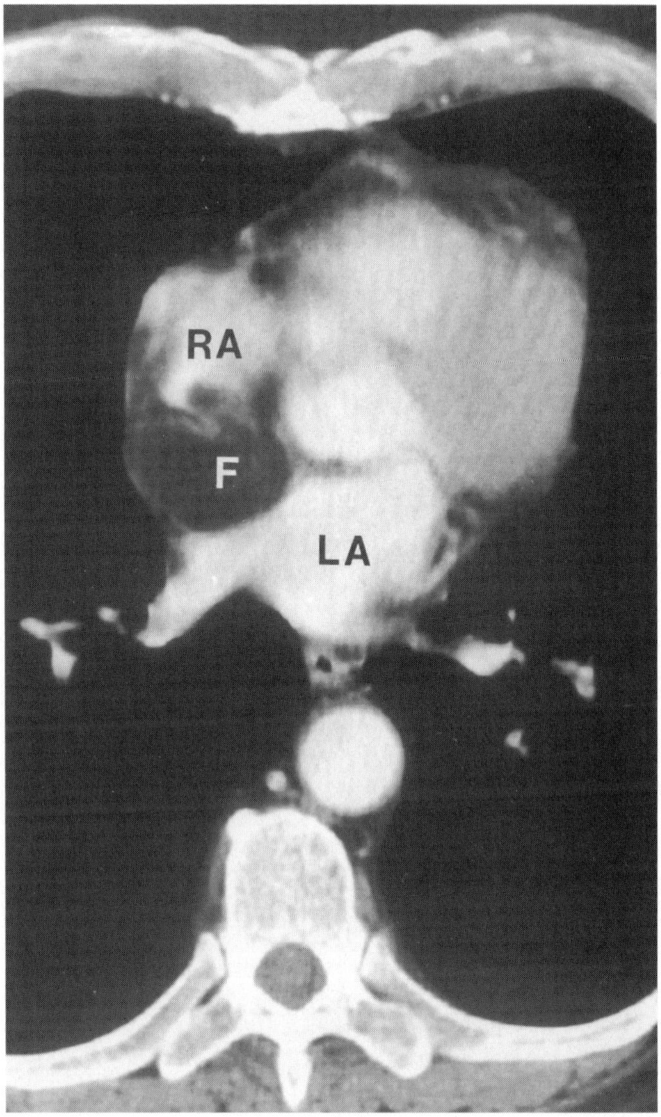

FIGURE 5.12 Lipomatous hypertrophy of the interatrial septum. Contrast-enhanced CT shows extensive fat deposition (F) within the interatrial septum between the right (RA) and left (LA) atria. (Figure courtesy of Matthew J. Fleishman, MD, Denver, CO.)

Normally, the pulmonary trunk measures about 3 cm in diameter and is slightly larger than the aorta in young adults, but it is the same size as or slightly smaller than the aorta in older patients. The **pulmonary arteries** divide into ascending and descending trunks and then lobar, segmental, and subsegmental branches. The left pulmonary artery arches above the left main bronchus, while the proximal right pulmonary artery courses in front of and slightly below the right main bronchus. The pulmonary arteries have approximately 17 divisions from the hilar region to the lung periphery and usually accompany the corresponding bronchi.

- **Pulmonary veins** are usually located in the periphery of the lobules and segments, whereas the arteries and bronchi have a central distribution within these same units. There are usually two major pulmonary veins on each side. The right upper and middle lobe veins join together to form the right superior pulmonary vein. The left upper lobe vein and lower lobe veins drain their respective lobes.

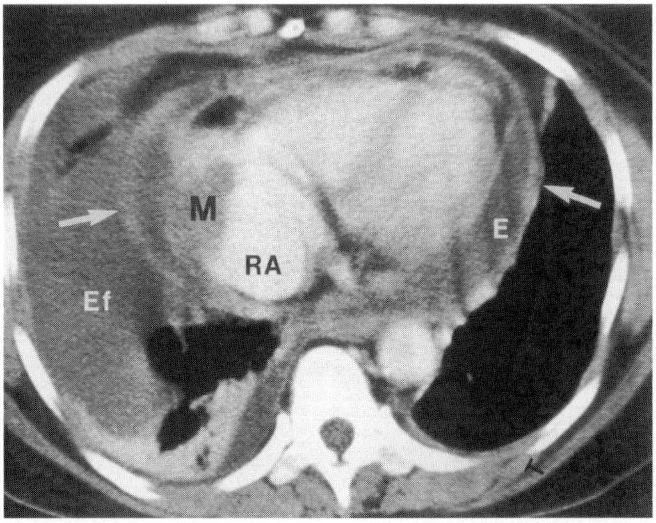

FIGURE 5.13 Angiosarcoma. Mass (M) in the right atrium (RA) invading the pericardium and right pleural space, causing a malignant pericardial effusion (E) with pericardial thickening *(arrows)* and a malignant pleural effusion (Ef). (From Slone RM, Gutierrez FR, Fisher AJ. *Thoracic Imaging: A Practical Approach.* New York: McGraw-Hill; 1999. With permission.)

- **Congenital anomalies** of the pulmonary arteries and veins are variable and can be isolated or associated with other defects. **Pulmonary artery sling** embryologically results from inadequacy of the proximal portion of the left sixth branchial arch. As a consequence, the left

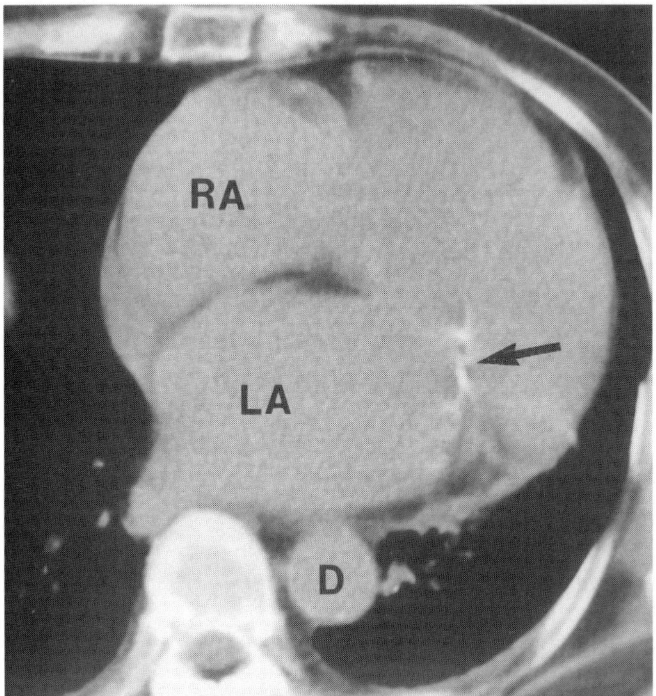

FIGURE 5.14 Mitral stenosis. Noncontrast CT shows enlargement of the left atrium (LA) and calcification of the mitral valve leaflets *(arrow)*. RA, right atrium; D, descending aorta.

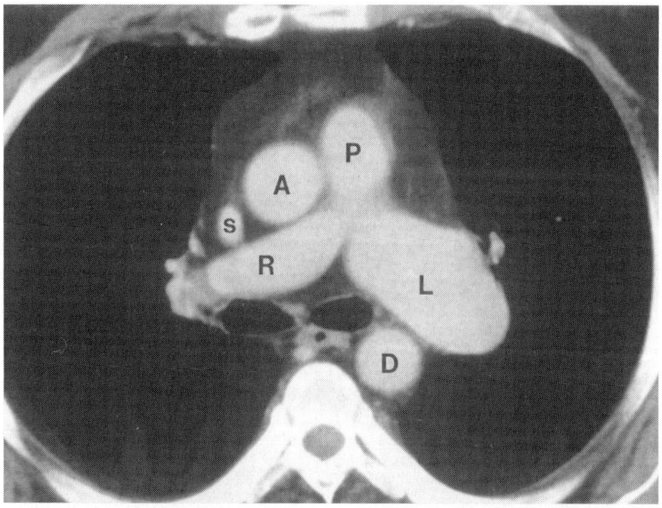

FIGURE 5.15 Pulmonary stenosis. Contrast-enhanced CT in a patient with pulmonary stenosis showing characteristic unilateral enlargement of the left pulmonary artery (L) but a normal-sized right pulmonary artery (R). P, pulmonary trunk; A, ascending aorta; S, superior vena cava; D, descending thoracic aorta.

pulmonary artery arises from the proximal right pulmonary artery and courses between the trachea and esophagus. **Pulmonary artery agenesis** can be isolated or associated with more complex syndromes such as tetralogy of Fallot. There is ipsilateral volume loss and shifting of the mediastinum. Enlarged collateral vessels are common. It is important to distinguish congenital from acquired causes such as a sequela from fibrosing mediastinitis, pulmonary thromboembolism, or postsurgical scarring. **Pulmonary artery hypoplasia** can be seen in the hypogenetic lung syndrome or scimitar syndrome (partial anomalous pulmonary venous return), unilateral hyperlucent lung, chronic pulmonary thromboembolism, and postoperative scarring.

- Pulmonary artery enlargement is most commonly the result of pulmonary artery hypertension, but other less common causes exist **(Differential 5.5).** In almost all cases, there is enlargement of the pulmonary trunk and both pulmonary arteries. Primary pulmonary hypertension occurs in young women and is idiopathic. Isolated left pulmonary artery enlargement can be seen as a result of the poststenotic jet in patients with pulmonary stenosis **(Fig. 5.15).**

5.5

ENLARGED PULMONARY ARTERIES

Pulmonary artery hypertension—severe lung disease (fibrosis, emphysema, pneumoconiosis, sarcoidosis), vasculitis, emboli (blood, tumor, fat), primary, Eisenmenger

Left-to-right shunt—ASD, VSD, PDA, endocardial cushion defect, anomalous pulmonary venous return

Pulmonary venous hypertension—CHF, fluid overload, renal failure, LA obstruction, constrictive pericarditis, mitral insufficiency or stenosis, TAPVR below the diaphragm

High-output heart disease—anemia, sickle cell, AV fistulas, polycythemia vera, pregnancy, thyrotoxicosis

Pulmonary valve stenosis—enlarged main and left PA, normal right

Behçet disease

Key: ASD, atrial septal defect; VSD, ventricular septal defect; PDA, patent ductus arteriosus; CHF, congestive heart failure; LA, left atrium; TAPVR, total anomalous pulmonary venous return; AV, arteriovenous; PA, pulmonary artery.

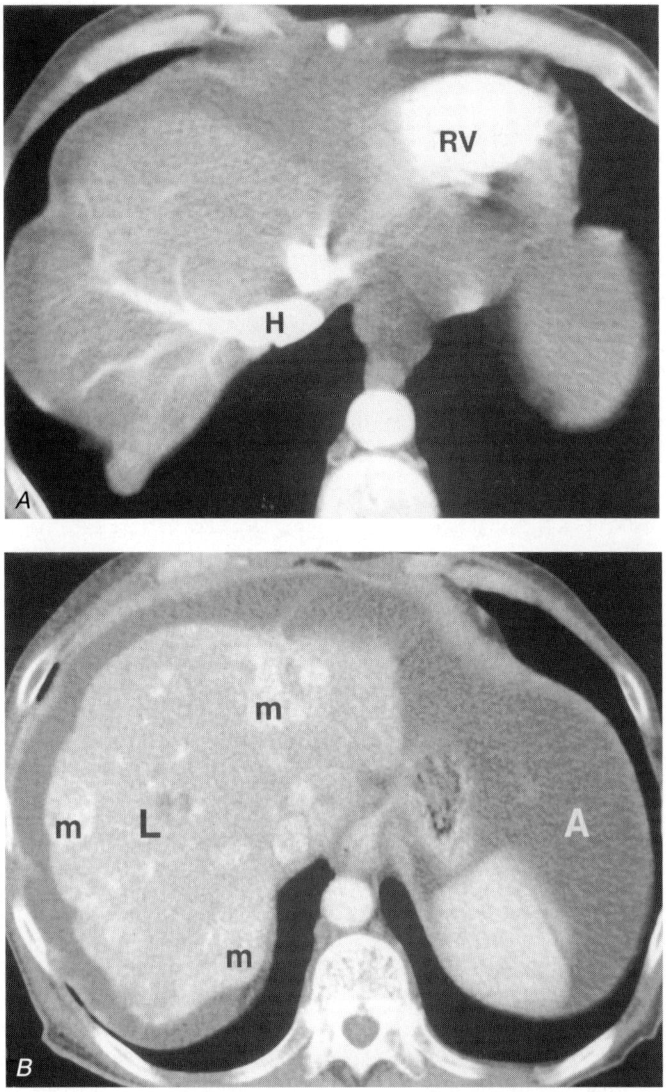

FIGURE 5.16 Carcinoid syndrome. *A*. Contrast-enhanced CT shows early opacification of the hepatic veins (H), implying tricuspid insufficiency. RV, right ventricle. *B*. Multiple high-attenuation metastases (m) are seen in the liver (L), which is also small and lobulated. A, ascites.

Eisenmenger syndrome results from a right-to-left cardiac shunt that ultimately can produce right heart failure from increasing pulmonary vascular resistance. The underlying cause of the shunt can be a septal defect, ventricular septal defect, or patent ductus arteriosus. Findings of pulmonary artery hypertension are present, with enlargement of the right heart, pulmonary trunk, and central pulmonary arteries and pruning of peripheral vessels.

Pulmonary Thromboembolism

- Deep venous thrombosis leading to pulmonary thromboembolism (PE) accounts for approximately 50,000 deaths per year in the United States, remaining undiagnosed in the majority of cases because of difficulties with clinical recognition. Recently, contrast-enhanced spiral CT has been effectively utilized in the diagnosis of PE, resulting in a reevaluation of the traditional diagnostic algorithm of clinical, scintigraphic, venographic, and angiographic criteria. Meticulous technique is required in patient selection, bolus delivery, data acquisition, image display, and observer experience in order to obtain optimal results. Breathing artifacts and suboptimal contrast enhancement are the usual causes of image degradation and diagnostic pitfalls.
- **Technique:** Scanning should start at the diaphragm and extend cephalad to the aortic arch. An optimal study requires suspended inspiration, although shallow respiration is tolerable in patients unable to hold their breath. A 5-mm **collimation** with a 3- to 4-mm reconstruction interval is adequate for visualizing the central and early-order arterial branches, but 3-mm sections at 2-mm reconstruction intervals are preferred to visualize subsegmental branches. A pitch of 1.5 to 2.0 allows maximum coverage while returning good resolution. A rapid bolus of **intravenous contrast** to produce peak enhancement of the pulmonary arteries is required. Typically, a flow rate of 3 mL/s and a total volume of 100 to 150 mL is used. The appropriate scan delay is dependent on the patient's cardiac output, but 20 s is adequate in most cases.
- Images should be viewed directly on a workstation, allowing image manipulation and multiplanar reconstructions in order to better appreciate flow and motion artifacts, which are common. The only bona fide evidence of PE on CT is the presence of an intraluminal defect **(Fig. 5.17).** Cutoff or nonfilling of pulmonary arteries is not as reliable a sign, particularly when only seen on a single image. Peripheral areas of oligemia, pleural-based triangular densities, and pleural effusions are ancillary signs that can help solidify the diagnosis. In cases of chronic PE, the thrombus may be peripheral **(Fig. 5.18).**
- **MRI angiography** is also being investigated for detection of pulmonary emboli. Breath-hold three-dimensional gradient-recalled echo images are acquired during the first pass of a gadopentetate dimeglumine contrast bolus with imaging in the coronal and sagittal planes. Major technical problems still remain to be solved, particularly artifacts from air-vessel interface and cardiac and respiratory motion.
- **Pulmonary artery aneurysms,** although rare, can be seen as a result of long-standing left-to-right shunts (particularly patent ductus arteriosus), pulmonary valvular stenosis, congenital absence of the

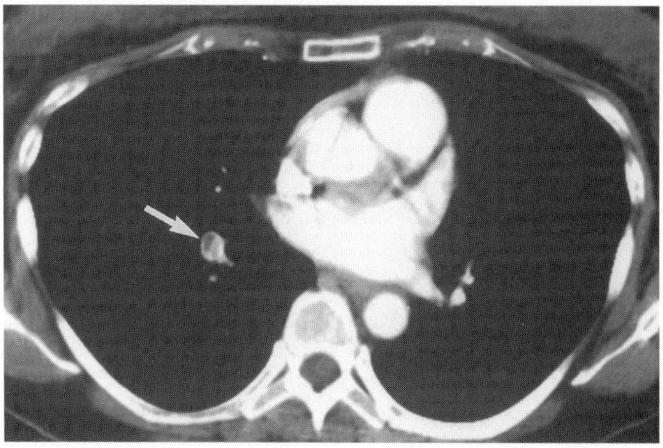

FIGURE 5.17 Acute pulmonary thromboembolism. Contrast-enhanced CT shows an enlarged, thrombosed right interlobar pulmonary artery branch *(arrow)* with a small amount of contrast peripherally.

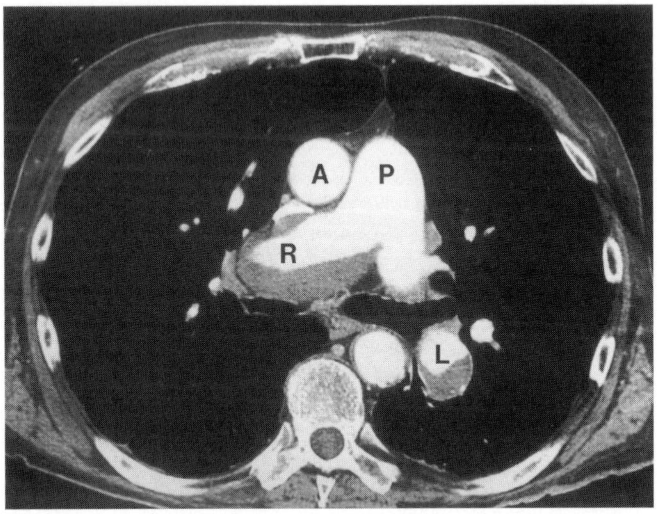

FIGURE 5.18 Chronic pulmonary thromboembolism. Contrast-enhanced CT shows marked enlargement of the right (R) and left (L) main pulmonary arteries in comparison to the normal size of the ascending aorta (A). Note the extensive circumferential mural thrombus in both. P, pulmonary trunk. (From Sagel SS, Slone RM. The lung. In Lee JKT, Sagel SS, Stanley RJ, Heiken JP (eds): *Computed Body Tomography with MRI Correlation*. Philadelphia: Lippincott-Raven, 1998. With permission.)

pulmonary valve, and acquired conditions such as Behçet disease and cystic medial necrosis. **Behçet syndrome** is a chronic vasculitis that involves veins, venules, capillaries, and, less frequently, arteries. Thrombosis or narrowing of the superior vena cava (SVC) is one of the most common manifestations. When the pulmonary arteries are involved, there is inflammation with disruption of the elastic fibers and, ultimately, aneurysm formation. Pseudoaneurysms of the pulmonary arteries can be seen as a complication of Swan-Ganz catheterization.

- **Pulmonary artery tumors** can be primary or metastatic. Primary tumors are extremely rare but are usually sarcomas arising from the vessel wall. A vast majority of cases are the result of bronchogenic carcinoma encasing the pulmonary arteries as they invade the hila and mediastinum **(Fig. 5.19).** Another common cause of pulmonary artery encasement is fibrosing mediastinitis from histoplasmosis.

Pulmonary Veins

- **Pulmonary venous anomalies** represent a small group of entities that, although rare, should be recognized and differentiated from diseases of the pulmonary parenchyma.
- **Partial anomalous pulmonary venous return** occurs when a pulmonary lobe drains into the right side of the circulation, usually a systemic vein. Anomalous venous drainage of the left upper lobe is usually an isolated congenital abnormality that has no clinical consequences. Anomalous drainage of the right pulmonary vein to the inferior vena cava (scimitar syndrome) can present as a left-to-right shunt in patients with volume loss of the right hemithorax and a peculiar comma-shaped density in the right lung base. Anomalous drainage of the right upper lobe is associated with a sinus venosus type of atrial septal defect. Left-lower-lobe pulmonary systemic drainage is associated with extralobar sequestration.

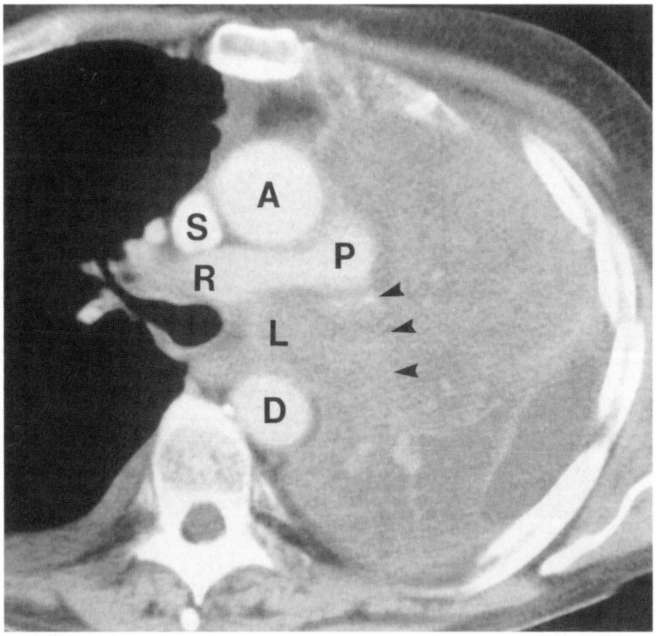

FIGURE 5.19 Bronchogenic carcinoma. Extensive mediastinal and left hilar invasion with occlusion of the left main bronchus (L) and pulmonary artery (arrowheads). There is complete opacification of the left hemithorax without volume loss or air bronchograms ("drowned lung"). A, ascending aorta; S, superior vena cava; R, right pulmonary artery; P, pulmonary trunk; D, descending aorta.

- **Pulmonary varices** represent focal dilatation of pulmonary veins just before they drain into the left atrium. They can be isolated or a sequela of chronic pulmonary venous hypertension, such as mitral valve disease. They are frequently first identified as a nodular density projecting below the hila since the lower-lobe veins are most commonly involved.
- **Pulmonary veno-occlusive disease** is a rare disorder with gradual narrowing and occlusion of the pulmonary veins of unknown etiology. A variety of insults such as viral infections and radiation have been proposed as the cause of endothelial proliferation and occlusion of small pulmonary veins that leads to pulmonary venous hypertension. High-resolution computed tomography (HRCT) can demonstrate interlobular septal thickening and areas of ground-glass attenuation. This entity should be differentiated from other causes of septal thickening.

5.4 AORTA

- CT of the aorta, particularly spiral CT angiography (CTA), has shown tremendous potential for evaluating aortic disease and may eventually surpass traditional angiographic methods. The aorta, with its large lumen perpendicular to the imaging plane, is well suited to CTA. There is a spectrum of clinical applications, including aneurysms, dissections, aortitis, and branch stenosis.
- **Technique:** Like pulmonary thromboembolism, CTA requires careful planning to optimize results, depending on the information desired. Technical guidelines vary depending on the equipment and software available. Before the start of the examination, the patient

should be coached on proper breath holding (suspended inspiration). Shallow respiration is allowed in critically ill patients unable to hold their breath. As a general rule, minor respiratory motion caused by shallow breathing does not significantly degrade image quality.

- The length and location of the aortic segment to be interrogated will determine the specific scanning parameters, but in general coverage should extend from 2 cm above the aortic arch to the superior aspect of the femoral heads. A 20-gauge or larger catheter placed in an antecubital vein will usually suffice to administer a total of 100 to 150 mL of intravenous contrast, with an injection rate of 3 mL/s. A test injection can be performed and a time-attenuation curve obtained so that a proper time delay can be selected. In general, time delays of 20 to 60 s are adequate. Collimation of 3 to 5 mm with overlapping reconstruction intervals is generally utilized. Depending on available software, multiplanar reformation (MPR), maximum-intensity projection (MIP), and shaded-surface display can be performed on an independent workstation.

Normal Anatomy

- The aorta begins at the level of the aortic valve and ends at the level of the iliac bifurcation in the pelvis. The **thoracic aorta** consists of the aortic root, which is composed of the aortic valve, annulus, and three sinuses of Valsalva. Just above the root is the tubular ascending aorta, which is mostly intrapericardial before ending at the level of the innominate artery, where the arch begins. The normal ascending aorta measures approximately 3.2 cm in diameter and is largest at the level of the sinuses of Valsalva. The diameter of the aortic arch measures approximately 2.5 to 3 cm, while the descending aorta measures about 2.5 cm. Slight variations can be encountered among different individuals, but in general the aorta should gradually taper in a consistent fashion along its entire length. One variation to this is an occasional area of narrowing (aortic isthmus) or dilatation (ductus diverticulum) just distal to the left subclavian artery that can be seen in young adults, both remnants from ductal circulation during intrauterine life. A prominent ductus diverticulum can give the false appearance of an aortic aneurysm or pseudoaneurysm at this level; therefore proper differentiation is important.

  The wall of the aorta measures several millimeters in thickness, although it tends to become thicker with advancing age. On nonenhanced scans, the aortic wall is not visible, since it has the same attenuation as the blood within it. In anemic patients, the aortic wall can appear hyperdense.

Anomalies of the Aortic Arch

- **Aberrant right subclavian artery** with a left-sided aortic arch is the most common congenital aortic anomaly, occurring in approximately 0.5 percent of the population. After arising as the most distal branch off the aortic arch, the right subclavian artery crosses behind the esophagus and up the right side of the superior mediastinum before heading to the right arm. Frequently, the proximal portion of the vessel has a diverticular dilatation, which can cause dysphagia from esophageal compression, particularly as it becomes atherosclerotic in elderly patients.

- A **right aortic arch** derives embryologically from the right fourth branchial arch instead of the left. The most common right arch seen in adults is associated with an aberrant left subclavian artery and is not associated with congenital heart defects. A less common variant corresponds to the mirror-image type of right aortic arch (left innominate, right common carotid, and right subclavian branches); this has a high association with congenital heart defects, most commonly tetralogy of Fallot.

- **Cervical aortic arch** is a condition in which the aortic arch (left or right) is a derivative of the second or third branchial arch instead of the fourth. The aortic arch is situated higher in the chest than usual, sometimes producing a pulsatile mass in the supraclavicular fossa. This condition is usually isolated and not associated with other congenital anomalies.

Acquired Conditions of the Aorta

- **Aortic aneurysms** are due to weakening caused by atherosclerosis, inflammation, trauma, or connective tissue disorders, leading to irreversible dilatation. ***True*** aortic aneurysms have all components of the wall present in the aneurysm. ***Pseudoaneurysms*** or false aneurysms do not contain all the elements of the wall and are usually associated with trauma, surgery, infections, or penetrating atherosclerotic ulcers.

  Aneurysms of the aorta can be focal, multifocal, or diffuse. About one-third of patients with an ascending aortic aneurysm have a concomitant infrarenal aneurysm, thus emphasizing the need to cover the entire aorta in evaluating aneurysms. Rupture and leak are the major complications and are a major cause of death if not diagnosed and treated appropriately. Aneurysmal size at diagnosis and rate of growth have important clinical and surgical implications. Most aneurysms involving the thoracic aorta are repaired when they exceed 5 to 6 cm in diameter. Although all segments of the aorta can be involved, the most frequent location of thoracic ather-

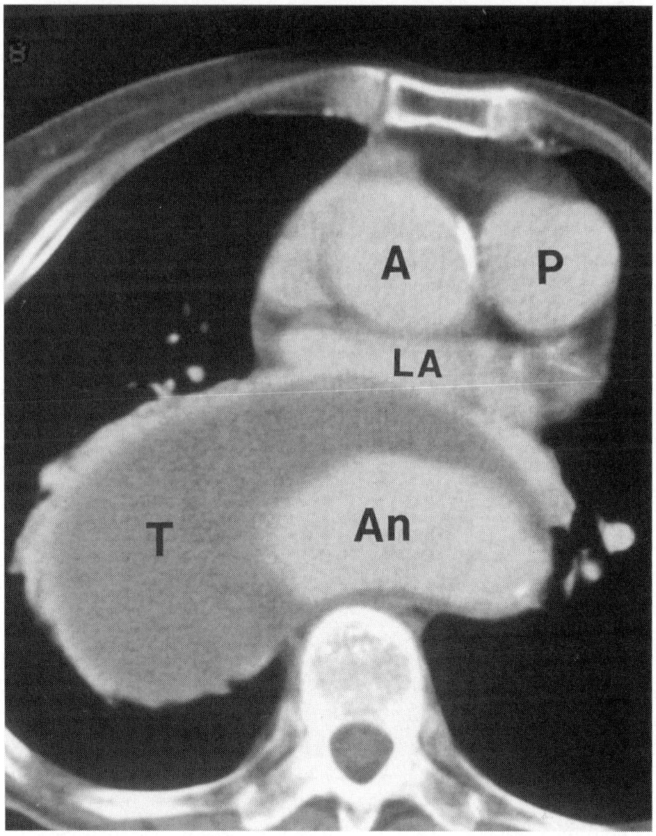

FIGURE 5.20 Large descending thoracic aortic aneurysm. CT shows a large aneurysm (An) protruding into the right hemithorax. Note large amount of thrombus (T) in the aneurysm wall. The aneurysm is seen compressing the posterior wall of the left atrium (LA). A, ascending aorta; P, pulmonary trunk.

osclerotic aneurysms is the proximal descending aorta **(Fig. 5.20).** Most true aneurysms are caused by atherosclerosis; cystic medial degeneration, mycotic, aortitis, and trauma are less common causes.

- **Abdominal aortic aneurysms** (AAA) are present in about 2 percent of patients over age 50. About 90 percent affect the infrarenal aorta, where an aneurysm is defined as a *luminal* diameter greater than 3 cm. CT findings of aortic aneurysm include (1) saccular or fusiform dilatation; (2) calcification in the aortic wall or, frequently, dystrophic calcification in mural thrombus; (3) intraluminal thrombus; (4) displacement or compression of adjacent structures. Thrombus is common and typically circumferential. Spiral technique with multiplanar three-dimensional reformatting can be very helpful in demonstrating the exact location of the aneurysm and its relationship to adjacent branch vessels.
- **Thoracic aneurysms** increase on average about 4 mm in size each year, while abdominal aneurysms grow approximately 3 mm per year. Aneurysms that increase in diameter more than 18 percent per year or more than 5 mm in a 6-month period are at high risk of rupture. In addition to rapid increase in size, the identification of high attenuation periaortic hematoma is indicative of aortic leak or impending rupture. The ***"aortic drape sign"*** is highly suggestive of a contained leak. This sign is present if the posterior aspect of the aorta cannot be identified as a distinct line from the adjacent structures and if the posterior aorta is closely applied to the spine and follows the contour of the vertebra on one or both sides. Frank bleeding may be seen around the aorta and adjacent retroperitoneal fascial planes. Ruptured aneurysms have a high mortality rate even after repair **(see discussion and figures in Sec. 10.7)**.
- **Aortic dissection** represents the most frequently occurring aortic catastrophe, presenting as an acute emergency two to three times more often than rupture of aortic aneurysms. Predisposing conditions are systemic hypertension, cystic medial degeneration, coarctation, bicuspid aortic valve, and pregnancy. After development of an ***entry point,*** blood gains access to the aortic wall (usually the tunica media), where it can extend along the long axis of the aorta, creating a ***false channel*** that can extend for a variable distance along the aorta. Multiple entry and reentry points can be present, thus allowing active flow along the false lumen.

  Depending on the location and extent of the disease, aortic dissections can be divided into two major groups with important prognostic and therapeutic implications. **Type A dissections** originate in the ascending aorta (an intrapericardial structure) and can extend along the aorta for variable lengths. Emergency surgery is the treatment of choice to prevent intrapericardiac rupture and tamponade **(see Sec. 5.6). Type B dissections** are limited to the descending aorta. The entry point is usually just distal to the left subclavian artery. Patients are usually managed medically by control of hypertension.
- **CT** is the imaging procedure of choice in the diagnosis of aortic dissection, not only because of its accuracy, ease of performance, and wide availability but also because it can provide information regarding other causes of chest pain and mediastinal widening. Familiarity with normal anatomic structures is important to avoid pitfalls **(Fig. 5.21).** In certain situations, precontrast images can be helpful in detecting a high-attenuation hematoma within the wall of the aorta or intimal calcification displacement **(Fig. 5.22).**

  CT findings of aortic dissection on noncontrast images include displacement of intimal calcification, high-attenuation thrombosed false lumen, and hemorrhagic pericardial or pleural effusion. Findings on contrast images **(Fig. 5.23)** include an intimal flap

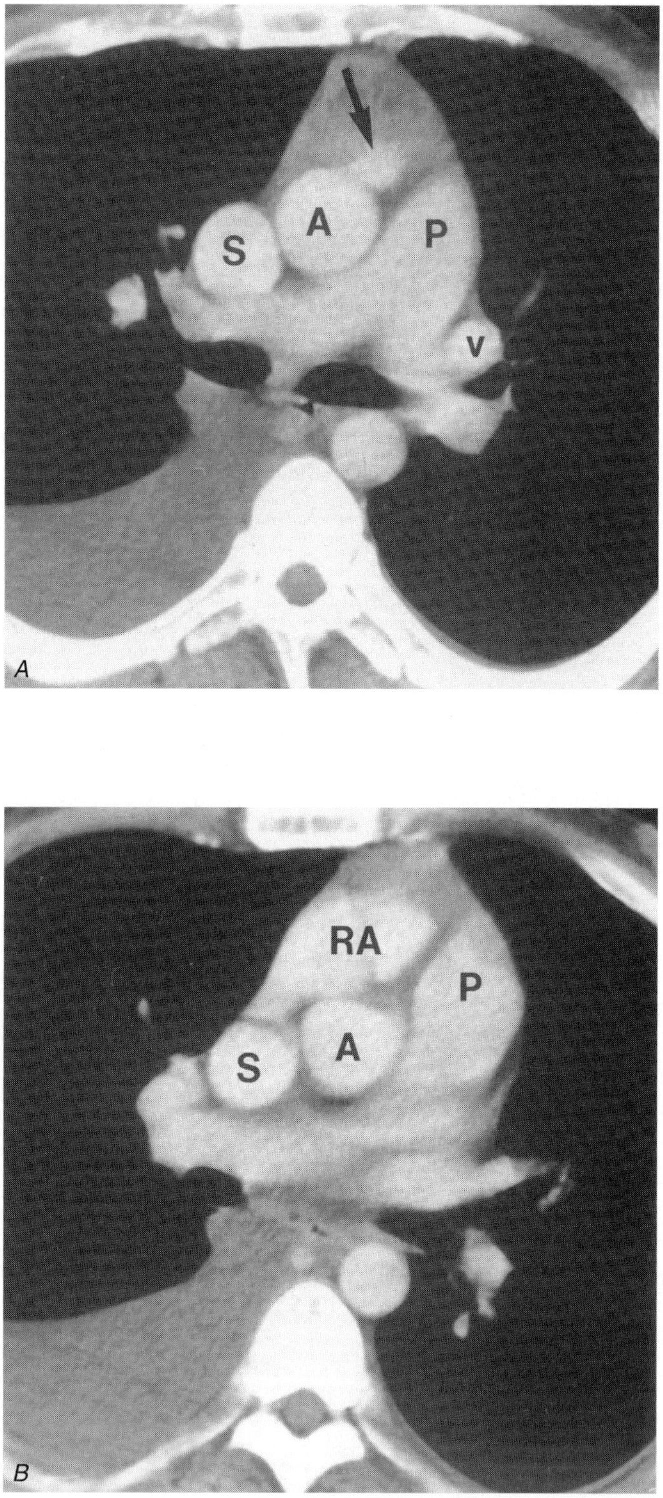

FIGURE 5.21 Prominent right atrial appendage mimicking dissection. A. Contrast-enhanced CT performed to investigate chest pain demonstrates a focal outpouching *(arrow)* apparently arising from the ascending aorta, suggesting a false lumen. *B.* Lower image demonstrates a large right atrial appendage (RA) wrapping in front of the ascending aorta as the cause of the apparent "dissection." Note moderate-size right pleural effusion. S, superior vena cava; P, pulmonary trunk; A, ascending aorta; v, left superior pulmonary vein.

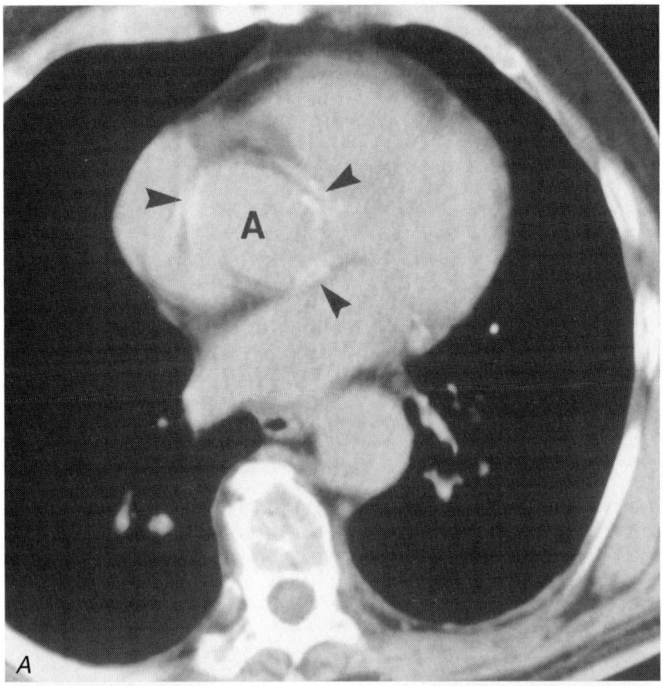

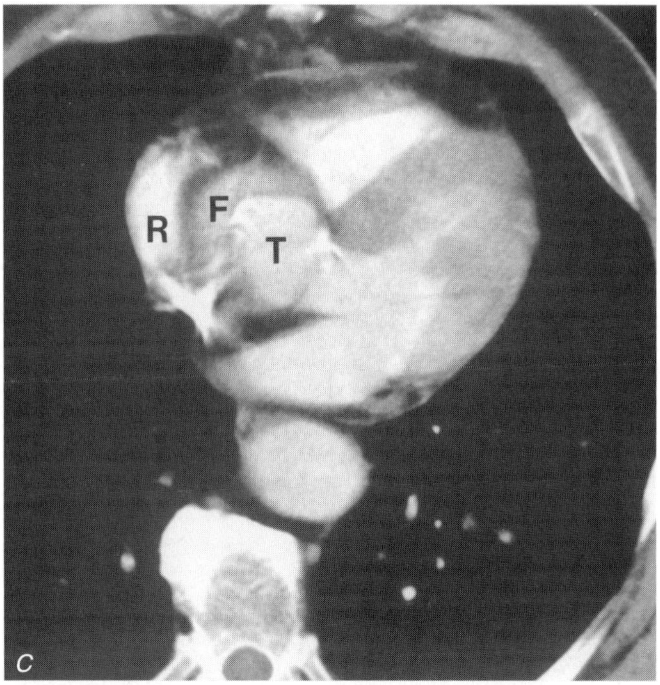

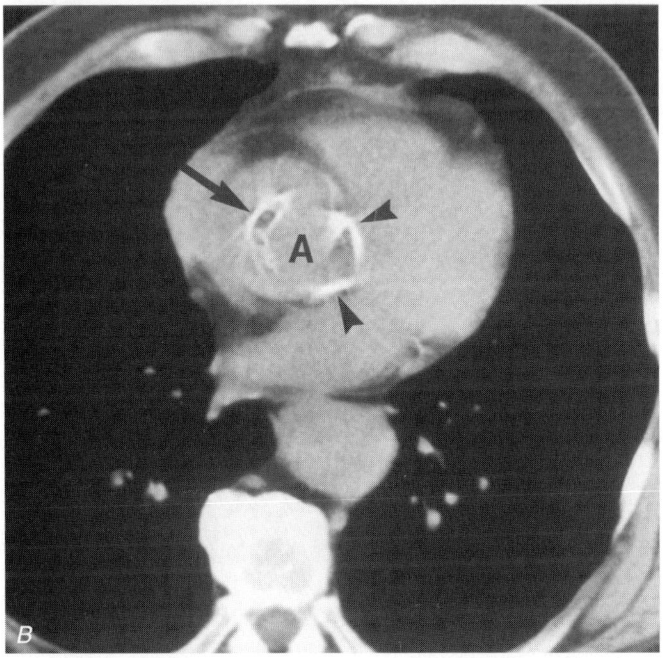

FIGURE 5.22 Type A aortic dissection. *A*. Contrast-enhanced CT in a 72-year-old patient demonstrates peripheral intimal calcification *(arrowheads)* in the aortic root (A). Three years later, the patient presented with chest pain. *B*. Noncontrast CT shows inward displacement of intimal calcification *(arrow)*. *C*. Contrast-enhanced CT shows the false (F) and true (T) lumen in the aortic root. R, right atrial appendage.

separating the false from the true lumen (the flap can extend into side branches), delayed opacification of the false lumen due to slow flow, compression and distortion of the true lumen by a thrombosed false lumen, and ischemia of organs with blood flow compromised by the false lumen.

- **Penetrating atherosclerotic ulcer of the aorta** represents an ulcerated atherosclerotic plaque that penetrates the internal elastic lamina, resulting in hematoma formation within the media of the aortic wall. Clinically, this resembles aortic dissection, but treatment can be quite different, particularly if surgery is necessary. The aortic graft required for penetrating atherosclerotic ulcers is often more extensive than for dissection. It is therefore important to recognize some fundamental differences between aortic dissection and an atherosclerotic ulcer. The natural history is variable and depends on proper diagnosis and treatment. The ulcer can extend through the media and even result in a saccular pseudoaneurysm. In about 8 percent of patients, transmural penetration leads to rupture.
- Patients with penetrating atherosclerotic ulcers are typically elderly patients with hypertension who present with acute chest or back pain. The classic CT finding is a localized intramural hematoma and mural ulcer involving the distal third of the descending thoracic aorta **(Fig. 5.24),** although any portion of the aorta can be involved. At times, there is extensive intramural hemorrhage extending proximal and distal to the ulcer.
- **Aortic branch occlusion** can be a result of severe atherosclerosis, embolization, dissection, vasculitis, or trauma. Good opacification and proper timing of the contrast bolus is crucial for proper diagnosis.

5.5 CAVAL SYSTEM

Superior Vena Cava

- The superior vena cava (SVC) is derived embryologically from the anterior cardinal venous system. It serves as a final tributary to many systemic veins from different parts of the body. A **persistent left SVC** is a congenital condition characterized by lack of involution of the left anterior cardinal vein system, resulting in a venous channel connecting the left brachiocephalic vein to the right atrium

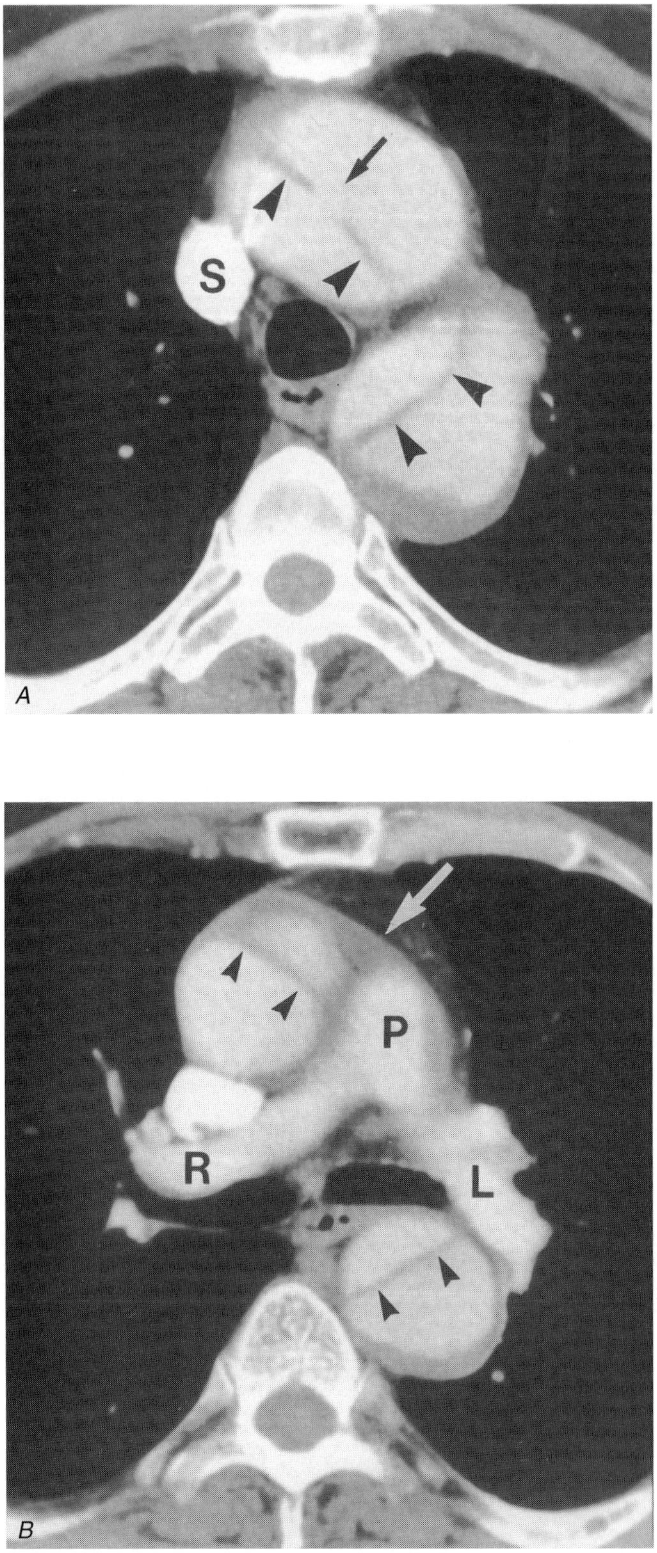

FIGURE 5.23 Type A aortic dissection. *A*. Contrast-enhanced CT showing an intimal flap *(arrowheads)* and entry point *(arrow)* at the level of the aortic arch. S, superior vena cava. *B*. Image at a lower level demonstrates involvement of the ascending aorta as well as a small amount of blood in the aortopulmonary pericardial recess *(arrow)*. Intimal flap *(arrowheads)* and mural thrombus are seen in the descending aorta. P, pulmonary trunk; R, right pulmonary artery; L, left pulmonary artery.

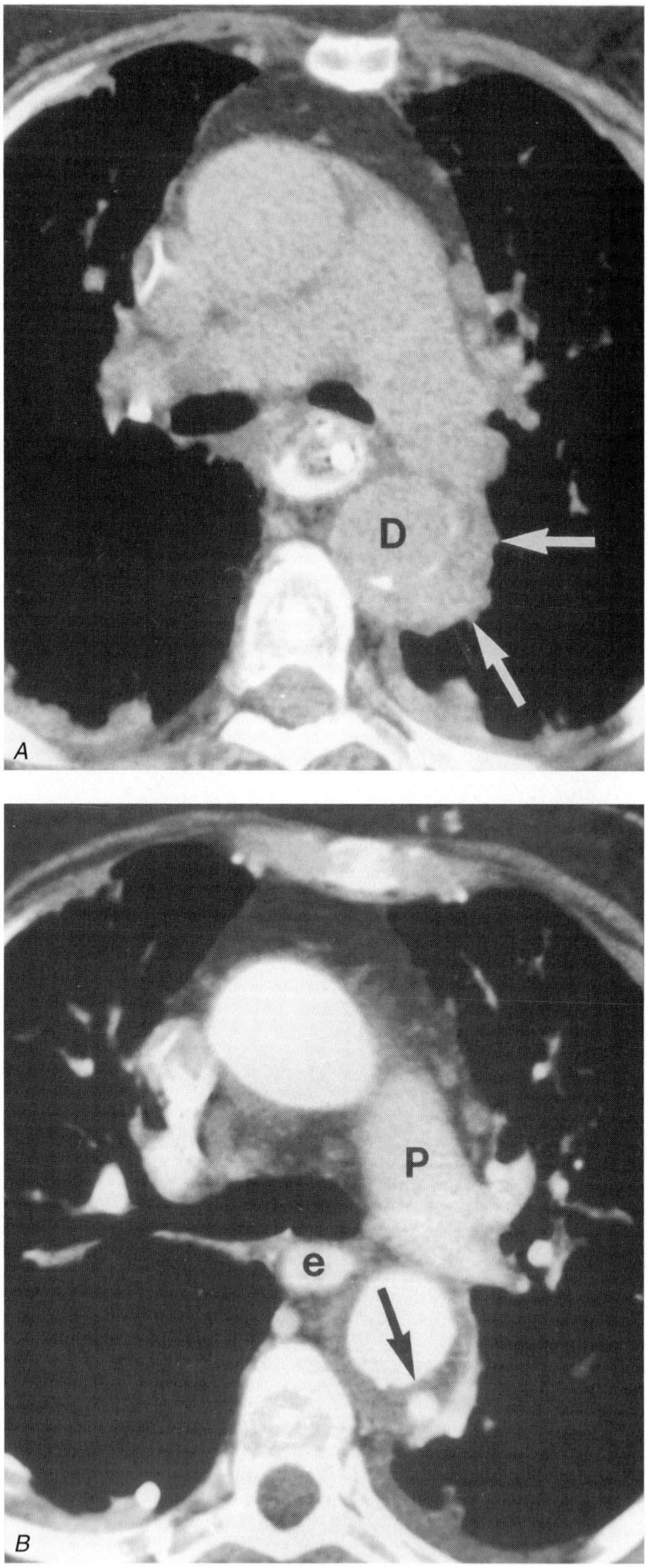

FIGURE 5.24 Penetrating atherosclerotic ulcer. A 75-year-old woman who developed back pain shortly after a right thoracotomy. *A*. Noncontrast exam demonstrating hematoma *(arrows)* in the descending aorta (D) peripheral to calcified intima. *B*. After contrast administration, a penetrating ulcer *(arrow)* becomes evident. P, pulmonary trunk; e, esophagus.

via the coronary sinus. In most cases, there is a right SVC with a connecting brachiocephalic vein **(Fig. 5.25).**

- There are many causes of **SVC obstruction.** Malignant neoplasms, particularly bronchogenic carcinoma, account for the vast majority. Other causes include metastatic adenopathy, fibrosing mediastinitis, and intraluminal thrombosis. CT can accurately determine the site and degree of SVC obstruction and identify collateral vessels associated with the obstruction. CT findings of venous obstruction are proximal enlargement of the vein with a low-attenuation central area representing thrombus. Care must be exercised to differentiate thrombosis from artifacts due to flow phenomena. In cases of SVC obstruction, an area of increased enhancement in the left lobe of the liver is frequently present. This is due to retrograde flow through portosystemic collateral vessels.
- The **inferior vena cava** (IVC) is formed by the confluence of the left and right common iliac veins at L4-L5 level. From this point, it ascends retroperitoneally to the right of the abdominal aorta and traverses the diaphragm before draining in the inferior aspect of the right atrium. **Caval transposition** or left-sided IVC is a condition characterized by a single left IVC that usually crosses to the right of the aorta at the level of the renal veins before draining to the right atrium. **Duplication of the IVC** results when a second, left-sided IVC originates from the left common iliac vein before ascending to the level of the left renal veins, where it usually terminates **(Fig. 5.26).** This condition must be differentiated from an enlarged left gonadal vein, which usually originates at the level of the left ovary or inguinal canal instead of the left common iliac vein.
- **IVC thrombosis** can be the result of bland thrombus or tumoral extension from kidney or liver neoplasms. CT findings include enlargement of the IVC and an intraluminal filling defect **(Fig. 5.27).**

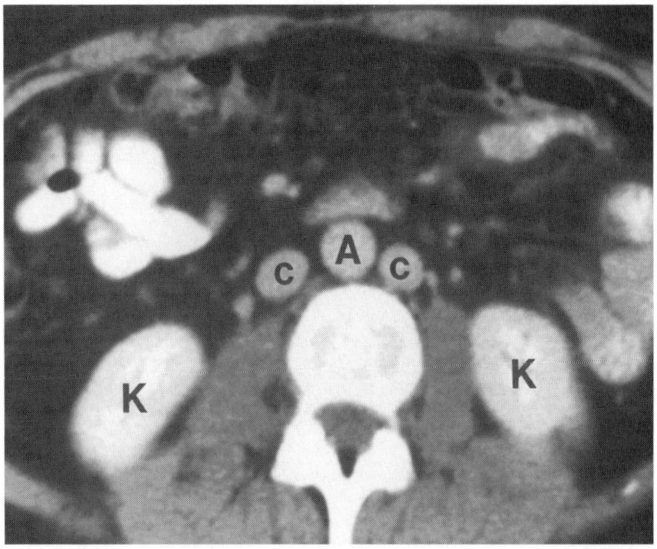

FIGURE 5.26 Duplicated inferior vena cava. Contrast-enhanced CT showing bilateral cava (c). A, abdominal aorta; K, kidneys. (Figure courtesy of Perry Pickhardt, MD.)

Care must be exercised not to confuse IVC thrombus with unopacified blood-flow artifacts on dynamic spiral CT scans, particularly at the level of the renal veins. More proximal venous thrombus may also be identified within the venous system **(Fig. 5.28).** Lack of formation of the suprarenal IVC describes **IVC interruption** with blood return mainly via the azygos or hemiazygos venous system **(Fig. 5.29).** This condition is usually isolated in adults but can be associated with polysplenia syndrome. Primary caval tumors are rare. **Leiomyosarcoma** of the IVC arises from the vessel wall. They can attain a large size and invade adjacent structures **(see Fig. 10.30).**

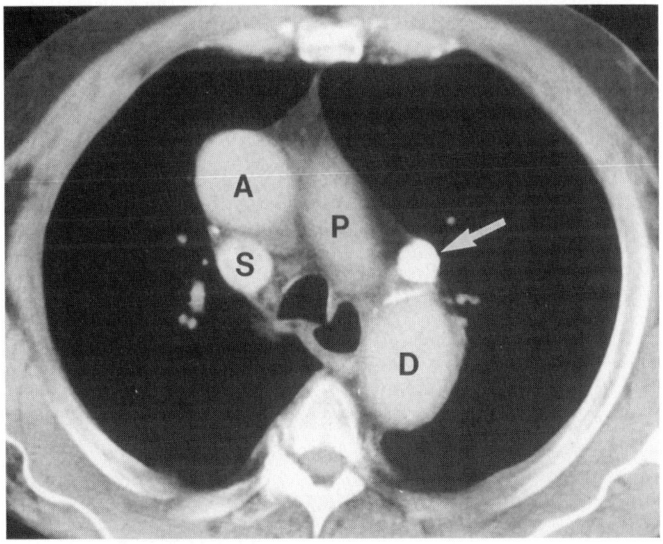

FIGURE 5.25 Persistent left superior vena cava. CT in a 65-year-old man shows a dense contrast enhancement of a left paramediastinal vessel *(arrow)* following injection of intravenous contrast in the left arm. Images at a higher level showed communication with the left brachiocephalic vein. Lower images showed drainage into the coronary sinus. A, ascending aorta; P, pulmonary trunk; S, superior vena cava; D, descending aorta.

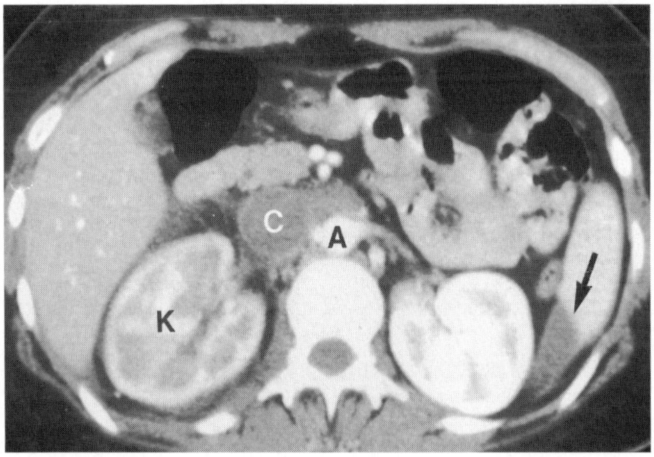

FIGURE 5.27 Thrombosis of the inferior vena cava. Contrast-enhanced CT demonstrating an enlarged, thrombosed inferior vena cava (C). Extension into the right renal vein caused a delayed cortical nephrogram in the right kidney (K) compared with the left. Note also splenic infarction *(arrow)*. A, abdominal aorta.

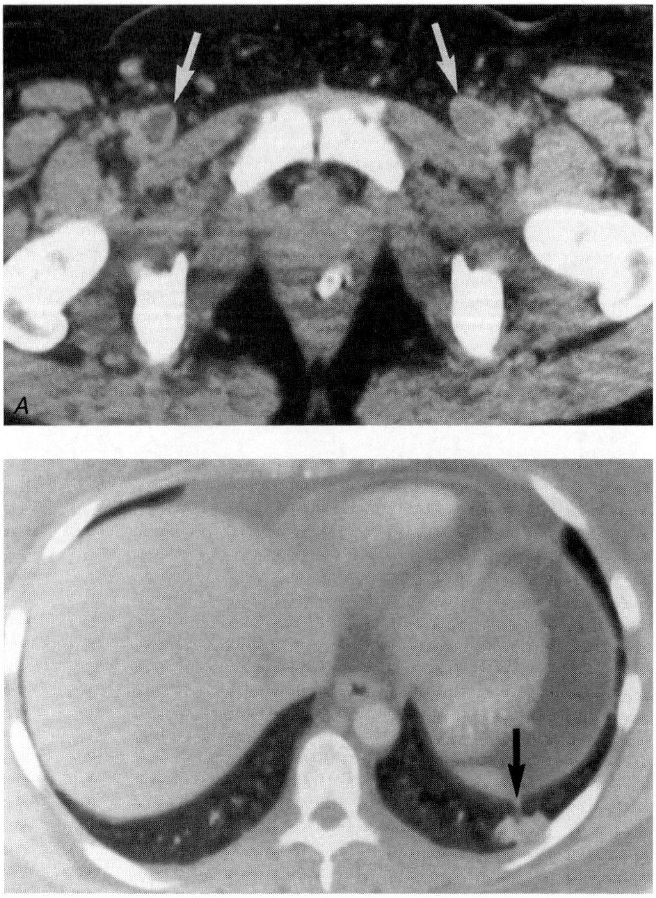

FIGURE 5.28 **Venous thrombosis and pulmonary infarction.** *A.* Bilateral femoral vein thrombosis *(white arrows)* in a patient with *(B)* pulmonary thromboembolism and infarction *(black arrow).*

5.6 CARDIOVASCULAR INTERVENTION AND SURGERY

- **Pulmonary thromboendarterectomy** is a viable treatment alternative for select patients with chronic pulmonary embolism. The disease must extend sufficiently proximal to permit surgical access. The procedure is performed by median sternotomy during deep hypothermia and circulatory arrest. The main pulmonary arteries are incised and an eversion endarterectomy is carried out into the segmental and subsegmental vessels. Reperfusion edema ranging from mild pulmonary edema to pulmonary hemorrhage is common and can occur up to 3 days following surgery.
- **Traumatic aortic transection** warrants emergent repair due to the high incidence of rupture and death. Tears typically occur in the region of the ligamentum arteriosum, just distal to the left subclavian artery. Repair is performed through a left thoracotomy. A median sternotomy is required for ascending aortic injuries.
- **Thoracic aortic aneurysms** are generally considered for surgical repair when their diameter exceeds 5 to 6 cm or there is a dramatic increase in size or symptoms over a short time. Significant aortic insufficiency calls for aortic replacement, even with small aneurysms. Descending thoracic aortic aneurysms are repaired through a left thoracotomy. There is a 10 percent mortality rate and 5 percent incidence of paraplegia. **Thoracoabdominal aneurysms** are repaired through a thoracoabdominal incision. Repair carries a 30 percent mortality and 15 percent rate of paraplegia. The celiac, superior mesenteric, and right renal arteries are often reanastomosed together as one pedicle.
- **Surgical repair** of an **AAA** usually involves end-to-end anastomoses of a Dacron graft to the aortic ends after aneurysmectomy. A portion of the aneurysm can be left in place or wrapped around the graft to isolate it from adjacent structures and prevent adhesions **(see Fig. 6.11).** Normally, postoperative gas resolves by 2 weeks and hematoma by 3 months. Postoperative complications include anastomotic leak, pseudoaneurysm formation, and graft infection.
- Recently, aortic aneurysms have been treated by nonsurgical percutaneous deployment of **endovascular stents (Fig. 5.30).** Advantages include decreased blood loss as well as reduction of depth and length of anesthesia, which permits a shorter hospitalization and a concomitant decrease in morbidity and mortality. Lack of long-term patency, leaking, and infection are problems related to these devices.
- **Type A aortic dissections** are repaired to prevent complications of aortic regurgitation, coronary occlusion, and pericardial tamponade rather than to "fix" the dissection. Planning the repair includes decisions regarding management of the aortic valve, coronary arteries, and transverse thoracic aortic arch. In patients with aortic insufficiency, the aortic valve can be replaced or the native valve resuspended. Coronary artery management can include reimplantation, or, if the coronaries are spared from involvement, the aortic valve can be repaired or replaced and an ascending aortic tube graft that begins above the coronary arteries can be inserted.
- The **Bentall procedure** is placement of a composite tube graft and valve conduit in the ascending aorta with a separate Dacron graft used to anastomose the right and left coronary orifices to the valve conduit. A valve-conduit repair is generally indicated in patients with Marfan syndrome because of the risk of degeneration and aneurysmal dilatation of the aortic segment containing the coronary ostia **(Fig. 5.31).**

Interventional Cardiology

- **Percutaneous techniques** applied to the coronary circulation include balloon angioplasty, laser ablation, atherectomy, and coronary stent placement. Balloon valvuloplasty is sometimes used for management of mitral and aortic stenosis.
- **Percutaneous transluminal coronary angioplasty** (PTCA) has become standard therapy for patients with coronary artery disease. PTCA works by fracturing the stenotic plaque and underlying intima and stretching the normal vessel wall. Indications include acute myocardial infarction (PTCA within 3 h), significant angina, or positive exercise testing in the presence of a 75 percent narrowing that is refractory to medical treatment. Although initially successful in more than 90 percent of patients, over one-third of these lesions have restenosed by 6 months. Success is lower with severe stenosis, dense atherosclerotic calcification, intraluminal thrombus, and right coronary lesions. Contraindications include left main and heavily calcified lesions as well as chronic occlusions, lesions spanning a bifurcation, and long-segment lesions.
- **Complications** occur in less than 10 percent, but include myocardial infarction and death. Emergent coronary artery bypass grafting is sometimes required in the event of complications. Endovascular **coronary stents** deployed immediately following angioplasty re-

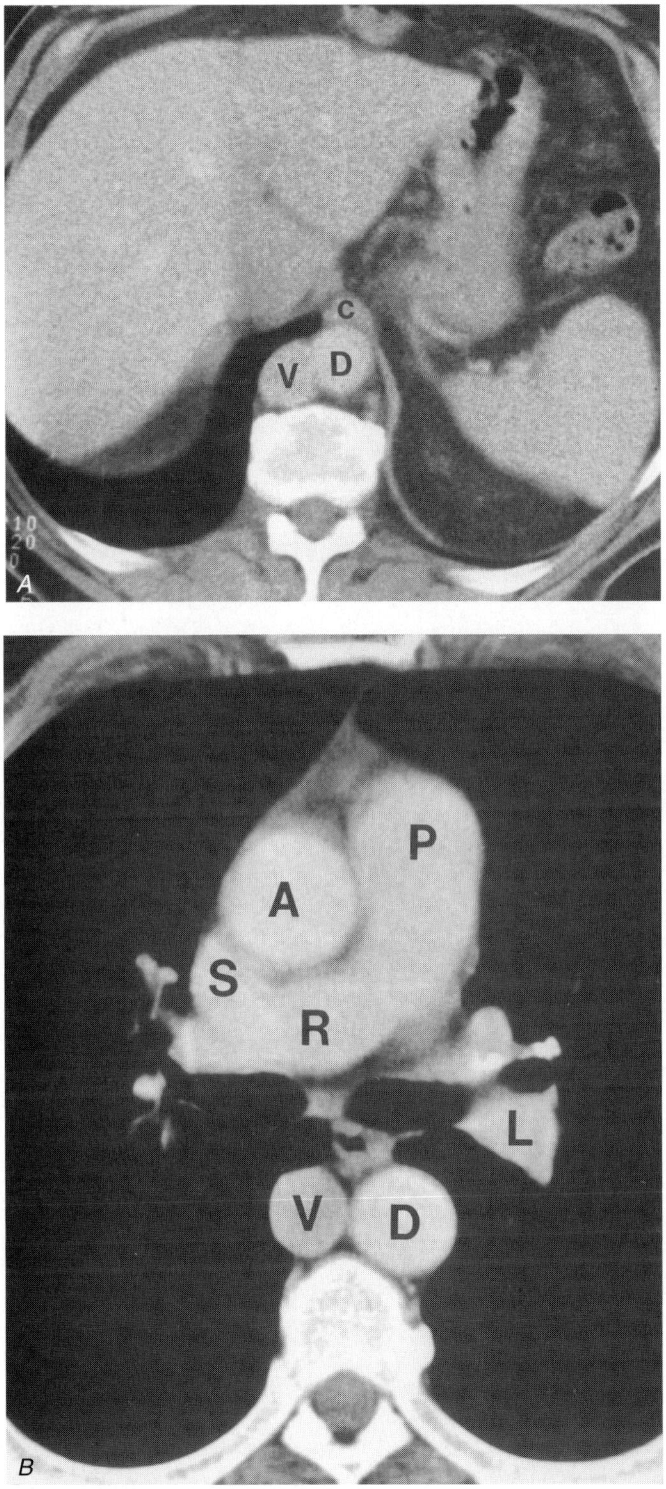

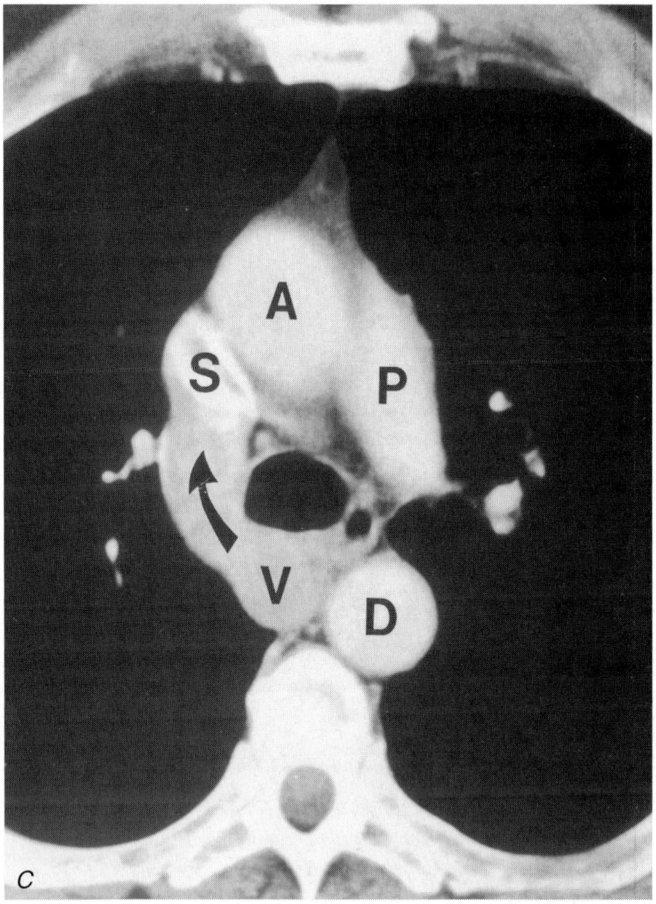

FIGURE 5.29 Interrupted inferior vena cava (IVC) with azygos continuation. *A*. An enlarged azygos vein (V) is seen to the right of the descending aorta (D). No suprarenal IVC was seen. c, crura of the left hemidiaphragm. *B*. The enlarged azygos vein can be followed as it ascends in front of the thoracic spine. Normal hilar anatomy can be seen at the level of the right main pulmonary artery (R). The left pulmonary artery (L) has passed above the left main bronchus while the right stays in front of the corresponding bronchus, excluding polysplenia. *C*. Above the carina, the azygos vein is seen draining *(arrow)* into the superior vena cava (S). A, ascending aorta; P, pulmonary trunk.

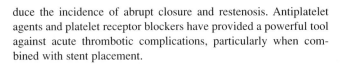

duce the incidence of abrupt closure and restenosis. Antiplatelet agents and platelet receptor blockers have provided a powerful tool against acute thrombotic complications, particularly when combined with stent placement.

Cardiac Surgery

- **Coronary artery bypass surgery** can improve patient survival but primarily improves quality of life in terms of pain-free survival. Coronary revascularization has the greatest benefit in patients with reduced ejection fractions and unstable angina. Specific indications include triple-vessel disease, double-vessel coronary artery disease with reduced ejection fraction, angina refractory to medical therapy, and left main and proximal left anterior descending coronary artery disease. At the present time, the "gold standard" for coronary revascularization is surgical anastomosis between the left internal thoracic artery and left anterior descending coronary artery. Due to intimal hyperplasia and atherosclerosis, the 10-year patency of saphenous vein grafts is about 50 percent, compared with 95 percent for internal thoracic artery grafts.
- A **left ventricular aneurysmectomy** can be performed in patients with poor ventricular function due to a dyskinetic or akinetic infarct segment. Indications include a large aneurysm with decreased cardiac output, congestive heart failure, and ventricular arrhythmias. Most aneurysms are anterolateral in position and associated

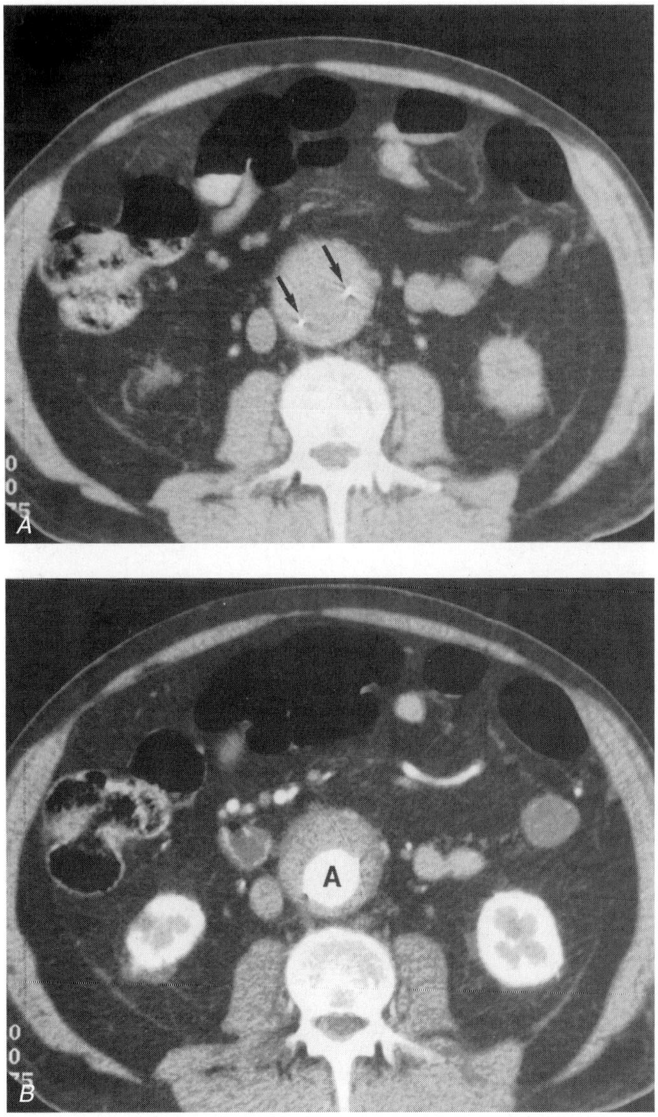

FIGURE 5.30 Endovascular stent. *A*. Precontrast images show a 5-cm abdominal aortic aneurysm. Metal wires mark the sides of the graft *(arrows)*. *B*. Arterial phase image shows complete opacification of the stent lumen but no evidence of contrast leaking around the stent. The space between the graft and vessel wall contains thrombosed blood.

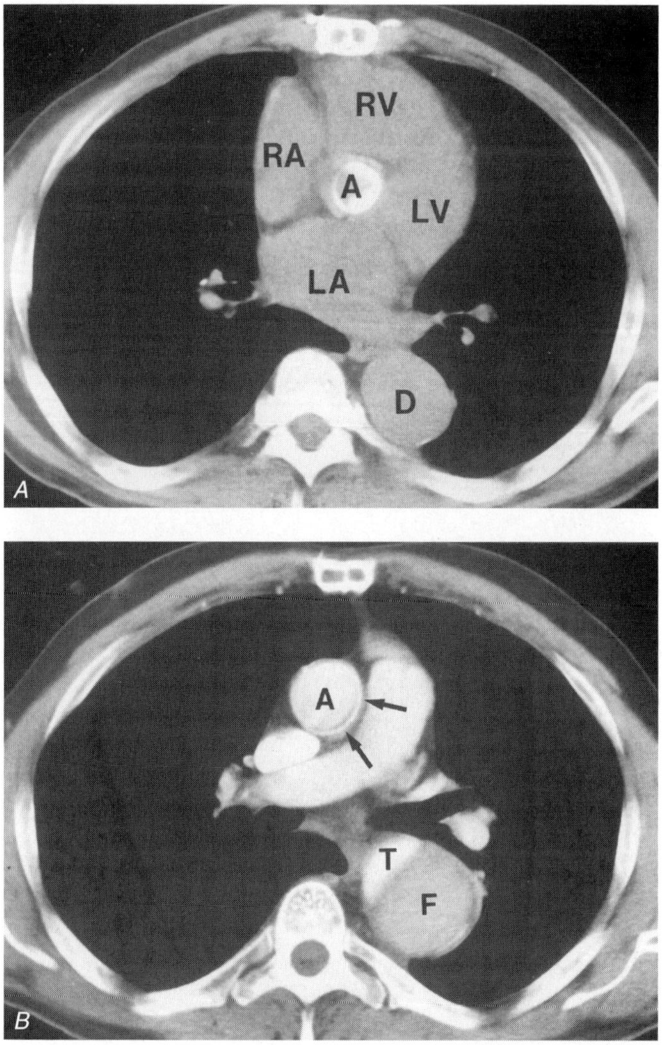

FIGURE 5.31 Repaired type A dissection. Bentall repair with valve-conduit in a patient with Marfan syndrome. *A*. Noncontrast image showing the prosthetic aortic valve (A). RV, right ventricle; RA, right atrium; LV, left ventricle; LA, left atrium; D, descending thoracic aorta. *B*. Contrast-enhanced CT at a higher level showing the high-density graft material *(arrows)*. There is contrast in the ascending aorta and true lumen (T) of the descending aorta. Note thrombosed false channel (F) in descending aorta.

organized thrombus is common. **Left ventricular reduction surgery,** termed a "Batiste partial left ventriculotomy" or "dynamic cardiomyoplasty," improves function by reducing left ventricular size. The procedure has gained acceptance as a viable surgical option in select patients with congestive failure.

- **Mitral valve repair** with commissurotomy, excision of thickened cordae, and placement of an annuloplasty ring is the procedure of choice for patients with mitral regurgitation. Congestive heart failure with prolapse of the central leaflet is the most common cause of mitral regurgitation in the United States. Repair is simple and has been so successful that surgery is now recommended in asymptomatic patients, although the functional results are not as satisfactory as valve replacement. **Mitral valve replacement** is more appropriate than repair in patients with mitral regurgitation caused by acute myocardial infarction with ventricular wall and papillary muscle damage. **Mitral stenosis** can often be managed with percutaneous balloon valvotomy. Surgical techniques also exist for repairing incompetent aortic valves. Repair of stenotic aortic valves is less successful.
- **Minimally invasive cardiac surgery** techniques are emerging for the treatment of heart disease. Coronary artery bypass grafting can be performed through a small anterior thoracotomy or thoracoscopy by dissecting the internal mammary artery and grafting to the anterior descending coronary artery. Catheter systems have also been developed for peripheral cardiopulmonary bypass and endoaortic clamping, thus facilitating less invasive bypass grafting, valve repair, replacement, and other cardiac procedures.

Bibliography

Baskin KM, Stanford W, Thompson BH, Tajik J, Heery SD, Hoffman EA. Helical versus electron-beam CT in assessment of coronary artery calcification (abstr). *Radiology* 1995;197(P):182.

Chung JW, Park JH, Im JG, Chung MJ, Han MC, Ahn H. Spiral CT angiography of the thoracic aorta. *Radiographics* 1996;16:811–824.

Clemente CD. *Grant's Anatomy,* 13th ed. Philadelphia: Lee & Febiger; 1985.

Coulden R. Functional cardiac CT. In: Miles K, Dawson P, Blomley M, eds. *Functional Computed Tomography.* St. Louis: Mosby–Year Book; 1997.

Ernst CB. Abdominal aortic aneurysm. *N Engl J Med* 1993;328:1167–1172.

Farmer DW, Lipton MJ, Higgins CB, Ringertz H, Dean PB, Sievers R, Boyd DP. In vivo assessment of left ventricular wall and chamber dynamics during transient myocardial ischemia using cine CT. *Am J Cardiol* 1985;55:560–567.

Goodman LR. CT of acute pulmonary emboli: Where does it fit? *Radiographics* 1997;17:1037–1042.

Halliday KE, Al-Kutoubi A. Draped aorta: CT sign of contained leak of aortic aneurysm. *Radiology* 1996;199:41–43.

Higgins CB. The heart and pericardium. In: Moss A, Gamsu G, Genant HK, eds. *Computed Tomography of the Body with Magnetic Resonance Imaging,* 2nd ed. Philadelphia: Saunders; 1992.

Moncada R, Baker M, Salinas M, Demos TC, Churchill R, Love L, Reynes C, Hale D, Cardoso M, Pifarre R, Gunnar RM. Diagnostic role of computed tomography in pericardial heart disease: Congenital defects, thickening, neoplasms, and effusions. *Am Heart J* 1983;103:263–282.

Moritz JD, Rotermund S, Deating DP, Oestmann JW. Infrarenal abdominal aortic aneurysms: Implications of CT evaluation of size and configuration for placement of endovascular aortic grafts. *Radiology* 1996;198:463–466.

Moshage WE, Achenbach S, Seese B, Bachmann K, Kirchgeorg M. Coronary artery stenoses: Three-dimensional imaging with electrocardiographically triggered, contrast agent–enhanced electron-beam CT. *Radiology* 1995;196:707–714.

Schiavone WA, Rice T. Pericardial disease: Current diagnosis and management methods. *Cleve Clin J Med* 1989;56:639–645.

Sebastià C, Pallisa E, Quiroga S, Alvarez-Castells A, Dominguez R, Evangelista A. Aortic dissection: Diagnosis and follow-up with helical CT. *Radiographics* 1999;19:45–60.

Shemesh J, Apter S, Rozenman J, Lusky A, Rath S, Itzchack Y, Motro M. Calcification of coronary arteries: Detection and quantification with double-helix CT. *Radiology* 1995;197:779–783.

Spodick DH. *The Pericardium: A Comprehensive Textbook.* New York: Marcel Dekker; 1997.

Welch TJ, Stanson AW, Sheedy PF 2d, Johnson CM, McKusick MA. Radiologic evaluation of penetrating atherosclerotic ulcer. *Radiographics* 1990;10:675–685.

Chapter 6

ALIMENTARY TRACT

Perry J. Pickhardt

6.1 Anatomy and Technique
6.2 Congenital Abnormalities
6.3 Stomach
6.4 Small Bowel
6.5 Colon and Rectum
6.6 Crohn Disease
6.7 Intussusception
6.8 Pneumatosis

6.1 ANATOMY AND TECHNIQUE

- Mucosal disease of the gastrointestinal (GI) tract is best evaluated by barium and endoscopic examinations. These diagnostic modalities, however, are limited by their inability to assess the extraluminal component of a given disease process. Consequently, **computed tomography (CT)** offers complementary information, since it is well suited to evaluate the mural and extramural component of alimentary tract pathology. In addition, CT is useful for many other applications in GI tract disease, including evaluation of palpable masses, staging of neoplasms, detection of disease recurrence, and evaluation of bowel obstruction, inflammatory conditions, or bowel perforation. Portions of the alimentary tract discussed in this chapter are the stomach, small bowel, and colon. The esophagus is covered in more detail in Chapter 4.

- The digestive system can be divided into three main components based on embryologic development: the foregut, midgut, and hindgut. Derivatives of the **foregut** include the pharynx, esophagus, stomach, proximal duodenum, pancreas, liver, and biliary tree. Arterial supply to the intra-abdominal foregut is via the **celiac axis.** Derivatives of the **midgut** include the distal duodenum, mesenteric small intestine, appendix, and proximal colon to the level of the distal transverse colon. The midgut derivatives are supplied by the **superior mesenteric artery (SMA).** Finally, the **hindgut** extends from the distal transverse colon to the rectum and is supplied by the **inferior mesenteric artery.** The abdominal portion of the GI tract is anatomically complex owing to a series of rotations and subsequent fixation that occur during development **(Fig. 6.1).**

- The **stomach** occupies the left upper abdominal quadrant and serves as a capacious reservoir bridging the esophagus and duodenum. The stomach can be divided into anatomic segments: The **cardia** of the stomach surrounds the esophagogastric junction; the **fundus** extends superiorly and laterally to the cardia and occupies the left subphrenic space; the gastric **body** extends inferiorly from the fundus to the level of the incisura that lies along the lesser curvature; the **antrum** is more anterior in location than the body and fundus and crosses the midline to the right side; finally, the antrum leads to the muscular **pylorus,** which communicates with the duodenal bulb. The stomach lies in close proximity to the left hepatic lobe anteromedially, the spleen posterolaterally, the pancreas posteriorly, and the transverse colon and jejunum inferiorly. On CT, the normal gastric wall should not exceed 5 mm. Pseudothickening is the result of incomplete distention and is especially common at the cardia, where a pseudomass can be seen in up to 40 percent of normal studies.

- The **duodenum** forms a C-shaped loop and is the only portion of small bowel fixed in the retroperitoneum. The **first portion** of the duodenum, however, remains peritonealized and extends posteriorly or posterolaterally relative to the antrum. This first portion is also referred to as the **duodenal bulb.** The descending **second portion** of the duodenum is retroperitoneal and has a cephalocaudal orientation. Medially, the second portion partially encompasses the pancreatic head and is the drainage site for the pancreatic and common bile ducts. The inferior **third portion** of the duodenum lies transversely and crosses the midline, passing between the aorta posteriorly and the SMA anteriorly. The ascending **fourth portion** terminates at the duodenojejunal flexure, which is stabilized by the suspensory **ligament of Treitz.** This landmark identifies the site where the midgut begins and the small bowel enters the peritoneal cavity.

- The **mesenteric small intestine,** comprising the jejunum and ileum, is the portion of small bowel that is suspended by a broad mesentery; it is affixed posteriorly in a diagonal orientation from the left upper to right lower abdomen. The **jejunum** comprises the proximal two-fifths of the small intestine and occupies the left upper abdomen. It often demonstrates a somewhat feathery fold pattern on barium studies or CT. The lower three-fifths of the mesenteric small intestine is the **ileum,** which terminates at the ileocecal valve and typically occupies the right lower quadrant and pelvis. Its fold pattern is more featureless than that of the jejunum. In general, assuming adequate distention, the small bowel wall should measure less than 3 mm on CT, and its luminal diameter should not exceed 2.5 cm.

- The **colon** can usually be traced throughout its entirety on CT because of the characteristic appearance of colonic haustra and mottled stool contents. Colonic anatomy reflects the counterclockwise rotation and fixation pattern that occurs during embryologic development. Knowledge of which portions of the colon are intraperi-

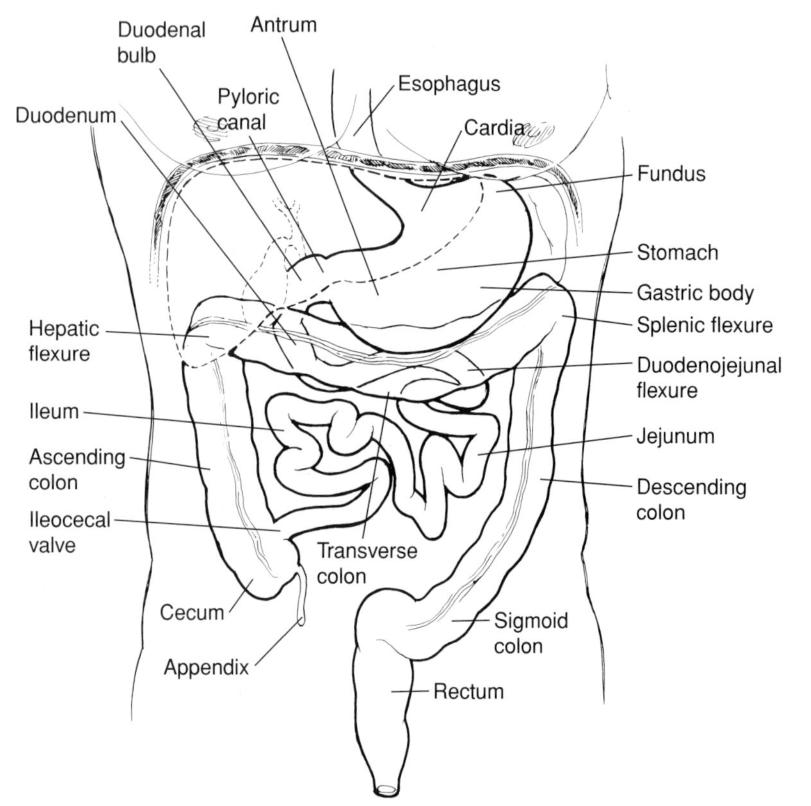

FIGURE 6.1 GI anatomy. Diagram of the major anatomic landmarks of the alimentary tract.

toneal and retroperitoneal can be important in CT interpretation. The **cecum** is a blind pouch that usually occupies the right iliac fossa, although the location of this intraperitoneal structure will vary depending on the length of its mesentery. The **ileocecal valve** connects the small and large intestines and is often identified on CT, particularly when lipomatous change is present (see **Fig. 6.17**). The vermiform **appendix** is a slender, blind-ending tubular structure extending off the medial aspect of the cecal tip, inferior to the ileocecal valve. Although the appendix varies widely in length, it averages approximately 8 cm. The appendiceal body and tip are most often directed into the pelvis or retrocecal region.

The **ascending colon** and **descending colon** are retroperitoneal segments and occupy the lateral aspects of the right and left anterior pararenal spaces, respectively. These segments are readily identified on axial CT because of their relative orientation to the imaging plane and surrounding retroperitoneal fat. The **transverse colon** is an intraperitoneal structure that bridges the ascending and descending colon, extending from the hepatic flexure to the splenic flexure. The location of the transverse colon in the peritoneal cavity is variable owing to the mobility afforded by the transverse mesocolon; it can lie anterior to the liver or as far inferior as the pelvis. The **transverse mesocolon** represents an important conduit for the spread of disease between the pancreas and transverse colon, while the **gastrocolic ligament** allows for a pathway between the stomach and transverse colon. The **sigmoid colon** is an S-shaped intraperitoneal segment that connects the descending colon and rectum. It is suspended by the **sigmoid mesentery** and is a frequent site of involvement for both inflammatory and neoplastic conditions.

- The **rectum** occupies the posterior aspect of the pelvis, conforming to the concave shape of the sacrum. Peritoneal investment in its superior aspect forms part of the rectovesical pouch in males and the rectovaginal pouch in females. The inferior two-thirds of the rectum is extraperitoneal and extends to the anal canal.
- **CT technique** for successful evaluation of the GI tract hinges on adequate intraluminal contrast to distend and opacify the specific hollow viscus being studied. **Unopacified bowel loops** continue to present a major source of diagnostic error in CT interpretation. Patients should have nothing by mouth for 8 hours prior to the examination to avoid the possibility that retained food will simulate pathology. Specific **oral contrast** regimens vary, but approximately 600 mL of dilute positive contrast beginning 60 to 90 minutes prior to scanning and followed by 200 to 300 mL immediately before scanning will usually suffice. Unless it is contraindicated, **intravenous (IV) contrast** should also be administered. Routine collimation and scan/reconstruction intervals ranging between 5 and 10 mm are satisfactory in most cases. Modifications in standard technique depend on the specific regions of concern, some of which are discussed in the paragraphs below.

Water may be given instead of dilute positive contrast immediately prior to scanning to improve visualization of the gastric and duodenal mucosa and submucosa (see **Fig. 6.6**). For gastric imaging, **effervescent agents** may also be given to maximize luminal distention. Repeat imaging with prone or decubitus positioning may be helpful to exclude a gastric pseudomass. In the setting of high-grade bowel obstruction, administration of oral contrast may unnecessarily delay imaging, since fluid within the distended loops serves as an effective contrast agent. When **appendicitis** is the major clinical concern, spiral technique with thin collimation (typically 5 mm) and contiguous or overlapping reconstruction intervals is useful. The appropriate combination of IV, oral, and rectal contrast in the setting of suspected appendicitis is an unsettled issue. **Rectal contrast**, either positive or air, can be helpful in cases of suspected rectosigmoid disease. **CT colonography** is a technique under active investigation using three-dimensional volume rendering to simulate endoscopy for the evaluation of polyps.

6.2 CONGENITAL ABNORMALITIES

- Congenital abnormalities of the GI tract that can be seen on CT include duplication cysts, true diverticula, and malrotation. **Duplication cysts** occur anywhere along the GI tract, with the ileum representing the single most common site. The CT appearance is that of a nonspecific cystic lesion, whereas ultrasound can suggest the specific diagnosis when the striated appearance of the bowel wall is resolved. Communication of the cyst with the adjacent true lumen is rare. Complications of duplication cysts include bowel obstruction from mass effect, peptic ulceration from ectopic gastric mucosa, and inflammation from ectopic pancreatic tissue. **Gastric diverticula** are relatively common and usually extend off the posterior aspect of the fundus, where they can simulate an adrenal mass on CT if not opacified with contrast (see **Fig. 11.13**). **Duodenal diverticula** are extremely common and only rarely cause symptoms. The typical location is along the inner aspect of the second or third portion of the duodenum. It is important not to confuse a duodenal diverticulum with an abscess, mass, or focal perforation. A **Meckel diverticulum** represents a remnant of the omphalomesenteric duct, usually occurring within 25 cm of the ileocecal valve. The primary complication of Meckel diverticulum is GI bleeding, which almost always occurs in young children. CT does not play a role in the diagnosis. Abnormalities of midgut rotation, or **malrotation**, can result in a variety of appearances. Nonrotation is most common, resulting in a left-sided colon and abnormal duodenal sweep, with small bowel occupying the right hemiabdomen **(Fig. 6.2)**. On CT, transposition of the superior mesenteric vessels may be present, with the SMA to the right of the vein. Although nonrotation is usually asymptomatic in adults, a predisposition to midgut volvulus exists because of the abnormal mesenteric fixation. On CT, the "whirl" sign of small bowel mesentery wrapped around the SMA axis in concentric rings is diagnostic of midgut volvulus **(Fig. 6.2)**.

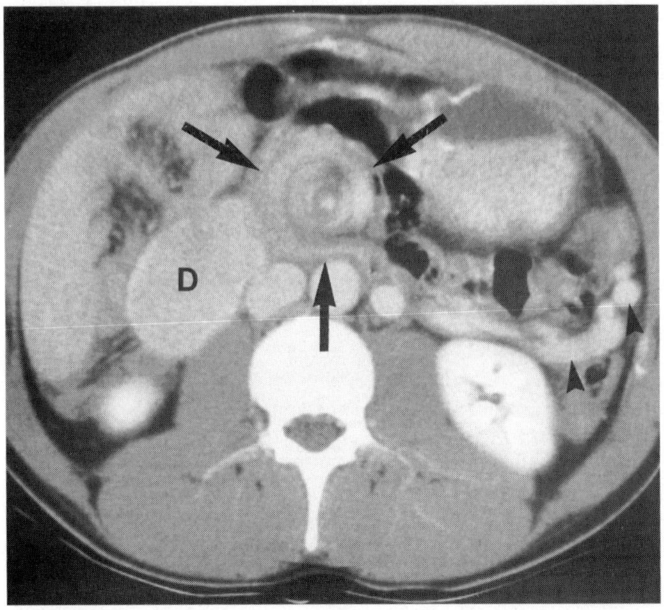

FIGURE 6.2 Malrotation with midgut volvulus. Contrast-enhanced CT in a 36-year-old man with abdominal pain of acute onset shows spiraled appearance of small bowel mesentery around SMA axis *(arrows)* from twisting due to midgut volvulus. The duodenum (D) is dilated and congested mesenteric vessels *(arrowheads)* are present. Fluid-filled small bowel occupies the right side of the abdomen and air-filled colon occupies the left, consistent with malrotation. (Case courtesy of Dr. Matthew Fleishman, Denver, CO.)

6.1 THICKENED GASTRIC WALL

Incomplete distention (pseudothickening)
Inflammation (gastritis)
- ***H. pylori*/peptic**
- **NSAID gastritis**
- **Alcohol**
- Pancreatitis—secondary stomach inflammation
- Corrosive ingestion
- Radiation
- Infection—CMV, tuberculosis, *bacterial, candidal, herpes*
- Zollinger-Ellison syndrome—gastrinoma
- Crohn disease
- *Vasculitis*

Tumor
- **Adenocarcinoma—** >90% of gastric malignancies
- **Lymphoma—**usually non-Hodgkin
- Direct ligamentous extension from colon or pancreas
- Metastasis—breast, melanoma

Gastric varices
Lymphoid hyperplasia
Infiltrative disease—eosinophilic gastritis, *amyloidosis*
Sarcoidosis
Ménétrier disease

Key: CMV, cytomegalovirus; NSAID, nonsteroidal anti-inflammatory drug.

6.3 STOMACH

- **Gastric wall thickening** is readily detected on CT and represents a nonspecific finding **(Differential 6.1).** Confident diagnosis of true wall thickening, whether focal or diffuse, requires adequate gastric distention by air or fluid to avoid the common pitfall of pseudothickening. Causes of gastric wall thickening include inflammation, infection, malignancy, infiltrative disease, Zollinger-Ellison syndrome, Ménétrier disease, sarcoidosis, and varices.
- Inflammation of the stomach, or **gastritis,** is usually depicted as diffuse gastric wall thickening on CT. *Helicobacter pylori gastritis*, gastritis associated with the use of nonsteroidal anti-inflammatory drugs (NSAIDs), and erosive gastritis from alcohol are the most common causes. A gastric ulcer is sometimes apparent on CT **(Fig. 6.3)** and is associated with *H. pylori* in up to 80 percent of cases. Secondary inflammation of the posterior aspect of the stomach is often present in the setting of acute **pancreatitis.** Bacterial causes other than *H. pylori* are rare but can progress to emphysematous gastritis, which carries a 60 to 80 percent mortality rate. Intramural gas is usually detectable on CT, especially within dependent portions of the stomach that are outlined by fluid. **Cytomegalovirus (CMV)** infection is an important cause of gastritis in immunosuppressed patients. Corrosive ingestion, especially with acidic agents, can result in extensive damage. Other causes of inflammatory gastric wall thickening are radiation gastritis, Crohn disease, tuberculosis, and vasculitis **(Fig. 6.4).**
- **Gastric neoplasms** arise from the mucosa, submucosa, or muscular wall **(Differential 6.2). Adenocarcinoma** accounts for over 90 percent of malignant gastric tumors. Wall thickening from adenocarcinoma usually measures greater than 10 mm and is more often focal than diffuse **(Fig. 6.5).** Tumors can be focal with a nodular,

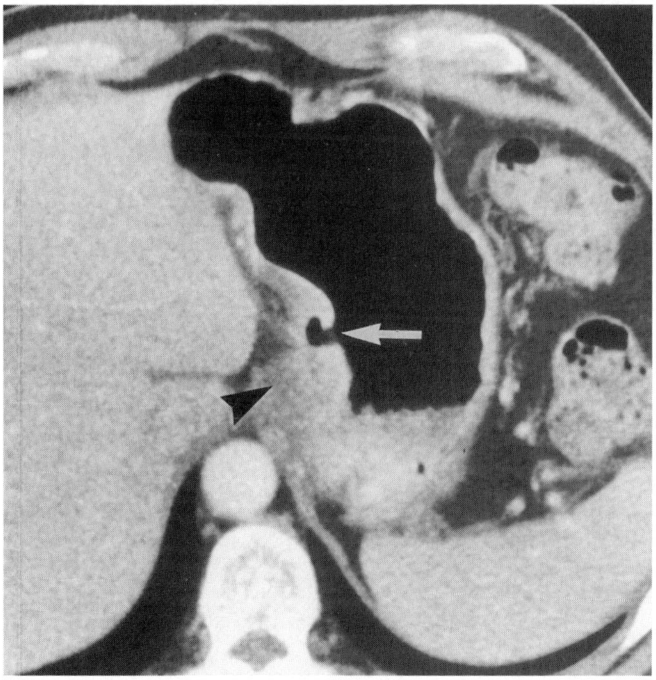

FIGURE 6.3 Benign gastric ulcer. Contrast-enhanced CT in a 52-year-old man reveals an extraluminal air collection *(arrow)* associated with gastric wall thickening along the lesser curvature and soft tissue infiltration of the adjacent fat *(arrowhead).*

6.2

GASTRIC MASS

Malignant tumor
- **Adenocarcinoma—** >90% of gastric malignancies
- **Lymphoma—**usually non-Hodgkin
- Metastases—melanoma, lung, breast, Kaposi sarcoma
- *Leiomyosarcoma*

Benign tumor
- Mesenchymal tumors—leiomyoma, lipoma, hemangioma
- Polyp—hyperplastic > adenomatous, hamartomatous

Bezoar—vegetable or hair
Surgery—fundoplication
Gastric varices
Ectopic pancreatic tissue
Hematoma—trauma, coagulopathy

lobulated, or polypoid appearance or diffusely infiltrative with rigid narrowing that is termed **linitis plastica.** Ulceration of the mass may be detected on CT; irregularity with marked thickening or a perceptible focal mass argues against benign ulcer disease. Direct ligamentous extension can result in hepatic, colonic, or pancreatic invasion. Cancers arising from the lesser curvature most often involve nodes in the gastrohepatic ligament and celiac axis, whereas cancers of the greater curvature favor omental nodes. Sensitivity and specificity for detection of metastatic nodal disease by CT depends on the size threshold used for abnormal nodal enlargement (see **Section 10.10**). Distant metastases may result from hematogenous, lymphatic, or intraperitoneal spread. CT is useful for detecting **local recurrence** in patients who have undergone subtotal gastrectomy for adenocarcinoma. The most common site for local recurrence is the celiac axis region, followed by the gastric stump or anastomosis. Prominent fluid distention of the afferent limb on CT suggests the possibility of afferent limb obstruction.

- **Lymphoma** represents approximately 5 percent of gastric malignancies. The stomach is the most common site for GI tract involvement in immunocompetent patients, accounting for 80 percent of

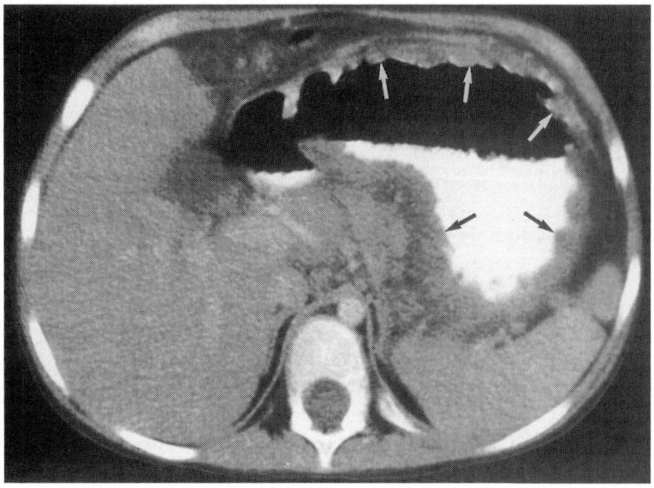

FIGURE 6.4 Gastric wall thickening in Behçet disease. Contrast-enhanced CT in an 8-year-old girl who presented with ocular inflammation, oral and genital ulcers, and GI bleeding. Diffuse nodular thickening of the gastric wall *(arrows)* is present. Colonic thickening was apparent at other levels. Endoscopy confirmed a vasculitic process.

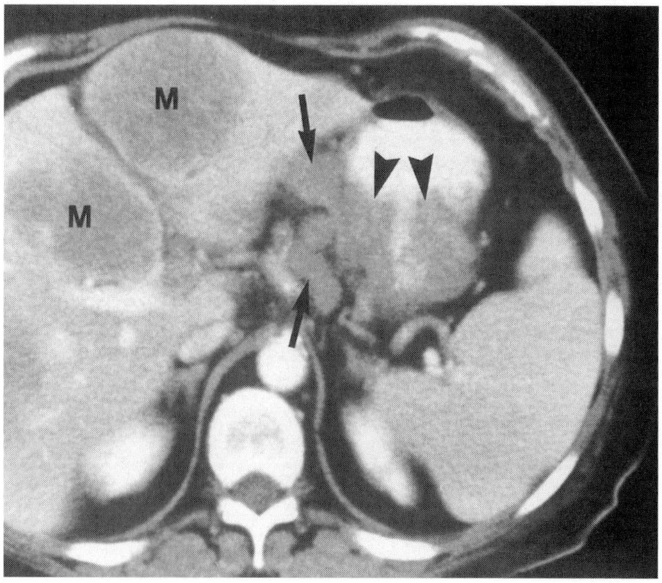

FIGURE 6.5 Gastric adenocarcinoma. Contrast-enhanced CT in a 74-year-old woman shows a large, irregular soft tissue mass involving the stomach *(arrowheads)*. Note metastatic disease involving the gastrohepatic lymph nodes *(arrows)* and liver (M).

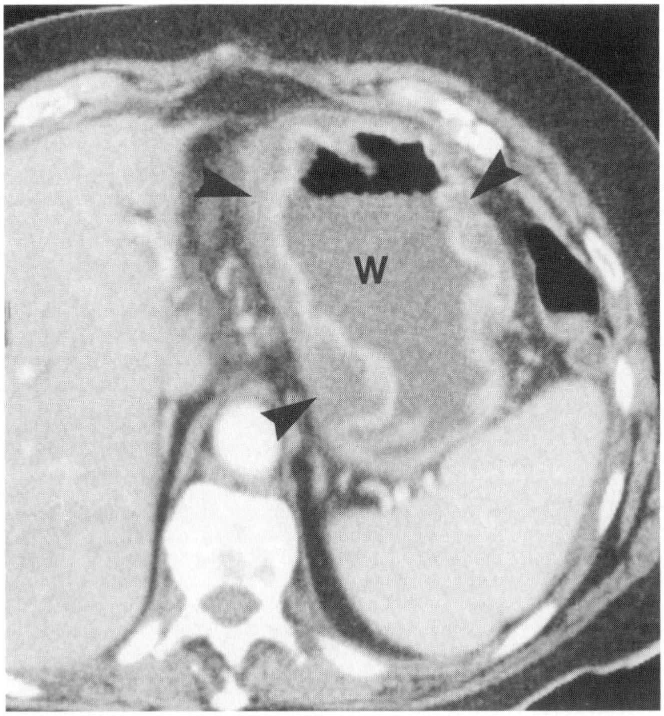

FIGURE 6.6 Gastric lymphoma. Contrast-enhanced CT in a 65-year-old woman shows diffuse low-attenuation submucosal thickening of the gastric wall *(arrowheads)*. Note how the use of water (W) as an oral contrast agent allows for the depiction of mucosal enhancement.

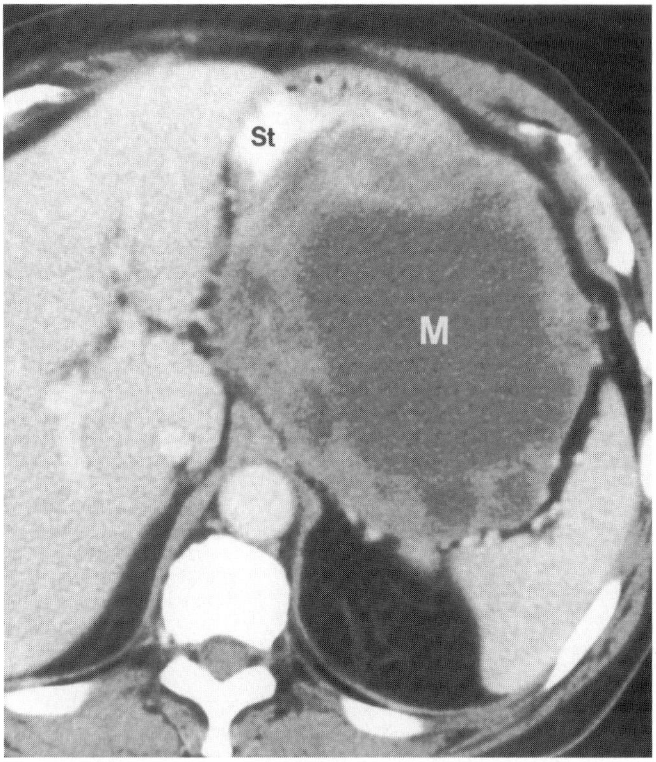

FIGURE 6.7 Malignant GI stromal tumor (leiomyosarcoma). Contrast-enhanced CT in a 63-year-old man shows a large heterogeneous mass (M) involving the posterior wall of the stomach. Note how the contrast-filled gastric lumen (St) is displaced anteriorly. Areas of low attenuation within the mass represent tumor necrosis.

cases. Over 90 percent of gastric lymphomas are of the **non-Hodgkin** variety and are usually part of a generalized process. Submucosal spread typically gives rise to diffuse wall thickening, often without significant luminal narrowing **(Fig. 6.6).** Ulceration of the mass or a focal polypoid lesion are less common features.

- **GI stromal tumors** are extramucosal mesenchymal neoplasms with either smooth muscle or neuroendocrine differentiation. **Leiomyomas** and **leiomyosarcomas** reflect smooth muscle differentiation and are the most common types. Leiomyoblastomas are rare and usually benign. On CT, these tumors are large, heterogeneous, and exophytic; they often demonstrate evidence of ulceration or necrosis at presentation **(Fig. 6.7).** Calcification is not uncommon. CT features associated with malignancy include size greater than 5 cm and central necrosis. GI stromal tumors with neuroendocrine features include neurofibromas and paragangliomas. Other benign mesenchymal neoplasms that can involve the stomach include lipomas and hemangiomas.
- **Gastric polyps** measuring greater than 1 cm in size are detected on CT if adequate distention is present. The majority of gastric polyps are **hyperplastic** or regenerative in nature and have no malignant potential. **Adenomatous** polyps are true neoplasms with a potential for malignant transformation that increases with increasing polyp size. Adenomatous polyps are associated with Gardner syndrome, although up to one-half of gastric polyps in this condition are non-adenomatous fundic gland polyps. **Hamartomatous** polyps are associated with Peutz-Jegher syndrome.
- **Metastatic disease** involving the stomach can result from direct ligamentous spread from adjacent organs such as the gallbladder, colon, and pancreas or from hematogenous dissemination from other primary malignancies **(Fig. 6.8).**
- Gastric wall thickening may result from processes other than neoplastic and inflammatory diseases. **Gastric varices** can be part of a complex of portosystemic collaterals in patients with portal hypertension or as an isolated finding in splenic vein thrombosis **(Fig. 6.9).** Gastric varices are usually located in the fundus and body. **Zollinger-Ellison syndrome** results from a pancreatic or duodenal gastrin-producing islet cell tumor and is associated with severe ulcer disease of the stomach and proximal small bowel. **Ménétrier disease** is an idiopathic protein-losing hyperplastic gastropathy; marked fold thickening is seen in the fundus and body but the antrum is typically spared. Infiltrative diseases involving the stomach include eosinophilic gastritis, amyloidosis, and sarcoidosis.
- **Gastric bezoars** represent undigested concretions that form a cast of the gastric lumen, usually from plant or hair material. The mass has a mottled appearance on CT due to air or contrast that fills interstices of the lesion **(Fig. 6.10).**

6.4 SMALL BOWEL

- **Thickening of the small bowel wall** is readily detected on CT and is an important indicator of underlying disease. In isolation, however, wall thickening is nonspecific and can result from a variety of

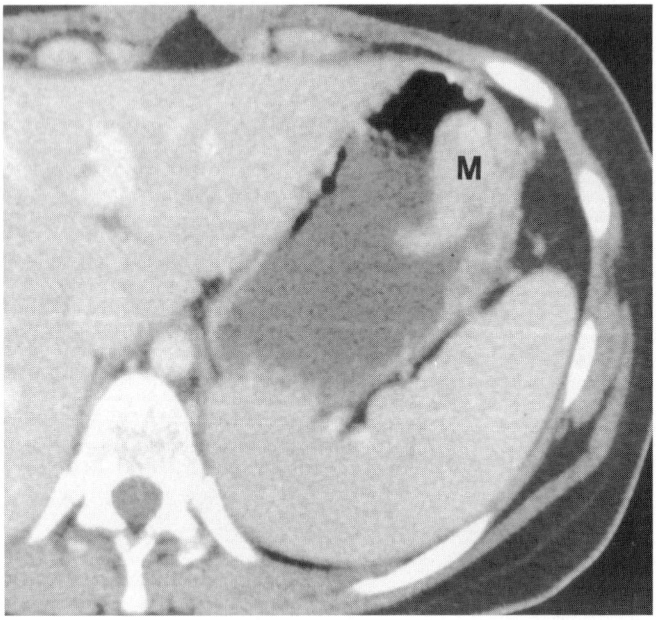

FIGURE 6.8 Gastric wall metastasis. Contrast-enhanced CT in a 23-year-old woman with abdominal pain shows a polypoid soft tissue mass (M) projecting from the greater curvature into the gastric lumen. No other lesions were present. The patient had been treated for a pelvic rhabdomyosarcoma in the past and a gastric metastasis was subsequently confirmed at endoscopy.

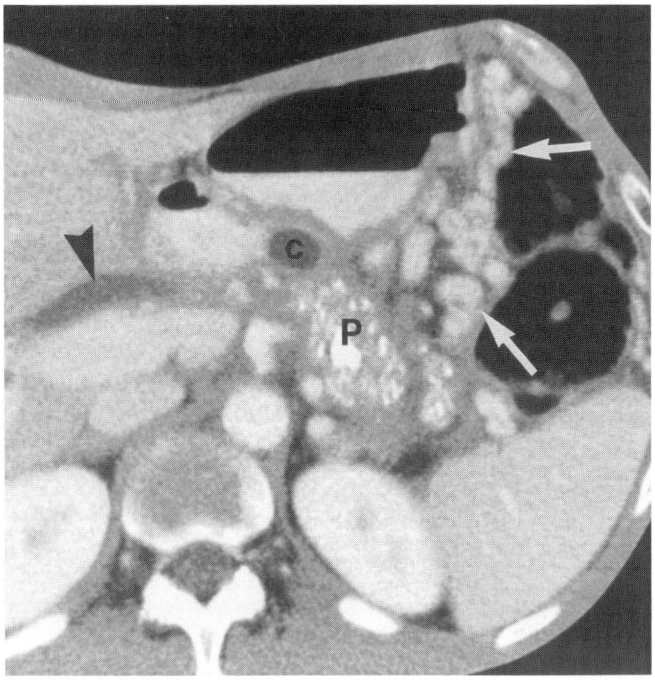

FIGURE 6.9 Gastric varices. Contrast-enhanced CT in a 44-year-old man with a history of chronic alcoholic pancreatitis shows multiple enhancing dilated vessels *(arrows)* along the posterolateral aspect of the stomach. Varices resulted from splenic vein thrombosis. Other sequelae of chronic pancreatitis seen here include coarse calcifications within the pancreas (P), dilatation of the common bile duct *(arrowhead)*, and a small pseudocyst (c).

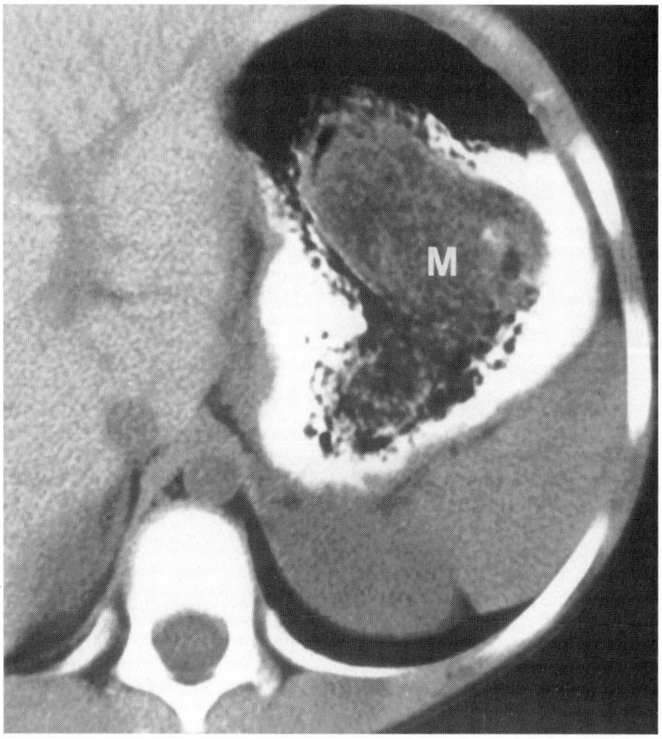

FIGURE 6.10 Gastric bezoar. Noncontrast CT in a 6-year-old girl with long hair shows a large mass (M) within the stomach that has a mottled appearance and conforms to the gastric contour. This was a trichobezoar.

diseases **(Differential 6.3).** Features that help modify the differential diagnosis include focal versus diffuse thickening, smooth versus nodular thickening, and associated findings such as lymphadenopathy and mesenteric disease. Broad categories of wall thickening include ischemia, infection, inflammation, neoplasia, noninflammatory edema, infiltrative diseases, hematoma, and lymphatic obstruction.

- **Acute mesenteric ischemia** can result from occlusive disease such as SMA thrombosis and embolism, or from nonocclusive low flow states. CT findings vary widely but bowel wall thickening from edema or hemorrhage is the most common abnormality. Lack of enhancement of an affected segment of bowel indicates infarction. Pneumatosis, sometimes with portal venous gas, may be present **(Fig. 6.11).** CT can demonstrate occlusion at the SMA origin in cases of **thrombosis**, which is usually associated with atherosclerotic calcification, whereas **embolic occlusion** typically occurs at branch points distal to the artery origin. Intraluminal thrombus is readily identified on CT in cases of superior mesenteric vein thrombosis. **Nonocclusive mesenteric ischemia** usually results from a hypotensive episode, often perioperative, in patients with underlying atherosclerotic disease **(Fig. 6.11).** Nonocclusive ischemia is also commonly seen in cases of severe trauma due to a hypotensive period followed by aggressive resuscitation resulting in reperfusion edema (see **Fig. 15.10**).
- A variety of **infectious processes** can result in thickening of the small bowel wall on CT. Parasitic infestation, as with giardiasis or strongyloidiasis, causes bowel wall thickening of the duodenum or jejunum, whereas bacterial infection, as with *Yersinia enterocolit-*

6.3 THICKENED SMALL BOWEL

Edema
- Congestive heart failure
- Hypoproteinemia—nephrotic syndrome, cirrhosis, malabsorption syndromes
- Venous congestion—thrombosis, mass (carcinoid)
- Lymphatic obstruction (secondary lymphangiectasia)—tumor, fibrosis, infection
- *Primary lymphangiectasia*
- *Angioneurotic edema*—C1 esterase inhibitor deficiency

Infection
- Proximal—giardiasis, strongyloidiasis, cryptosporidiosis
- Distal—yersiniosis, salmonellosis, CMV
- Diffuse—MAI, Whipple disease, CMV

Inflammation (enteritis)
- Crohn disease
- Vasculitis—HSP, Behçet disease, scleroderma
- Radiation—small bowel very radiosensitive
- Graft-versus-host disease
- Zollinger-Ellison syndrome
- Duodenitis—*H. pylori*/peptic, pancreatitis
- *Mastocytosis*

Tumors
- Lymphoma
- Carcinoid
- Metastases
  - Hematogenous—melanoma, breast, lung, Kaposi sarcoma
  - Peritoneal seeding—ovarian, GI malignancies

Ischemia
- Occlusive—thromboembolism
- Nonocclusive

Hematoma
- Trauma, coagulopathy, vasculitis

Infiltrative
- Eosinophilic enteritis
- *Amyloidosis*
- *Abetalipoproteinemia*

Key: CMV, cytomegalovirus; HSP, Henoch-Schönlein purpura; MAI, *Mycobacterium avium-intracellulare*.

ica or *Salmonella,* results in distal ileal disease. GI tuberculosis also favors the ileocecal region, but diffuse enteric involvement can also be seen **(Fig. 6.12).** CMV, *Mycobacterium avium-intracellulare* (MAI), and cryptosporidiosis should all be considered in the setting of AIDS with diffuse thickening of the small bowel wall. MAI often resembles Whipple disease on CT, with thickening of the small bowel wall associated with low-attenuation lymphadenopathy.

- Noninfectious **inflammatory processes** are another major disease category causing thickening of the small bowel wall. A target or double-halo appearance of the bowel wall in cross section on CT, with enhancement of the mucosal and serosal surfaces separated by low-attenuation submucosal edema, usually indicates inflammatory and not neoplastic disease **(Fig. 6.13).** Idiopathic regional enteritis, or **Crohn disease,** is an important cause of bowel inflammation (see **Section 6.6**). **Vasculitis** associated with Henoch-Schönlein purpura, Behçet disease, scleroderma, or other autoimmune disorders can result in thickening of the small bowel wall from edema and hemorrhage **(Fig. 6.13).** Wall thickening from **radiation enteritis** is the result of an obliterative endarteritis. **Graft-versus-host disease** in bone marrow transplant recipients can cause bowel wall inflammation and thickening. **Mastocytosis** is a rare systemic disease that often involves the small bowel with proliferation of mast cells in the lamina propria, resulting in wall thickening from histamine release.

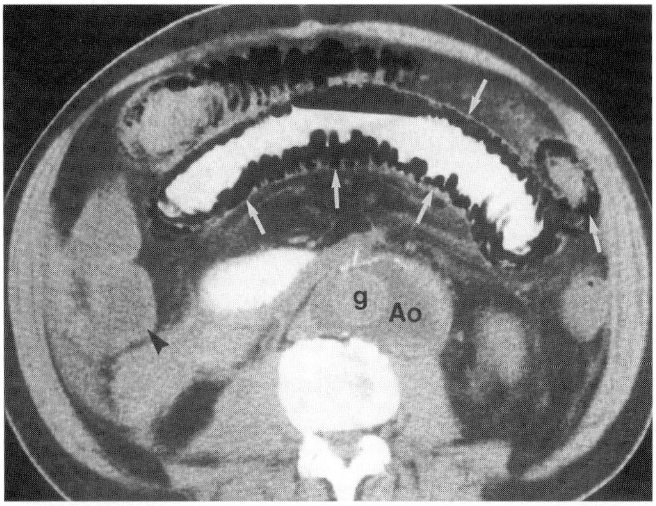

FIGURE 6.11 Acute mesenteric ischemia with pneumatosis. Noncontrast CT in a 74-year-old man with severe abdominal pain following aortic aneurysm repair shows gas within the walls of dilated small bowel loops *(arrows)*. Note how intraluminal contrast is displaced by pneumatosis, even along dependent portions of the bowel. Bowel wall thickening is present in loops without pneumatosis *(arrowhead)*. Synthetic graft (g) is present within the dilated native aorta (Ao). (Case courtesy of Dr. Matthew Fleishman, Denver, CO.)

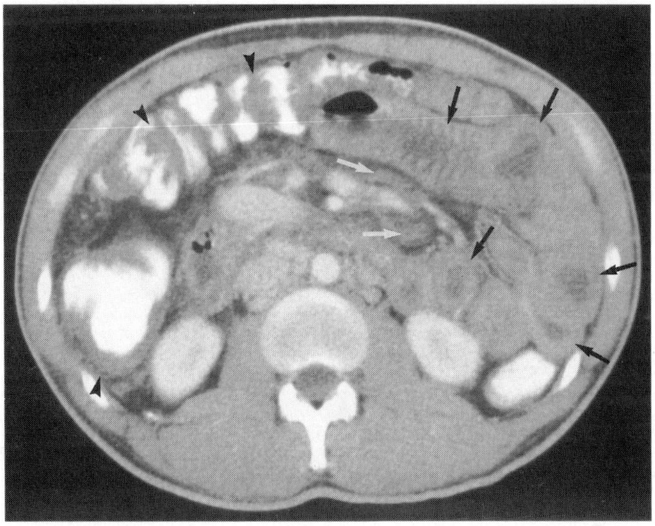

FIGURE 6.12 Intestinal tuberculosis. Contrast-enhanced CT in a 40-year-old man with a 1-year history of abdominal pain and diarrhea shows diffuse wall thickening of the small bowel *(black arrows)* and right colon *(arrowheads)*. Mesenteric soft tissue infiltration and lymphadenopathy *(white arrows)* are present. Diagnosis was confirmed on endoscopy.

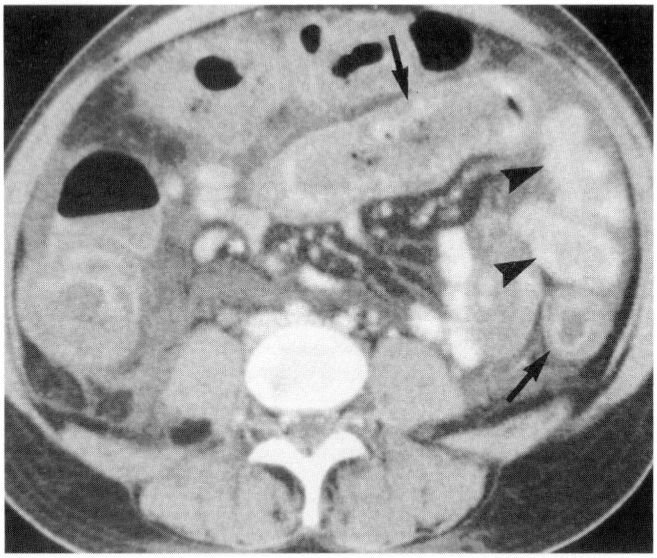

FIGURE 6.13 Bowel wall thickening in Wegener granulomatosis. Contrast-enhanced CT in a 26-year-old man with GI bleeding and a recent diagnosis of Wegener granulomatosis shows diffuse bowel wall thickening, mesenteric inflammation, and ascites. Some loops demonstrate a target appearance or mural striation *(arrows),* whereas other loops show diffuse high-attenuation wall thickening *(arrowheads).* Hemorrhagic necrosis and edema from vasculitis were confirmed after surgery.

- **Small bowel neoplasms** are depicted by CT as focal mass lesions or wall thickening, occasionally with associated ulceration, intussusception, obstruction, or mesenteric involvement **(Differential 6.4).** The small bowel is the second most common site of GI **lymphoma** after the stomach, although this order is reversed in immunosuppressed states such as AIDS and solid organ transplantation **(Fig. 6.14).** As with all extranodal disease, **non-Hodgkin lymphoma** predominates over Hodgkin disease. A common pattern on CT is focal, circumferential wall thickening with

6.4
SMALL BOWEL MASS

Malignant tumor
- **Lymphoma**
- Adenocarcinoma
- Metastases
  - Hematogenous—melanoma, breast, lung, Kaposi
  - Peritoneal seeding—ovarian, GI malignancies
- *Leiomyosarcoma*

Benign tumor
- **Leiomyoma**
- **Carcinoid** (can be benign or malignant)
- Lipoma
- Hemangioma
- Adenoma
- *Neurofibroma*

Polyps—adenomatous, hamartomatous, inflammatory
Duplication cyst
Hematoma

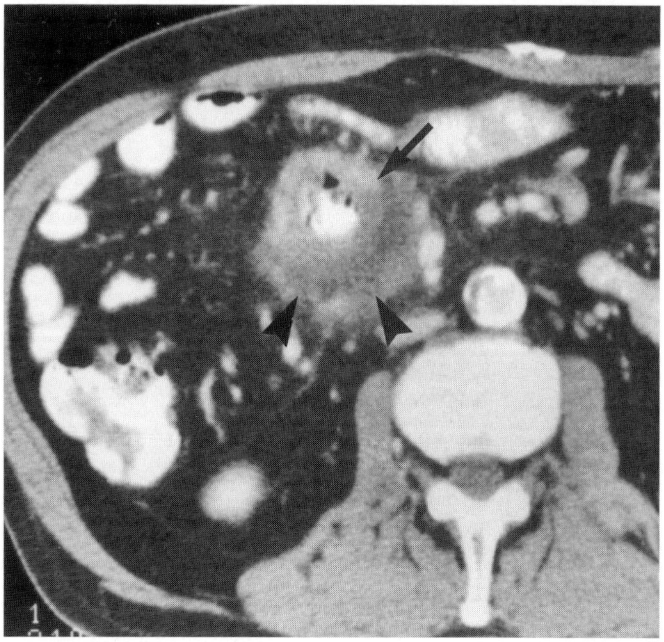

FIGURE 6.14 Small bowel lymphoma. Contrast-enhanced CT in a 67-year-old man with abdominal pain shows circumferential wall thickening of an ileal loop *(arrow)* with mild luminal excavation. Infiltration of surrounding mesenteric fat *(arrowheads)* was due to focal perforation, confirmed at surgery. The patient had undergone heart transplantation 4 years earlier. (From Pickhardt PJ, Siegel MJ. Abdominal manifestations of posttransplantation lymphoproliferative disorder. *AJR* 1998;171:1007–1013. With permission.)

aneurysmal dilatation and luminal excavation. Obstruction is uncommon despite large tumor size. Associated lymphadenopathy is a common finding. **Carcinoid** is the most common primary small bowel tumor. This neuroendocrine neoplasm actually involves the appendix more commonly but is usually asymptomatic. The desmoplastic nature of the tumor can be appreciated on CT and is depicted as a stellate, retractile mesenteric mass that tethers and thickens adjacent small bowel loops. **(Fig. 6.15).** Punctate calcification within the mesenteric mass is a common associated finding, seen in approximately 70 percent of cases. The actual primary tumor within the small bowel wall is seldom recognized on CT. Patients with liver metastases may demonstrate the **carcinoid syndrome,** which is caused by the systemic effect of vasoactive amines and is characterized by diarrhea, flushing, asthma, and endocardial fibroelastosis affecting the right heart.

- **Adenocarcinoma** of the small bowel is rare and tends to occur in the duodenum or jejunum. Duodenal adenocarcinoma most often arises in villous tumors of the periampullary region **(Fig. 6.16). GI stromal tumors** of the small bowel resemble those of the stomach. Leiomyomas represent the most common benign neoplasm of the small bowel. Other benign tumors include lipoma, hemangioma, and neurogenic tumors. **Metastatic disease** can involve the small bowel by either hematogenous spread or intraperitoneal seeding. Tumors commonly associated with hematogenous spread include melanoma, breast, lung, and Kaposi sarcoma.

- Many miscellaneous entities can result in bowel wall thickening. Causes of **noninflammatory edema** include congestive heart failure, nephrotic syndrome, hypoalbuminemia, and angioneurotic

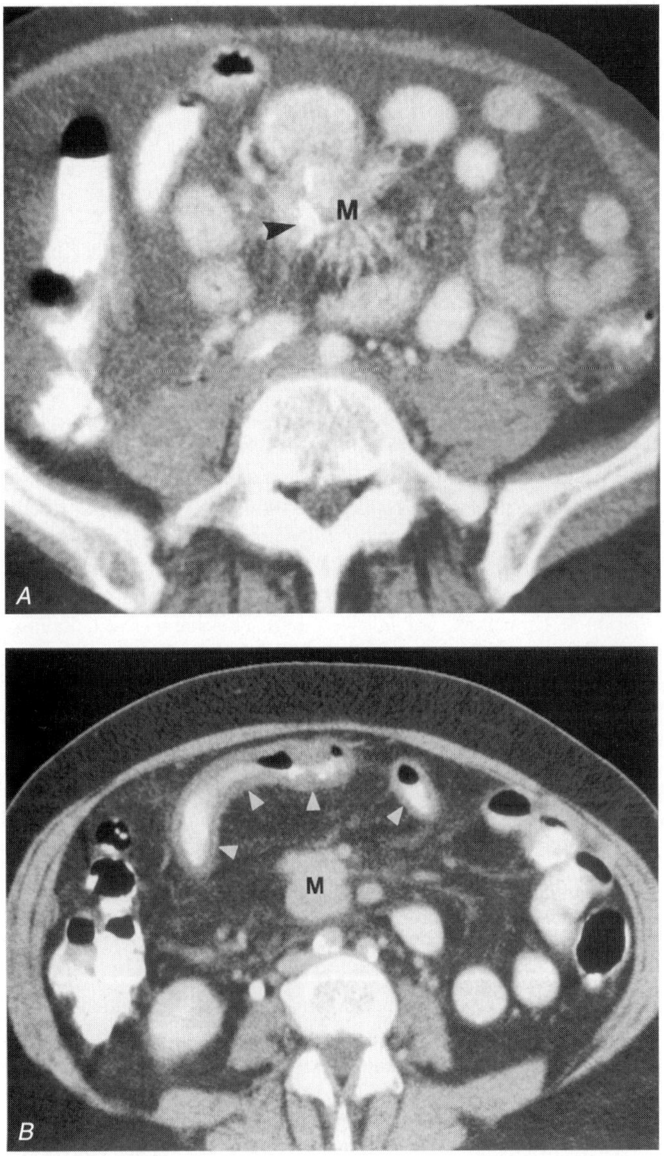

FIGURE 6.15 Small bowel carcinoid tumor. *(A)* Contrast-enhanced CT in a 70-year-old man with carcinoid syndrome shows a stellate mesenteric mass (M) with associated calcification *(arrowhead)*. Ascites was due to right-sided heart failure and diffuse hepatic metastases. *(B)* Contrast-enhanced CT in a 67-year-old woman shows a mesenteric soft tissue mass (M) and circumferential wall thickening of adjacent small bowel loops *(arrowheads)*.

edema. The malabsorption syndromes are an important cause of hypoalbuminemia, leading to thickening of the small bowel folds; celiac disease is the most common entity in this category. **Infiltrative diseases** include eosinophilic enteritis, amyloidosis, and abetalipoproteinemia. Intramural small bowel **hematoma** can occur in the setting of trauma, coagulopathy, and vasculitis. **Lymphatic disease** resulting in wall thickening can be congenital in nature (primary lymphangiectasia) or due to infiltration by tumor, infection, or fibrosis (secondary lymphangiectasia).

- CT is useful when there is clinical suspicion of **small bowel obstruction** and is often able to identify the level of obstruction, suggest the underlying cause **(Differential 6.5),** and assess for

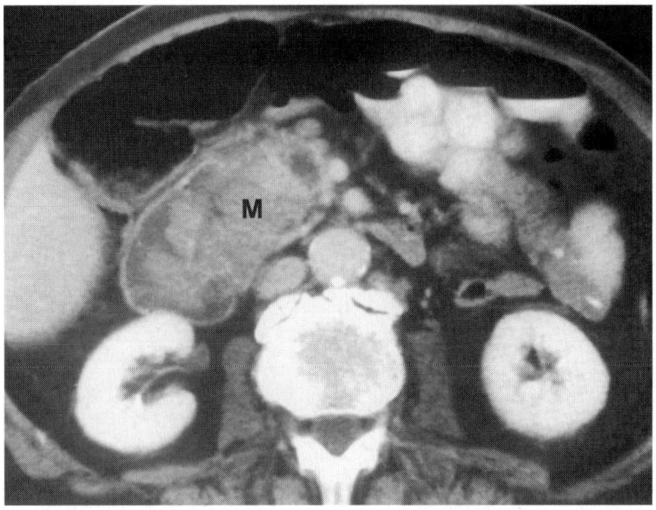

FIGURE 6.16 Duodenal villous adenocarcinoma. Contrast-enhanced CT in a 90-year-old man with nausea and emesis shows a large soft tissue mass (M) arising from the periampullary region and expanding the duodenum. The frond-like appearance suggests a villous tumor and the size favors malignancy. (Case courtesy of Dr. Matthew Fleishman, Denver, CO.)

evidence of strangulation. The diagnosis of obstruction is based on the presence of dilated bowel proximal to a **transition point,** where bowel becomes normal in caliber **(Fig. 6.17).** CT is valuable for identifying cases of **closed-loop obstruction,** where a segment of bowel is occluded at two points **(Fig. 6.18).** A fixed, radial distribution of dilated small bowel loops with convergence of the mesenteric vessels to the point of obstruction is characteristic.

6.5 DILATED BOWEL

Obstruction
- **Adhesions—**surgery, peritonitis, radiation
- **Hernia—**95% external
- **Inflammation—**diverticulitis, appendicitis, abscess
- **Tumor—**colon carcinoma, serosal metastases
- Intussusception—lead mass, celiac disease, scleroderma
- Volvulus—sigmoid, cecal, midgut, *transverse*
- Foreign body—gallstone, ascariasis
- Stricture—Crohn disease, radiation, ischemic
- Hematoma—trauma, coagulopathy, vasculitis
- Fecal impaction

Adynamic ileus
- **Recent surgery,** peritonitis, medications, pancreatitis, electrolyte imbalance, abdominal infection, gastroenteritis

Idiopathic pseudo-obstruction
- Small bowel—scleroderma, *primary neuromuscular*
- Colon—Ogilvie syndrome

Celiac disease (nontropical sprue)—small bowel dilatation

Toxic colitis
- UC, PMC, Crohn disease, ischemia, amebiasis, CMV

Laxative abuse—colonic dilatation

Chagas disease—colonic dilatation

Key: CMV, cytomegalovirus; PMC, pseudomembranous colitis; UC, ulcerative colitis.

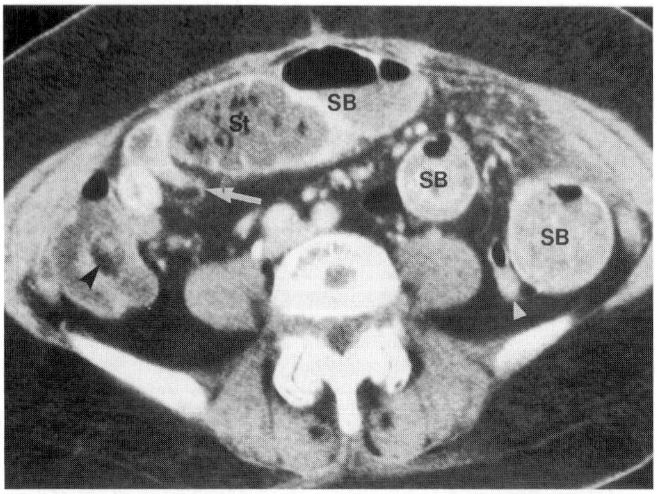

FIGURE 6.17 High-grade small bowel obstruction. Contrast-enhanced CT in a 72-year-old woman with a history of prior abdominal surgery demonstrates multiple dilated small bowel loops (SB) and normal caliber colon *(white arrowhead).* A transition point *(arrow)* without an associated mass is present and was due to an adhesion. Fecal-appearing material near the transition point in the distal ileum represents "small bowel stool" (St) and usually indicates high-grade obstruction. Note the normal fatty appearance of the ileocecal valve *(black arrowhead).*

Identification of a closed-loop obstruction is important because treatment is surgical, owing to the high incidence of strangulation.

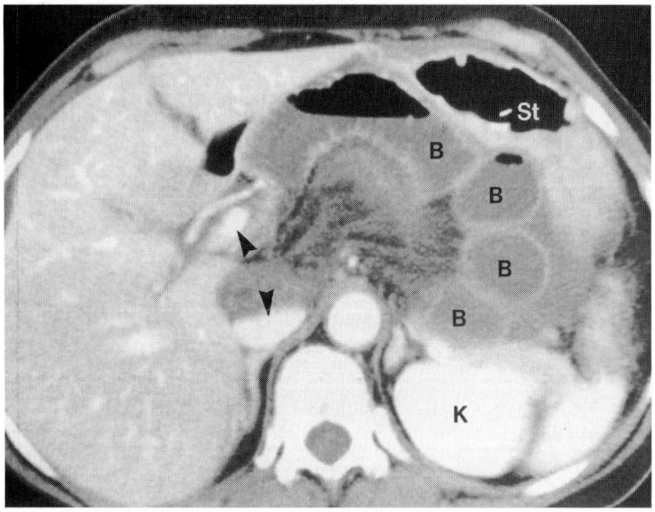

FIGURE 6.18 Internal hernia with closed-loop obstruction. Contrast-enhanced CT in a 48-year-old woman with a sudden onset of epigastric pain shows herniation of fluid-filled small bowel loops (B) into the lesser sac. The stomach (St) is displaced anteriorly. Features of a closed-loop obstruction include a radial arrangement of herniated loops and convergence of mesenteric vessels toward the foramen of Winslow, which is located between the inferior vena cava and the portal vein *(arrowheads).* Ascites, mesenteric infiltration, and bowel wall thickening are concerning for vascular compromise. K, left kidney.

CT signs of **strangulation** include increased bowel wall attenuation on unenhanced images, bowel wall thickening, pneumatosis, delayed and persistent wall enhancement, and lack of enhancement. In some cases of high-grade small bowel obstruction, CT may demonstrate the presence of fecal-appearing intraluminal material proximal to the transition point, the **"small bowel stool" (Fig. 6.17).**

- Postoperative **adhesions** are the single most common cause of all small bowel obstruction **(Fig. 6.17).** An abrupt transition without an apparent cause, such as an inflammatory mass or neoplasm (see **Fig. 6.33**), is the typical appearance on CT. **Hernias** are another common cause of obstruction and are well evaluated by CT **(Figs. 6.18 and 6.19).** Abnormal protrusion through fascial defects can be internal or external, with the latter accounting for about 95 percent of cases. Inguinal herniation accounts for about 75 percent of all **external hernias.** Other types of external hernias include ventral, umbilical, femoral, incisional, lumbar, parastomal, spigelian, sciatic, and obturator **(Fig. 6.19). Internal hernias** are less common and include paraduodenal and foramen of Winslow types among others. The feared complication of hernias is incarceration, leading to obstruction and strangulation **(Fig. 6.18).** Other causes of small bowel obstruction include intussusception, volvulus, postinflammatory stricture, hematoma, and gallstone ileus. The characteristic findings of gallstone ileus—ectopic gallstones, small bowel obstruction, and pneumobilia **(Rigler triad)—**are more often detected by CT than by conventional radiography.

6.5 COLON AND RECTUM

- **Acute appendicitis** remains the most common cause of acute abdominal pain requiring surgery in the United States and affects approximately 6 percent of the population. Although traditionally considered a clinical diagnosis, a high rate of false-positive appendectomies was accepted in the past. Currently, both CT and ultrasound are being performed more frequently in patients with suspected appendicitis, especially among the elderly, children, and women of reproductive age, where the rate of misdiagnosis is highest. CT examination performed with spiral technique and relatively thin collimation yields a high sensitivity and specificity (well above 90 percent) regardless of the particular contrast regimen employed. Advantages of performing CT include earlier diagnosis, identification of complications, and a reduction in the number of unnecessary operations.

  CT findings in acute appendicitis consist of an abnormal appendix that measures greater than 6 mm in diameter and has a thickened enhancing wall, associated with periappendiceal inflammation and cecal changes **(Fig. 6.20).** Inflammation of the periappendiceal fat ranges from mild stranding to phlegmon or abscess formation. The presence of an appendicolith supports the diagnosis but is not in itself diagnostic. Variants to be aware of include distal (or tip) appendicitis, where the proximal segment is normal, and chronic or recurrent appendicitis. Other inflammatory and neoplastic conditions affecting the ileocecal region can mimic appendicitis **(Differential 6.6).**

- **Mucocele** of the appendix can result from simple luminal obstruction leading to distention or, rarely, from a mucinous neoplasm. CT findings are characteristic—an oblong, low-attenuation mass impressing on the medial aspect of the cecum at the level of the appendiceal orifice **(Fig. 6.21).** Rim calcification is occasionally seen. Rupture of the extremely rare mucinous cystadenocarcinoma of the appendix can result in recalcitrant gelatinous ascites, referred to as **pseudomyxoma peritonei** (see **Fig. 10.6**).

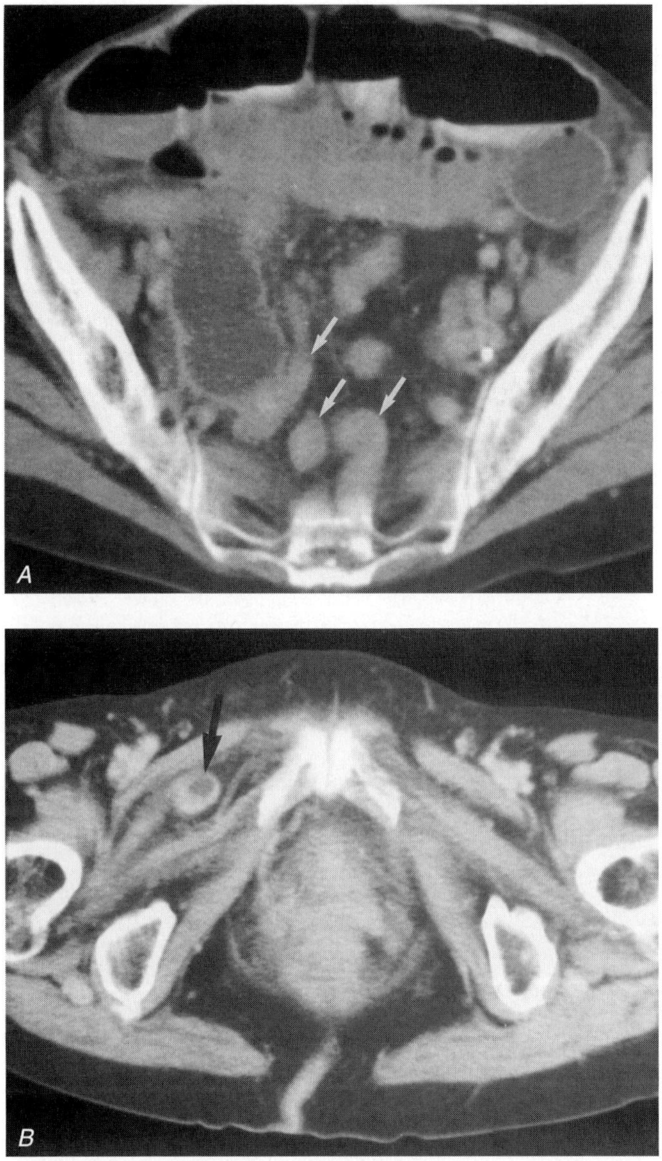

FIGURE 6.19 **Small bowel obstruction due to obturator hernia.** Contrast-enhanced CT in an 81-year-old woman shows *(A)* multiple dilated small bowel loops with air-fluid levels. The presence of decompressed small bowel loops *(arrows)* suggests a transition point. A more caudal section *(B)* through the pelvis demonstrates a knuckle of bowel *(arrow)* herniating between fascicles of the obturator externus muscle, representing the cause of obstruction.

- Colonic inflammation, or **colitis,** has both infectious and noninfectious causes **(Differential 6.7).** CT demonstrates nonspecific wall thickening, often with a double-halo or target appearance and stranding of the pericolonic fat. Its utility, however, lies in the detection of extraluminal complications, such as abscess.
- **Pseudomembranous colitis (PMC)** typically occurs in the setting of diarrhea following a recent course of antibiotics; it results from a toxin produced by *Clostridium difficile*. Patients often present with nonspecific abdominal pain and the diagnosis of PMC may be first suggested on CT, especially in cases where sigmoidoscopy is normal. Typical CT manifestations of PMC include prominent colonic wall thickening, intramural low attenuation, and involvement of the entire colon **(Fig. 6.22).** Disease is occasionally confined to the right colon. The CT appearance of intraluminal contrast trapped between thickened haustra in PMC constitutes the **accordion sign.** Inflammation of the pericolonic fat and ascites are present in up to one-half of cases.

  Other **infectious etiologies** of colitis include viral, bacterial, fungal, and parasitic pathogens. **CMV colitis** occurs in immunocompromised individuals and results in marked low-attenuation colonic wall thickening similar in appearance to that of PMC **(Fig. 6.23). Histoplasmosis** is another opportunistic infection that can

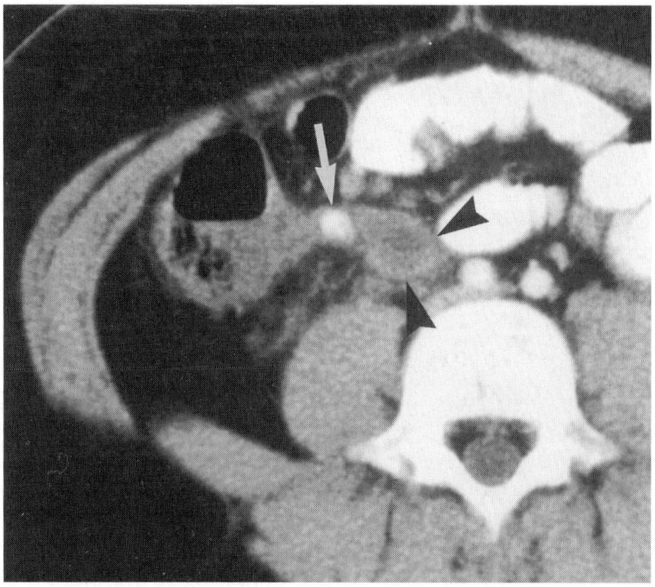

FIGURE 6.20 **Appendicitis.** Contrast-enhanced CT in a 10-year-old girl shows a dense appendicolith *(arrow)* and dilated, enhancing appendix *(arrowheads)* with associated soft tissue infiltration of periappendiceal fat.

6.6

THICKENED ILEOCECAL REGION

Inflammation
- **Crohn disease**
- **Appendicitis**
- Diverticulitis—ileal, cecal
- Ulcerative colitis—backwash ileitis
- Radiation
- Neutropenic colitis—cecal

Infection—yersiniosis, salmonellosis, TB, CMV, amebiasis
Tumor—lymphoma, carcinoid, cecal adenocarcinoma, metastasis
Mucocele
Hematoma—trauma, coagulopathy, vasculitis
Ischemia—thromboembolic disease

Key: CMV, cytomegalovirus; TB, tuberculosis.

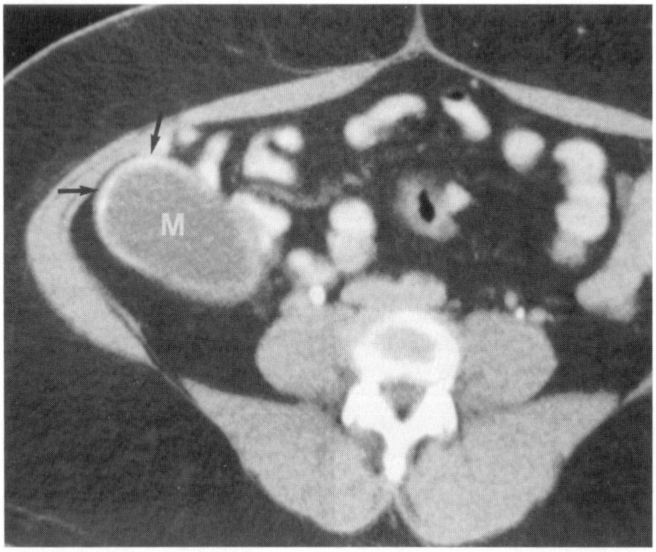

FIGURE 6.21 Mucocele of the appendix. Contrast-enhanced CT in a 58-year-old woman shows an ovoid cystic mass (M), which impressed upon the medial aspect of the cecum on other images. Note rim calcification *(arrows)*.

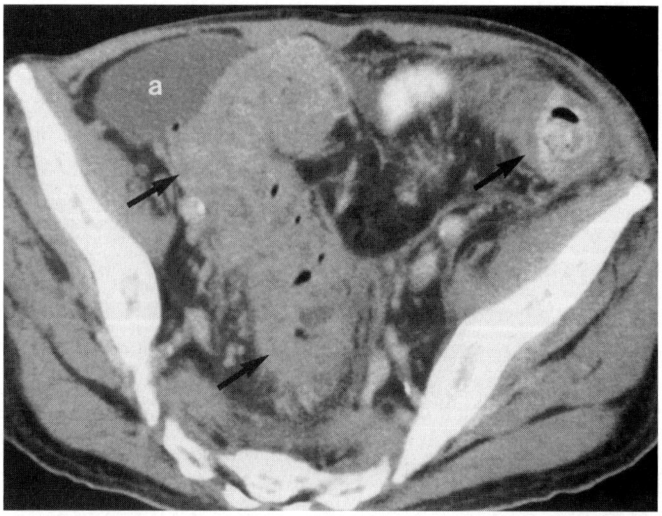

FIGURE 6.22 Pseudomembranous colitis. Contrast-enhanced CT in a 64-year-old man with abdominal pain shows marked colonic wall thickening *(arrows)*, ascites (a), and inflammatory stranding of the pericolonic fat. The entire colon was similarly involved. The patient denied diarrhea but had been taking antibiotics recently. Stool sample was positive for *Clostridium difficile* toxin.

involve the colon in such patients, but this process is typically more localized. Yersiniosis, salmonellosis, tuberculosis, and amebiasis have a predilection for the right colon.

- Causes of **noninfectious colitis** include inflammatory bowel disease, vasculitis, neutropenic colitis, radiation colitis, and ischemia. Diverticulitis, strictly speaking, consists primarily of pericolonic inflammation and is considered separately.

6.7 THICKENED COLON

Inflammation
  Diverticulitis
  Ulcerative colitis
  Crohn disease
  Typhlitis
  Vasculitis
  Radiation
Infection
  Pseudomembranous colitis—*C. difficile*
  Bacterial—TB, *Yersinia, Salmonella, Shigella, E. coli*
  Viral—CMV
  Fungal—histoplasmosis
  Parasitic—amebiasis, schistosomiasis
Ischemia—classically splenic flexure and descending colon
Tumor
  Adenocarcinoma
  Lymphoma
  Metastases—serosal > hematogenous
Toxic colitis—UC > PMC, Crohn, ischemia, amebiasis, CMV
Hematoma—trauma, coagulopathy, vasculitis
Amyloidosis
Angioneurotic edema—C1 esterase inhibitor deficiency

Key: CMV, cytomegalovirus; PMC, pseudomembranous colitis; UC, ulcerative colitis.

- **Ulcerative colitis (UC)** is an idiopathic inflammatory condition that invariably involves the rectum and demonstrates contiguous extension proximally to involve the colon for a variable length. On CT, mild to moderate circumferential colonic wall thickening of the affected segment is the major finding and usually measures less than 10 mm. In severe cases, patients may present acutely with life-threatening **toxic colitis** due to extensive inflammation **(Fig. 6.24);** enema examination is contraindicated in these patients because of the risk of perforation. ***Toxic colitis,*** which is a more appropriate

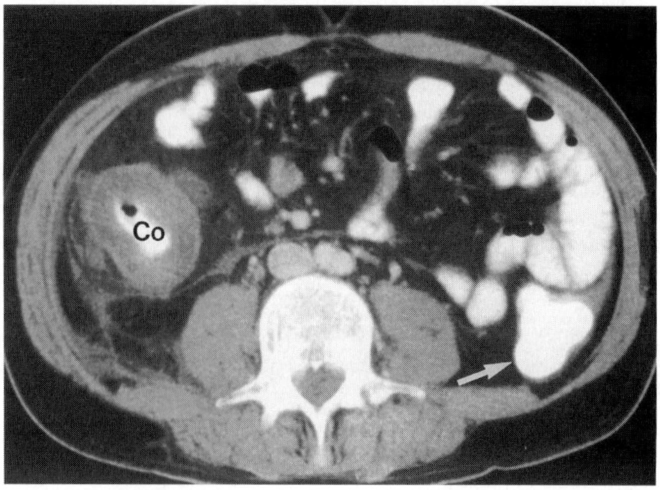

FIGURE 6.23 CMV colitis. Contrast-enhanced CT in a 41-year-old HIV-positive man with right-lower-quadrant pain demonstrates prominent low-attenuation wall thickening of the right colon (Co) with stranding of the pericolonic fat. Note normal left colon *(arrow)*.

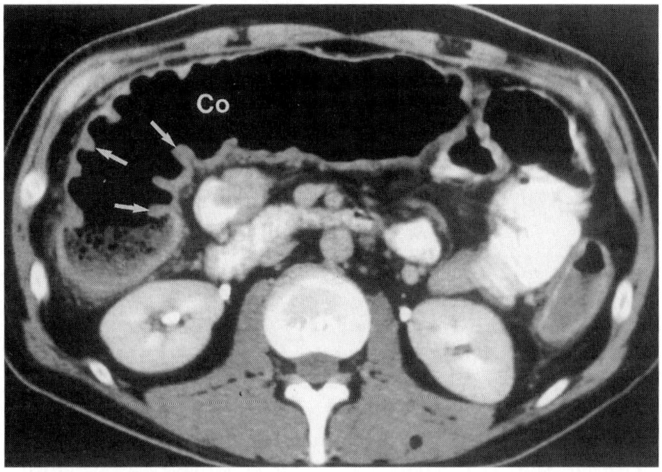

FIGURE 6.24 Toxic colitis. Contrast-enhanced CT in a 34-year-old with history of ulcerative colitis who presented acutely with fever, leukocytosis, and abdominal pain shows massive colonic distention (Co) with haustral-fold thickening *(arrows).*

term than ***toxic megacolon,*** since dilatation is not always present, is also related to other disease processes **(Differential 6.7).** In long-standing UC, a target appearance of the rectum and colon with central low attenuation reflects submucosal fat deposition or edema, often associated with proliferation of the perirectal fat. Patients with UC are at increased risk for colonic adenocarcinoma, but, unlike the case in Crohn disease, extraluminal inflammatory complications are unusual, since it is predominantly a mucosal disease.

- **Vasculitis** from Behçet disease, lupus, Wegener granulomatosis, or other vasculitides can result in colonic thickening from edema or hemorrhage (see **Fig. 6.13**). **Neutropenic colitis,** or typhlitis, manifests radiographically with prominent wall thickening of the right colon, with or without pneumatosis **(Fig. 6.25). Radiation** colitis can present clinically in an acute or chronic form and results from an obliterative endarteritis; CT shows modest wall thickening. **Crohn disease** involvement of the colon, also referred to as granulomatous colitis, is covered in more detail in **Section 6.6.**
- **Ischemic colitis,** unlike mesenteric ischemia, is typically a self-limited disease affecting older patients that can be managed conservatively. Approximately one-third of patients experience a more fulminant course of disease. Surgical intervention is reserved for cases where necrosis and perforation are likely. Arterial insufficiency is the most frequent underlying cause; venous thrombosis is responsible in a minority of cases. On CT, mild to moderate wall thickening involving the splenic flexure and descending colon is the classic appearance **(Fig. 6.26);** other colonic segments are less frequently affected. Pneumatosis and portal venous gas usually signify more severe ischemia. Stricture formation after the healing phase is relatively common and can occur even in uncomplicated cases.
- Because **colonic diverticulitis** is an extraluminal process, CT is an ideal method for detecting and staging its extent. Diverticulosis of the sigmoid colon is extremely common among older adults and manifests itselfs on CT as multiple rounded extraluminal air-filled outpouchings, often associated with muscular hypertrophy of the colonic wall. Diverticular inflammation, or diverticulitis, usually presents with left-lower-quadrant pain, fever, and leukocytosis. CT has been shown to be useful in confirming the diagnosis and, more

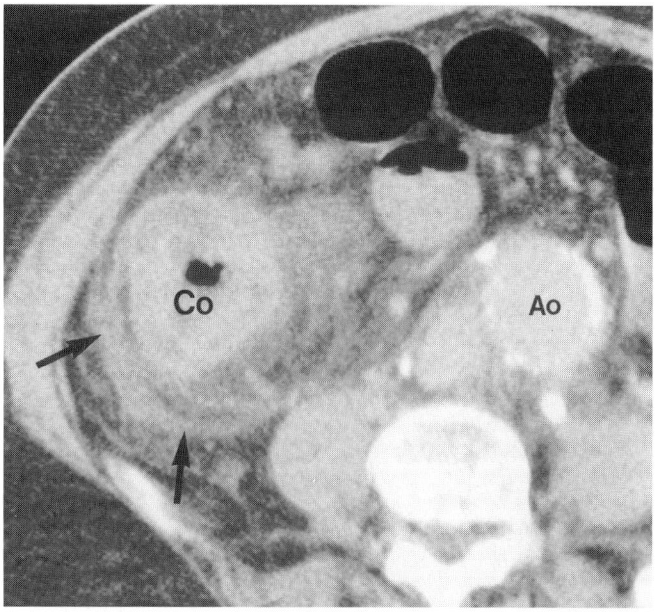

FIGURE 6.25 Neutropenic colitis. Contrast-enhanced CT in a 62-year-old man with fever, right-lower-quadrant pain, and diarrhea shows marked inflammatory changes involving the right colon (Co) and pericolonic fat *(arrows).* The patient was pancytopenic from recent chemotherapy for acute myelogenous leukemia. Dilated small bowel loops reflect adynamic ileus and/or obstruction. Incidentally noted is an abdominal aortic aneurysm (Ao).

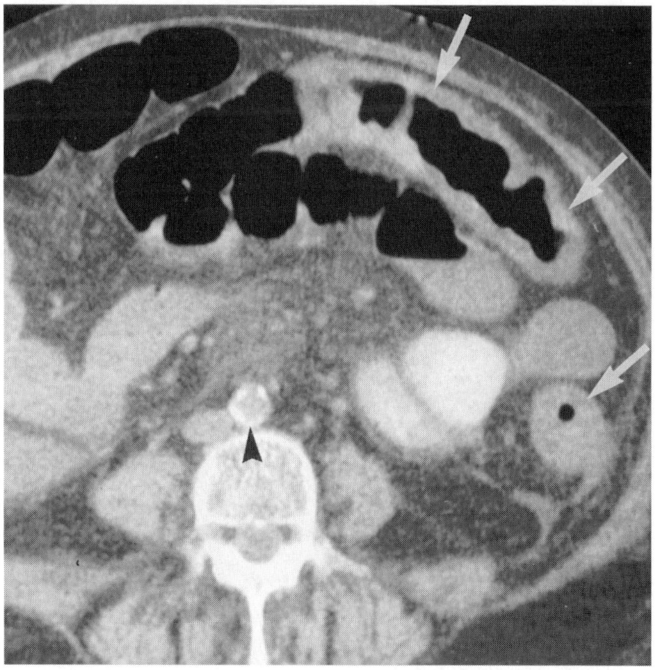

FIGURE 6.26 Ischemic colitis. Contrast-enhanced CT in a 76-year-old woman shows moderate wall thickening near the splenic flexure *(arrows).* Diffuse atherosclerotic changes were present throughout the aortoiliac system *(arrowhead).*

importantly, determining which patients will benefit from conservative therapy and which will require more invasive intervention.

CT findings of diverticulitis consist of stranding and increased density of the pericolonic fat associated with the presence of diverticula and wall thickening **(Fig. 6.27).** A focal extraluminal fluid collection signifies peridiverticular abscess and usually requires drainage, either surgically or percutaneously under CT guidance **(Fig. 6.28).** In cases where sigmoid resection is necessary, preoperative percutaneous abscess drainage has decreased surgical morbidity by allowing for primary bowel anastomosis, thus avoiding a two-stage surgical procedure. CT may also demonstrate fistula formation, most commonly involving the bladder—a colovesical fistula **(Fig. 6.28).** The main differential diagnostic considerations in diverticulitis are Crohn disease and perforated adenocarcinoma. The CT features of each disease overlap significantly **(Fig. 6.29).** Correct diagnosis usually requires a combination of clinical history, follow-up imaging, endoscopy, or surgery.

Right-sided diverticulitis is a difficult clinical diagnosis and accounts for up to 5 percent of cases. If the diagnosis is suggested from the CT findings, unnecessary surgery may be avoided. Patients usually present with symptoms resembling acute appendicitis. CT findings are analogous to those of sigmoid diverticulitis, although coexisting noninflamed diverticula are often absent.

- **Colonic neoplasms** range from incidental benign lesions to aggressive malignancies **(Differential 6.8).** Benign colonic tumors rarely require imaging unless complications arise. Adenomatous polyps may be seen incidentally on CT if large enough and if adequate luminal distention is present. Most submucosal tumors will have a nonspecific appearance on CT with the exception of **colonic lipomas,** where a specific diagnosis can be made **(Fig. 6.30).**

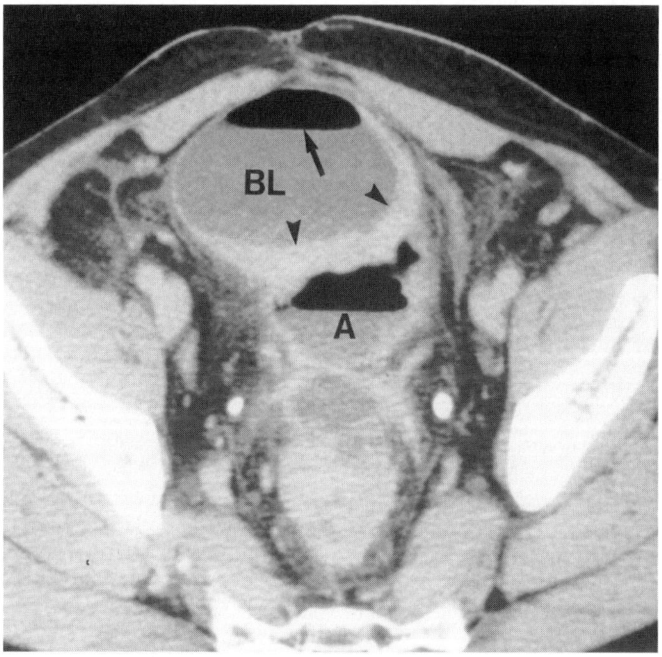

FIGURE 6.28 Peridiverticular abscess and colovesical fistula. Contrast-enhanced CT in a 53-year-old man with a 1-day history of pneumaturia superimposed upon several weeks of intermittent fever and abdominal pain. An extraluminal air-fluid collection with an enhancing rim represents a peridiverticular abscess (A). Air *(arrow)* within the bladder (BL) and thickening of the posterior wall *(arrowheads)* are due to colovesical fistula. Sigmoid diverticulitis was apparent on other levels.

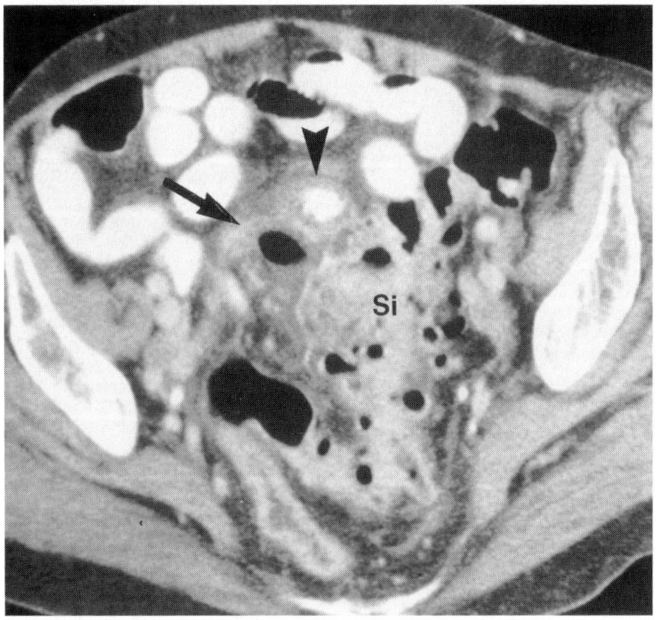

FIGURE 6.27 Sigmoid diverticulitis. Contrast-enhanced CT in an 84-year-old woman with fever, leukocytosis, and abdominal pain shows diverticulosis of the sigmoid colon (Si) and inflammatory stranding around a focus of extraluminal air *(arrow).* The inflammatory process also thickens an adjacent small bowel loop *(arrowhead).*

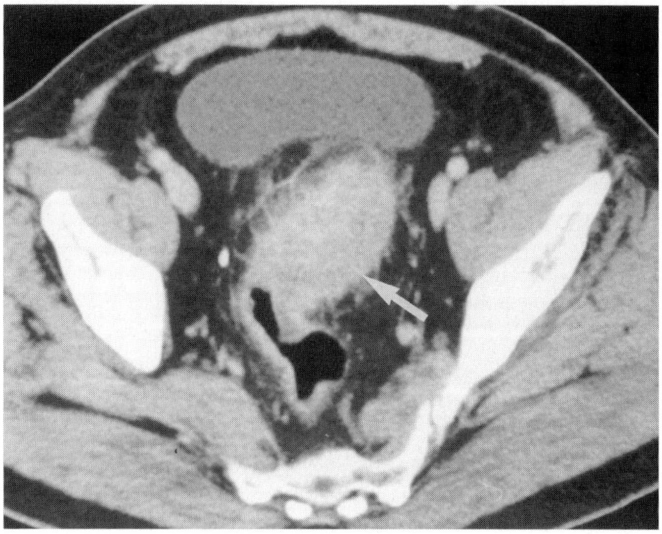

FIGURE 6.29 Diverticulitis simulating adenocarcinoma. Contrast-enhanced CT in a 62-year-old man shows mass-like soft tissue thickening of the sigmoid colon *(arrow)* with mild infiltration of the sigmoid mesentery. The diagnosis of carcinoma was favored, but this was diverticulitis.

6.8

COLONIC MASS

Polyps
- **Adenomatous—**tubular, tubulovillous and villous types, familial adenomatous polyposis syndromes
- Hamartomatous—Peutz-Jegher, Cowden, juvenile polyps
- Hyperplastic—typically <5 mm
- Inflammatory—Cronkhite-Canada

Tumors
- **Adenocarcinoma**
- Lymphoma—typically immunocompromised
- Metastases
- Carcinoid
- Mesenchymal tumors—lipoma, leiomyoma, hemangioma

Mucocele
Hematoma—trauma, coagulopathy, vasculitis
Infection—ameboma, histoplasmoma

- **Adenocarcinoma** of the colon and rectum represents the most common GI malignancy. The majority of these tumors arise in the sigmoid colon and rectum, but any colonic segment can be involved. CT is routinely used for the preoperative staging of colorectal cancer. Factors affecting prognosis include extension of the primary tumor into or through the muscularis propria, regional lymph node involvement, and metastatic disease. Adenocarcinoma is often depicted on CT as an eccentric, lobulated soft tissue mass or as a region of circumferential wall thickening and luminal narrowing (**Figs. 6.31** and **6.32**). Pericolonic soft tissue infiltration can represent local tumor extension or secondary inflammation.

  The liver is the most common site for hematogenous spread of adenocarcinoma. CT is important for the detection of hepatic metastases. Other findings in colon cancer include mesenteric lymphadenopathy, peritoneal seeding, proximal bowel obstruction, and

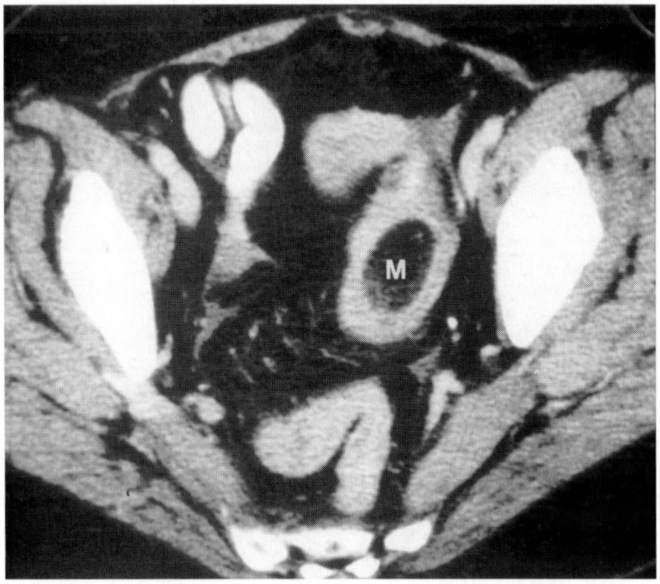

FIGURE 6.30 Colonic lipoma. Contrast-enhanced CT in a 58-year-old woman shows a sigmoid mass (M) of homogeneous fat density.

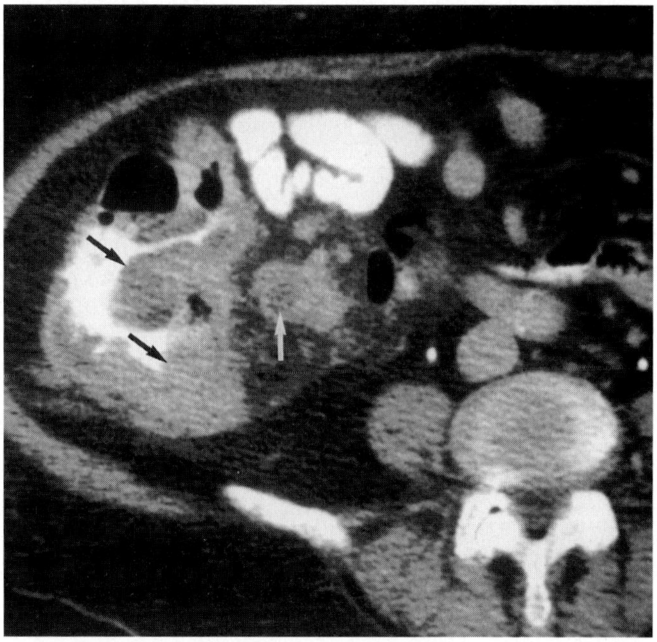

FIGURE 6.31 Colon carcinoma. Contrast-enhanced CT in an 81-year-old woman shows irregular wall thickening of the ascending colon *(black arrows)*. Soft tissue infiltration of the mesentery and low-attenuation mesenteric lymphadenopathy *(white arrow)* proved to be local extension of tumor at surgery.

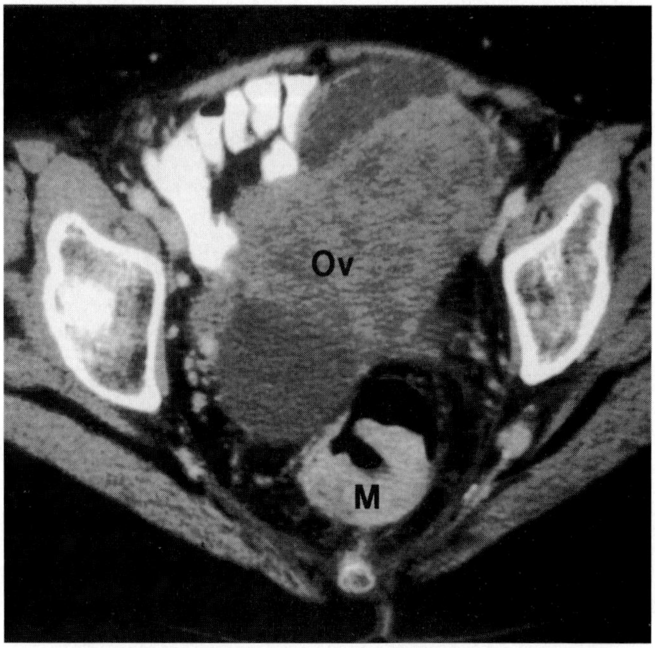

FIGURE 6.32 Rectal carcinoma. Contrast-enhanced CT in a 78-year-old woman with weight loss and persistent diarrhea shows a polypoid soft tissue mass (M) involving the posterior rectum. The large solid and cystic pelvic mass anterior to the rectum proved to be an ovarian adenofibroma (Ov) at surgery.

low-attenuation mesenteric collections due to necrosis or superimposed abscess **(Fig. 6.33).** Overall, CT has a relatively low accuracy rate for preoperative staging, ranging from 50 to 75 percent. Difficulties arise in predicting the degree of mural extension, involvement of normal-sized lymph nodes, and detection of small peritoneal deposits. CT demonstrates greater utility in detecting tumor recurrence, which typically appears as a soft tissue mass or thickening at the anastomotic site. CT, however, is not specific for recurrence, because postoperative fibrosis can have a similar appearance. A progressively enlarging soft tissue mass near the anastomosis on follow-up studies should be regarded as recurrence until disproven. Some centers perform FDG-positron emission tomography imaging to evaluate for recurrence.

- Colonic or rectal **lymphoma** is uncommon and has an appearance similar to that of small bowel involvement **(Fig. 6.34).** An increased prevalence of colonic involvement can be seen with congenital or acquired immunocompromised states. **Metastatic disease** involving the colon is most often due to serosal implants from peritoneal spread of tumor and commonly affects the sigmoid colon. Other routes of metastatic involvement include extension of a gastric primary lesion through the gastrocolic ligament and spread of pancreatic cancer via the transverse mesocolon to involve the transverse colon.
- **Colonic dilatation** on CT can reflect true mechanical obstruction in the cases of tumor, stricture, volvulus, inflammatory processes, hematoma, and fecal impaction (see **Differential 6.5**). Sigmoid or cecal **volvulus** can result from redundancy in the supplying mesentery and may demonstrate a "whirl" sign or beak on CT from the twisted mesenteric segment **(Fig. 6.35).** Volvulus of the transverse colon also occurs but is rare. Nonobstructive causes of colonic dilatation include adynamic ileus, colonic pseudo-obstruction (Ogilvie syndrome), laxative abuse (cathartic colon), Chagas disease, and toxic megacolon (see **Fig. 6.24**). **Ogilvie syndrome** occurs in elderly patients and is frequently associated with cathartics and anticholinergic medication. **Chagas disease** results in megacolon owing to injury of the colonic ganglion cells by parasitic infection with *Trypanosoma cruzi;* similar involvement of the esophagus resembles achalasia.

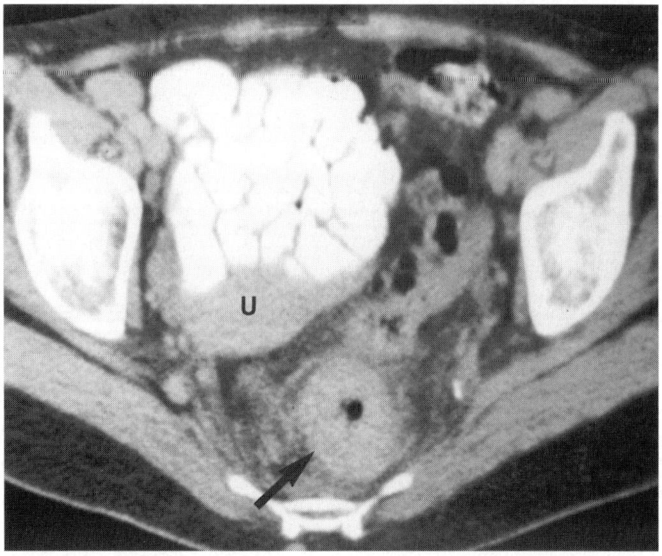

FIGURE 6.34 Rectal lymphoma. Contrast-enhanced CT in a 63-year-old woman with GI bleeding shows circumferential thickening of the rectal wall *(arrow)* and perirectal stranding. There was no evidence of obstruction despite significant luminal narrowing. U, uterus.

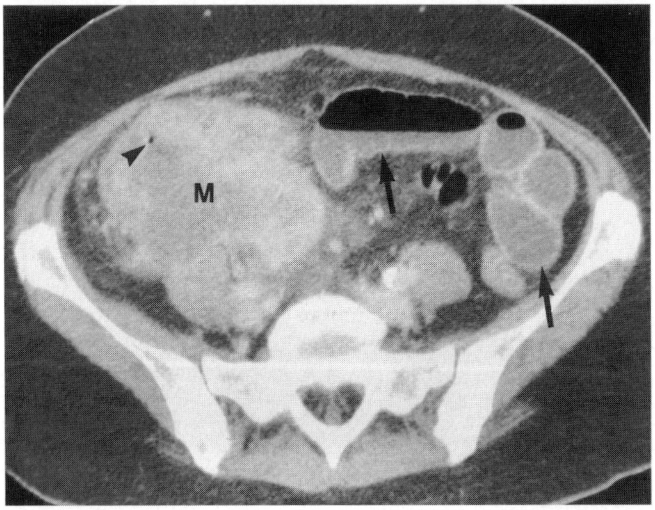

FIGURE 6.33 Perforated colon carcinoma causing small bowel obstruction. Contrast-enhanced CT in a 66-year-old woman with fever, nausea, and abdominal pain shows a complex cecal mass (M) and multiple dilated small bowel loops *(arrows)*. Note small gas bubble in mass *(arrowhead)*. Attempted percutaneous drainage of a presumed abscess revealed a predominantly solid mass, which proved to be cecal cancer on biopsy.

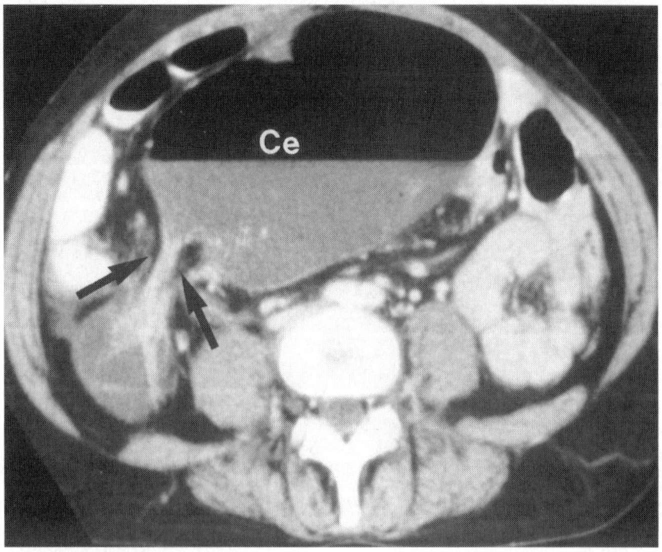

FIGURE 6.35 Cecal volvulus. Contrast-enhanced CT in a 54-year-old woman with abdominal pain shows an air-fluid level and massive dilatation of the cecum (Ce), which has twisted on its mesenteric attachment and now occupies the midabdomen. Note beaking at the site of volvulus *(arrows)*. The cecum extended well into the left upper abdomen.

6.6 CROHN DISEASE

CT plays an important role in the management of Crohn disease, since it allows for the evaluation of extraluminal disease. Any portion of the GI tract can be affected, but the terminal ileum and proximal colon are most often involved. Overall, the colon is involved in approximately one-half of patients, and disease may initially be confined to the colon in 25 percent. CT features include segmental wall thickening and fibrofatty proliferation of the surrounding mesenteric fat **(creeping fat).** The presence of skip lesions or discontinuous disease involvement with intervening normal bowel strongly suggests the diagnosis **(Fig. 6.36).** CT findings of colonic involvement are similar to those of small bowel disease, with wall thickening that is typically more pronounced than that seen with ulcerative colitis. Vascular engorgement of the supplying mesenteric vessels combined with prominent spacing between vessels from fibrofatty proliferation gives rise to the **comb sign** on CT. Other complications associated with Crohn disease include sinus tract formation, fistulous communication with adjacent structures, bowel obstruction, and mesenteric phlegmon or abscess formation **(Fig. 6.37).** CT is the procedure of choice for the diagnosis of intra-abdominal abscess from Crohn disease. Percutaneous abscess drainage can be performed with US or CT guidance.

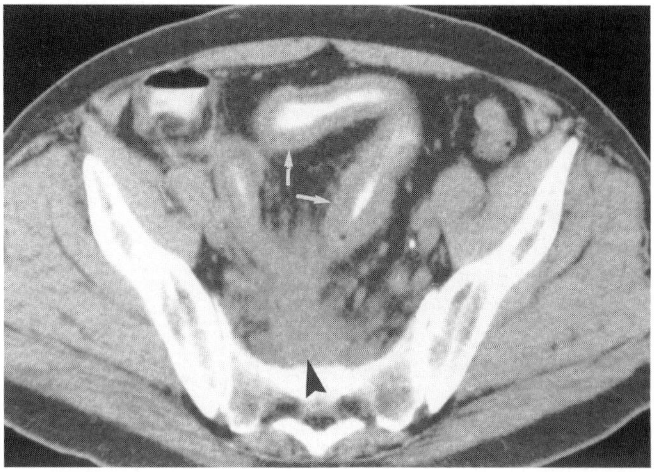

FIGURE 6.37 Crohn disease. Noncontrast CT in a 51-year-old man with Crohn disease shows a long segment of ileal wall thickening and luminal narrowing *(arrows)* as well as prominent presacral soft tissue *(arrowhead)*. Differentiation between phlegmon and abscess is difficult without IV contrast.

6.7 INTUSSUSCEPTION

- Intestinal **intussusception** represents the telescoping of one bowel segment into another. The small bowel, large bowel, or both may be involved. In children from ages 3 months to 3 years, the vast majority of intussusceptions are idiopathic, involve the ileocecal region, and can usually be successfully reduced by enema under fluoroscopy. Intussusception in older children and adults, however, is usually due to a pathologic **lead mass.** Such causes include benign and malignant tumors, celiac disease, scleroderma, bowel wall hemorrhage, and an inverted Meckel diverticulum. Direct demonstration of the receiving intussuscipiens surrounding both the intussusceptum and its associated mesenteric fat and vessels is a characteristic finding on CT **(Fig. 6.38).** A lead mass, when present, is sometimes detected on CT.

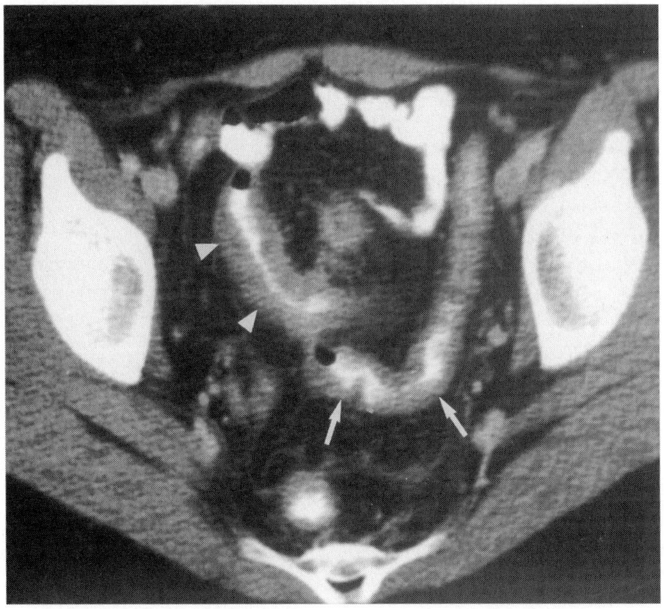

FIGURE 6.36 Crohn disease with skip lesions. Contrast-enhanced CT in a 37-year-old woman with Crohn disease demonstrates a long segment of wall thickening and luminal narrowing of both the distal ileum *(arrowheads)* and sigmoid colon *(arrows)*. Intervening bowel segments were not involved. Note also proliferative changes of mesenteric fat.

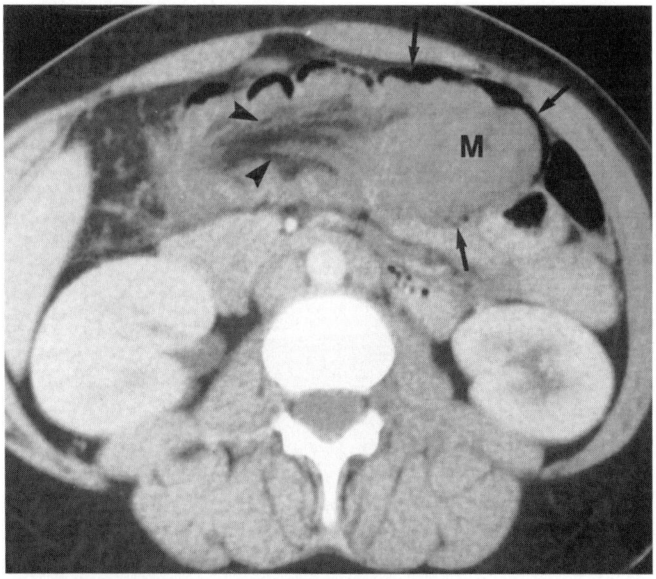

FIGURE 6.38 Intussusception. Contrast-enhanced CT in a 39-year-old woman with a history of cocaine abuse who presented acutely with crampy abdominal pain. Colocolic intussusception is present with intussusceptum (M) and mesenteric fat and vessels *(arrowheads)* extending into the transverse colon (intussuscepiens; *arrows*). The lobulated appearance of the intussusceptum suggests a pathologic lead mass, which proved to be a cecal hematoma at surgery.

6.9

PNEUMATOSIS INTESTINALIS (AIR IN BOWEL WALL)

Idiopathic—cystic, asymptomatic, often sigmoid colon
Bowel necrosis
  Acute mesenteric ischemia
  Necrotizing enterocolitis—premature infants
  Typhlitis
  Ischemic colitis
Mucosal disruption
  Recent bowel surgery or endoscopy
  Perforated ulcer or diverticulum
  Inflammatory bowel disease
  Infectious colitis or enteritis
Increased mucosal permeability
  Collagen vascular disease—scleroderma, SLE
  Corticosteroids
  Graft-versus-host disease
  Organ transplantation
Pulmonary disease—COPD, cystic fibrosis

Key: COPD, chronic obstructive pulmonary disease; SLE, systemic lupus erythematosus.

6.8 PNEUMATOSIS

- **Pneumatosis intestinalis** refers to the presence of intramural intestinal gas and has many causes, including an innocuous cystic form, bowel necrosis, mucosal disruption, increased mucosal permeability, and pulmonary disease **(Differential 6.9).** CT is more sensitive and specific than conventional radiography for the diagnosis of pneumatosis, since it can directly demonstrate gas within dependent portions of bowel wall **(Fig. 6.39).** Repeat imaging with decubitus or prone positioning may be necessary on occasion to confirm the presence of pneumatosis. The more benign idiopathic form tends to involve the colon with a multicystic appearance caused by many discrete subserosal air cysts **(Fig. 6.39),** whereas causes related to underlying ischemia or mucosal disruption often appear more curvilinear. The presence of portal venous gas is not necessarily indicative of transmural infarction and may just reflect mucosal disruption. Pneumoperitoneum can be associated with any cause of pneumatosis. Although findings of bowel ischemia on CT will sometimes help determine the significance of pneumatosis, correlation with the patient's clinical status is essential because of the large overlap in imaging findings among the various etiologies.

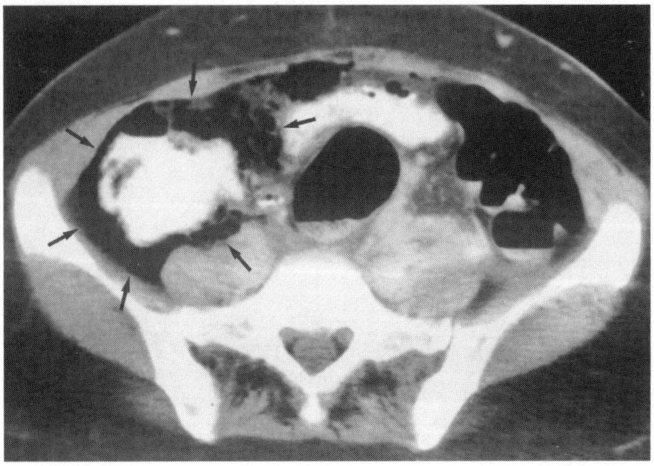

FIGURE 6.39 Benign pneumatosis coli. Contrast-enhanced CT in a 46-year-old woman obtained because unsuspected pneumoperitoneum was detected on chest radiography. Innumerable subserosal air cysts surround the ascending colon *(arrows)*. Free intraperitoneal air was confirmed at other levels (see **Fig. 10.7**), which slowly resolved spontaneously over the next several days.

Bibliography

Balthazar EJ. CT of small-bowel obstruction. *AJR* 1994;162:255–261.

Buckley JA, Fishman EK. CT evaluation of small bowel neoplasms: Spectrum of disease. *Radiographics* 1998;18:379–392.

Curtin KR, Fitzgerald SW, Nemcek AA Jr, Hoff FL, Vogelzang RL. CT diagnosis of acute appendicitis: Imaging findings. *AJR* 1995;164:905–909.

Fishman EK, Urban BA, Hruban RH. CT of the stomach: Spectrum of disease. *Radiographics* 1996;16:1035–1054.

Frager D, Medwid SW, Baer JW, Mollinelli B, Friedman M. CT of small-bowel obstruction: Value in establishing the diagnosis and determining the degree and cause. *AJR* 1994;162:37–41.

Gore RM, Balthazar EJ, Ghahremani GG, Miller FH. CT features of ulcerative colitis and Crohn's disease. *AJR* 1996;167:3–15.

Koehler RE, Memel DS, Stanley RJ. Gastrointestinal tract. In: Lee JKT, Sagel SS, Stanley RJ, Heiken JP (eds): *Computed Body Tomography with MRI Correlation,* 3rd ed. Philadelphia: Lippincott-Raven; 1998:637–700.

Megibow AJ. The gastrointestinal tract. In: Haaga JR (ed): *Computed Tomography and Magnetic Resonance Imaging of the Whole Body,* 3rd ed. St. Louis: Mosby–Year Book; 1994:855–895.

Pear BL. Pneumatosis intestinalis: A review. *Radiology* 1998;207:13–19.

Philpotts LE, Heiken JP, Westcott MA, Gore RM. Colitis: Use of CT findings in differential diagnosis. *Radiology* 1994;190:445–449.

Rao PM, Rhea JT, Novelline RA, McCabe CJ, Lawrason JN, Berger DL, Sacknoff R. Helical CT technique for the diagnosis of appendicitis: Prospective evaluation of a focused appendix CT examination. *Radiology* 1997;202:139–144.

Ros PR, Buetow PC, Pantograg-Brown L, Forsmark CE, Sobin LH. Pseudomembranous colitis. *Radiology* 1996;198:1–199.

Wills JS, Lobis IF, Denstman FJ. Crohn disease: State of the art. *Radiology* 1997;202:597–610.

Winter TC, Ager JD, Nghiem HV, Hill RS, Harrison SD, Freeny PC. Upper gastrointestinal tract and abdomen: Water as an orally administered contrast agent for helical CT. *Radiology* 1996;201:365–370.

Chapter 7

LIVER AND BILIARY SYSTEM

Christopher J. Gordon

7.1 Anatomy and Physiology
7.2 Diffuse Disease and Cirrhosis
7.3 Hepatic Infection
7.4 Benign Masses
7.5 Malignant Hepatic Neoplasms
7.6 Hepatic Vascular Phenomena
7.7 Gallbladder and Biliary Disease
7.8 Hepatic Biopsy and Surgery

7.1 ANATOMY AND PHYSIOLOGY

- The **liver** is the largest solid abdominal organ. It occupies much of the right upper quadrant and performs a variety of essential functions. These include filtering drugs and toxins from the blood, storing glycogen, cholesterol metabolism, hormonal regulation, secreting bile salts, and synthesizing substances such as albumin, coagulation factors, and complement.
- A **dual blood supply** protects the liver from ischemia and infarction. Approximately 25 percent of hepatic blood flow is from the hepatic artery, which delivers oxygenated blood, and 75 percent from the portal vein, which delivers nutrients from the splanchnic bed. Venous outflow is via the right, middle, and left hepatic veins, which drain into the inferior vena cava (IVC) near the hepatic dome. These veins divide the liver into segments that are both surgically and structurally important. Venous blood from the caudate drains directly into the IVC.
- The **right hepatic lobe** is separated from the left by the interlobar fissure, which extends from the gallbladder fossa to the middle hepatic vein. The right lobe is further subdivided into anterior and posterior segments by the right hepatic vein. The **left hepatic lobe** is divided into medial and lateral segments by the fissure for the ligamentum teres. These four segments are further divided into superior and inferior portions by a transverse plane through the organ created by the right and left portal veins. The caudate is situated between the fissure for the ligamentum venosum and the IVC.
- The liver is a complex organ with normal variation in the sizes of lobes and the hepatic vasculature. Middle and left hepatic veins share a common trunk in 70 percent of cases. Accessory draining veins are common. The most common morphologic variant is a Riedel's lobe, which is hypertrophy and caudal extension of the anterolateral portion of the right lobe. It can extend to the iliac crest and is more common in women.
- A variety of **CT techniques** can be used to image the liver. Spiral CT allows short image-acquisition time and avoids respiratory and motion misregistration; consequently, both hepatic arterial and portal venous phases of contrast enhancement can be imaged. This "dual-phase" hepatic imaging is commonly performed in evaluating patients with cirrhosis, primary hepatic tumors, and hypervascular hepatic metastasis. This permits depiction of transiently enhancing lesions that might otherwise be missed on routine monophasic images.

  With less than 30 s of breath holding, the entire liver can be imaged. A dual-phase scan uses infusion of 150 mL of intravenous (IV) contrast at a rate of 4 mL/s. Scanning begins 20 s after the start of the contrast bolus for arterial-phase images and 50 s later for the portal venous–phase images. Patients with poor cardiac function often require longer delays owing to poor transit of administered contrast.
- There are many causes of liver lesions **(Differential 7.1) (Fig. 7.1).** Most hepatic lesions are of low density as compared with enhanced liver and will be seen on routine portal venous–phase imaging **(Differential 7.2)**; however, delayed imaging can prove beneficial in selected instances. Hepatocytes take up about 5 percent of administered contrast, so scans obtained 4 to 6 h after injection can show small or isoenhancing metastases. Cavernous hemangiomas over a few centimeters in size can demonstrate "fill-in" with contrast over a few minutes. Additionally, cholangiocarcinoma occasionally demonstrates increased attenuation 10 to 15 min following administration of intravenous contrast. Hypervascular hepatic lesions (**Differential 7.3**) are best imaged with both early arterial and portal venous phases.

7.2 DIFFUSE DISEASE AND CIRRHOSIS

- The liver has a wide range of normal appearances owing to its complex architecture and normal variability. Diffuse hepatic disease can have a variety of appearances, but in some cases hepatomegaly may be the only clue to underlying liver disease. Normal hepatic size is roughly 1300 to 1500 gr with an attenuation of 55 ± 15 HU with-

7.1

LIVER LESION

Cyst
Malignant tumors
- **Metastases—**lung, breast, colon, many others
- **Hepatocellular carcinoma**
- Cholangiocarcinoma
- Fibrolamellar carcinoma
- Lymphoma
- Hepatoblastoma—children
- *Angiosarcoma*
- *Kaposi sarcoma*—AIDS
- *Hemangioendothelioma*—children

Benign tumors
- **Hemangioma**
- Focal nodular hyperplasia
- Regenerating nodule—cirrhosis
- Adenoma
- Biliary cystadenoma

Abscess—pyogenic, amebic, fungal
Hematoma—posttraumatic, underlying lesion (adenoma)
Hamartoma

out IV contrast. Splenic attenuation is usually 5 to 10 HU less than that of the liver on precontrast CT. Hepatomegaly **(Differential 7.4)** can be due to many causes.

- **Multifocal hepatic disease** can have a variety of appearances, ranging from benign calcified granulomas to diffuse low-density lesions. The causes of the majority of these lesions will be benign or malignant neoplasms, vascular lesions, or infection **(Differential 7.5).** The radiologic appearance as well as clinical and laboratory information will help to narrow the diagnostic considerations. Use of an appropriate imaging protocol can increase the detection of multifocal hepatic disease. Patients with primary carcinomas that may appear hypervascular need to have arterial phase imaging. These lesions may easily be missed on routine portal venous images.

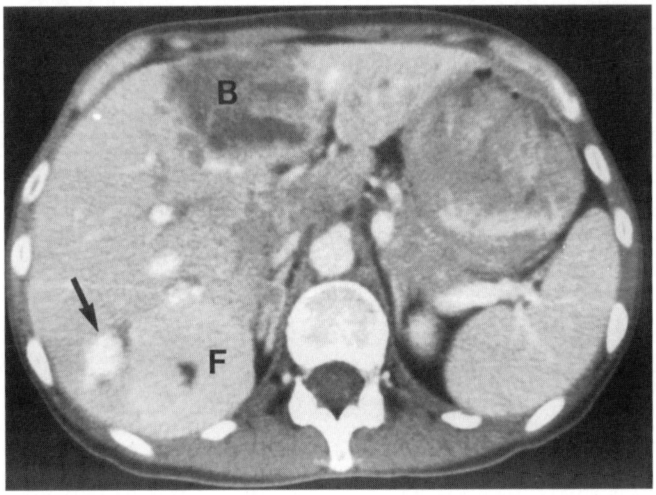

FIGURE 7.1 Multiple liver neoplasms. Contrast-enhanced CT shows three distinct liver lesions, including a low-density metastases from breast carcinoma (B), a densely enhancing cavernous hemangioma *(arrow),* and focal nodular hyperplasia (F) with a central scar.

7.2

LOW-DENSITY LIVER LESION POSTCONTRAST

Tumors
- **Metastases**
- "Giant" hemangioma >5 cm
- Cystic masses—biliary cystadenoma/cystadenocarcinoma, *lymphangioma*
- Cholangiocarcinoma
- Regenerating nodules

Cyst
Focal fatty infiltration—periligamentous, pericholecystic, perihilar, geographic
Abscess
Hematoma—posttraumatic, underlying lesion (adenoma)

- **Hepatic calcifications** are seen in a wide array of hepatic conditions, ranging from old, healed granulomatous diseases to benign and malignant hepatic neoplasms **(Differential 7.6).** Hepatic calcifications from healed granulomatous diseases such as histoplasmosis and tuberculosis are common. Benign hepatic calcifications are usually small and often multiple. The presence of other calcified granulomas in the spleen or lung is a clue to prior systemic granulomatous infection. *Pneumocystis carinii,* CMV, and toxoplasmal infection can also give rise to calcified granulomas, often in an immunocompromised host.
- **Increased and decreased hepatic attenuation** have specific differential diagnoses. Diffuse calcifications and multiple low-attenuation lesions are other patterns of diffuse disease often seen with infection and neoplasm. Patients with anemia can have slightly decreased hepatic attenuation. High-density liver parenchyma (on noncontrast images) has a limited differential diagnosis **(Differential 7.7).**
- **Thorotrast,** or thorium dioxide, was an angiographic contrast agent used until the late 1950s. An alpha-emitting agent taken up by the reticuloendothelial system, Thorotrast caused high-dose liver parenchymal radiation and exposed patients can develop hepatic

7.3

HYPERVASCULAR LIVER LESION

Malignant tumors
- **Hepatocellular carcinoma**
- **Vascular metastases—**carcinoid, melanoma, islet cell, renal cell, breast, sarcomas
- *Hemangioendothelioma*—children
- *Angiosarcoma*

Benign tumors
- **Hemangioma**
- Adenoma
- Focal nodular hyperplasia
- Regenerating nodules

Focal fat-sparing—simulates enhancing mass
Vascular phenomena—transient hepatic attenuation difference (THAD)
Arteriovenous malformation
Hepatic artery aneurysm—trauma or inflammation

7.4

HEPATOMEGALY

Fatty infiltration—obesity, alcohol, steroids, diabetes, chemotherapy, hyperalimentation, pregnancy
Metastases—lung, breast, colon, many others
Primary tumor—hepatocellular carcinoma, giant hemangioma (>5 cm), adenoma, *hepatoblastoma, hemangioendothelioma, angiosarcoma*
Hepatic congestion—heart failure, constrictive pericarditis, tricuspid valve disease, Budd-Chiari syndrome, veno-occlusive disease
Hepatitis—A, B, C
Hemochromatosis
Storage diseases
Lymphoma
Cirrhosis
Myeloproliferative disease—myelofibrosis, polycythemia vera
Mononucleosis—Epstein-Barr virus
Riedel lobe
Others—sarcoid, schistosomiasis, extramedullary hematopoiesis, polycystic disease, Wilson disease, amyloidosis, malaria, tuberculosis, histoplasmosis, chronic granulomatous disease of childhood

7.6

HEPATIC CALCIFICATIONS

Old healed granulomatous disease—tuberculosis, histoplasmosis, coccidioidomycosis
Metastases—colon, breast, stomach, ovarian, melanoma, osteosarcoma, thyroid, teratoma, also following radiation or chemotherapy
Primary tumor
Fibrolamellar carcinoma—30% calcify
Hepatocellular carcinoma—occasional calcification
Hemangioma—phleboliths are uncommon
Hepatoblastoma—most frequent childhood hepatic malignancy
Hemangioendothelioma—children
Cholangiocarcinoma
Hydatid cyst—*Echinococcus granulosus*—25% calcify
Chronic abscess—pyogenic, amebic, fungal
Calcified gallbladder
Old hematoma—posttraumatic, underlying lesion (adenoma)
Mimic—lipoidal embolization (focal); hemochromatosis, hemosiderosis, Thorotrast (diffuse)
Regenerating nodules—rarely calcify
Chronic granulomatous disease of childhood

angiosarcoma, cholangiocarcinoma, and hepatocellular carcinomas. Residual high attenuation is seen within the spleen, abdominal lymph nodes, and hepatic parenchyma in a reticular pattern that is predominant within the periphery **(Fig. 7.2).** There is evidence to suggest that this is not due to residual contrast but rather to calcification in tissues exposed to Thorotrast. Markedly dense spleen and lymphatic foci help narrow the differential diagnosis. Low-attenuation foci within the liver on precontrast CT or regions of marked enhancement following IV contrast administration suggest underlying neoplasia.

- **Hemochromatosis,** an uncommon autosomal recessive disease, results in increased intestinal absorption of iron. If it is left untreated, excess iron accumulates within hepatocytes and patients can present with the classic triad of cirrhosis, diabetes mellitus (30 percent), and increased skin pigmentation (90 percent; bronze diabetes). Other findings include splenomegaly (50 percent) and arthropathy (50 percent). Iron deposition within the myocardium can result in impaired cardiac function and cardiomyopathy. One-quarter of patients with untreated hemochromatosis develop hepatocellular carcinoma; otherwise they tend to have a preserved life span.
- **Hemosiderosis** is similar to hemochromatosis, but, in contrast the iron is deposited within the reticuloendothelial system, sparing the pancreas. Hemosiderosis is generally due to iron overload from multiple transfusions for chronic anemia. The increased hepatic iron content is manifest by increased CT attenuation of the liver, 80 to 140 HU. The distribution of increased attenuation may not be uniform. The ferromagnetic properties of iron allow MRI to detect iron deposition within the viscera. Gradient echo images accentuate the T2 effects of iron, and involved organs appear dark. The liver, pancreas, and myocardium have decreased T2-weighted signal in hemochromatosis **(Fig. 7.3),** whereas the pancreas and heart are spared in hemosiderosis.
- **Wilson disease** is a rare autosomal recessive disorder of copper metabolism due to decreased levels of circulating ceruloplasmin. Toxic accumulation results from impaired excretion of copper, with resultant deposition in the liver, eye (Kayser-Fleischer rings), and basal ganglia resulting in *hepatolenticular degeneration.* Children can present with hepatic manifestations such as hepatomegaly, hepatitis, or cirrhosis; neurodegenerative changes are more commonly seen in adults. Diagnosis is made on clinical, biochemical, and biopsy findings. CT can reveal a normal, increased, or decreased hepatic attenuation depending on the degree of associated fatty infiltration. The majority of patients have normal hepatic attenuation.
- **Amiodarone** is a medication used in the treatment of cardiac arrhythmias. It contains iodine and has a long half-life of 90 days. Deposition of amiodarone within the liver occurs because it is excreted into bile. In addition to hepatobiliary concentration, amio-

7.5

MULTIPLE LIVER LESIONS

Metastases—lung, breast, colon, many others
Cysts
Hemangioma
Hepatocellular carcinoma
Focal nodular hyperplasia
Regenerating nodules
Caroli disease
Adenomatosis

7.7

HIGH-DENSITY LIVER PRECONTRAST

Amiodarone—iodine deposition
Primary hemochromatosis
Hemosiderosis
Storage diseases—more often low-density
Wilson disease—copper deposition
Gold—treatment of rheumatoid arthritis
Thorotrast

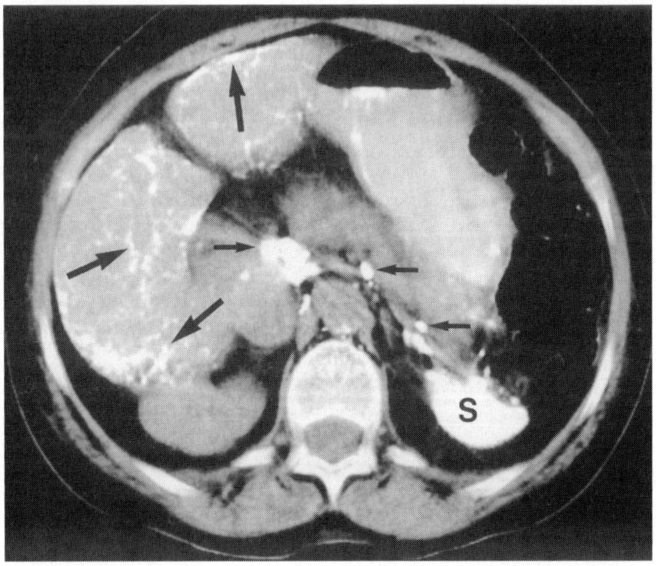

FIGURE 7.2 Thorotrast. Noncontrast CT demonstrates reticular high density throughout the hepatic parenchyma *(large arrows)*. Residual high attenuation is also noted within an atrophied spleen (S) as well as multiple peripancreatic lymph nodes *(small arrows)*. Subsequent hepatic MRI failed to demonstrate an underlying hepatic neoplasm. This 63-year-old female gave a history of prior Thorotrast administration for cerebral angiography in the 1950s.

darone can have pulmonary toxicity, causing areas of ground-glass attenuation and eventually pulmonary fibrosis. CT demonstrates hepatic attenuation of greater than 80 HU on precontrast CT **(Fig. 7.4).** Normal attenuation in the spleen and lymph nodes distinguishes this condition from Thorotrast exposure. An appropriate clinical history will confirm the diagnosis.

- **Sarcoidosis** is a multisystem disorder characterized by the formation of noncaseating granulomas. The lungs and mediastinal lymph nodes are involved in the overwhelming majority of patients. The abdominal organs are involved less commonly, the liver in 25 percent and the spleen in 50 percent. Patients can present with abdominal pain or organomegaly. Homogeneous hepatosplenomegaly is the most frequent finding. Granulomas can be too small to be detected by CT, but multiple roughly 2-cm low-attenuation nodules are sometimes demonstrated. Abdominal or pelvic involvement with sarcoidosis can precede the development of disease in the thorax by several years.
- **Amyloidosis** is a group of disorders in which there is extracellular deposition of an insoluble fibrillary protein termed *amyloid.* The primary type is uncommon and is seen in association with immunoglobulin disorders. The familial form is also uncommon. Secondary amyloidosis accounts for the majority of cases and is often present in association with inflammatory processes.
- **Fatty infiltration** (steatosis) is the most common cause of a low-density liver **(Differential 7.8).** The most common causes for fatty liver include obesity, steroid use, and alcohol use **(Differential 7.9).** Because of the different enhancement patterns of the liver and spleen, precontrast CT images of the upper abdomen have greater sensitivity for detection of fatty change than contrast-enhanced images. Normal hepatic attenuation is 5 to 10 HU greater than that of the spleen. Fatty infiltration can be suspected when splenic attenuation is 10 HU greater than that of the liver on precontrast CT and 25 HU greater on contrast-enhanced CT **(Fig. 7.5).** Nodular fatty infiltration can be difficult to distinguish from primary or secondary hepatic neoplasm, although focal fatty infiltration has no mass effect on adjacent parenchyma or vessels. Fatty change may be very irregular in appearance or focal on both precontrast CT and contrast-enhanced CT images but there is no architectural distortion **(Fig. 7.6) (Differential 7.10).** In difficult cases, MRI with in-phase and opposed-phase imaging can be useful in distinguishing fatty infiltration from tumor or confluent hepatic fibrosis.

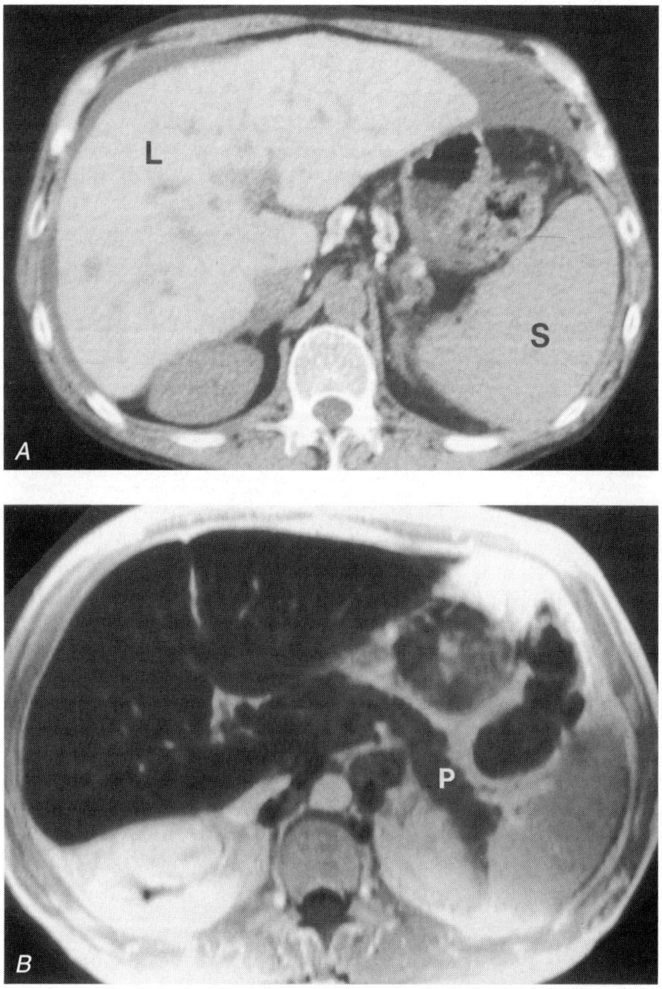

FIGURE 7.3 Hemochromatosis. *A.* Noncontrast CT shows increased hepatic attenuation (L) compared to the spleen (S). *B.* MRI using an in-phase two-dimensional FLASH technique shows complete signal dropout in the liver and pancreas (P) as a result of iron deposition.

- **Cirrhosis** causes approximately 25,000 deaths each year in the United States and is the eighth leading cause of death. Hepatitis, alcoholism, and parasitic infections are the most common etiologies and vary by location. In the western hemisphere, 70 percent of cirrhosis is due to alcohol abuse. The remainder is due to chronic hepatitis or idiopathic causes. In Asia and Africa, chronic viral hepatitis is the most prevalent cause, and other causes include chronic biliary obstruction, hepatic veno-occlusive disease, chronic

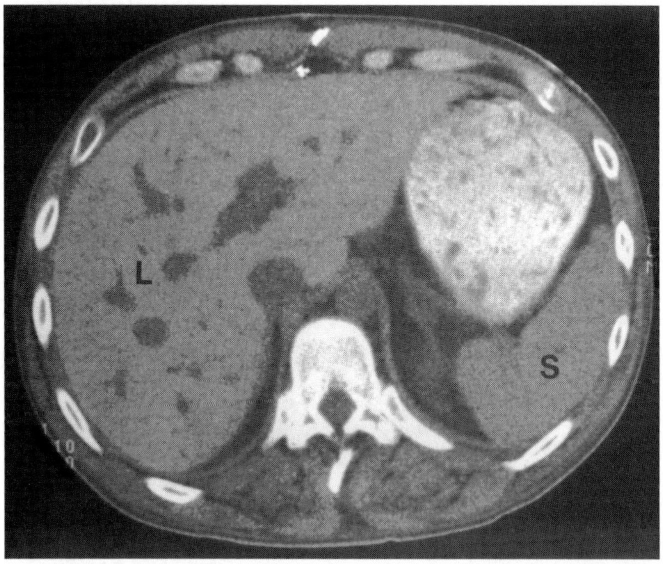

FIGURE 7.4 Amiodarone. Noncontrast CT in a patient taking amiodarone shows homogeneous increased attenuation of the hepatic parenchyma in comparison with the normal spleen (S). Note clear visualization of intrahepatic vessels.

congestive heart failure, and metabolic disorders such as hemochromatosis and Wilson disease.

The disease is characterized by diffuse parenchymal destruction, fibrosis, and regeneration in the setting of chronic liver disease. On gross inspection, three morphologic appearances have been described. Micronodular regeneration appears as 1- to 5-mm regenerative nodules, often seen in a setting of alcohol abuse. Macronodular cirrhosis has variably sized nodules measuring up to several centimeters in diameter. Chronic viral hepatitis is often the cause of macronodular regeneration. Mixed regeneration has prominent features of both the micronodular and macronodular patterns and can be seen with chronic biliary obstruction. There is enlargement of the liver in early cirrhosis with variable degrees of fatty infiltration. The liver becomes more normal in size as it scars, with a shrunken and nodular liver noted late in the disease.

- **Clinical features** that can be seen in the cirrhotic patient include weight loss, malaise, jaundice, urticaria, and low-grade fevers. More severe manifestations include coagulopathy, bleeding from esophageal varices, ascites, and hepatic encephalopathy. **Treatment** of cirrhosis is often directed toward the complications of late cirrhosis, such as esophageal varices and ascites. Transesophageal sclerotherapy is attempted for bleeding esophageal varices, and patients who fail can be treated with a transjugular intrahepatic portosystemic shunt (TIPS). The treatment of conditions known to precede the development of cirrhosis can aid in limiting progression of disease. Chelating agents in Wilson disease and hemochromatosis are examples. Hepatic transplantation is an effective treatment for cirrhosis and has resulted in improved survival for selected patients.

CT is often used to give morphologic information about the hepatic parenchyma and vasculature, evaluate the effects of portal hypertension, and assess for the development of hepatocellular carcinoma **(Fig. 7.7).** Early in the disease, the liver can have a variety of appearances, ranging from normal to fatty infiltration and/or hepatomegaly. With disease progression, the liver can develop a nodular contour with regenerating nodules and heterogeneous attenuation due to irregular fibrosis and fatty infiltration **(Fig. 7.8).** Later in the disease, there is a decrease in the size of the right hepatic lobe and the medial segment of the left lobe, with enlargement of the caudate and lateral segment of the left hepatic lobe. Inhomogeneous enhancement following contrast administration is also seen late in the disease. With pseudocirrhosis **(see Fig. 7.19),** there will be a history of treated liver metastases and splenomegaly.

Late in the disease, portal hypertension develops, with several imaging findings. CT can often demonstrate enlargement of the su-

7.8

LOW-DENSITY LIVER PRECONTRAST

Fatty liver—diffuse, geographic, focal, multinodular
Hepatic congestion—heart failure, tricuspid valve disease, constrictive pericarditis, Budd-Chiari syndrome, veno-occlusive disease
Diffuse metastases—lung, breast, colon, many others
Amyloidosis
Storage diseases

7.9

FATTY LIVER

Obesity
Steroids
Alcohol
Cirrhosis
Cystic fibrosis
Pregnancy
Chemotherapy—cytotoxic agents
Intravenous hyperalimentation
Diabetes mellitus
Hyperlipidemia
Storage diseases

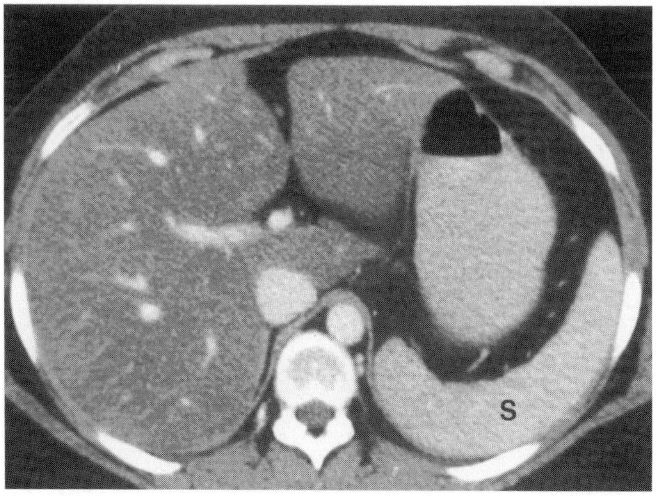

FIGURE 7.5 Hepatic steatosis. Contrast-enhanced image of the upper abdomen shows diffuse decreased hepatic attenuation. Note marked difference in attenuation between the liver and the spleen (S).

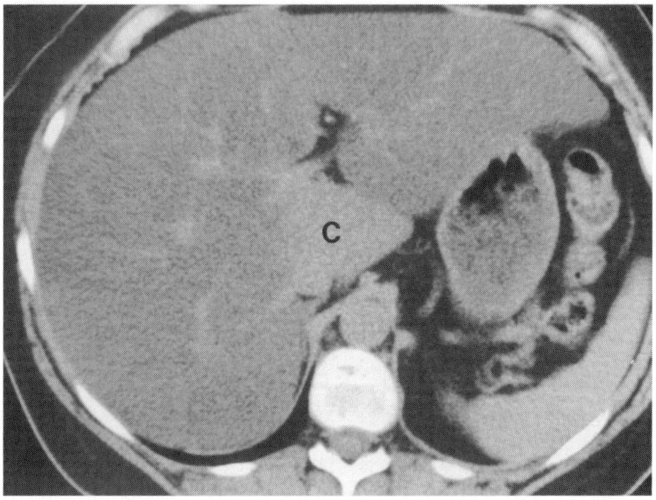

FIGURE 7.6 Focal fat sparing. A 49-year-old woman with fatty replacement of the liver sparing the caudate (C).

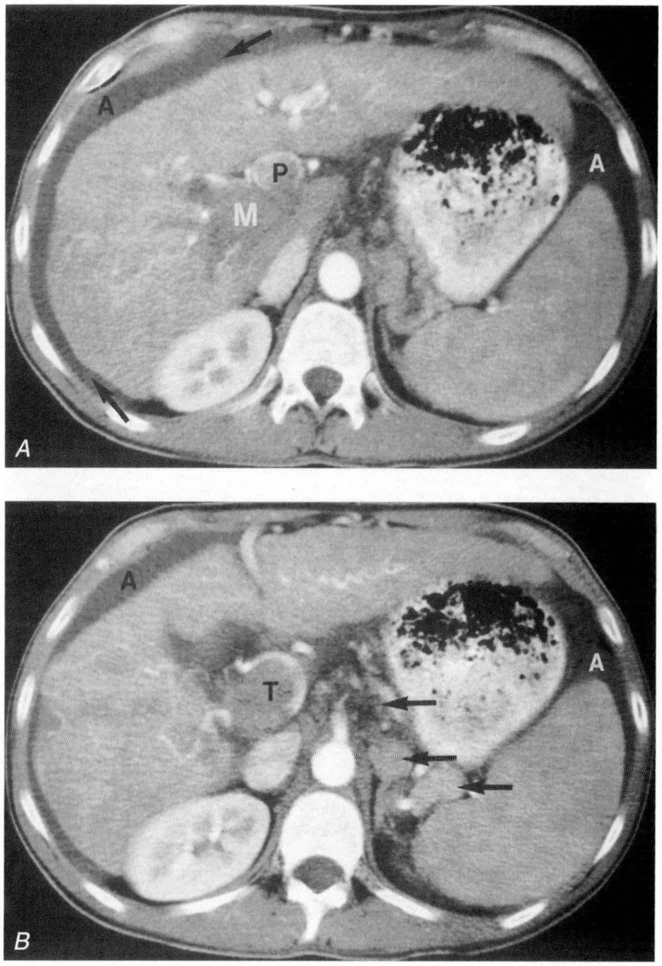

FIGURE 7.7 Cirrhosis. Patient with long-standing cirrhosis. *A*. There is a subtle nodular contour to the hepatic surface *(arrows)* and a focal mass (M) with invasion into the portal vein (P). Hepatocellular carcinoma was found on biopsy. Perihepatic and perisplenic fluid is present (A). *B*. Same patient, different level, demonstrating multiple varices *(arrows)* and paraumbilical collateral. Tumor thrombus (T) can be seen within the enlarged portal vein. A, ascites.

perior mesenteric, splenic, and portal veins; gastroesophageal varices; splenomegaly; ascites; and collaterals in the left gastric, retroperitoneal, and paraumbilical regions. Recruitment of retroperitoneal collaterals from the splenic vein can result in spontaneous splenorenal shunting.

- **Regenerating nodules** are most commonly seen in cirrhosis of a viral etiology. Regenerating nodules represent hyperplastic foci of hepatocytes and hepatic stroma. Cirrhotic patients have increased levels of various hormones and growth factors because of their altered hepatic clearance. Some authors believe that these increased levels of growth factors stimulate the development of regenerating nodules, which are multiple and range in size from 0.3 to 1.0 cm. CT typically shows multiple foci of increased attenuation on precontrast CT. With contrast-enhanced CT, regenerating nodules can blend with enhancing parenchyma and often become invisible.

7.10
LOW-DENSITY LIVER LESION PRECONTRAST

Cyst
Focal fatty infiltration
Malignant tumor
- **Metastases**
- Hepatocellular carcinoma
- Cholangiocarcinoma
- Lymphoma

Benign tumor
- **Hemangioma**
- Focal nodular hyperplasia
- Adenoma

Abscess
- Pyogenic
- Amebic—*Entamoeba histolytica*
- Fungal—*Candida, Cryptococcus*
- Parasitic—hydatid disease, schistosomiasis

Hematoma—posttraumatic, underlying lesion (adenoma)
Biloma—posttraumatic, intervention
Infarct
Radiation therapy—leads to local fatty replacement

7.3 HEPATIC INFECTION

- **Hepatitis** can be divided into acute and chronic forms. Acute hepatitis can be caused by many viral agents including hepatitis A to E, Epstein-Barr virus, and cytomegalovirus (CMV). Hepatitis B (HBV) is transmitted either parenterally or by sexual contact. Hepatitis C (HCV) is transmitted parenterally. Chronic hepatitis is the persistence of abnormalities for more than 6 months and can be found with HBV and HCV infection. Hepatitis can have nonspecific imaging findings of hepatomegaly, gallbladder wall thickening, and low periportal attenuation. CT is better suited to survey for the complications of chronic hepatitis, namely development of hepatocellular carcinoma (HCC) in HBV and cirrhosis in HCV.
- **Pyogenic abscess.** Seeding of the hepatic parenchyma via the he-

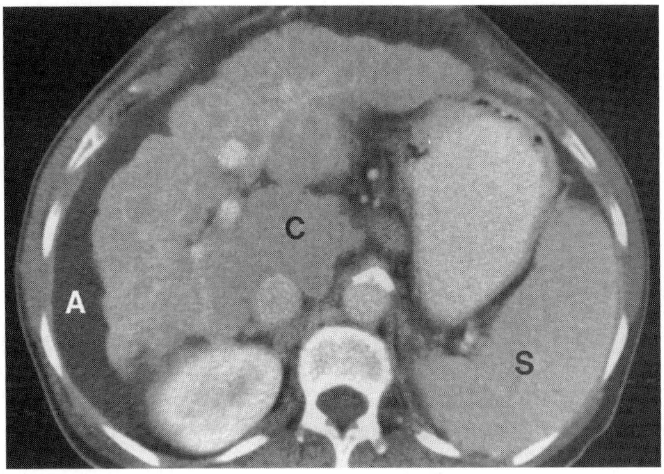

FIGURE 7.8 Cirrhosis. Contrast-enhanced CT in a patient with a history of alcohol abuse, demonstrating a nodular hepatic surface, caudate enlargement (C), ascites (A), and splenomegaly (S).

patic artery, portal vein, bile ducts, trauma, or direct extension can result in the formation of a hepatic abscess. Focal accumulation of pathogens and inflammatory cells leads to hepatic necrosis. The pyogenic variety accounts for 85 percent of hepatic abscesses in the United States. The remainder are amebic and fungal. *Escherichia coli* is the most frequently cultured organism. Cholangitis with biliary obstruction from benign or malignant causes can precipitate the development of a pyogenic abscess. Patients can present with fevers, malaise, sepsis, and abdominal discomfort; however, many have only vague constitutional symptoms, without the usual features of pyogenic abscess.

CT characteristically demonstrates a single or multiloculated low-attenuation lesion (0 to 40 HU) with peripheral enhancement **(Fig. 7.9)**. Gas can be seen in about 20 percent of these lesions. The sensitivity for detection is highest with helical CT following bolus administration of contrast. Treatment of small lesions can be with antibiotics alone; larger lesions may require percutaneous or surgical drainage.

- **Fungal abscess.** Colonization of the liver with fungi almost always occurs in the setting of an immunocompromised host. At autopsy, hepatic involvement with *Candida albicans* is present in half of the patients with leukemia or lymphoma. Fungal microabscesses can also be caused by *Aspergillus* and *Cryptococcus.* CT shows multiple round hypodense lesions distributed throughout the hepatic parenchyma. Some lesions can have a target appearance with a central area of high attenuation. The spleen and kidneys can be similarly affected.
- **Amebic abscesses** are uncommon in the United States and usually occur in patients with a travel history to an endemic area. *Entamoeba histolytica* is the causative agent, and superinfection with pyogens can occur in up to 20 percent. Symptoms are usually not as severe as in those with pyogenic abscesses. CT typically reveals a solitary fluid-attenuation mass in the right hepatic lobe with a well-defined, enhancing wall. Foci of gas can be present within the lesion, and ipsilateral pneumonitis with pleural effusion is common. Abscess erosion through the diaphragm and pleura is a rare but known complication of amebic abscess. Treatment with metronidazole is often curative; drainage is usually reserved for lesions adjacent to the pericardium, those of large size, and in cases of poor response to medication.
- ***Echinococcus granulosus*** causes the majority of hydatid disease in humans. *Echinococcus multilocularis,* the least common variety, can have an aggressive appearance mimicking malignant tumor. Human disease is caused by the larval forms of these parasites. The CT findings in both diseases are similar. Well-demarcated unilocular or multilocular fluid-density lesions with or without enhancement of the cyst wall are common. Curvilinear or coarse calcification within the cyst wall can be present with *Echinococcus granulosus* infection **(Fig. 7.10)**. An amorphous appearance with central calcification is more suggestive of *E. multilocularis* disease.

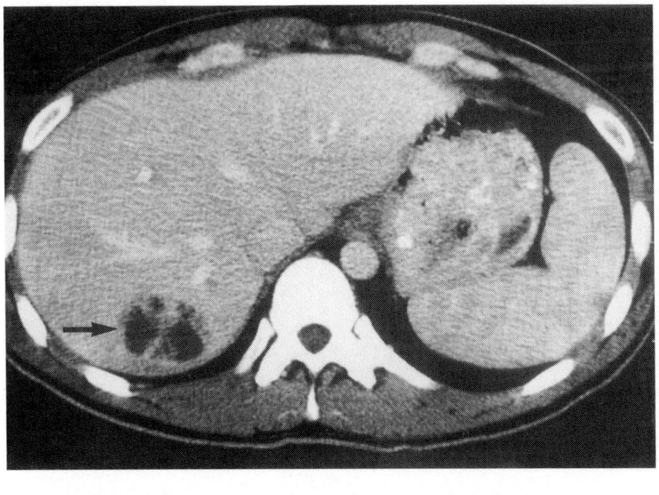

FIGURE 7.9 Hepatic abscess. Fluid-attenuation abscess *(arrow)* in the posterior segment of the right hepatic lobe in a patient with appendicitis. Note the thin septations within the abscess.

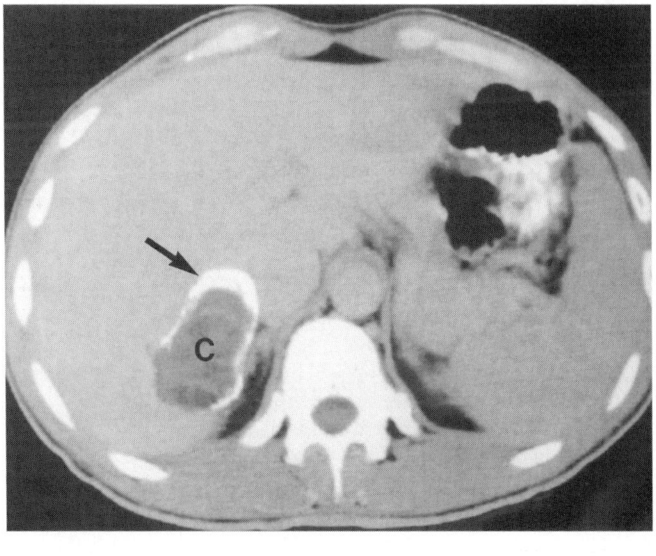

FIGURE 7.10 Echinococcal cyst. Fluid-density cyst (C) with dense rim calcification *(arrow)* in a patient with *Echinococcus granulosus* infection.

MRI can demonstrate a rim surrounding the cyst, with low T1 and T2 signal consistent with fibrous tissue. Treatment is with drainage.

- **Schistosomiasis.** Two species of schistosomes cause significant hepatic disease in humans: *Schistosoma japonicum* and *Schistosoma mansoni*. Their eggs embolize to the terminal branches of the portal veins and incite a granulomatous reaction in the liver. Both are associated with an increased risk of HCC. Broad fibrous septa are formed in the hepatic parenchyma as a result of infection with *S. japonicum*. *S. mansoni* elicits more periportal fibrosis. Calcification can be seen with *S. japonicum* but not *S. mansoni*. Prolonged disease can eventually lead to presinusoidal portal hypertension.
- ***Pneumocystis carinii*** pneumonia (PCP) is most commonly seen in the immunocompromised host, usually in association with AIDS. Extrapulmonary involvement with *P. carinii* can occur with no clinical or radiographic evidence of concurrent PCP. CT demonstrates multifocal low-density lesions with a propensity to calcify in a stippled central or peripheral curvilinear fashion. Calcifications can occur in a variety of locations including hepatic, adrenal, renal, splenic, nodal, and mesenteric. Other causes of calcifications in this distribution include *Mycobacterium avium-intracellulare* (MAI) and CMV infection. A less common appearance for *P. carinii* infection is that of multiple low-attenuation nodules (usually in the liver and spleen, although any visceral organ may be affected).

7.4 BENIGN MASSES

- **Hepatic cysts** can be congenital or acquired **(Differential 7.11).** Infection, trauma, and parasitic disease are common causes of acquired hepatic cysts. Congenital cysts are more common and appear as small, well-circumscribed lesions near water attenuation that do not enhance following contrast administration. Larger lesions can demonstrate septations. Multiple cysts **(Fig. 7.11)** are often seen in the context of autosomal dominant polycystic kidney disease (ADPCKD).
- **Polycystic liver disease** is an uncommon disorder where multiple hepatic cysts are present in the absence of ADPCKD or other disorder. Multiple hepatic cysts associated with ADPCKD are far more common than polycystic liver disease. The presence of multiple, usually bilateral, renal cysts in ADPCKD helps to distinguish between these two entities. Patients are asymptomatic and the cysts are found incidentally. Multiple fluid-attenuation cysts of varying sizes are seen throughout the hepatic parenchyma **(Fig. 7.12).** The cysts may show thin septation with no enhancement. These cysts do not affect hepatic function and no treatment is necessary.

7.11

LIVER CYST

Epithelial
Traumatic—hematoma or biloma
Autosomal dominant polycystic kidney disease
Cystic metastasis—ovarian, gastric primaries
Abscess—pyogenic, amebic, fungal
Von Hippel-Lindau disease
Biliary cystadenoma or cystadenocarcinoma
Choledochal cyst
Hydatid disease—Echinococcus granulosus
Caroli disease
Lymphangioma

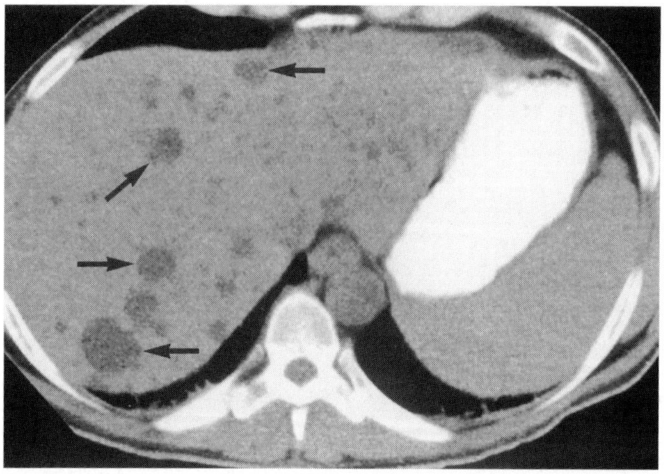

FIGURE 7.11 Hepatic cysts. Multiple fluid-attenuation cysts *(arrows)* in all hepatic segments in a patient with autosomal dominant polycystic kidney disease.

- **Cavernous hemangioma** is the most common benign hepatic neoplasm and second most common hepatic mass, exceeded only by metastases. Many are solitary, but up to 10 percent are multiple. Large, thin-walled vascular spaces make up the lesion, with variable amounts of fibrous septa and fat. Most hemangiomas are less than 5 cm in size and cause no symptoms. Larger lesions can be complicated by arteriovenous shunting, mass effect, and hemorrhage. Consumptive coagulopathy and thrombocytopenia from platelet sequestration is known as the Kasabach-Merritt syndrome.

  CT findings are variable depending upon the size of the lesion and the phase of contrast enhancement. With precontrast CT, these lesions are often isodense with blood. After IV contrast administration, some portion of the lesion characteristically enhances to the same degree or greater than the aorta. Small lesions can show complete enhancement and be missed on portal venous phase imaging. In larger lesions, there is usually globular enhancement in some portion of the periphery. On delayed images, all the patent vascular

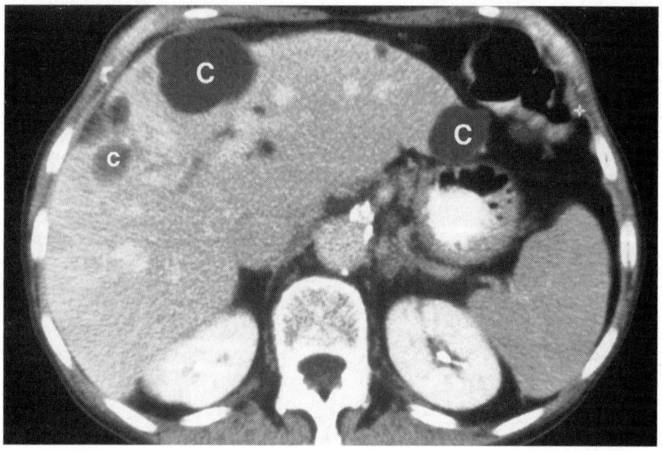

FIGURE 7.12 Polycystic liver disease. Multiple fluid attenuation cysts (C) of varying sizes in the hepatic parenchyma. Note the absence of renal cysts.

elements are opacified. This leads to "filling in" of the lesion, so that it becomes isodense to surrounding hepatic parenchyma **(Fig. 7.13).** Areas of fibrosis will remain hypodense. The ability of MRI to provide serial spoiled gradient-echo images following gadolinium administration is helpful in distinguishing hepatic hemangioma from other lesions. Nuclear medicine red blood cell scintigraphy can also be used to confirm the diagnosis of hemangioma.

- **Focal nodular hyperplasia (FNH)** is the second most common benign neoplasm of the liver. Often solitary and more common in women, it is usually discovered incidentally in the third to fifth decades. FNH is a hypervascular, well-marginated hepatic tumor that often contains a stellate central scar **(Differential 7.12).** The tumor is usually peripheral and can be multiple. It does not contain bile ducts, which helps to distinguish it from a hepatic adenoma.

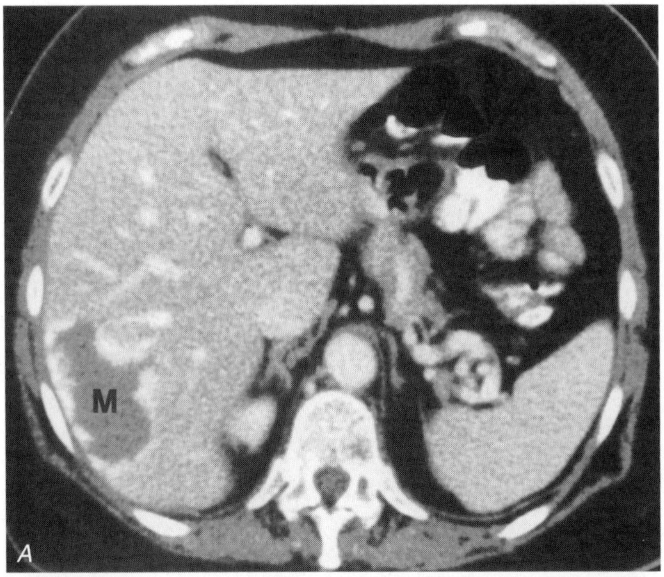

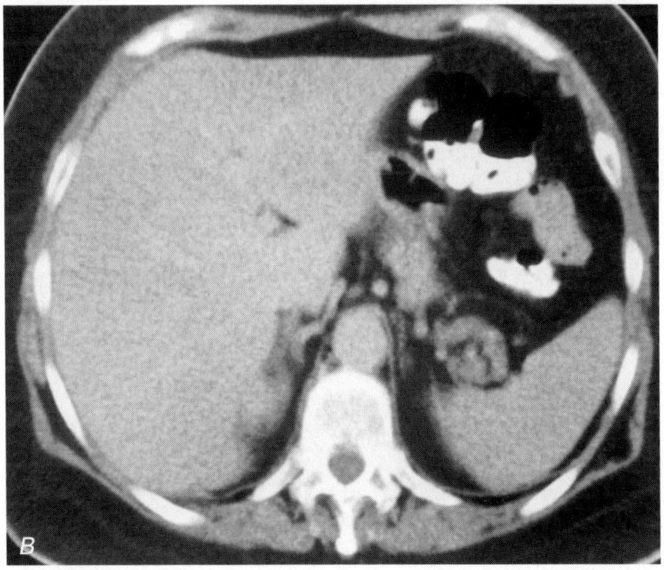

FIGURE 7.13 Cavernous hemangioma. *A*. Arterial phase contrast-enhanced CT shows intense peripheral enhancement of a low-density mass (M). *B*. Delayed image shows complete filling in of the lesion.

7.12

LIVER LESION WITH CENTRAL SCAR

Focal nodular hyperplasia
Fibrolamellar hepatocellular carcinoma
Hemangioma
Adenoma

FNH shows intense but brief enhancement on arterial phase CT **(Fig. 7.14).** A spoke-wheel pattern of enhancement can be seen, but this is not specific for FNH **(see Fig. 7.21).** On MRI, the scar can show high signal on T2-weighted images, whereas a hepatoma is usually low in T2 signal. The presence of Kupffer cells causes FNH to accumulate sulfur colloid on scintigraphy equal to or greater than that of the hepatic parenchyma in about 60 percent of cases. No treatment is necessary.

- **Hepatic adenomas** were true pathologic curiosities before the advent of oral contraceptives. These benign tumors, which are less common than focal nodular hyperplasia, are seen in young women of childbearing age who have used oral contraceptives. Hepatic adenomas can also be seen in patients with glycogen storage diseases and in men taking anabolic steroids.

  Adenomas are hypervascular lesions with discernible capsules. They are low in intensity on T1-weighted MR images and high in intensity on T2 sequences. The appearance on CT is variable owing to the propensity of these lesions to hemorrhage **(Fig. 7.15).** It is common for adenomas to be multiple. Some tumors may demonstrate fatty change. Large areas of infarction and hemorrhage are common, and it can be difficult to distinguish them from HCC. A "nodule-in-nodule" appearance may be seen with both hepatic ade-

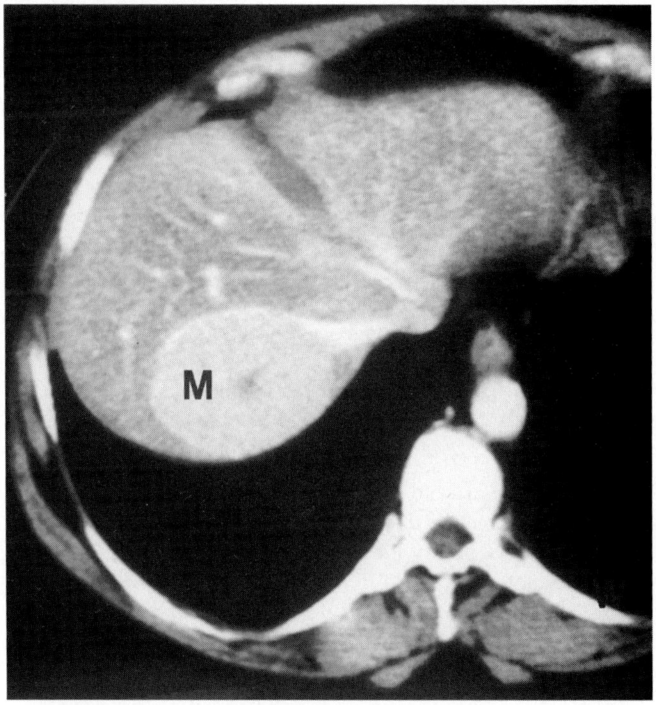

FIGURE 7.14 Focal nodular hyperplasia. Arterial phase image demonstrating intense enhancement in a well-marginated hepatic mass (M) with central low density representing scar.

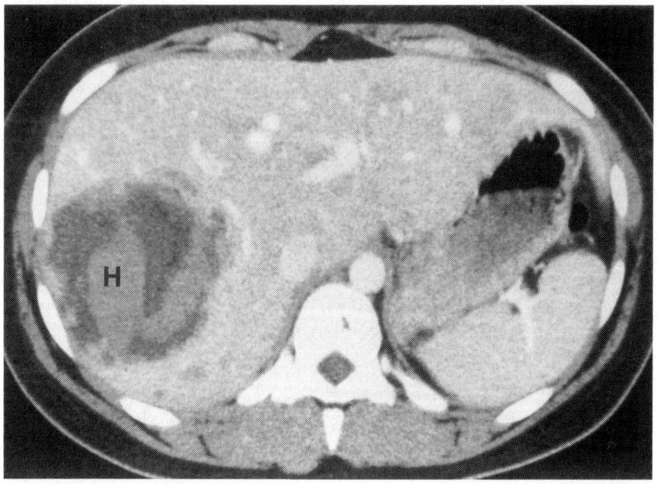

FIGURE 7.15 Adenoma with spontaneous hemorrhage. Contrast-enhanced CT in a 25-year-old woman presenting with abdominal pain. There is a complex mass in the liver with varied attenuation representing hemorrhage (H) within the tumor. A few smaller adenomas are also present.

noma and HCC. Adenomas contain bile ducts on biopsy, distinguishing them from focal nodular hyperplasia, and they do not accumulate sulfur colloid, appearing as cold defects on liver-spleen scintigraphy. Surgical excision is often required owing to their propensity for hemorrhage with increasing size.

- The **mesenchymal hamartoma** likely represents a rare developmental abnormality rather than a true neoplasm. It presents in children usually before the age of 2, with a slight male predominance. The presenting feature is an abdominal mass and most are found in the right hepatic lobe; calcification is unusual. There is no elevation of alpha-fetoprotein. CT demonstrates varying amounts of cystic and solid (mesenchymal) components. Imaging features, laboratory data, and patient age suggest the diagnosis, which can be confirmed by biopsy.

- **Inflammatory pseudotumor** is a rare benign lesion that demonstrates changes of chronic inflammation within a fibrous stroma on histologic examination. Variable amounts of plasma cells and spindle cells are present, with no anaplasia. Diagnosis is usually made by biopsy. Symptoms include fever, fatigue, abdominal pain, weight loss, nausea, and vomiting. CT findings are variable, with all lesions appearing as hypodense on precontrast CT. Following contrast administration, lesions can remain hypodense, become isodense, or even become hyperdense. The imaging findings are nonspecific and biopsy is required for diagnosis.

- **Hepatic teratomas** are rare benign lesions with imaging and histologic features similar to those of hepatoblastoma. This lesion presents in the first year of life as an abdominal mass, sometimes with elevated alpha-fetoprotein. Teratomas are usually several centimeters in diameter when discovered and have variable amounts of fat and calcification. Fatty change is not specific for this tumor.

7.5 MALIGNANT HEPATIC NEOPLASMS

- **Metastases** account for the majority of malignant hepatic neoplasms in the noncirrhotic liver. Primary carcinomas of the breast, lung, pancreas, and colon comprise the bulk of hepatic metastases **(Fig. 7.16).** Alterations in hepatic enzymes, pain, weight loss, and tumor markers suggest the diagnosis clinically.

  The CT appearance ranges from solitary, well-defined lesions to diffusely infiltrative disease. The most common appearance is a hypodense mass with peripheral enhancement on routine portal venous phase imaging. Some lesions can be isodense or even hyperdense, and calcification can occur in some cases **(Fig. 7.17).** Hypervascular metastases may not be demonstrated on routine exams and dual-phase imaging is necessary to detect the early enhancement of these lesions in the hepatic arterial phase **(Fig. 7.18).** This technique is particularly helpful in imaging small lesions. The appearance of metastases can be altered by various treatment regimens **(Fig. 7.19).**

- **Hepatocellular carcinoma (HCC)** is the most common primary malignant hepatic epithelial neoplasm. It usually develops in the setting of chronic liver disease such as cirrhosis, hemochromatosis, and glycogen storage diseases. Predisposing factors for eastern and African cultures are hepatitis and exposure to aflatoxin B. In the western hemisphere, cirrhosis is due to alcohol abuse, toxin exposure, and chronic hepatitis. Clinical features include pain, mass, weight loss, and alpha-fetoprotein elevation.

  CT features overlap to some extent with those of adenomas and FNH. Most HCCs appear as a heterogeneously enhancing irregular mass with ill-defined margins. Hepatocellular cancers usually enhance during the arterial phase **(Figs. 7.20 and 7.21)** on CT but do not take up superparamagnetic iron oxide on MRI. HCC can present as a solitary mass with or without encapsulation or as multifocal or diffuse disease. Necrosis, hemorrhage, vascular invasion, and regional spread are common. Clues to the diagnosis include the presence of lymphadenopathy, portal vein invasion **(Fig. 7.7),** and small peritumoral "satellite" lesions.

- **Fibrolamellar carcinoma** is a slow-growing variant of hepatocellular carcinoma. It is often seen in younger patients (below 35 years of age) and has a better prognosis than HCC. Unlike HCC, it occurs in patients without underlying chronic liver disease. The usual presentation is a large mass, and up to 60 percent have a central fibrous scar with low T2 signal on MRI. The tumor can be pedunculated or

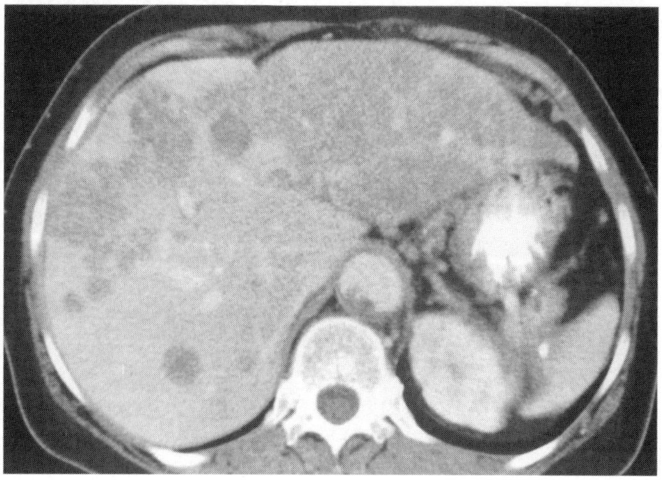

FIGURE 7.16 Hepatic metastasis. Multiple low-attenuation lesions of varying sizes throughout the liver parenchyma in a patient with metastatic lung carcinoma.

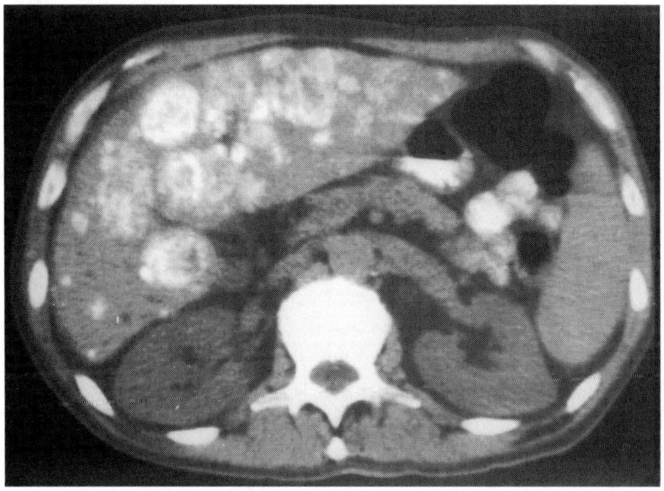

FIGURE 7.17 Calcified metastases. Noncontrast CT demonstrating multiple calcified metastases from mucinous colon cancer.

contain dystrophic calcification. The presence of calcification aids in the diagnosis, as untreated HCC rarely contains calcification. The tumor is of low density with variable enhancement. Most lesions are well demarcated from adjacent hepatic parenchyma and rarely demonstrate hemorrhage or necrosis. Many lesions can be resected, but recurrence occurs in up to 50 percent. Roughly 25 percent of patients will have extrahepatic disease at the time of diagnosis.

- **Intrahepatic cholangiocarcinoma** is the second most common primary malignant hepatic neoplasm. It occurs in the fifth to sixth decade with a slight male predominance. It is associated with intrahepatic cholelithiasis, *Clonorchis sinensis* infection, Thorotrast exposure, and Caroli disease. Symptoms of abdominal pain and a palpable mass do not occur until late in the disease.

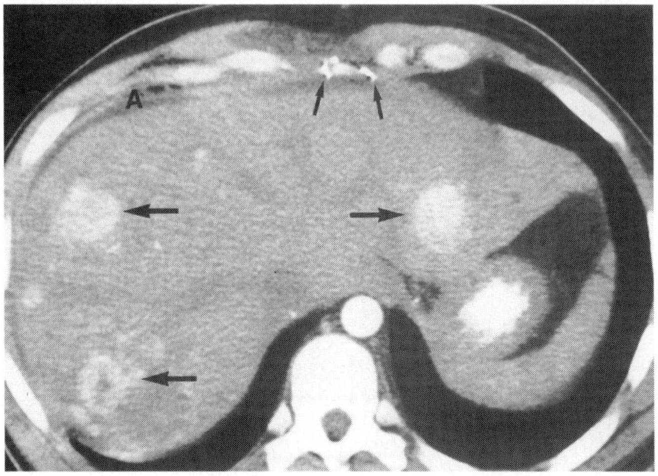

FIGURE 7.18 Hypervascular metastases. Arterial phase image demonstrating multiple hypervascular metastases *(large arrows)* in a patient with carcinoid and carcinoid syndrome. Median sternotomy wires *(small arrows)* are from tricuspid valve replacement for endocardial fibroelastosis. A small amount of perihepatic ascites (A) is present.

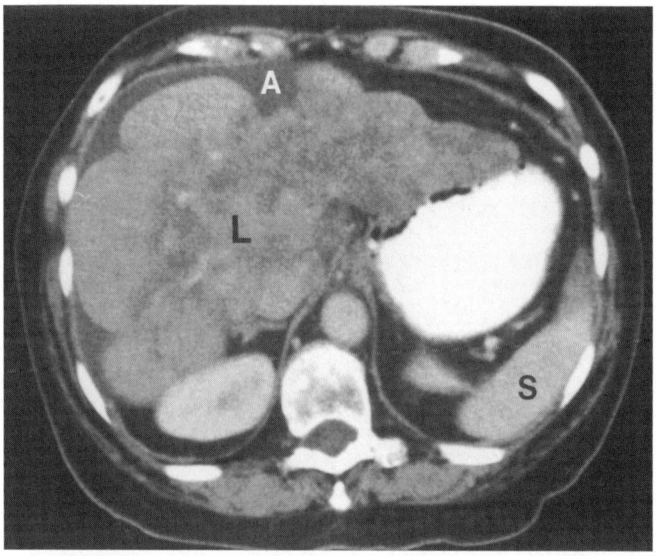

FIGURE 7.19 Pseudocirrhosis. Contrast-enhanced CT in a 69-year-old woman following chemotherapy for metastatic breast cancer. The liver is irregular and heterogeneously enhancing, with nodular margins simulating cirrhosis. Note the small spleen (S) and ascites (A). The subtle sclerotic areas in the vertebral body are bone metastases.

Two features of enhancement may suggest the diagnosis of intrahepatic cholangiocarcinoma. First, mild to moderate peripheral enhancement with washout on later images is known as the peripheral washout sign. The second finding often seen with intrahepatic cholangiocarcinoma is delayed enhancement of central areas of the tumor **(Fig. 7.22).** Small areas of necrosis, hemorrhage, mucin, and calcification can be present. Biliary dilatation near the tumor is present in 20 percent of cases. This lesion can commonly encase vascular structures, but actual invasion is unusual.

- **Hepatic lymphoma.** Secondary involvement of the liver with lymphoma occurs in half of all cases of Hodgkin and non-Hodgkin disease. Primary lymphoma arising in the liver is rare. Secondary lymphoma is usually diffusely infiltrative and does not cause significant architectural distortion. Primary lymphoma often presents as a focal mass but may appear as diffuse disease. CT usually demonstrates multiple homogeneous low-attenuation masses, but diffuse infiltration can present as hepatomegaly with little alteration in parenchymal density or architectural distortion **(Fig. 7.23).** Lack of parenchymal distortion in diffuse disease makes both CT and MRI insensitive for lesion detection.

- **Angiosarcoma** is the most common primary sarcoma of the liver. This malignant vascular tumor is often accompanied by a history of exposure to polyvinyl chloride, arsenic, or Thorotrast. It is more common in men and can be associated with systemic diseases such as von Recklinghausen disease and hemochromatosis. Most lesions are unresectable at diagnosis; 60 percent present with metastatic disease. Chemotherapy can extend the median survival from 6 to 13 months.

  CT demonstrates a single or multiple low-density masses with progressive peripheral enhancement and areas of high or low attenuation corresponding to recent or remote hemorrhage, respectively. Without features of prior Thorotrast exposure, accurate diagnosis of

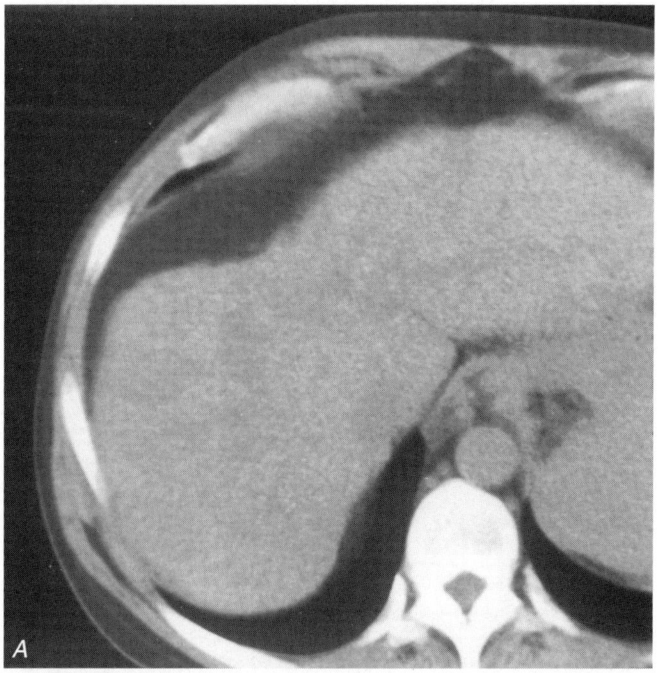

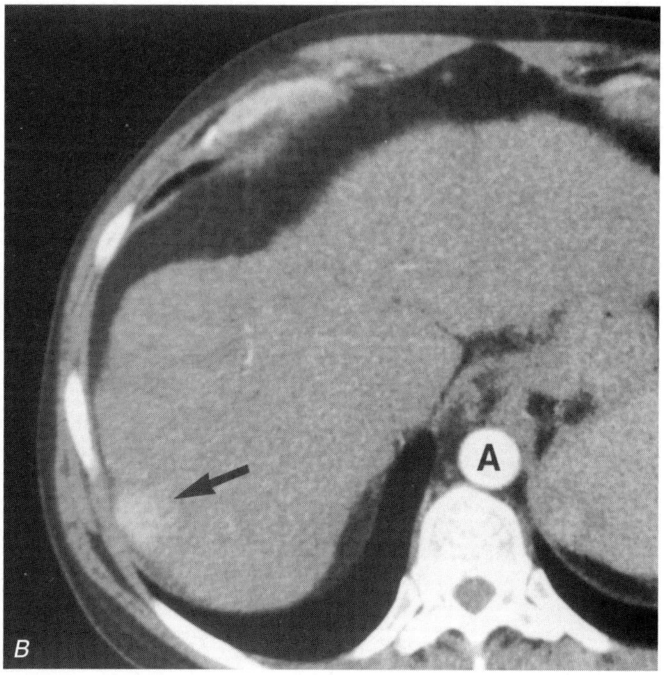

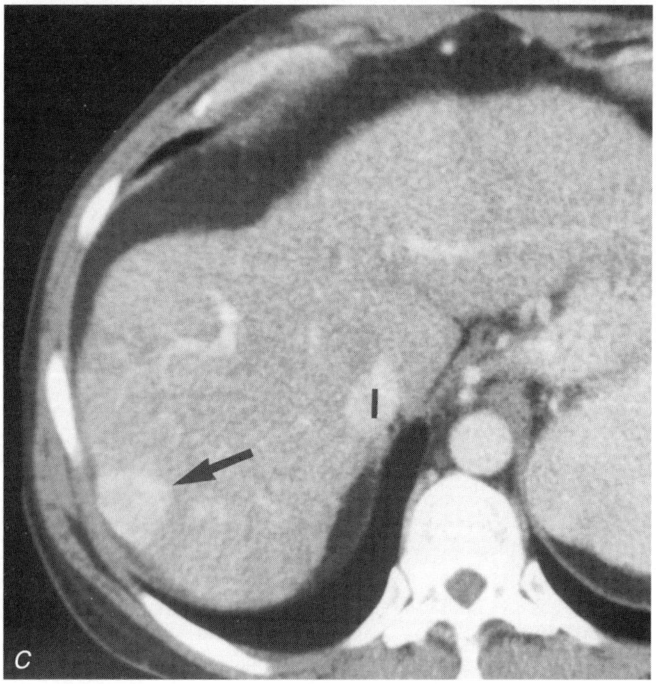

FIGURE 7.20 Hepatocellular carcinoma. Triple-phase CT. *A*. Precontrast image. *B*. Arterial phase shows dense opacification of the aorta (A) and an arterial blush in the right lobe *(arrow)*. *C*. Portal venous phase shows enhancement of the tumor *(arrow)*. I, inferior vena cava.

angiosarcoma can be impossible because of the overlap in appearance with hepatic hemangiomas. Spontaneous hemoperitoneum and hemorrhagic ascites occasionally occur. Percutaneous biopsy can lead to massive bleeding; open biopsy is preferred.

- **Epithelioid hemangioendothelioma** is a malignant vascular neoplasm. It is more common in women, with an average age at presentation of 45. The name stems from the epithelioid appearance of the neoplastic cells on light microscopy. Twenty percent of patients have no symptoms, while many present with abdominal pain, jaundice, weakness, anorexia, and hepatomegaly. Imaging demonstrates multiple low-attenuation lesions, which can have subcapsular growth and marked enhancement. Enlargement of uninvolved hepatic parenchyma is suggestive of this lesion, but it is indistinguishable from metastatic disease. Biopsy often demonstrates perivascular involvement and will often yield the correct diagnosis.

- **Kaposi sarcoma** is a rare vascular neoplasm often seen in AIDS patients. Involvement of the liver is not usually symptomatic and is unrelated to mortality. The disease is multifocal and CT demonstrates multiple small hypodense lesions that are slow to fill with contrast. Kaposi sarcoma is indistinguishable from multiple hemangiomas and peliosis hepatis; it requires no treatment. The differential in these patients includes metastases, microabscesses, and bacillary angiomatosis. One clue to the diagnosis is concurrent cutaneous involvement with Kaposi sarcoma.

- **Hepatoblastoma** is a rare, typically malignant hepatic neoplasm that occurs in children less than 5 years of age. The majority are less than 24 months, with a mean age at diagnosis of about 16 months. This lesion has a male (2:1) predominance with clinical features of anorexia and weight loss in the presence of an enlarging abdomen. Serum alpha-fetoprotein is usually elevated, and some tumors produce human chorionic gonadotropin, which can cause precocious puberty in males.

  Hepatoblastoma **(Fig. 7.24)** is usually solitary, right-lobe-predominant, and hypodense with areas of chunky calcification (50 percent). Multiple lesions and diffuse disease occur much less frequently. Following contrast administration, the lesion enhances less than normal liver. Vascular invasion can be present. The best prognostic indicator is resectability rather than histologic classification. Therefore imaging of the chest and abdomen is essential in the detection of lung metastases and regional lymph node disease.

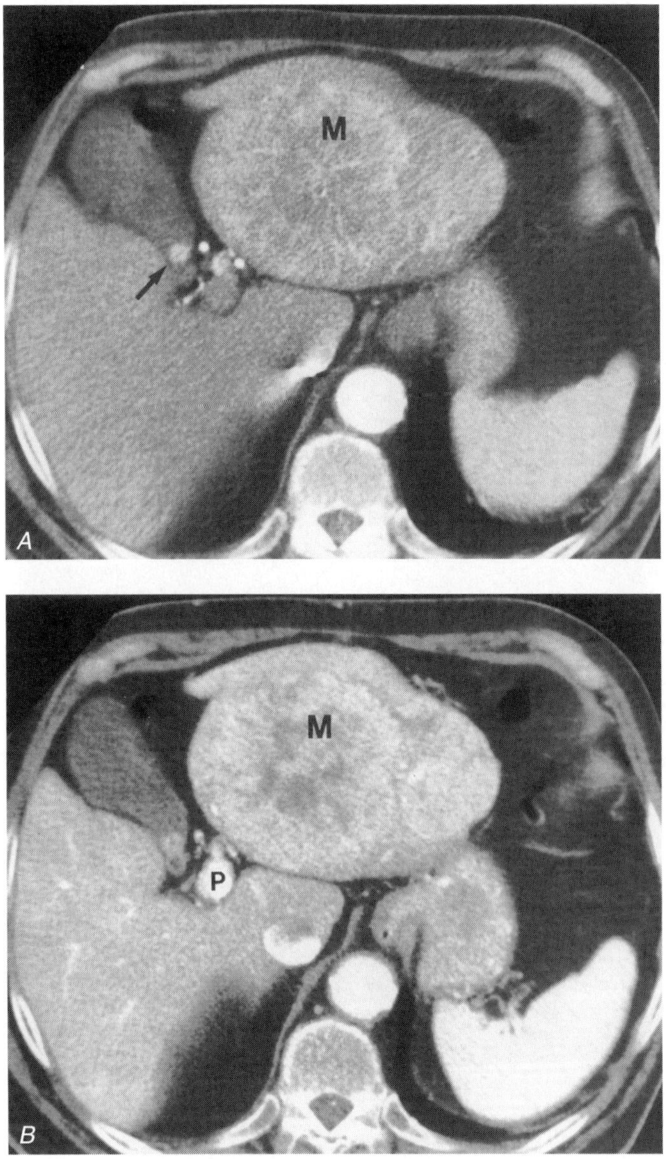

FIGURE 7.21 Hepatocellular carcinoma. *A*. Arterial-phase CT with heterogeneous enhancement (spoke-wheel pattern) in a large mass (M) in the left hepatic lobe. *B*. Portal venous phase showing portal vein (P). Arrow, gallstone.

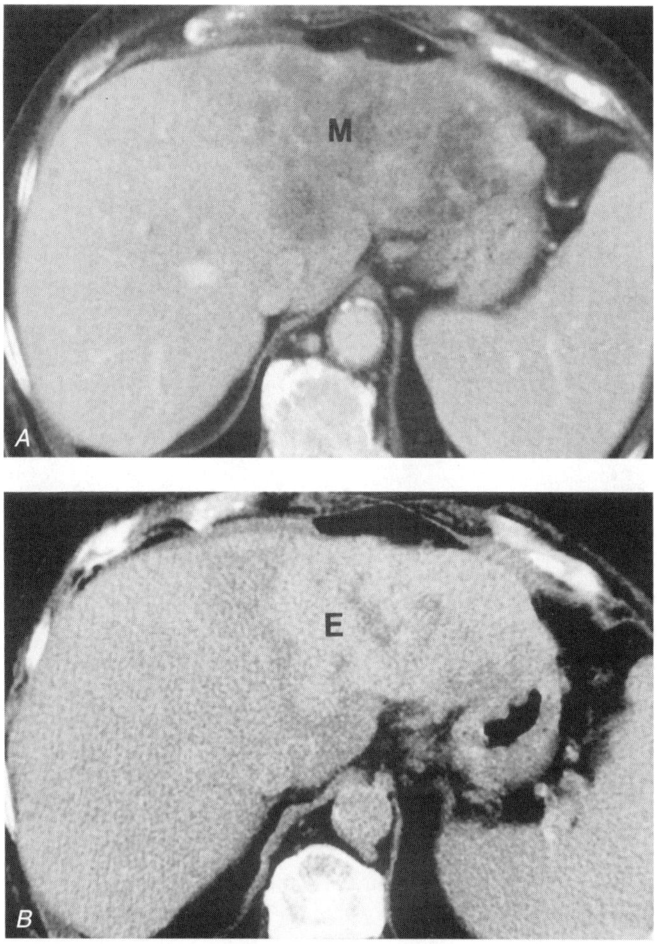

FIGURE 7.22 Intrahepatic cholangiocarcinoma. *A*. Portal venous phase CT demonstrates a large low-attenuation mass (M) in the left hepatic lobe. *B*. Delayed enhancement (E) 10 min following contrast administration.

- **Infantile hemangioendothelioma** is the most common hepatic tumor in the first 6 months of life. Half of these lesions become clinically apparent in the first month, with girls affected more than boys. Congestive heart failure can occur in up to 25 percent due to arteriovenous shunting. Cutaneous hemangiomas are seen in 40 percent of affected patients. Large or multiple lesions can cause Kasabach-Merritt syndrome.

  Classic imaging findings are a well-defined low-attenuation mass with nodular peripheral enhancement that "fills in" on delayed imaging. Areas without enhancement can represent infarction or fibrosis. Variable amounts of fibrosis can be present, depending on the age of the lesion. Calcification and hemorrhage are not uncommon.

- **Undifferentiated embryonal sarcoma** is a highly malignant lesion with slight female predominance that presents in older children. Clinically there is an abdominal mass with or without pain and, rarely, elevation of alpha-fetoprotein. Imaging typically demonstrates both cystic and solid components of this aggressive tumor. MRI shows low T1 intensity and high intensity on T2-weighted images. Some tumors demonstrate a pseudocapsule, which, when present, has low signal intensity on both T1- and T2-weighted sequences.

7.6 HEPATIC VASCULAR PHENOMENA

- **Passive congestion** occurs in the setting of right heart failure, usually from tricuspid regurgitation or constrictive pericarditis. Hepatojugular reflux may be present on physical exam. Hepatocytes are compromised by both sinusoidal congestion and decreased cardiac output. Variable degrees of atrophy and centrilobular necrosis may be present. CT demonstrates dilatation of the inferior vena cava and hepatic veins. The liver may have mottled enhancement with contrast-enhanced CT. Reflux of intra-

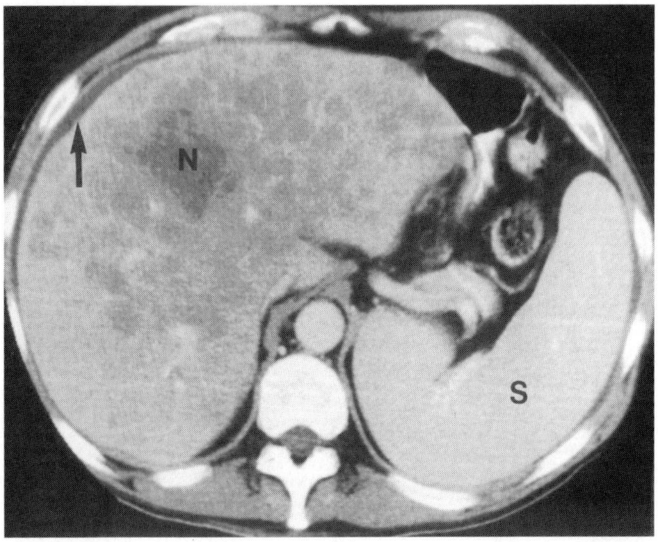

FIGURE 7.23 **Hepatic lymphoma.** A 61-year-old male with a history of B-cell lymphoma being treated with chemotherapy for a mesenteric nodal mass. Innumerable hepatic nodules are seen throughout the left hepatic lobe and anterior segment of the right hepatic lobe. A focal region of necrosis (N) is present. A small rim of perihepatic fluid is also present *(arrow)*. S, splenomegaly.

venously administered contrast into the dilated hepatic veins is not uncommon. With chronic congestion there is necrosis and fibrosis, which can lead to the rare condition of "cardiac cirrhosis."

- **Portal hypertension** is often manifest by the presence of multiple portosystemic collaterals. Common areas for collateral development include the distal esophagus as well as the paraumbilical, retroperitoneal, and hemorrhoidal regions. Portal hypertension can be divided into three subtypes: prehepatic, intrahepatic, and posthepatic. Prehepatic portal hypertension occurs in the setting of portal or splenic vein occlusion **(Fig. 7.25)**. Intrahepatic portal hypertension is caused by cirrhosis, metastases, and parasitic infection such as schistosomiasis in endemic areas. Portal hypertension can occur from posthepatic causes such as congestive heart failure, tricuspid insufficiency or regurgitation, or constrictive pericarditis. Occlusion of the hepatic veins (known as Budd-Chiari syndrome) is also a cause of posthepatic portal hypertension. CT can demonstrate increased size of the portal vein (>13 mm), splenomegaly, portal vein thrombosis, ascites, and enlargement in the size of the splenic and mesenteric veins (>10 mm). Portosystemic collaterals can be found in characteristic locations.

- **Budd-Chiari/hepatic veno-occlusive disease** is the result of venous outflow obstruction from occlusion of the hepatic veins. Patients may present with upper abdominal pain and ascites **(Fig. 7.26)**. The disease in Asian cultures is often secondary to membranes or webs in the hepatic veins, and segmental hepatic involvement is common. In Western cultures, occlusion of the major hepatic veins or inferior vena cava by tumor or thrombus is often the cause. Bland thrombus can result from hypercoagulable states, such as polycythemia, systemic disease, and pregnancy. Tumor thrombus from primary hepatic, renal, and adrenal lesions can cause Budd-Chiari syndrome.

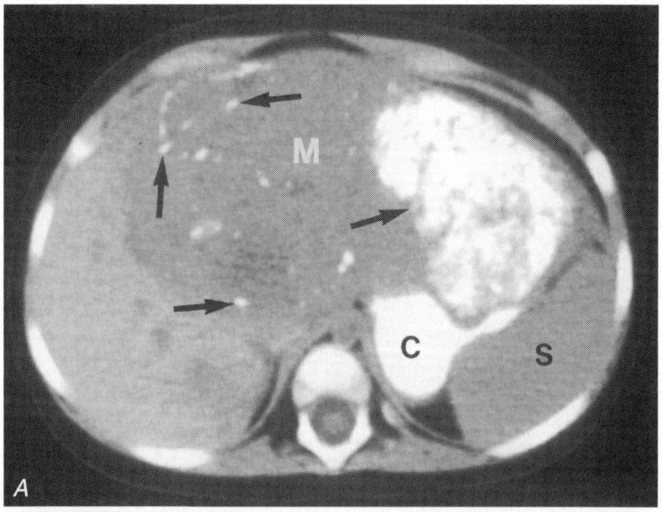

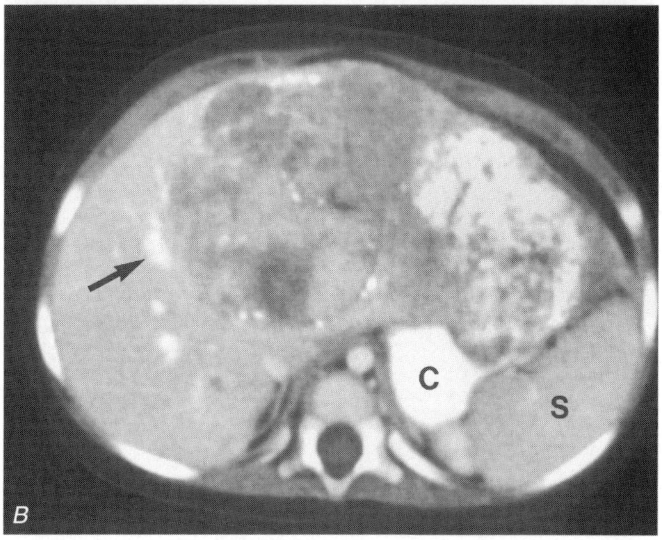

FIGURE 7.24 **Hepatoblastoma.** A 1-year-old girl with a palpable abdominal mass. *A*. Noncontrast CT image reveals a large and heterogeneous left hepatic mass (M) with both punctate and flocculent calcifications *(arrows)*. *B*. Following intravenous contrast administration, there is marked heterogeneous enhancement of the mass abutting and bowing the middle hepatic vein toward the right *(arrow)*. S, spleen; C, oral contrast within stomach. (Case courtesy of Dr. Jeffrey Friedland, Denver, CO.)

CT demonstrates coarse hepatic attenuation with nonvisualization of the hepatic veins. Following contrast administration, there is inhomogeneous hepatic enhancement due to sinusoidal congestion, hepatocyte atrophy, and necrosis. The caudate lobe has venous drainage directly into the inferior vena cava and may show compensatory enlargement and homogeneous enhancement.

- **Portal venous gas** has historically been regarded as an ominous sign and is often seen in the context of bowel ischemia or obstruction. Portal venous gas can be idiopathic or iatrogenic or it may result from such causes as perforated diverticulum or gastric ulcer, pancreatitis, endoscopy, or surgery **(Differential 7.13)**.

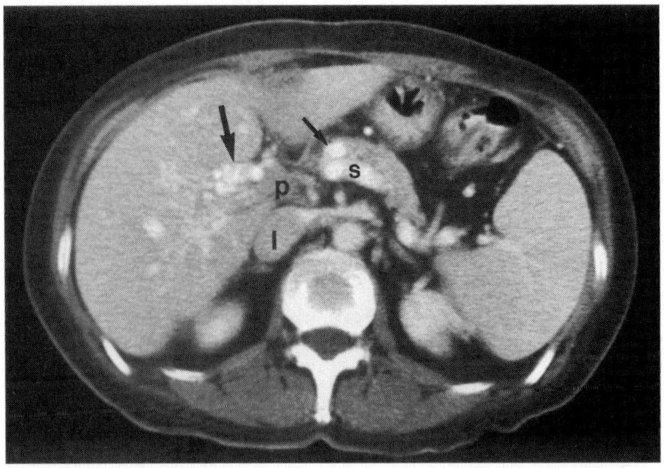

FIGURE 7.25 Cavernous transformation of the portal vein. Contrast-enhanced CT shows multiple small vessels in the porta hepatis *(large arrow)*. S, splenic vein; small arrow, superior mesenteric vein; P, thrombosed portal vein; I, inferior vena cava.

- **Transient hepatic attenuation difference (THAD)** is a vascular phenomenon of hepatic enhancement that has been described for over 20 years. THAD is seen in hepatic arterial phase images as lobar or segmental increased attenuation that becomes isodense during the portal venous phase or delayed imaging **(Fig. 7.27).** The pathophysiology has been attributed to two likely causes: (1) shunting of hepatic arterial blood into a portal segment and (2) occlusion or stricture of a portal vein by tumor or bland thrombus, which would cause decreased or delayed contribution of portal blood to hepatic enhancement.
- **Hepatic infarction** is an uncommon condition, since the dual blood supply of the liver is relatively protective. Approximately 25 percent of hepatic blood flow is provided by the hepatic artery, which delivers oxygenated blood, and 75 percent by the portal vein, which delivers blood and nutrients from the splanchnic bed. Occlusion of the hepatic artery alone will not cause hepatic infarction in an otherwise normal patient. The combination of hepatic artery occlusion and decreased or absent portal venous flow are required to cause hepatic infarction. Hepatic infarction can be seen with hepatic transplantation, sickle cell disease, shock, sepsis, intra-arterial chemotherapy, and oral contraceptive use. The ideal contrast-enhanced CT appearance of hepatic infarction is a well-defined wedge-shaped area of decreased attenuation abutting the capsular surface. The shape and location of hepatic infarction is variable, but the lesions should not significantly enhance on delayed images.
- **Peliosis hepatis** is a rare condition associated with chronic disease or malignancy. Tuberculosis and the use of anabolic steroids or oral contraceptives are known to precede the development of peliosis hepatis. In patients with **AIDS,** peliosis is now a more common finding. In this setting, an infection with *Rochalimaea* species must be suspected. Treatment with antibiotics such as erythromycin is often curative. CT demonstrates multiple cystic spaces throughout the liver parenchyma, with a tendency to become isodense with hepatic parenchyma following contrast administration. Histologically, these cystic spaces represent blood-filled areas of sinusoidal dilation.

7.13

PORTAL VENOUS GAS

Mesenteric ischemia, necrosis, or infarction
Pneumobilia (mimic)
Bowel obstruction
Necrotizing enterocolitis—children
Diverticulitis, intra-abdominal abscess
Inflammatory bowel disease—following barium enema or colonoscopy
Recent bowel surgery
Toxic megacolon—ulcerative colitis; Crohn disease, cytomegalovirus, ischemia, pseudomembranous colitis, amebiasis

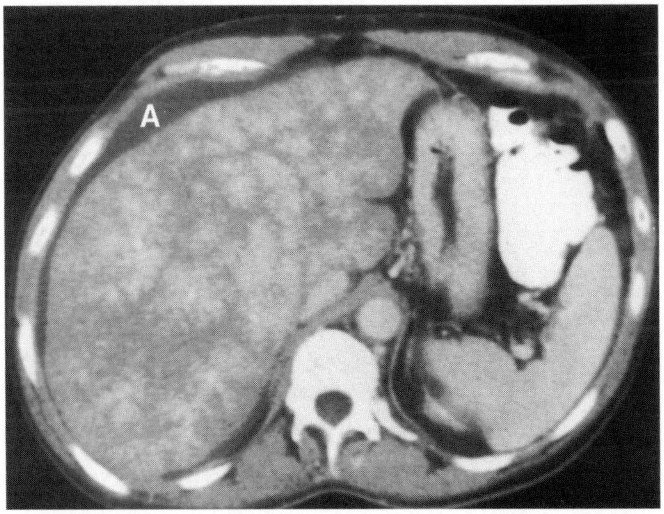

FIGURE 7.26 Budd-Chiari syndrome. Contrast-enhanced CT shows mottled hepatic enhancement and ascites (A).

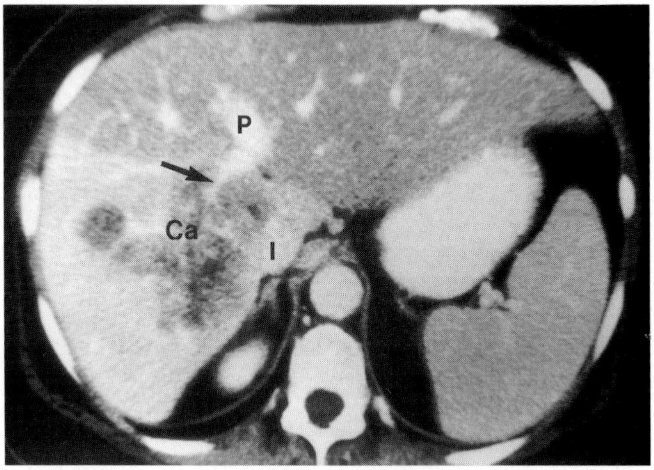

FIGURE 7.27 Transient hepatic attenuation difference (THAD). Contrast-enhanced CT in a patient with a hepatocellular carcinoma (Ca) invading the right portal vein *(arrow)*, leading to differential perfusion of the right and left hepatic lobes. P, left portal vein; I, inferior vena cava.

7.7 GALLBLADDER AND BILIARY DISEASE

Anatomy, Physiology, and Technique

- The **gallbladder** serves as a reservoir for bile awaiting transport to the duodenum to aid digestion. Bile is formed in the liver at a rate of 1.5 L/day. The dominant conjugated form aids lipid metabolism. The gallbladder has a muscular wall that contracts upon stimulation with cholecystokinin, which is released following the ingestion of food. The cystic artery, arising from the hepatic artery, possesses few anastomoses, predisposing the gallbladder to ischemia.
- The intrahepatic **bile ducts** can be seen on CT as low-attenuation foci adjacent to portal vein radicals. These ducts are solely on one side of the vascular structures, distinguishing them from periportal tracking of fluid, which is present on both sides of the vessels. The intrahepatic biliary radicals form right and left hepatic ducts, which have a confluence near the hilum, becoming the common hepatic duct (CHD). The CHD can be seen as a water-attenuation structure anterior to the portal vein at the hepatic hilum. The common bile duct (CBD) normally measures less than 6 to 8 mm, and there is usually tapering of the intrapancreatic segment. The CBD can be up to 1 cm in size in older patients or those who have undergone prior cholecystectomy. The very thin (1-mm) duct wall normally enhances following IV contrast administration and can be appreciated on routine CT. The cystic duct joins the CBD, which subsequently traverses the pancreatic head to empty into the duodenum at the ampulla of Vater with its sphincter of Oddi.
- Biliary pathology can be identified on routine abdominal CT; however, dedicated biliary technique requires thinner collimation, such as spiral CT technique with contiguous 5-mm collimation and a pitch of 1 to 1.5. For duct evaluation, 1- to 3-mm reconstructions are required. Negative (water) oral contrast or no oral contrast can aid in detecting distal choledocholithiasis; in these patients, IV contrast is also withheld. Rarely, contrast material that is excreted in bile is administered to obtain a CT cholangiogram.

Congenital Abnormalities

- **Choledochal cysts** are dilatations of the extrahepatic biliary tree thought to arise from reflux of pancreatic enzymes into the distal duct. Choledochal cysts infrequently present with the classic triad of right-upper-quadrant pain, jaundice, and a palpable mass. Choledochal cysts are depicted as cystic lesions adjacent to the portal vein and can be difficult to distinguish from gastrointestinal duplication cysts. There can be mild intrahepatic biliary dilatation. Complications include stone formation and cholangiocarcinoma.
- **Choledochoceles** are dilatations of the terminal portion of the common bile duct that often herniate into the duodenum. CT can demonstrate a cystic lesion interposed between the pancreatic head and the duodenum. Generally, dilatation of the proximal duct is not seen unless pancreatitis or an obstructing calculus is present. The differential diagnosis includes pancreatic pseudocysts, gastrointestinal duplication cysts, and gastric or duodenal diverticuli.
- **Caroli disease** is a rare entity consisting of saccular intrahepatic biliary dilatation. It is often associated with medullary sponge kidney, congenital hepatic fibrosis, and infantile polycystic kidney disease. These patients develop cholangitis, intrahepatic stones, abscesses, or cholangiocarcinoma. CT shows multiple interconnected hepatic cystic lesions **(Fig. 7.28)**. Rarely, the "central dot sign" of dilated ducts encasing portal triads can be observed, although this is better demonstrated on sonography.

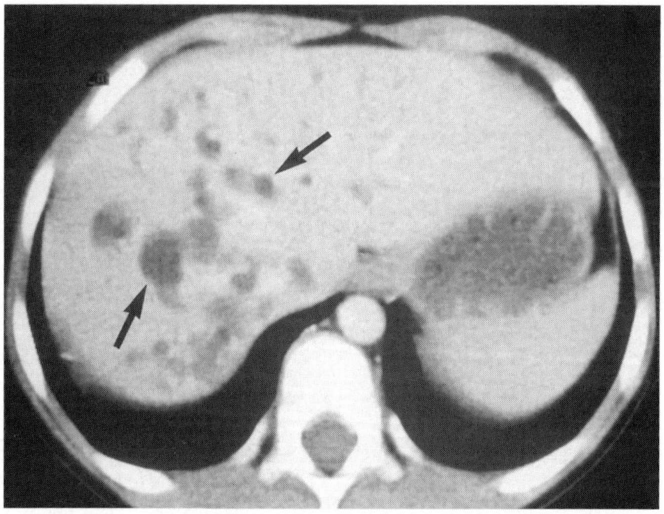

FIGURE 7.28 Caroli disease. Saccular intrahepatic biliary dilatation in a 35-year-old woman with Caroli disease. Multiple interconnected cysts *(arrows)* are the hallmark of this disease.

Cholelithiasis and Biliary Obstruction

- **Biliary dilatation** is depicted as linear fluid attenuation structures tracking adjacent to the portal veins on CT. The dilated bile ducts are observed on one side of the vessel only and extend to the hepatic periphery **(Fig. 7.29)**. This is in contradistinction to periportal edema or peribiliary cysts that surround the portal structures. Causes of dilatation include choledocholithiasis, cholangitis, benign strictures, cholangiocarcinoma, pancreatic head masses, and ampullary stenosis **(Differentials 7.14 and 7.15)**.

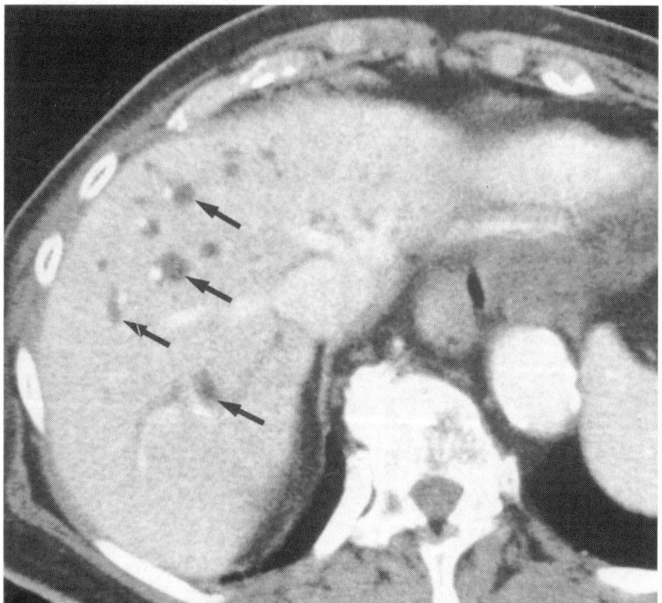

FIGURE 7.29 Intrahepatic biliary dilatation. Contrast-enhanced CT in an 85-year-old woman with choledocholithiasis shows enlarged intrahepatic bile ducts *(arrows)* adjacent to vessels.

7.14

INTRAHEPATIC BILIARY DILATATION

Obstructing stone
Pancreatic head mass
Stricture—prior surgery, inflammation, idiopathic
Sclerosing cholangitis
Caroli disease
Periportal edema (mimic)
Periportal adenopathy—hepatic, pancreatic, gastric, lymphomatous primaries
Infectious cholangitis—bacterial, parasitic, viral (HIV)
Hepatic fibrosis

- **Pneumobilia,** or air within the biliary tree, is usually the result of surgery or instrumentation but can also result from fistulas (gallstone ileus) or infection **(Differential 7.16).** Pneumobilia tends to be more central and confluent than portal venous gas, although the two can be difficult to differentiate. The distinction can be significant, as portal venous gas can be associated with bowel ischemia.
- **Cholelithiasis** (gallstones) is a very common cause of abdominal discomfort, typically seen in obese women of childbearing age. Predisposing factors include hemolytic states such as sickle cell disease, cholestasis, strictures, parasites, inflammatory bowel disease, and genetic predilection. Stones can vary in composition, the most common consisting of cholesterol alone or cholesterol combined with calcium carbonate or bilirubinate. Pigmented stones are soft and frequently intrahepatic.

  About 65 percent of gallstones can be seen on CT, depending on calcium content. Only one-quarter are homogeneously of high attenuation on CT. Gallstones are typically seen as high-attenuation or calcific foci layering dependently within the fluid-attenuation bile of the gallbladder. Gallstones can contain nitrogen gas from negative internal pressure, demonstrable as the "Mercedes-Benz sign" **(Fig. 7.30). Choledocholithiasis** with an obstructing stone in the distal common bile duct can be demonstrated and may be a source of biliary obstruction and pain. In this setting, CT demonstrates biliary dilatation, wall thickening, and potentially the distal stone **(Figs. 7.31 and 7.32).** Ultrasound is the modality of choice for detecting cholelithiasis; Magnetic resonance cholangiopancreatography is the best noninvasive method for detecting choledocholithiasis.
- **Biliary sludge** represents calcium bilirubinate granules or cholesterol crystals and can increase bile attenuation on CT. Hemobilia, mucus, parasitic infestations, and tumors can have an appearance similar to that of high-attenuation bile **(Differential 7.17).**
- **Bilomas** are the sequelae of iatrogenic or traumatic biliary injury. They can be free-flowing or loculated portal, intrahepatic, or perihepatic collections. While intra-abdominal fluid collections are present about 10 percent of the time following laparoscopic cholecystectomy, few persist or become symptomatic. Image-guided drainage is indicated for infected or persistent bilomas.

7.15

DILATED COMMON BILE DUCT WITHOUT OBSTRUCTION

Aging
Prior biliary surgery
Recent gallstone passage
Type I choledochal cyst

7.16

PNEUMOBILIA

Sphincterotomy
Recent gallstone passage
Cholecystoenterostomy or choledochoenterostomy—Whipple procedure
Emphysematous cholecystitis—diabetics
Trauma—generally penetrating
Gallstone ileus
Enteric fistula—cholecystitis, perforated ulcer, or cancer

Inflammation

- **Acute cholecystitis** is typically the result of cystic duct obstruction from a stone impacted in the cystic duct. Symptoms include pain, fever, and right-upper-quadrant tenderness with leukocytosis and a **Murphy sign** of inspiratory arrest upon palpation of the gallbladder fossa. Sonography is the preferred modality for diagnosis. On CT, the gallbladder is usually distended **(Differential 7.18)** with a thick wall **(Differential 7.19)**, cholelithiasis, pericholecystic fluid, and soft tissue stranding **(Fig. 7.32).** A perforation or hepatic abscess can be evident **(Fig. 7.33).**
- Other forms of gallbladder inflammation include acalculous, chronic, and emphysematous cholecystitis. **Acalculus cholecystitis** is seen in debilitated, postoperative, and posttraumatic patients or those receiving total parenteral nutrition. **Chronic cholecystitis** involves cholelithiasis and thickening of the gallbladder. **Emphysematous cholecystitis** is seen in the elderly and in diabet-

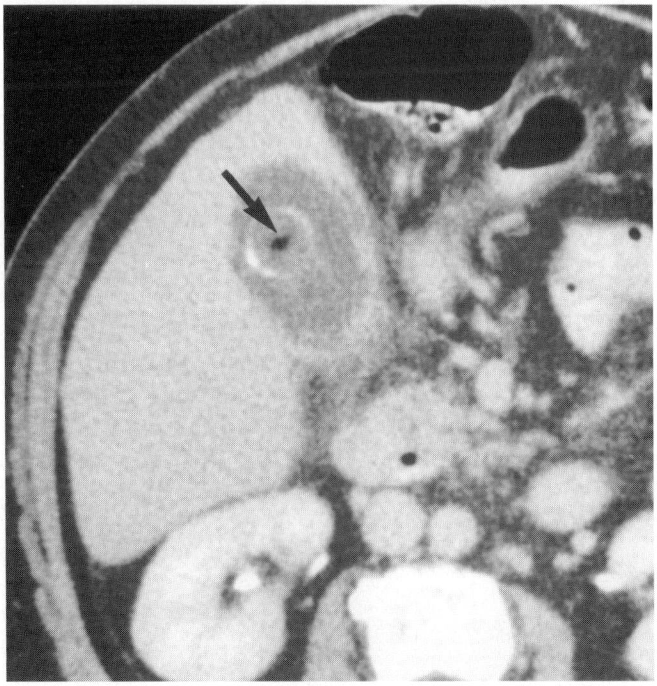

FIGURE 7.30 Gallstone containing gas. A 63-year-old woman with cholecystitis and gas density within a calcified gallstone *(arrow).*

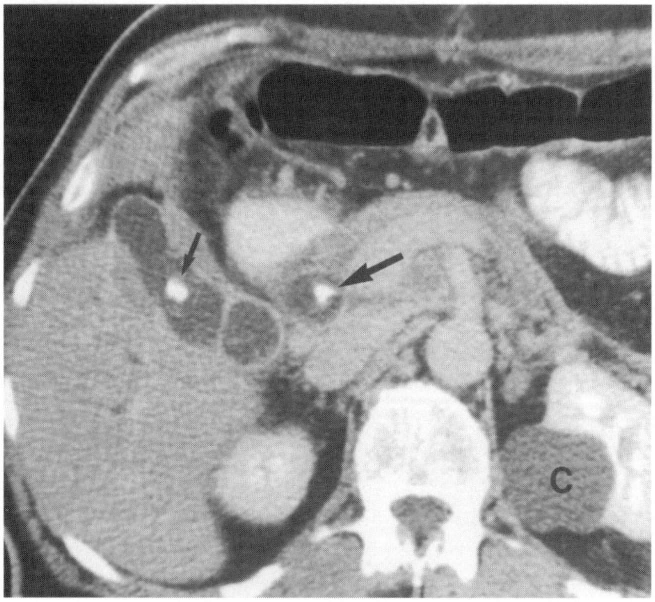

FIGURE 7.31 Choledocholithiasis. A 50-year-old woman with cholecystitis, cholelithiasis *(small arrow)*, and choledocholithiasis. There is a calcified choledocholith in the dilated common bile duct *(large arrow)*. C, renal cyst.

ics; *Clostridium perfringens* is the infectious agent. Patients can have a normal white blood cell count and can lack focal tenderness. Gas can be seen within the gallbladder wall and lumen **(Fig. 7.34).** Treatment is surgical, since there is high morbidity and mortality.

- **Adenomyomatosis** is a hyperplastic cholecystosis causing segmental or diffuse thickening of the gallbladder wall. A localized form can simulate gallbladder cancer. It is best diagnosed sonographically.

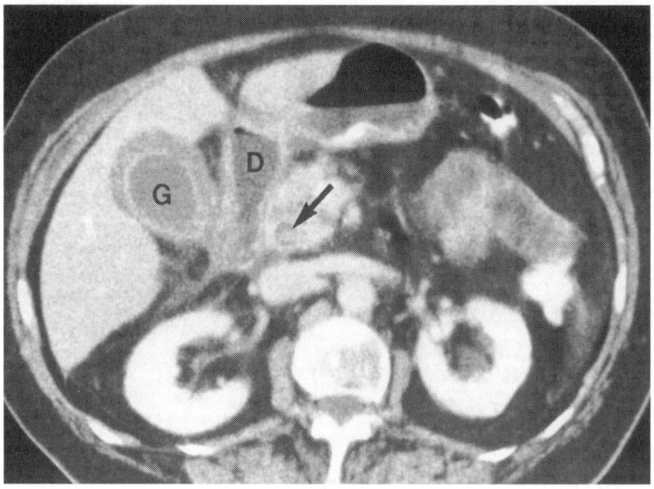

FIGURE 7.32 Acute cholecystitis and choledocholithiasis. Diffuse thickening of the gallbladder wall (G) and a stone *(arrow)* in the common bile duct. D, fluid-filled duodenum.

7.17

HIGH-ATTENUATION BILE

Vicarious excretion of contrast
Cholelithiasis
Milk of calcium
Hematobilia—trauma

- **Mirrizi syndrome** is an uncommon cause of biliary obstruction in which a stone impacted in the cystic duct or gallbladder compresses the adjacent common bile duct. This can simulate choledocholithiasis on CT.
- **Sclerosing cholangitis** is a chronic inflammatory condition of the biliary tree, with jaundice, pain, pruritus, and occasionally fever. It has an association with inflammatory bowel disease. There is segmental stricturing and dilatation of both intra- and extrahepatic ducts with a "pruned tree" appearance. Thickening of the ductal wall can be indistinguishable from **AIDS cholangitis** due to infection by *Cryptosporidium,* CMV, or HIV.
- **Recurrent pyogenic (Oriental) cholangiohepatitis** is a common disease in Asia due to *Clonorchis sinensis* infestation. It is clinically characterized by intermittent bouts of fever, abdominal pain, and jaundice. Dilated intrahepatic ducts contain sludge or pigment stones, best demonstrated on noncontrast images. Hepatic abscesses are a relatively common complication; pancreatitis is a less common sequela.

Neoplasia

- **Cholangiocarcinoma** is a tumor of the bile ducts that invades the hepatic parenchyma, metastasizes to local lymph nodes and the lung, and can cause proximal biliary obstruction. It is usually an adenocarcinoma and carries the eponym of Klatskin tumor when it occurs at the confluence of the right and left hepatic ducts. Approximately one-quarter of these tumors are intrahepatic, half occur near the hepatic hilum, and the remaining quarter arise within the CBD. There are associations with ulcerative colitis, sclerosing cholangitis, infestation with *C. sinensis,* and choledochal cysts, although most cholangiocarcinomas are sporadic.

  On CT, cholangiocarcinoma appears as an infiltrating, mildly enhancing mass, usually near the hepatic hilum, although it can be more peripheral. Delayed (10 to 20 min) contrast enhancement can be demonstrated on CT in about 40 percent **(Fig. 7.22).** This is because of retained contrast material within the tumor's fibrous stroma. Cholangiocarcinoma is otherwise indistinguishable from other solid hepatic neoplasms. Extrahepatic tumors can be depicted as large obstructing masses but are often very subtle, seen simply as CBD wall thickening or small polypoid masses.

7.18

ENLARGED GALLBLADDER

Fasting or hyperalimentation
Biliary obstruction—cholecystolithiasis or pancreatic head mass
Pancreatitis
Diabetes
Drugs—narcotics, anticholinergics
AIDS

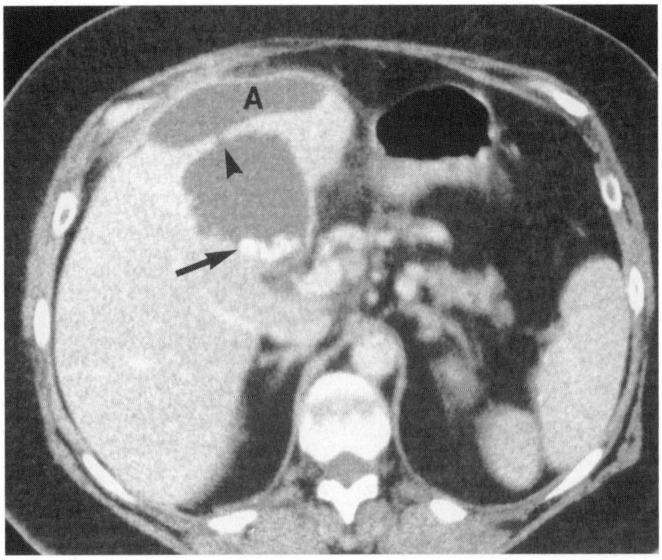

FIGURE 7.33 Acute cholecystitis with abscess. A 63-year-old woman with cholelithiasis *(arrow)*, cholecystitis, perforation *(arrowhead)*, and abscess (A). Note adjacent stranding of perihepatic fat.

- **Gallbladder cancer** follows colorectal, pancreatic, gastric, and esophageal primaries as the fifth most frequent abdominal malignancy. It is a disease of the elderly, with predisposing factors including cholelithiasis, porcelain gallbladder, inflammatory bowel disease, familial polyposis, and chronic cholecystitis. Symptoms include abdominal pain, anorexia, and jaundice. A thickened or irregular gallbladder wall, polypoid mass, or replacement of the lumen can be signs of malignancy **(Fig. 7.35).** Lymphadenopathy, hepatic metastases, or direct invasion is present in over half the cases at presentation. Peritoneal spread and omental disease are often identified. Metastases to the gallbladder are uncommon; most are from melanoma.

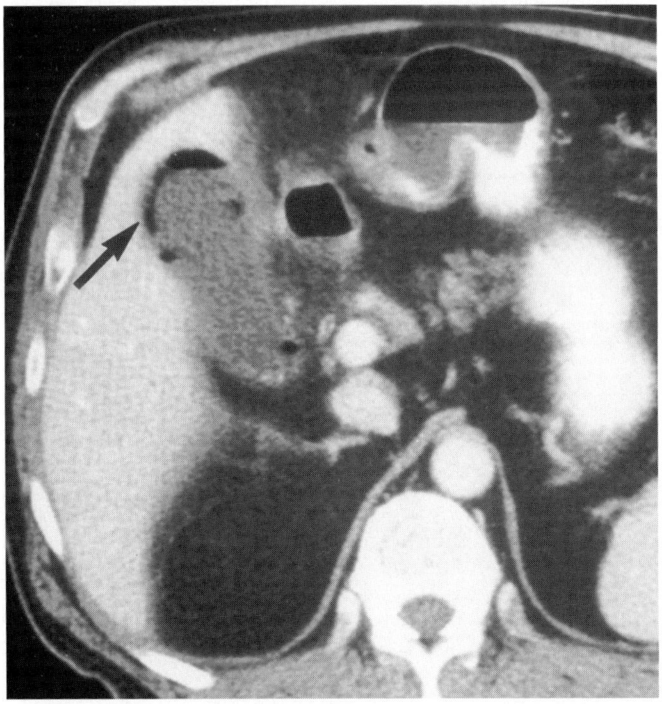

FIGURE 7.34 Emphysematous cholecystitis. Gas within the gallbladder wall *(arrow)* in a 64-year-old diabetic man.

7.19

GALLBLADDER WALL THICKENING

Focal
- **Inflammatory polyp**
- **Adenomyomatosis**
- **Gallbladder carcinoma**
- **Adherent stone/sludge**
- Metastasis—melanoma
- Benign tumors—adenoma, papilloma, carcinoid
- Varices
- *Ectopic mucosa*

Diffuse
- **Incomplete distention**
- **Ascites**
- **Cholecystitis**
- **Adjacent inflammation—**hepatitis, pancreatitis, peptic ulcer
- Gallbladder carcinoma
- AIDS
- Adenomyomatosis

- The term **porcelain gallbladder** refers to dystrophic calcification occurring in the gallbladder wall or within dilated Rokitansky-Aschoff sinuses. Patients are usually asymptomatic unless there is associated cholelithiasis, and most cases are detected as an incidental finding. Elective cholecystectomy is performed, as one-quarter of these patients develop gallbladder carcinoma. A porcelain gallbladder is readily demonstrated on CT as segmental or complete calcification of the gallbladder wall **(Fig. 7.36).** An internal gallbladder mass is highly suspicious for carcinoma.

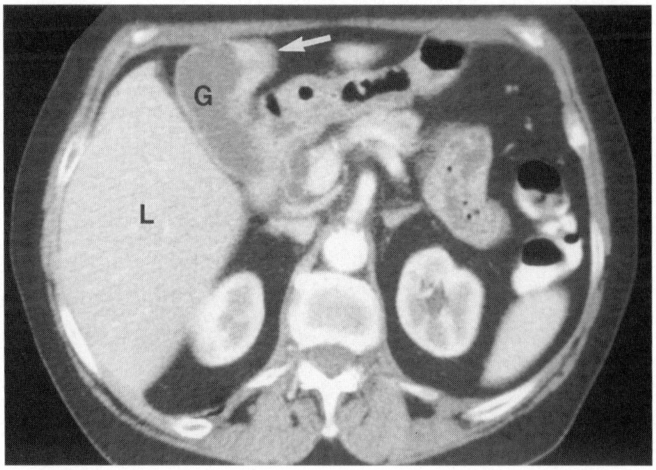

FIGURE 7.35 Gallbladder carcinoma. Contrast-enhanced CT demonstrates eccentric irregular thickening of the gallbladder wall *(arrow)*. G, gallbladder; L, liver.

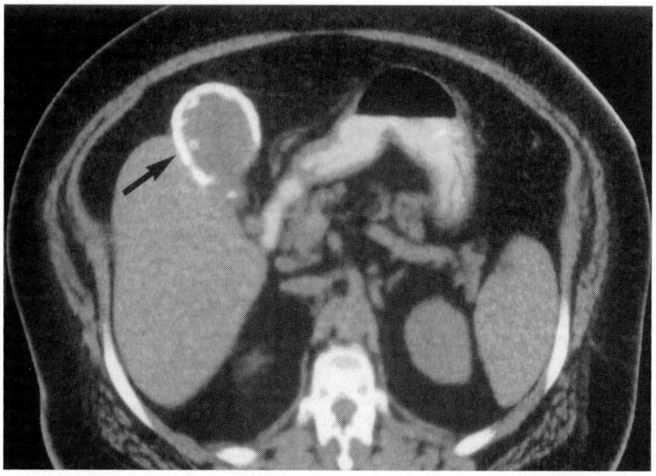

FIGURE 7.36 Porcelain gallbladder. Densely calcified gallbladder wall *(arrow)* in an asymptomatic patient.

- **Biliary cystadenoma and cystadenocarcinoma** are rare biliary neoplasms typically occurring in middle-aged women. Generally, the tumor is intrahepatic, but it can be centered at the hepatic hilum. Biliary cystadenomas and cystadenocarcinomas are depicted on CT as well-defined cystic masses that can be unilocular or multiseptate. Often there is thickening of the focal wall as well as enhancing septations or mural nodules, which aid in distinguishing these neoplasms from simple hepatic cysts. Biliary cystadenomas are excised because of their malignant potential.
- **Rhabdomyosarcoma of the biliary tree** is a rare malignancy occurring in young children. It follows choledochal cysts as the second most common cause of biliary obstruction in this age group. Symptoms are usually fever, jaundice, and lethargy. Local invasion is common and the prognosis is grim. CT demonstrates a soft tissue tumor in the region of the porta hepatis or CBD. Biliary dilatation and hepatic parenchymal invasion are readily depicted.
- **Other rare biliary neoplasms** include lymphoma, sarcoma, granular cell myoblastoma, carcinoid, and benign stromal tumors.

7.8 HEPATIC BIOPSY AND SURGERY

- **Biopsy** is often required to interrogate lesions with a nonspecific appearance on imaging studies, particularly to confirm a suspected diagnosis of metastases. Although ultrasound can be used for guidance in most cases, CT is sometimes required. A coaxial technique in which a larger guiding needle is placed in or very near the lesion in question facilitates multiple successive passes into the lesion with a smaller biopsy needle **(Fig. 7.37).**
- **Partial hepatectomy.** Partial resection of a hepatic lobe can be performed for a number of conditions, including primary hepatic tumor, metastases, and traumatic injuries **(Fig. 7.38).** Primary hepatic neoplasms amenable to surgical intervention include HCC, cholangiocarcinoma, hepatic adenoma, and hepatoblastoma, among others. Patients with limited metastatic deposits from colorectal carcinoma can benefit from hepatic segmentectomy or lobectomy.
- **Cryotherapy.** Subzero temperatures to ablate abnormal hepatic tissues are used with intraoperative ultrasound in patients with hepatic metastasis who do not qualify for surgical resection. During hepatic cryotherapy, sonography demonstrates the formation of an ice ball, which is hyperechoic. Follow-up CT of a successfully treated cryolesion will reveal concavity of the hepatic surface for lesions near the liver capsule. Smaller lesions may disappear, while larger lesions can persist as low-attenuation foci. The presence of small gas bubbles in the cryolesion can be seen on CT for weeks following ablation. Development of an abscess within the cryolesion is manifest by an

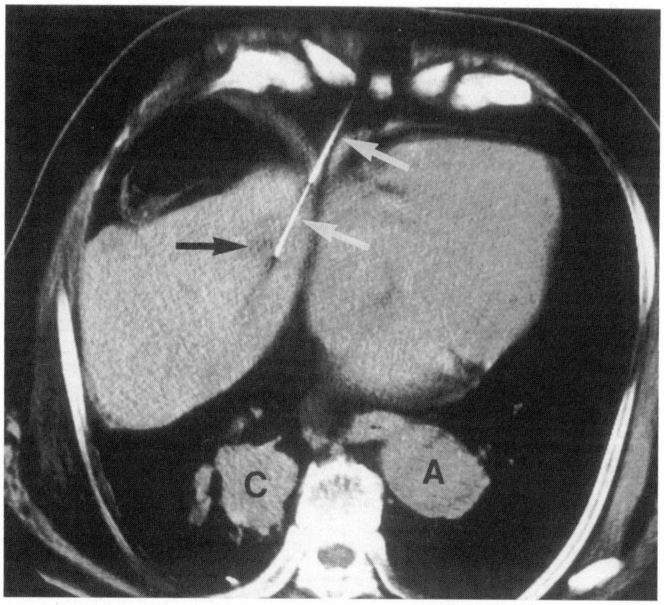

FIGURE 7.37 Biopsy technique. Percutaneous subxyphoid hepatic biopsy technique using coaxial needle *(white arrows)* combined with gantry tilt in a patient with lung carcinoma (C) and a hypodense hepatic metastasis *(black arrow).* Note the beam-hardening artifact at the needle tip and the two different calibers of the needle from coaxial technique *(white arrows).* A, aorta.

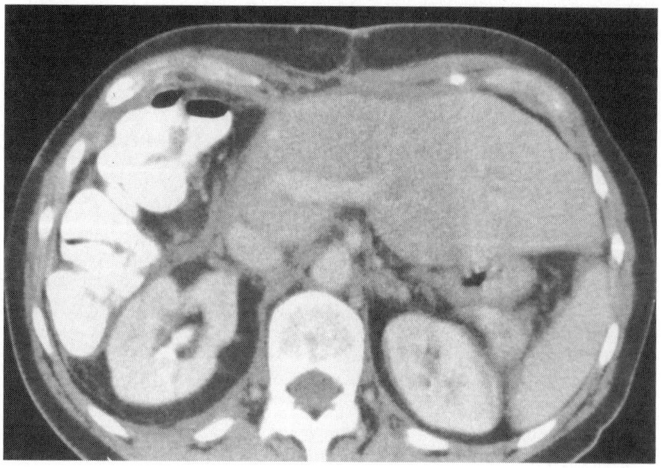

FIGURE 7.38 Right hepatectomy. Contrast-enhanced CT in a 58-year-old woman after right hepatectomy for metastatic ovarian carcinoma.

increase in the size and number of gas bubbles. Inadequate treatment of the cryolesion is suspected when the cryolesion measures smaller than the original lesion or when adjacent tumor is demonstrated.

Bibliography

Baker ME, Pelly R. Hepatic metastases: Basic principles and implications for radiologists. *Radiology,* 1995;197:329–337.

Baron RL, Freeny PC, Moss AA. The liver. In: Moss AA, Gamsu G, Genant HK (eds.): *Computed Tomography of the Body with Magnetic Resonance Imaging*. Philadelphia: WB Saunders; 1992, pp. 735–821.

Baron RL. The biliary tract. In: Moss AA, Gamsu G, Genant HK (eds.): *Computed Tomography of the Body with Magnetic Resonance Imaging*. Philadelphia: WB Saunders; 1992: pp. 823–868.

Baron RL. Liver: normal anatomy, imaging techniques, and diffuse diseases. In: Haaga JR et al. (eds.): *Computed Tomography and Magnetic Resonance Imaging of the Whole Body*. St. Louis: Mosby-Year Book, Inc.; 1994: pp. 945–977.

Brown JJ, Naylor MJ, Yagan N. Imaging of hepatic cirrhosis. *Radiology,* 1997;202:1–16.

Brown JJ, Wippold IJ. *Practical MRI*. Philadelphia: Lippincott-Raven; 1996.

Burgener FA, Kormano M. *Differential Diagnosis in Computed Tomography.* New York: Thieme; 1996.

Heiken JP. Liver. In: Lee JKT et al. (eds.): *Computed Body Tomography with MRI Correlation*. Philadelphia: Lippincott-Raven; 1998, pp. 701–778.

Herbener TE. The gallbladder and biliary tract. In: Gay SM (ed.): *Computed Tomography and Magnetic Resonance Imaging of the Whole Body.* St. Louis: Mosby-Year Book, Inc.; 1994, pp. 978–1036.

Ito K et al. CT of acquired abnormalities of the portal venous system. *RadioGraphics* 1997;17:897–917.

Jabra AA, Fishman EK, Taylor GA. Hepatic masses in infants and children: CT evaluation. *AJR* 1992;158:143–149.

McGahan JP, Stein M. Complications of laparoscopic cholecystectomy: Imaging and intervention. *AJR* 1995;165:1089–1097.

McLoughlin RF, Saliken JF, McKinnon G, Wiseman D, Temple W. CT of the liver after cryotherapy of hepatic metastases: Imaging findings. *AJR* 1995;165:329–332.

Mergo PJ et al. Diffuse disease of the liver: Radiologic-pathologic correlation. *RadioGraphics,* 1994;14:1291–1307.

Miller FH et al. Using triphasic helical CT to detect focal hepatic lesions in patients with neoplasms. *AJR* 1998;171:643–649.

Moss AA, Gamsu G, Genant HK. *Computed Tomography of the Body with Magnetic Resonance Imaging*. Vol. 1-3, 2nd ed. Philadelphia: WB Saunders; 1992, p. 434.

Semelka RC, Ascher SM, Reinhold C. *MRI of the Abdomen and Pelvis*. New York: Wiley-Liss; 1997.

Slone RM, Fisher AJ. *Pocket Guide to Body CT Differential Diagnosis*. New York: McGraw-Hill; 1999.

Soyer P et al. Imaging of intrahepatic cholangiocarcinoma:1. peripheral cholangiocarcinoma. *AJR* 1995;165:1427–1431.

Soyer P et al. Carcinoma of the gallbladder: Imaging features with surgical correlation. *AJR* 1997;169:781–785.

Sutton D. *Textbook of Radiology and Imaging*. New York: Churchill Livingstone; 1998.

Chapter 8

SPLEEN

Andrew J. Fisher

8.1 Anatomy, Physiology, and Technique
8.2 Diffuse Disease
8.3 Splenic Cysts
8.4 Benign Lesions
8.5 Malignant Lesions

8.1 ANATOMY, PHYSIOLOGY, AND TECHNIQUE

- The **spleen** forms part of the reticuloendothelial system, filtering blood-borne cellular elements and playing an important immunologic function. It serves as a blood reservoir and assists in iron metabolism following red blood cell breakdown. The spleen is attached to the adjacent stomach by the gastrosplenic ligament and to the left kidney by the splenorenal (lienorenal) ligament. The pancreatic tail is contained within the splenorenal ligament, allowing pancreatic pathology to spread directly to the spleen. The splenic surface is smooth, although there may be prominent splenic clefts and lobulations **(Fig. 8.1).** Analogous to the liver, there is a small portion of the lateral splenic surface—termed the *bare area*—without a visceral peritoneal covering.

  The spleen is composed of red, white, and marginal pulp. Arterial supply is via the splenic artery arising from the celiac axis. Venous drainage is by the splenic vein, which courses adjacent to the posterior pancreatic surface and joins the superior mesenteric vein to form the portal vein. Lymphatic drainage is to hilar nodes and subsequently to celiac chain lymph nodes.

- **Splenules** are round foci of normal splenic tissue generally found near the splenic hilum, with attenuation and enhancement similar to that of the spleen. Failure of embryologic mesodermal buds to coalesce can yield this accessory splenic tissue. Rarely, splenules may be located within the pancreatic tail or bowel wall, mimicking pathology. Splenules are found in approximately one-quarter of the population and may grow following splenectomy. Not surprisingly, they can contain pathologic processes similar to those arising within the spleen itself.

  Splenosis, characterized by multiple deposits of splenic tissue in the abdomen or at distant sites such as the thorax, may be seen following trauma **(see Fig. 3.18).** When they are located within the thorax, these lesions can simulate other causes of pulmonary nodules, including metastatic disease. On computed tomography (CT), splenosis has a nonspecific appearance: there are small foci of soft tissue attenuation that enhance in a similar fashion to normal splenic tissue. Scintigraphy with heat-damaged red blood cells can confirm the diagnosis.

  The spleen is relatively mobile on its mesentery. This is evidenced by the alteration in splenic position seen following nephrectomy, with the spleen frequently occupying the renal fossa. When the splenorenal ligament fails to fuse with the retroperitoneum, the spleen may assume ectopic intra-abdominal positions. This is termed **"wandering spleen."** This ligamentous laxity is generally found in female patients and can simulate an abdominal neoplasm.

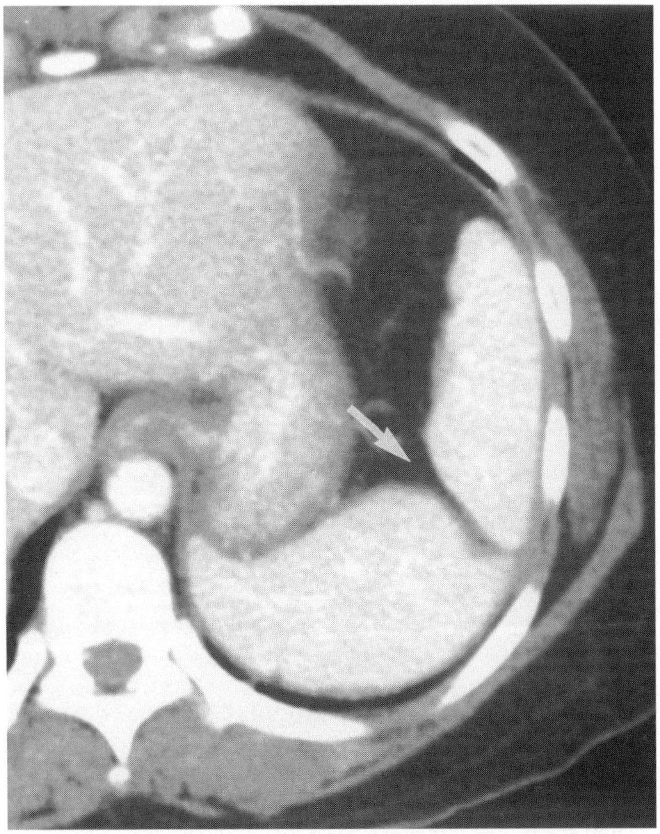

FIGURE 8.1 Splenic cleft. A 47-year-old man with right-sided abdominal pain. CT shows a prominent cleft *(arrow)* within the spleen, a normal variant.

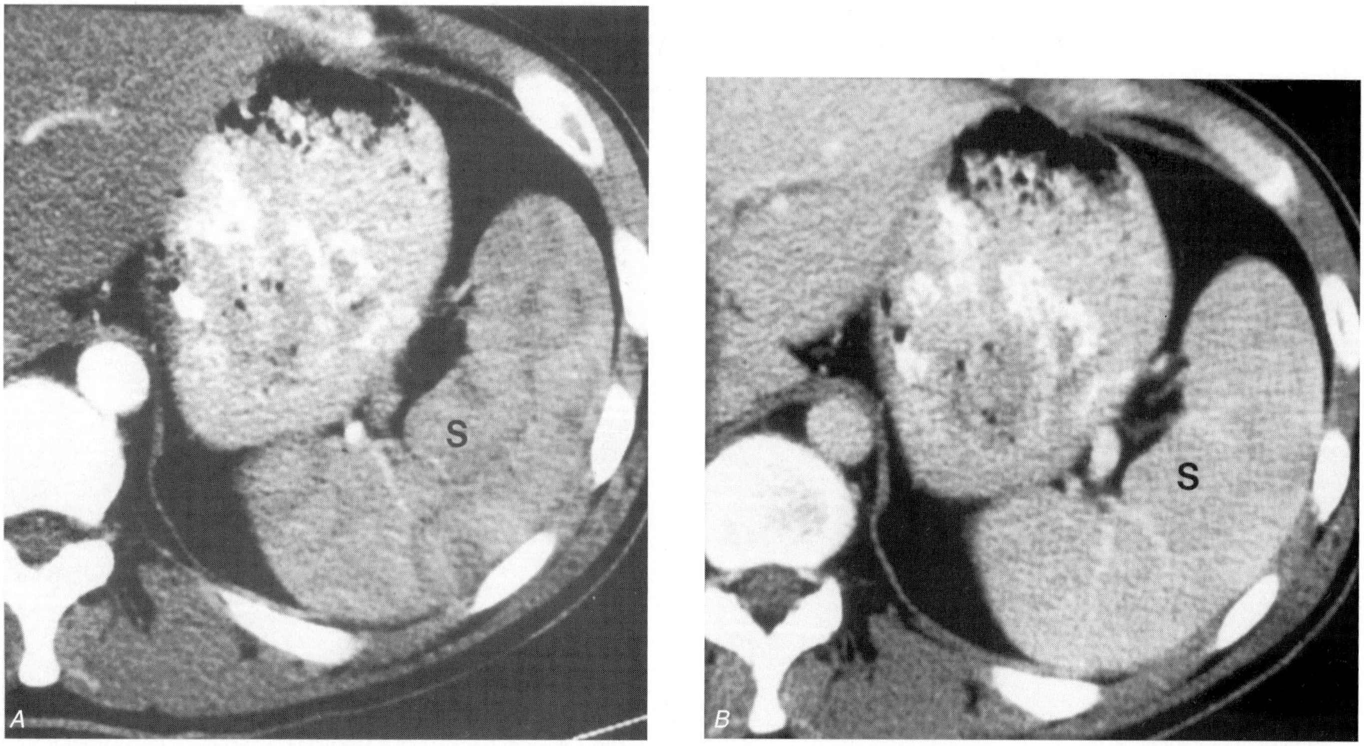

FIGURE 8.2 Splenic enhancement. Arterial-*(A)* and equilibrium-*(B)* phase CT images following IV contrast administration demonstrate initial parenchymal heterogeneity, which becomes homogeneous on scans obtained 40 s later. There is wide variation in the normal arterial-phase appearance of the spleen (S).

Occasionally, torsion of the spleen around its vascular pedicle can occur, resulting in parenchymal infarction and producing acute left-upper-quadrant pain.

- **CT technique** for the spleen is conventional. Slice thickness is generally 5 to 8 mm and intravenous (IV) contrast is administered. The attenuation of the splenic parenchyma without IV contrast is 40 to 60 HU, approximately 10 HU less than the hepatic attenuation. Differential flow through the splenic parenchyma, likely within the unique splenic cords of the red pulp, can yield bizarre and heterogeneous enhancement during the arterial phase of CT imaging **(Fig. 8.2).** During this phase, the presence of pathology cannot reliably be determined. Splenic enhancement becomes homogeneous 1 min following IV contrast administration, corresponding to the typical portal venous phase of imaging. Persistent lesions during this phase can reliably be interpreted as abnormal.

8.2 DIFFUSE DISEASE

- The spleen normally weighs 100 to 250 g and has a maximum cephalocaudal span of 13 cm. **Splenomegaly** can be determined by an increased cephalocaudal span or, more accurately, by an increased splenic index. The splenic index is calculated using a formula based on multiplying the three-dimensional measurements (length × width × height). The normal index is 120 to 480 cm^3. Numerous conditions can produce splenomegaly, including lymphoma and leukemia (particularly chronic myelocytic leukemia, or CML), mononucleosis, and other infections **(Fig. 8.3),** cirrhosis with portal hypertension, splenic vein thrombosis, glycogen and other storage diseases such as Gaucher disease, sarcoidosis, polycythemia vera, myelofibrosis, and hemolytic anemias **(Differential 8.1).**

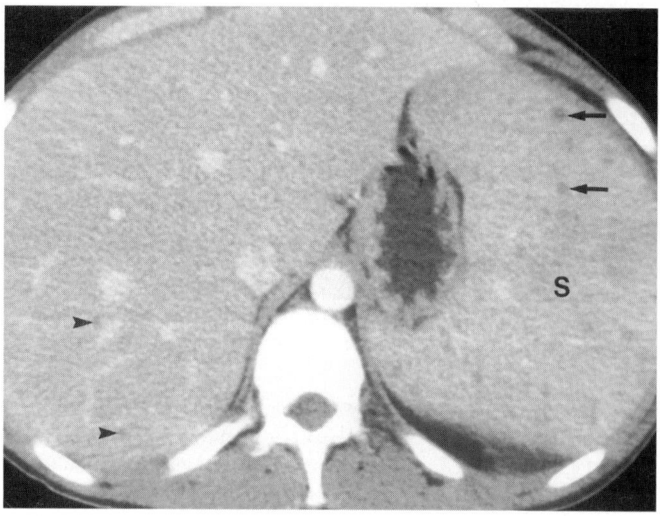

FIGURE 8.3 Splenomegaly. There is diffuse splenomegaly in this patient with candidal microabscesses in both the spleen (S; *arrows)* and liver *(arrowheads)*. The splenic cephalocaudal span was 16 cm.

8.1

SPLENOMEGALY (>13-CM CEPHALOCAUDAL SPAN)

Tumor
- **Lymphoma**
- Leukemia—particularly chronic myelocytic
- Metastases—melanoma, breast, lung, ovary, colon

Congestion—portal venous hypertension, splenic venous thrombosis
Hemolytic anemia
Infection—especially mononucleosis
Sarcoidosis
Extramedullary hematopoiesis—myelofibrosis, polycythemia vera
Storage diseases
Chronic granulomatous disease of childhood
Collagen vascular disease—lupus
Amyloidosis

- The spleen may be **small** or **absent** in heterotaxy syndromes (asplenia, polysplenia) or following surgery, trauma, infarction, or irradiation **(Differential 8.2). Asplenia,** also known as the *Ivemark syndrome,* is congenital absence of the spleen in association with a midline liver and other abnormalities of the biliary and cardiovascular systems.
- **Splenic surgery** may be indicated for traumatic injury **(Section 15.5),** neoplasm of the spleen, or pancreatic tail and other less common pathologies. The entire spleen is resected, although small foci of splenic tissue (splenosis) may occasionally appear following splenectomy. However, this is more common after splenic trauma. Complications following splenectomy include abscess, increased risk of infection due to encapsulated organisms, and pseudoaneurysm formation **(Fig. 8.4).**
- **Polysplenia** is characterized by multiple small, right-sided splenules as well as cardiac and vascular anomalies, including azygos continuation of the inferior vena cava (IVC). The liver is usually right-sided in these patients.
- **Sickle cell disease** can produce splenomegaly and generally leads to splenic infarction and "autoamputation." Acute sequestration of a significant amount of blood products can cause rapid splenic enlargement and a falling hematocrit. The spleen may demonstrate diffusely increased attenuation from hemosiderin or calcium deposition **(Differential 8.3) (Fig. 8.5).** Other findings may include a small, calcified spleen; cardiomegaly from increased cardiac output; characteristic osseous changes of diffuse sclerosis and infarcts; and prior cholecystectomy for cholecystitis due to hemolysis, which forms pigmented stones or sludge.

8.2

SMALL SPLEEN

Splenule
Trauma (rupture/fragmentation)
Infarction—sickle cell disease
Polysplenia
Hypoplasia
Radiation
Atrophy

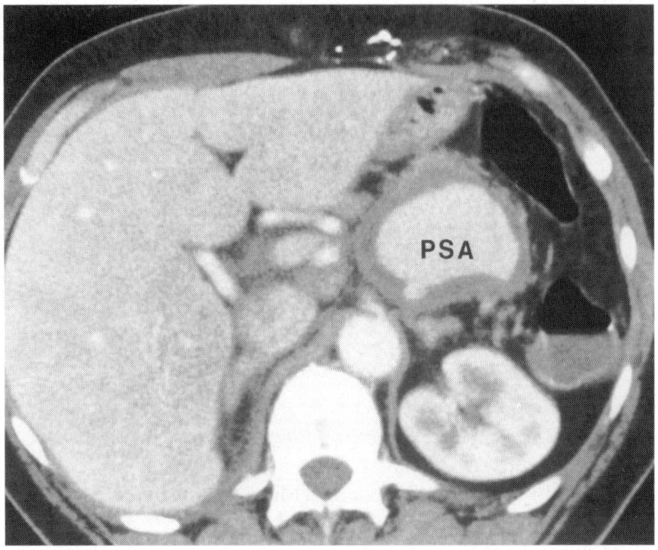

FIGURE 8.4 Splenic artery pseudoaneurysm. CT in a 68-year-old woman postsplenectomy. A large pseudoaneurysm (PSA) is present in the left midabdomen with central enhancement equal to that of the aorta. The low-attenuation rim represents thrombus.

Other conditions such as hemochromatosis, hemosiderosis, and prior **Thorotrast** exposure can cause diffusely increased splenic attenuation. Accumulation of Thorotrast colloidal particles also occurs in the liver and abdominal lymph nodes. Thorotrast has a long biological half-life and emits energetic alpha particles. Thorotrast has a rare but fatal link with splenic angiosarcomas.

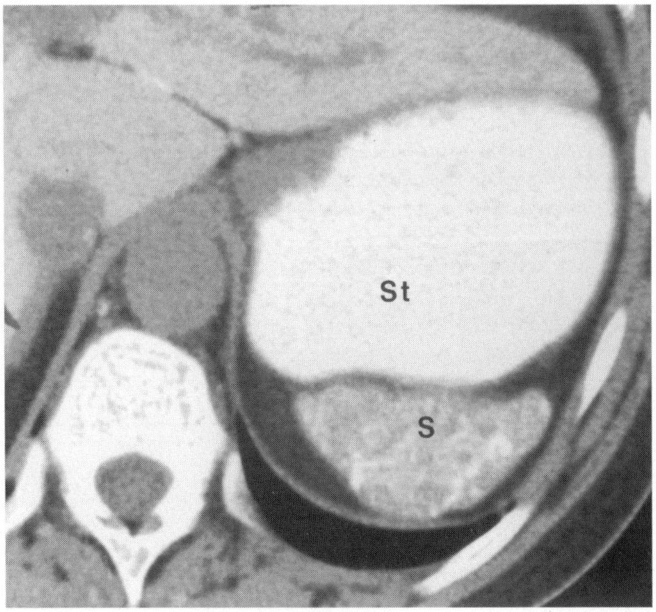

FIGURE 8.5 Splenic sickle cell disease. Noncontrast CT scan in a 49-year-old man with sickle cell disease demonstrates a small, partially calcified spleen (S). St, stomach.

8.3

SPLENIC CALCIFICATIONS

Atherosclerotic splenic artery
Healed granulomatous disease—tuberculosis, histoplasmosis
Sickle cell disease
Cyst with rim calcification
Hemangioma
Infarction
Dense spleen (mimic)—hemochromatosis, Thorotrast

8.3 SPLENIC CYSTS

- **Splenic cysts** are uncommon and usually asymptomatic. Hemorrhage, rupture, or superimposed infection can precipitate an attack of acute symptoms. Uncommonly, cysts may become large enough to cause pain or abdominal fullness. Splenic cysts may be classified as pseudocysts, true epithelial cysts, or parasitic cysts **(Differential 8.4).**
- **Splenic pseudocysts** are the most common cause of splenic cysts. They typically result from prior trauma leading to liquefaction of an intraparenchymal hematoma **(Fig. 8.6).** Pancreatic pseudocysts can rarely dissect along the splenic vascular pedicle and occasionally into the parenchyma.
- **True splenic cysts,** termed ***primary cysts,*** contain an epithelial lining. They are less common than pseudocysts and are generally asymptomatic.
- **Echinococcal cysts** (hydatid disease) result from parasitic infestation with *Echinococcus granulosus* or, less commonly, *Echinococcus multilocularis (alveolaris).* Humans are accidental intermediate hosts, acquiring the parasite from contaminated food. Patients are usually asymptomatic or present with focal pain, mass, or fullness. Acute pain, urticaria, and anaphylaxis occurs in some patients when the cyst ruptures. Patients usually have peripheral eosinophilia. Echinococcal cysts most commonly occur in the liver and spleen, although hematogenous dissemination may lead to cystic lesions in the pulmonary parenchyma and in the brain.

The various types of splenic cysts are very difficult to differentiate on CT. All appear as well-marginated, spherical, water-attenuation masses that do not enhance following IV contrast. Septations are more common in true cysts, while calcifications are more common in pseudocysts and parasitic cysts **(Fig. 8.7).** Dissecting pancreatic pseudocysts may coexist with other sequelae of pancreatitis, but in many cases their connection with the pancreatic parenchyma is not obvious and they are indistinguishable from other splenic cysts. Hemorrhagic cysts can demonstrate fluid-fluid or fluid-debris levels.

Echinococcal cysts are usually larger than true epithelial cysts. Also, echinococcal cysts frequently demonstrate crescentic or circumferential calcification. Internal septations and layering "sand" are other diagnostic clues. Reports have warned that percutaneous puncture can precipitate an anaphylactic reaction, although the risk of anaphylaxis is now thought to be negligible.

- **Cystic splenic metastases** are uncommon. The most common primary types are melanomas as well as lung, breast, ovarian, and gastrointestinal carcinomas.

8.4

SPLENIC CYST

Posttraumatic
Congenital—epithelial
Abscess—pyogenic, candidal, Pneumocystis carinii, MAI
Metastases
Hemangioma
Lymphangioma
Hamartoma
Hydatid—Echinococcus granulosus
Dissecting pancreatic pseudocyst

Key: MAI, *Mycobacterium avium-intracellulare.*

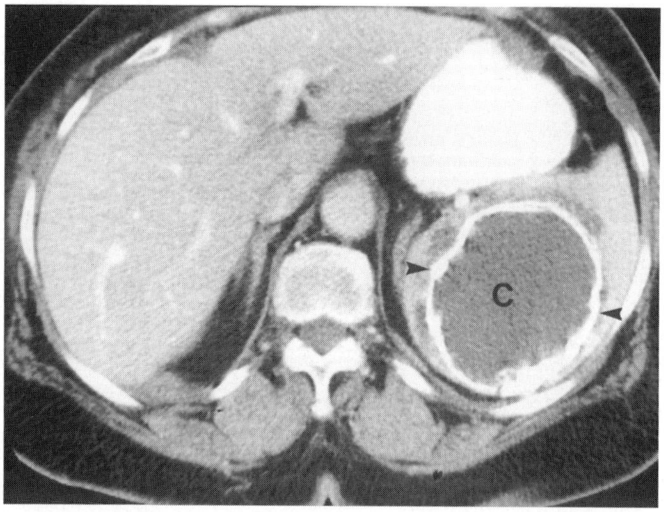

FIGURE 8.6 Posttraumatic splenic cyst. IV contrast–enhanced CT in an 84-year-old woman demonstrates a large splenic cyst (C). This has a thick rind of calcification (arrowheads). The patient gave a history of prior left-sided trauma.

8.4 BENIGN LESIONS

- **Hemangiomas** are the most common benign splenic tumors **(Differential 8.5).** They can be isolated or associated with other an-

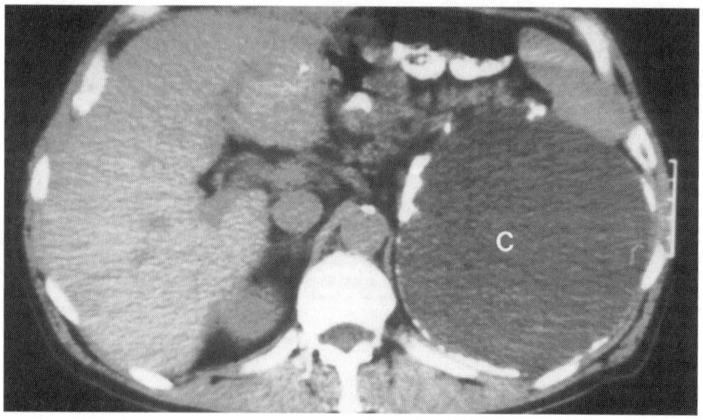

FIGURE 8.7 Echinococcal cyst. A large cyst (C) replaces the majority of the posterior aspect of the spleen. A partially calcified wall is present.

8.5

SPLENIC LESION

Benign tumor
  Hemangioma
  Lymphangioma
  Hamartoma
Malignant tumor
  Lymphoma
  Leukemia—particularly chronic myelocytic
  Metastases—melanoma, breast, lung, ovarian, colon, gastrointestinal
  Angiosarcoma and rare neoplasms
Cyst
Infarct
Abscess—pyogenic, candidal, *Pneumocystis carinii,* MAI
Hematoma
Sarcoid
Inflammatory pseudotumor
Peliosis
Arteriovenous malformation

Key: MAI, *Mycobacterium avium-intracellulare.*

giomatous lesions in Klippel-Trenaunay-Weber syndrome (cutaneous, gastrointestinal, and soft tissue hemangiomas, sometimes with unilateral limb hypertrophy). Like splenic cysts, hemangiomas are typically incidental findings; however, they can hemorrhage spontaneously, precipitating an acute presentation.

The **CT** characteristics of splenic hemangiomas are similar to those of hepatic hemangiomas. Although they are of low attenuation on precontrast images, there is often peripheral or heterogeneous enhancement following IV contrast administration **(Fig. 8.8).** However, splenic hemangiomas demonstrate this pattern of enhancement less commonly than hepatic hemangiomas. The lesions may, in fact, appear solid or even avascular with markedly delayed enhancement. This appearance is common in patients with Klippel-Trenaunay-Weber syndrome. Multiple hemangiomas may present in a single patient **(Fig. 8.9).**

- **Hamartomas** are rare, benign splenic tumors composed of normal histologic elements and are usually discovered as incidental findings. They are solid lesions that can contain cystic or necrotic regions. In some splenic hamartomas, hemosiderin deposition leads to increased attenuation on noncontrast CT.

- **Pyogenic splenic abscesses** can occur in the setting of septicemia, endocarditis, immunocompromised status, and IV drug abuse. Direct penetrating trauma can also produce an intrasplenic abscess. Although surgery was previously the treatment of choice, percutaneous drainage and antibiotic therapy are now routinely employed.

  CT typically demonstrates a complex cystic mass, often with septations or an irregular wall. When a pseudocapsule is present, the cystic mass will have an enhancing rim. Intralesional gas is uncommon, although it is a specific finding for abscess **(Fig. 8.10).** When the pyogenic source is hematogenous dissemination, abscesses can also be present in the liver or kidneys.

- **Fungal microabscesses** are common in immunocompromised patients with AIDS and in patients undergoing aggressive chemotherapy or bone marrow transplantation. *Candida* species are the most common organisms. Treatment is with systemic antifungal agents.

  Small fungal microabscesses can be difficult to detect with CT; consequently, thin collimation is required if this entity is suspected.

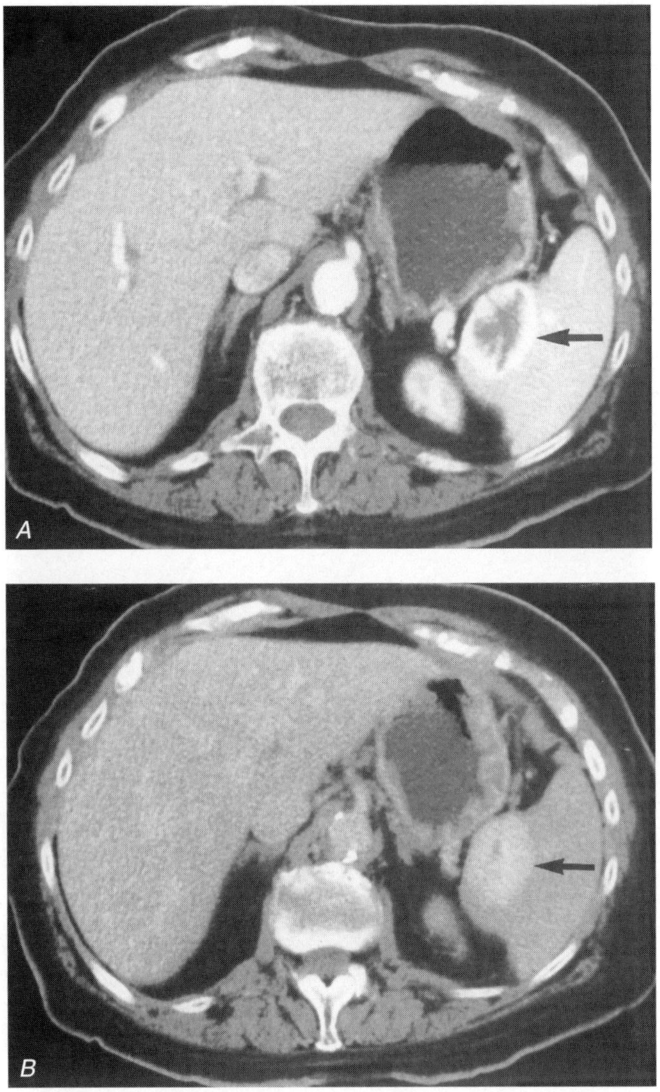

FIGURE 8.8 Splenic hemangioma. Arterial-*(A)* and portal venous-*(B)* phase CT images demonstrate an oval splenic lesion *(arrow)* that has a dense rim of enhancement. This hemangioma subsequently "fills in" on delayed images.

The characteristic pattern is that of numerous, randomly distributed, low-attenuation foci that become more apparent after IV enhancement **(Fig. 8.11,** also **Fig. 8.3).** The lesions are generally 1 cm or smaller in size. A central high-attenuation focus may be present, yielding a "wheel-within-a-wheel" pattern. Similar findings can also be present in the liver and kidneys.

- **Tuberculosis (TB)** can involve the spleen from hematogenous dissemination. Data from autopsy series indicate that splenic involvement is present in over 80 percent of such patients. Also, 30 percent of AIDS patients with abdominal tuberculosis have splenic manifestations. CT findings include mild splenomegaly, with tiny regions of decreased attenuation, similar to fungal microabscesses, distributed throughout the splenic parenchyma. Other abdominal findings of tuberculosis include low-attenuation adenopathy, high-attenuation ascites, peritoneal nodules, and thickened ileocecal bowel loops. In chronic disease, calcified granulomata persist.

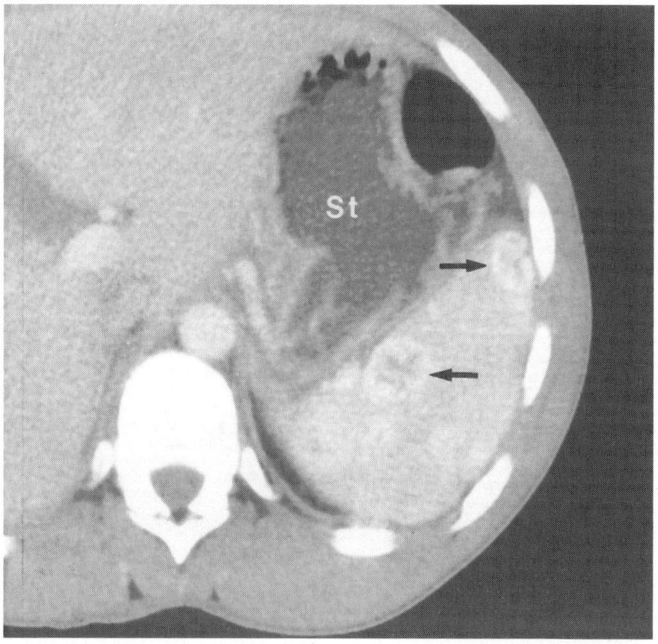

FIGURE 8.9 Multiple splenic hemangiomas. A 36-year-old man with HIV. Multiple peripherally enhancing splenic lesions *(arrows)* are readily identified. St, stomach.

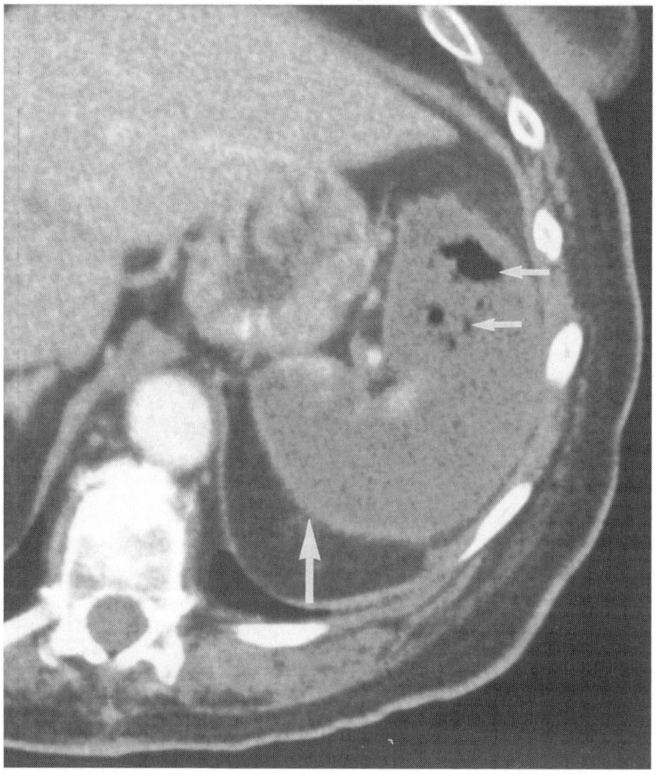

FIGURE 8.10 Splenic abscess. An 83-year-old woman with abdominal pain, chills, and leukocytosis. There is diffuse low attenuation throughout the splenic parenchyma, with several gas bubbles *(small arrows)* confirming the diagnosis of splenic abscess. Other regions of the spleen had normal enhancement, and a "rim sign" of preserved capsular flow *(large arrow)* is noted.

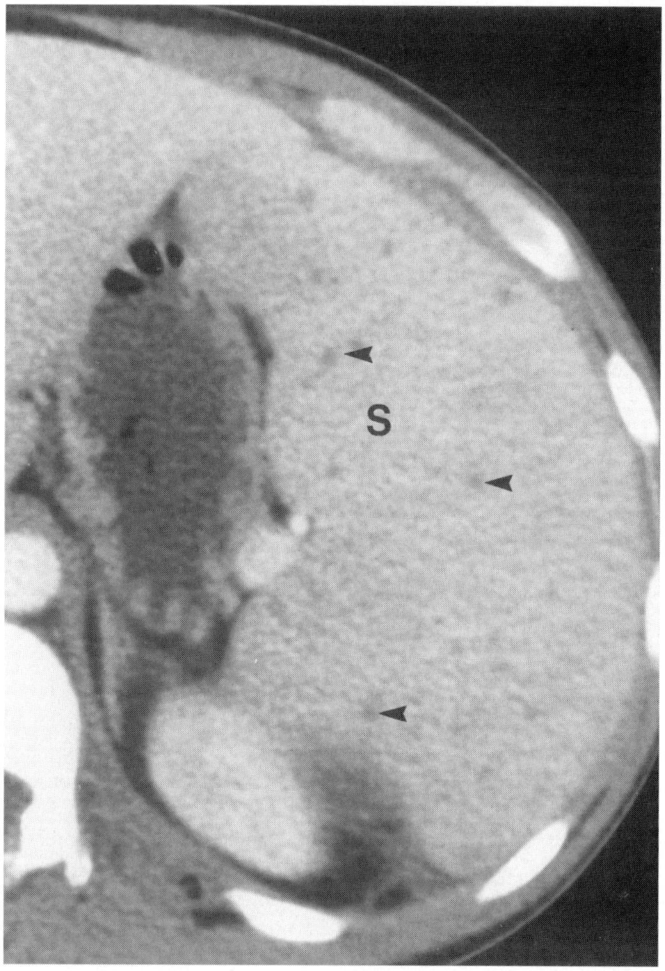

FIGURE 8.11 Splenic microabscesses from *Candida*. A 21-year-old man with fever, night sweats, and recent chemotherapy for lymphoma. Contrast-enhanced CT shows splenomegaly (S) and numerous punctate, low-attenuation foci within the spleen compatible with microabscesses *(arrowheads)*. The patient had candidemia on concurrent hematologic evaluation.

- ***Mycobacterium avium-intracellulare*** (MAI) can likewise involve the spleen, particularly in immunocompromised patients. In these cases, there is often marked splenic enlargement, low-attenuation adenopathy, and jejunal wall thickening **(Fig. 8.12).**
- ***Pneumocystis carinii*** rarely involves the spleen, although the prevalence has been increasing with the enlarging AIDS population. Splenic PCP is typically secondary to hematogenous dissemination. Like TB and MAI, *Pneumocystis carinii* can cause splenomegaly with focal low-attenuation parenchymal lesions. The lesions are generally small, ranging from 0.5 to 2 cm. These may calcify over time and be indistinguishable from other granulomatous processes.
- **Calcified splenic granulomas** are the sequelae of prior exposure to *Histoplasma, M. tuberculosis,* or other organisms. Over time, the lesions become punctate calcific foci **(Fig. 8.13).** There are often similar findings in the liver. Noncalcified splenic granulomas can be incidentally demonstrated when the acute phase of infection is imaged. These lesions are of no clinical significance.

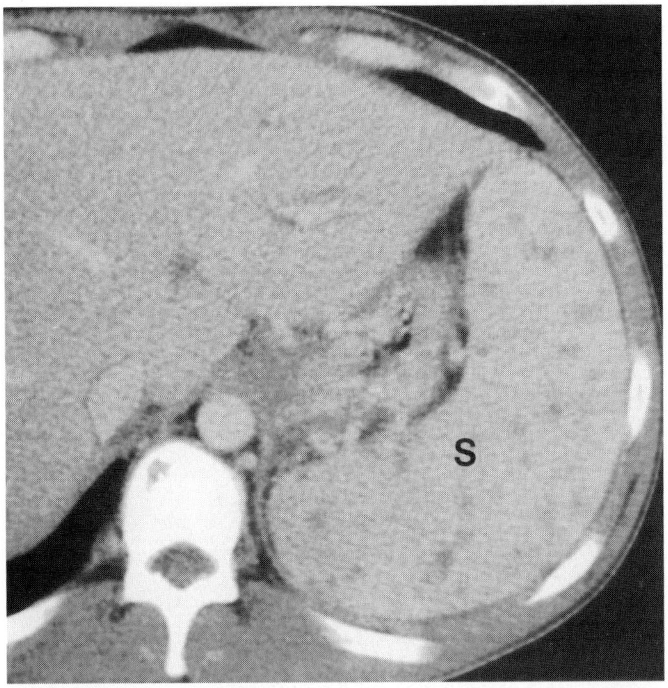

FIGURE 8.12 Splenic microabscesses from MAI. A 36-year-old man with HIV. There are multiple low-attenuation foci within the spleen (S) indistinguishable from candidal microabscesses. There was lymphadenopathy in the splenic hilum and retrocrural regions.

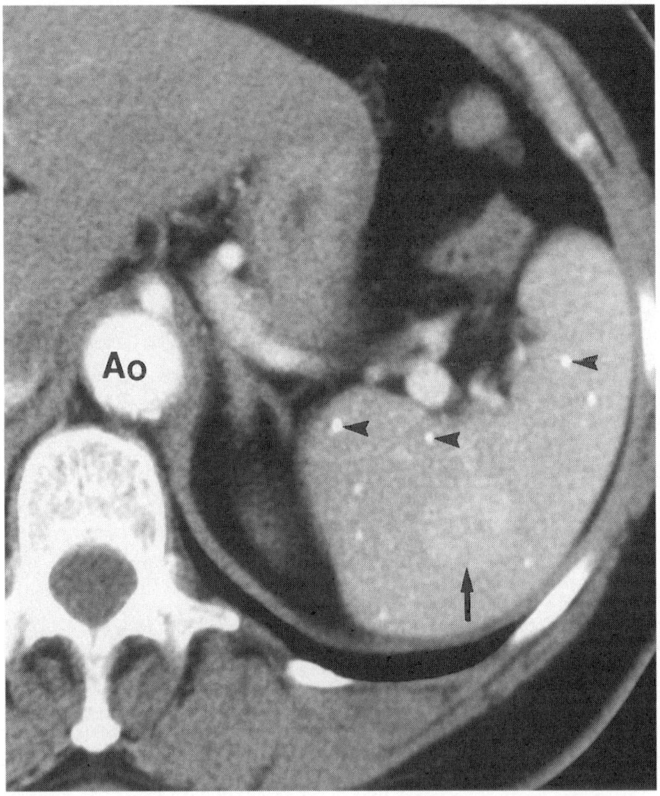

FIGURE 8.13 Calcified splenic granulomas. Multiple punctate calcifications *(arrowheads)* are present within the splenic parenchyma, representing old healed granulomatous disease. Incidental note is made of a faintly enhancing splenic lesion, likely a hemangioma *(arrow)*. Ao, aorta.

- **Sarcoidosis** can also lead to splenic granulomas. Splenic involvement occurs in about one-third of patients with sarcoidosis. There is associated pulmonary disease in the vast majority of cases. Other abnormal findings that occur in patients with sarcoidosis include splenomegaly (present in one-quarter of patients), hepatomegaly, low-attenuation splenic nodules, and retroperitoneal or hepatic hilar lymphadenopathy **(Fig. 8.14).**

- **Splenic infarction** is the result of local vascular compromise. Typical etiologies include thromboembolic processes, inflammatory diseases, or neoplastic processes affecting the splenic vasculature. Collagen vascular disease is an uncommon cause, and practical considerations are limited to lupus erythematosus or polyarteritis nodosa. Spontaneous splenic infarcts may be seen in AIDS patients. Global infarction is common in patients with sickle cell disease.

  CT findings are characteristic, showing peripheral wedge-shaped lesions that point to the hilum. These lesions are almost always of low attenuation. If there is a substantial hemorrhagic component, the lesions may have focal or diffuse increased attenuation. The infarcted parenchyma does not enhance after IV contrast administration; however, there may be thin, peripheral enhancement of the splenic surface owing to preserved capsular vessels, resulting in the "rim sign" **(Fig. 8.15).** When the infarction is due to embolic phenomena, other organs, particularly the kidneys, show similar findings. With time, the infarcted area may undergo calcification or may contract, leaving only a capsular contour abnormality, the resulting scar.

- **Lymphangiomas** of the spleen are rare. They are benign malformations that contain multiple, endothelium-lined cysts. The multiseptate cystic mass is nonenhancing and well delineated. Calcifications of the peripheral rim may also be present. These multiloculated cystic masses are benign but may infiltrate adjacent structures, necessitating wide excision. This lesion tends to recur if it is incompletely resected.

- **Inflammatory pseudotumor of the spleen** is distinctly rare. It is a localized collection of inflammatory, fibroblastic, and granulomatous cellular infiltrate. On CT, the lesion is a low-attenuation, well-demarcated mass that may gradually enhance following IV contrast administration. Calcifications may be present, and a central scar from focal fibrosis can be seen.

8.5 MALIGNANT LESIONS

- **Primary neoplasms** of the spleen are rare with the exception of lymphoma. Histologic evaluation shows splenic involvement in approximately 25 percent of patients with Hodgkin disease and 35 percent of those with non-Hodgkin disease. Patients with splenic involvement are generally older or have AIDS-related lymphoma.

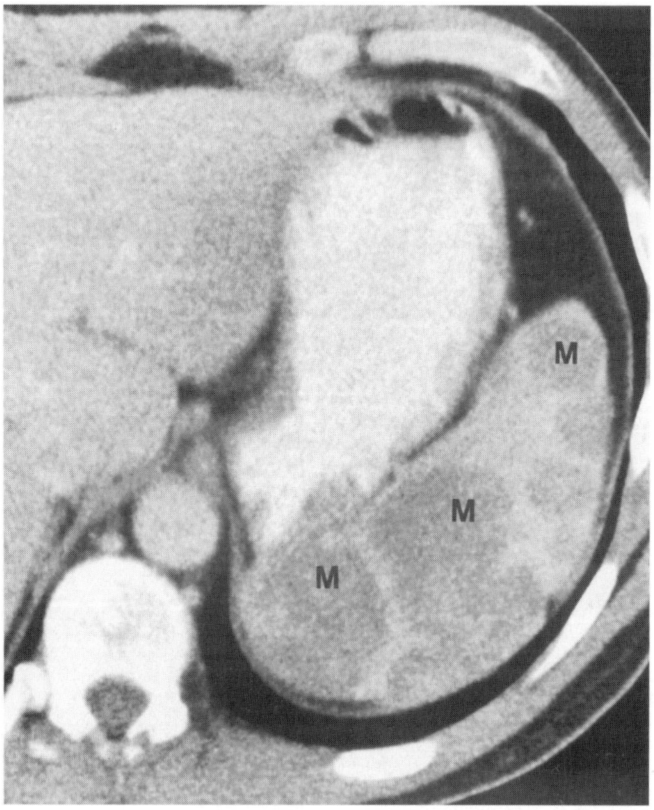

FIGURE 8.14 Splenic sarcoidosis. Numerous hypoenhancing splenic masses (M) are seen in this 46-year-old man with known sarcoidosis. The spleen is of normal size.

They may present with splenic rupture following minor or unrecognized trauma. Splenic lymphoma almost always has associated adenopathy, a diagnostic clue to the etiology of splenomegaly.

CT is of limited value in detecting lymphoma within the spleen; more than 50 percent of cases have diffuse disease or nodules much less than 1 cm in size; they are visible only as diffuse splenic enlargement. Even a normal-sized organ can harbor lymphoma. When lymphoma deposits are detected by CT, they are focal, low-attenuation nodules that demonstrate minimal enhancement following IV contrast administration **(Fig. 8.16).** Leukemia can have an identical appearance.

- **Angiosarcoma** is a rare splenic tumors, yet it is the most common nonlymphomatous primary malignancy of the spleen. The only documented predisposing condition is prior Thorotrast administration. Clinically, the tumor is rapidly progressive and the prognosis is grave. On CT, the lesion appears as a heterogeneous and densely enhancing tumor. It may involve the majority of the splenic parenchyma or be evident as multinodular disease. Rapid growth is common on interval exams. Metastases commonly occur in the liver.
- **Metastases** to the spleen arise most commonly from melanoma (up to 35 percent of melanoma patients) as well as primary tumors of the lung or breast. Other primaries that involve the spleen or splenic capsule include ovarian, pancreatic, endometrial, and gastrointestinal malignancies. Metastatic foci may appear as solitary or multiple

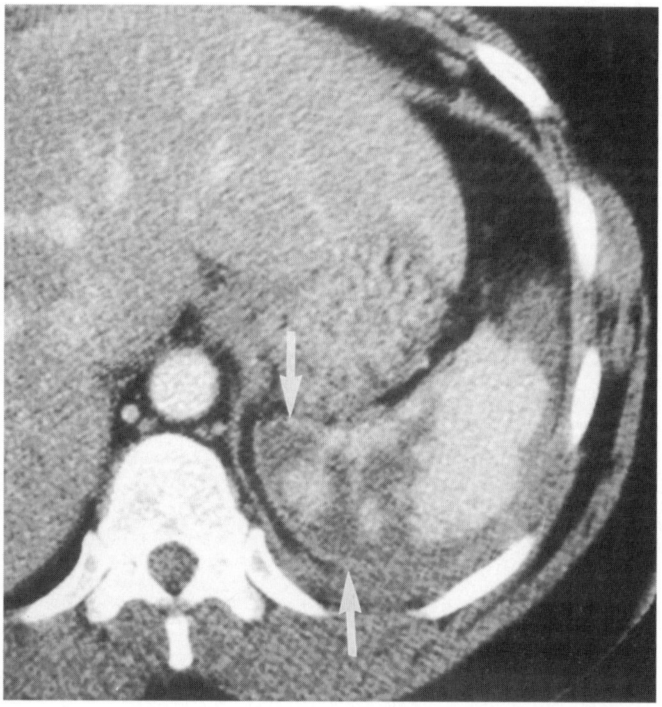

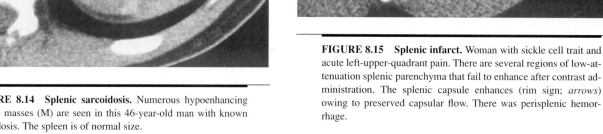

FIGURE 8.15 Splenic infarct. Woman with sickle cell trait and acute left-upper-quadrant pain. There are several regions of low-attenuation splenic parenchyma that fail to enhance after contrast administration. The splenic capsule enhances (rim sign; *arrows*) owing to preserved capsular flow. There was perisplenic hemorrhage.

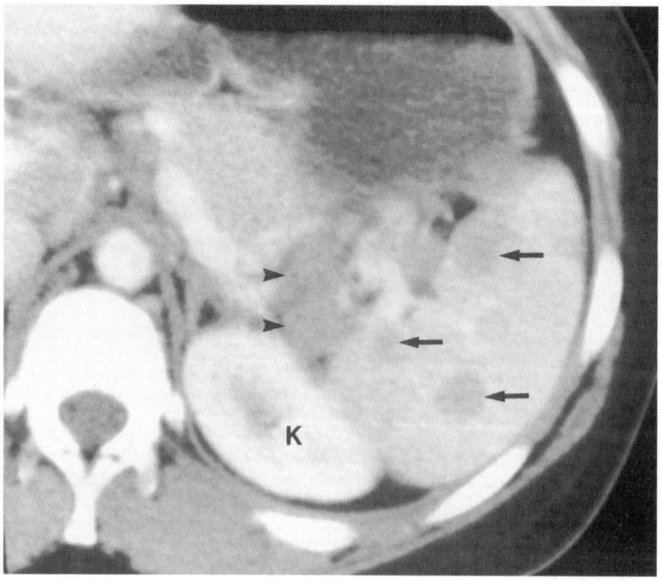

FIGURE 8.16 Splenic lymphoma. A 24-year-old who was treated for lymphoma 4 years prior to presentation with abdominal pain. There are multiple discrete low-attenuation foci within the spleen *(arrows)*, which demonstrate decreased enhancement compared to the normal parenchyma. Lymphadenopathy is noted in the hilum *(arrowheads)*. K, left kidney.

low-attenuation parenchymal lesions that enhance less than surrounding splenic tissue **(Fig. 8.17).** Isolated splenic metastases are uncommon; usually, other metastatic sites are evident, often in the liver.

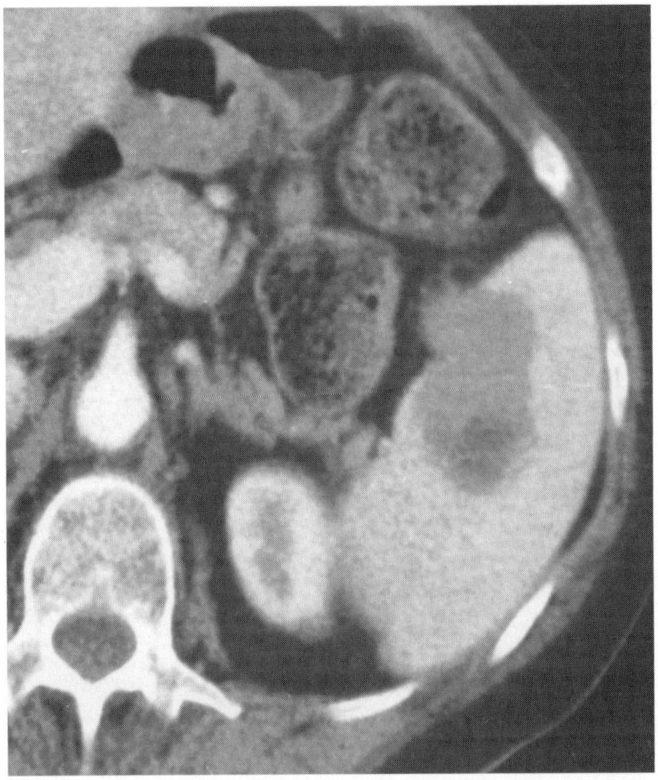

Figure 8.17 Splenic metastasis. A 61-year-old woman with ovarian cancer. A solid and cystic mass is present in the spleen. This lesion and an additional hilar mass were ovarian metastases.

Bibliography

Burgener FA, Kormano M. *Differential Diagnosis in Computed Tomography*. New York: Thieme; 1996.

Ito K et al. MR imaging of acquired abnormalities of the spleen. *AJR* 1997;168:697–702.

Rabushka LS, Kawashima A, Fishman EK. Imaging of the spleen: CT with supplemental MR examination. *Radiographics* 1994;14:307–332.

Slone RM, Fisher AJ. *Pocket Guide to Body CT Differential Diagnosis*. New York: McGraw-Hill; 1999.

Urban B, Fishman EK. Helical CT of the spleen. *AJR* 1998;170:997–1003.

Urrutia M, Mergo PJ, Ros LH, Torres GM, Ros PR. Cystic masses of the spleen: Radiologic-pathologic correlation. *Radiographics* 1996;16:107–129.

Warshauer DM, Koehler RE. Spleen. In: JKT Lee, Sagel SS, Stanley RJ, Heiken JP, (eds.): *Computed Body Tomography with MRI Correlation*, 3rd ed. Philadelphia: Lippincott-Raven; 1998:845–872.

Chapter 9

PANCREAS

Andrea M. Fisher and Perry J. Pickhardt

9.1 Anatomy, Physiology, and Technique
9.2 Congenital Abnormalities
9.3 Pancreatitis
9.4 Cystic Lesions
9.5 Solid Tumors
9.6 Fatty Replacement
9.7 Pancreatic Surgery

9.1 ANATOMY, PHYSIOLOGY, AND TECHNIQUE

- The **pancreas** is an elongated, lobulated gland lying in the anterior pararenal space of the retroperitoneum; it has both exocrine and endocrine functions. It is composed of four anatomic segments: the head, neck, body, and tail. The pancreatic head lies medial to the second portion of the duodenum and anterior to the inferior vena cava (IVC). The uncinate process is the inferomedial extension of the pancreatic head; the superior mesenteric vein (SMV) lies in a groove on its anteromedial surface. The pancreatic neck lies anterior to the junction of the SMV and the splenic vein as they join to form the portal vein. The proximal body arches over the superior mesenteric artery (SMA) and is separated from it by a fat plane. The distal body and tail lie anterior to the splenic artery and vein. The tail of the pancreas extends toward the splenic hilum within the splenorenal ligament.

  The root of the transverse mesocolon extends across the inferior border of the pancreatic body and constitutes a potential pathway for spread of disease processes between the pancreas and the transverse colon. The root of the small bowel mesentery also originates near the inferior aspect of the pancreas and allows for extension of pancreatic disease to the mesenteric small bowel.

- **Embryologically,** the pancreas originates from two buds arising from primitive gut epithelium. The larger dorsal pancreatic anlage forms the body and tail of the pancreas. The smaller ventral pancreatic anlage makes up the head and uncinate process and is closely related to the common bile duct (CBD). During development, the primitive duodenum rotates and becomes C-shaped, also rotating the ventral bud and the CBD in the process. Later, the parenchyma and ductal systems of the dorsal and ventral buds fuse in a characteristic manner.

  The **main pancreatic duct** (of Wirsung) is formed by the peripheral portion of the embryologic dorsal duct and the entire ventral pancreatic duct. Together with the distal CBD, the main pancreatic duct enters the duodenum at the **major papilla of Vater.** The normal width of the main pancreatic duct is less than 3 mm. The **accessory duct** (of Santorini), which derives from the central segment of the embryologic dorsal duct, enters the duodenum at the **minor papilla,** which is located cephalad to the major papilla. The minor papilla is often not patent and the accessory duct usually atrophies to some degree.

  The pancreas receives its **blood supply** from branches of the splenic artery, common hepatic artery, gastroduodenal artery, pancreaticoduodenal arcades, and SMA. Venous drainage is chiefly into the splenic vein, which serves as a useful landmark for locating the pancreatic body and tail, as these parallel the vein anteriorly. **Peripancreatic lymph nodes** include splenic, superior pancreatic, celiac, pyloric, pancreaticoduodenal, and superior mesenteric groups as well as lymph nodes along the common bile duct in the hepatoduodenal ligament.

- The pancreas serves both exocrine and endocrine functions. The **exocrine pancreas** forms the majority of the gland. It consists of closely packed secretory acini, which drain into a branched ductal system. Alkaline, enzyme-rich fluid, which is secreted into the duodenum via the main pancreatic duct, neutralizes the acidic chyme from the stomach. Pancreatic enzymes include trypsin and chymotrypsin, lipase, and amylase, which degrade proteins, lipids, and carbohydrates, respectively. Pancreatic exocrine secretion occurs continuously and is regulated by hormonal and nervous system controls.

  The **endocrine cells** migrate from the duct system during embryogenesis and aggregate around capillaries to form isolated clumps of cells, known as **islets of Langerhans.** They are scattered throughout the gland but are most numerous in the pancreatic tail. The various islet cells produce different hormones. For example, alpha cells secrete glucagon, beta cells produce insulin, and delta cells make somatostatin. These hormones play an important role in carbohydrate metabolism.

- **Computed tomography (CT) technique** for the pancreas varies depending on the diagnostic question. In evaluating pancreatitis, a routine examination with intravenous (IV) contrast using 5- to 8-mm collimation should be performed through the entire abdomen and pelvis to assess for fluid collections, inflammation, necrosis, and hemorrhage. Scanning commences 40 s after the start of the contrast bolus (150 mL at 3 mL/s). Although positive oral contrast is useful, patients with acute pancreatitis are treated with bowel rest; thus, oral contrast is often withheld in severe cases.

  To **exclude a pancreatic tumor,** a dual-phase protocol should be used, with IV contrast administered at a high rate (4 to 5 mL/s). Water is used as a negative oral contrast agent, particularly if multiplanar reconstructions are being considered, since its low attenuation will not interfere with the depiction of enhanced vessels. The pancreatic phase consists of 3- to 5-mm sections, starting approximately 40 s after initiation of the contrast bolus. The venous phase follows at 70 s with 5-mm collimation through the pancreas and liver to improve detection of hypoenhancing pancreatic masses or hypodense hepatic metastases.

9.2 CONGENITAL ABNORMALITIES

- **Pancreas divisum** is a common anatomic variant of the pancreas. It results from failure of the dorsal and ventral pancreatic anlagen to fuse during development. The embryologic dorsal pancreatic duct drains into the minor papilla and the shorter ventral pancreatic duct drains with the common bile duct into the major papilla. Pancreas divisum is present in 4 to 10 percent of adults but is seen in up to one-fourth of patients with recurrent idiopathic pancreatitis. Inability of the smaller minor papilla to drain the entire dorsal pancreas has been postulated to account for recurrent pancreatitis in these patients. CT may demonstrate a fat cleft between the dorsal and ventral pancreas or, rarely, the separate ductal drainage itself.
- **Annular pancreas** is a rare developmental anomaly that likely results from a bifid ventral pancreatic bud which fuses with the dorsal bud at both ends, thus encircling the duodenum. The majority of cases coexist with duodenal atresia or stenosis and present early in life, but some patients present later on with obstructive symptoms. On CT, an annular pancreas is depicted as circumferential soft tissue thickening around the second portion of the duodenum that matches the attenuation and enhancement characteristics of the rest of the pancreas **(Fig. 9.1)**. Demonstration of a duct that encircles the duodenum on endoscopic retrograde cholangiopancreatography (ERCP) is diagnostic of annular pancreas.
- **Ectopic** pancreatic tissue or pancreatic rests are found in up to 5 percent of autopsies. Characteristic locations include the gastric antrum and proximal duodenum, where they appear as submucosal nodules on barium studies, often with a central umbilication. Pancreatic rests are occasionally found within the jejunum, ileum, duplication cysts, and Meckel diverticulum.

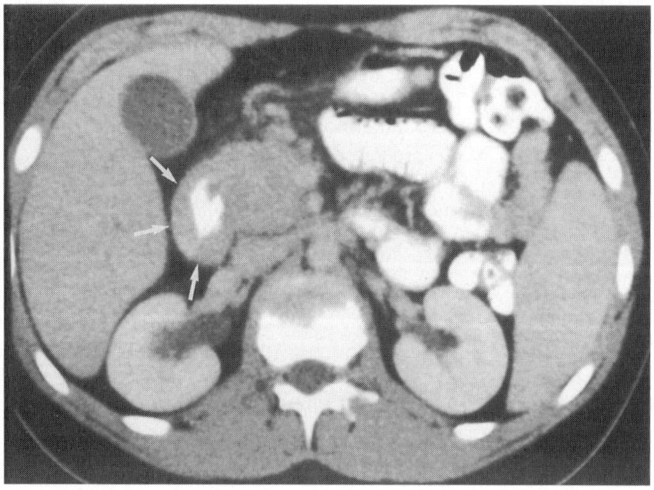

FIGURE 9.1 Annular pancreas. Contrast-enhanced CT in a 13-year-old boy shows narrowing of the contrast-filled duodenum by circumferential soft tissue thickening *(arrows)*, which appears similar to the rest of the pancreas. Annular pancreas was confirmed on endoscopic retrograde cholangiopancreatography. (Case courtesy of Dr. Marilyn Siegel, St. Louis, MO.)

9.3 PANCREATITIS

- **Acute pancreatitis** remains a challenging clinical entity despite its relatively high frequency of occurrence. Delay in diagnosis and underestimation of disease severity continue to result in significant morbidity and mortality. Advances in CT imaging have had a major impact on the diagnosis and management of acute pancreatitis, especially in severe disease. Alcohol abuse and biliary tract disease (particularly gallstone pancreatitis) account for over 80 percent of cases in the United States. Other causes include trauma, ERCP, medications, infection, metabolic abnormalities, and mechanical duct obstruction **(Differential 9.1)**; over 10 percent of cases have no discernible cause. Pancreatitis results from premature activation and leakage of pancreatic enzymes and subsequent autodigestion of the pancreas and adjacent tissues. The inflammatory exudate consists of varying combinations of edematous fluid, leukocyte infiltration, hemorrhage, and fat necrosis.
- The **clinical presentation** of acute pancreatitis is often nonspecific and ranges from mild abdominal discomfort to severe systemic illness with metabolic derangement, hypotension, sepsis, or death. The Ranson criteria, a battery of clinical parameters, were developed as an indicator of morbidity and mortality. A rise in the number of positive criteria correlates with a poorer clinical outcome. More recently, the APACHE II score was developed as another measure of disease severity. Mild edematous pancreatitis accounts for the majority of cases and typically responds well to supportive care, whereas necrotizing pancreatitis is associated with a mortality rate that may exceed 20 percent.

  A spectrum of local and systemic complications can be seen in the acute setting. Local pancreatic and peripancreatic complications include fluid collections, abscesses, biliary obstruction, and vascular insults, such as hemorrhage, thrombosis, and pseudoaneurysm formation. Systemic complications include shock, acute respiratory distress syndrome (ARDS), disseminated intravascular coagulation, renal failure, and electrolyte imbalances. Multiple-system organ failure is also common.
- **CT** has become the study of choice for imaging acute pancreatitis, providing information that is vital for prognosis and appropriate pa-

9.1 PANCREATITIS

Alcohol
Cholelithiasis (gallstone pancreatitis)
Trauma
Idiopathic—>10 %
Ductal obstruction—tumor, choledochocele, ductal anomaly, ascariasis
ERCP
Infection—mumps, measles, AIDS, CMV
Drugs—AZT, thiazides, and sulfonamides
Hyperlipidemia
Hypercalcemia
Hereditary pancreatitis

Key: ERCP, endoscopic retrograde cholangiopancreatography; CMV, cytomegalovirus; AZT, azidothymidine.

tient management. Grading of the severity of disease on CT appears to correlate with clinical outcome, although no single imaging-based grading system has demonstrated superiority. Of paramount importance is the distinction between edematous and necrotizing pancreatitis.

- Patients with **edematous pancreatitis** typically have an uneventful recovery with supportive therapy. The pancreas may be normal on CT in cases of mild disease. When CT findings are present, the gland may be slightly enlarged, with mild infiltration of the peripancreatic fat and obscuration of the pancreatic margins **(Fig. 9.2)**. CT imaging is usually not required in such cases unless the diagnosis is uncertain, the patient's symptoms worsen, or the patient fails to respond to conservative therapy.

  CT plays a more important role with increasing severity of pancreatitis. The local inflammatory changes seen with mild disease become much more pronounced in severe pancreatitis **(Fig. 9.3)**. In addition, acute pancreatic and peripancreatic fluid collections are commonly present. On CT, fluid can be seen dissecting along retroperitoneal and mesenteric fascial planes, sometimes extending to involve the kidneys, transverse colon, stomach, spleen, or small bowel. Significant pancreatic ascites is present in a minority of cases.

- Contrast-enhanced CT is particularly useful in patients with **necrotizing pancreatitis.** Pancreatic necrosis is depicted as a region that lacks the contrast enhancement seen with viable pancreatic tissue **(Fig. 9.4)**. The degree of necrosis on CT is predictive of clinical outcome; patients with extensive necrosis that involves over 50 percent of the gland have a mortality rate approaching 30 percent. An area of pancreatic necrosis can become infected and form an abscess.

- **Abscesses** typically occur within days to weeks from the onset of symptoms and result from superinfection of pancreatic necrosis, hemorrhage, or fluid collection. Infection should be considered in a patient with severe pancreatitis and a deteriorating clinical course. CT evaluation to rule out abscess is warranted in this setting, since the mortality rate of untreated abscesses approaches 100 percent. Therapy may consist of percutaneous drainage or open surgical debridement. Unfortunately, pancreatic or peripancreatic abscesses are often indistinguishable from uninfected collections on CT. Diagnostic ultrasound or CT-guided needle aspiration of such collections offers a rapid answer and can play an important role in management decisions. The presence or development of gas bubbles within a focal pancreatic or peripancreatic collection is more suggestive of abscess **(Fig. 9.5)** but is present in the minority of cases. Retroperitoneal gas is less commonly due to fistula formation with the gastrointestinal tract.

- **Vascular complications** of acute pancreatitis include pseudoaneurysm formation, hemorrhage, and venous thrombosis. **Pseudoaneurysms** can be seen in the setting of acute or chronic pancreatitis and result from erosion into peripancreatic arteries by the proteolytic inflammatory exudate. A pseudocyst can also erode

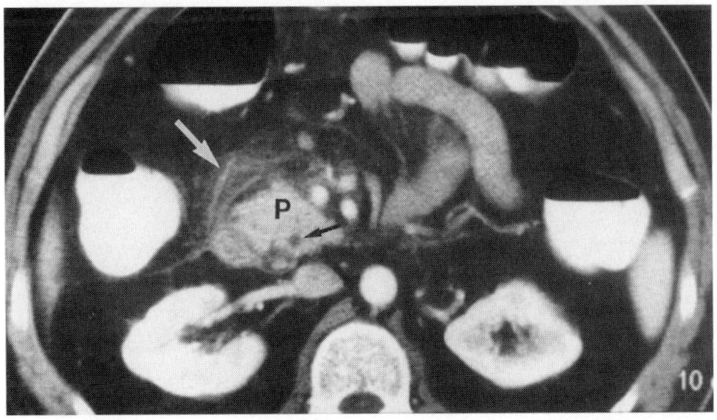

FIGURE 9.2 Mild edematous pancreatitis. Contrast-enhanced CT shows soft tissue infiltration of the fat *(white arrow)* surrounding the head of the pancreas (P). Note normal caliber common bile duct *(black arrow)*.

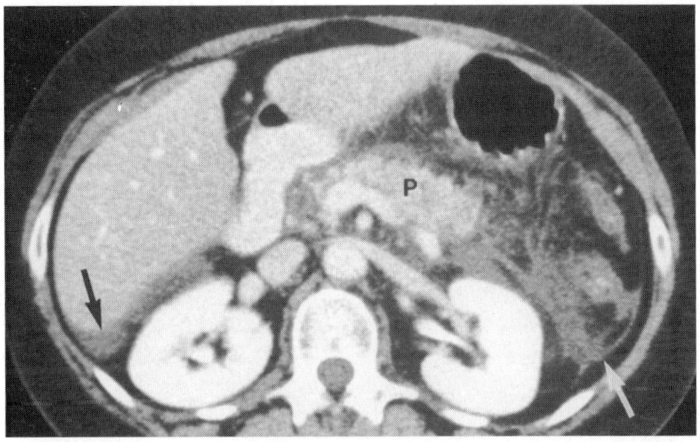

FIGURE 9.3 Severe edematous pancreatitis. Contrast-enhanced CT in a 39-year-old woman shows diffuse peripancreatic inflammation that extends along the left pararenal space *(white arrow)*. The pancreas (P) enhances normally. Note small amount of ascites *(black arrow)* adjacent to the liver.

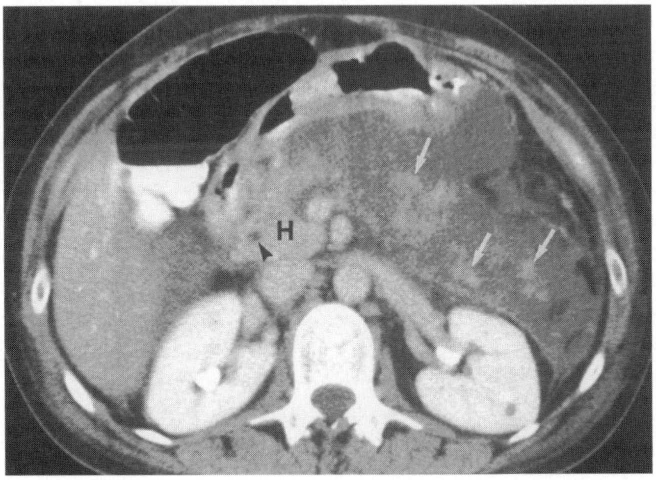

FIGURE 9.4 Necrotizing pancreatitis. Contrast-enhanced CT in a 38-year-old woman with alcoholic pancreatitis shows extensive necrosis of the pancreatic body and tail with only small islands of parenchymal enhancement remaining *(arrows)*. The pancreatic head (H) has more viable tissue. The common bile duct *(arrowhead)* is well seen.

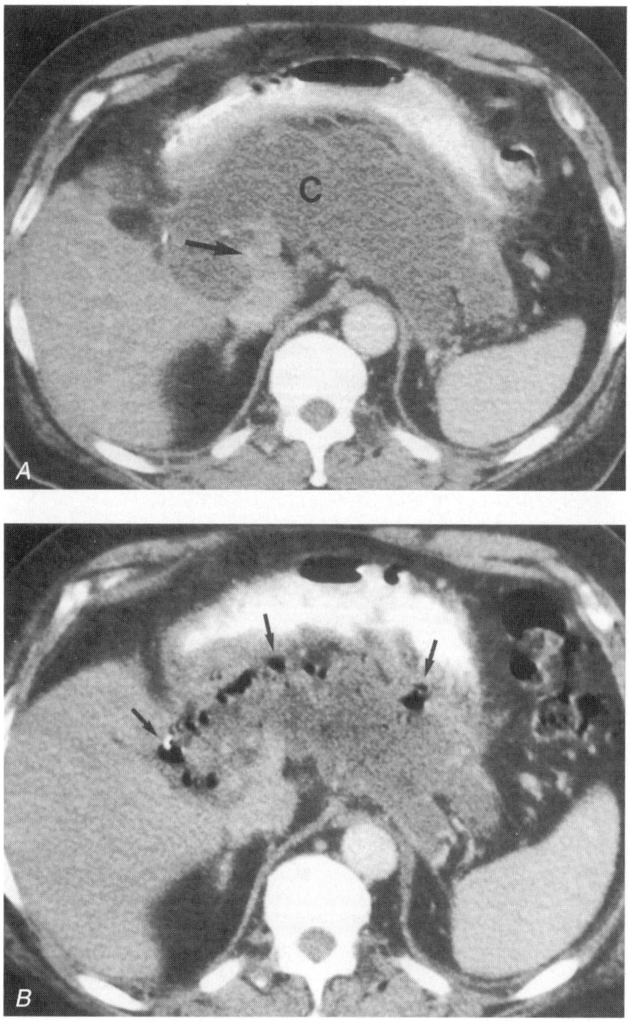

FIGURE 9.5 Pancreatic abscess. *A*. Contrast-enhanced CT in a 17-year-old with severe pancreatitis demonstrates a large fluid collection (C) that replaces nearly the entire pancreas. A small amount of enhancing parenchyma remains in the head *(arrow)*. *B*. Follow-up CT 1 week later, after the onset of fever and worsening abdominal pain, shows interval development of gas bubbles *(arrows)* within the fluid collection. Purulent material was aspirated under ultrasound guidance.

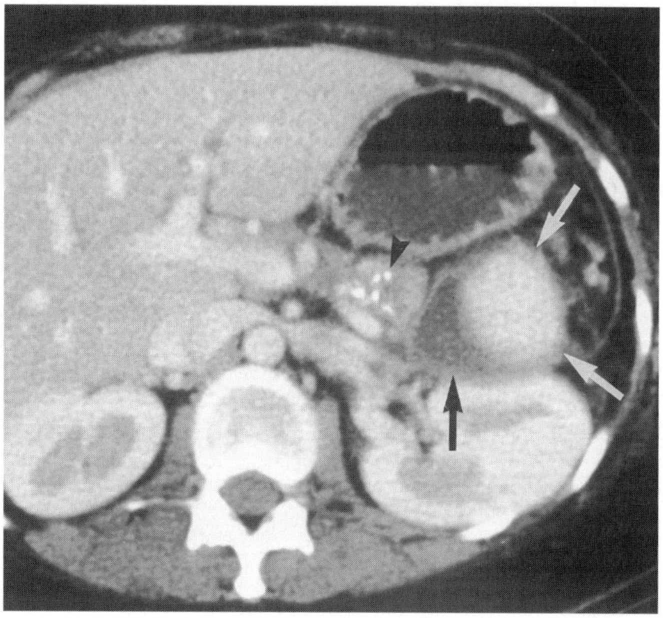

FIGURE 9.6 Splenic artery pseudoaneurysm. Contrast-enhanced CT in a 35-year-old woman with chronic pancreatitis secondary to alcohol abuse shows a densely enhancing lesion *(white arrows)* near the pancreatic tail, consistent with a splenic artery pseudoaneurysm. Note low-attenuation thrombus peripherally *(black arrow)* and parenchymal calcification *(arrowhead)* from chronic pancreatitis.

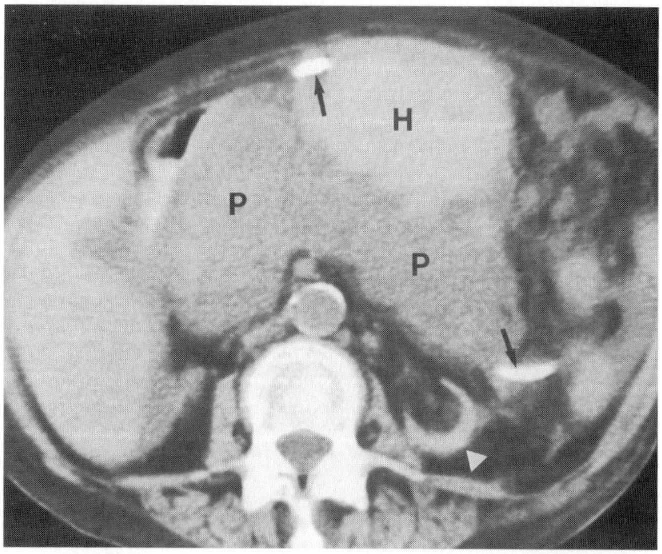

FIGURE 9.7 Necrotizing pancreatitis with hemorrhage. Noncontrast CT in a 63-year-old woman with severe necrotizing pancreatitis (P) shows a large, ill-defined region of higher attenuation anterior to the pancreas (H), representing hemorrhage. Drainage catheters are in place *(arrows)*. Intravenous contrast was withheld due to acute-on-chronic renal failure. Note atrophic left kidney *(arrowhead)*.

into a vessel and form a large pseudoaneurysm that is at high risk for rupture. The splenic artery is most often involved, followed by the gastroduodenal artery. Dynamic contrast-enhanced CT can readily detect pseudoaneurysms by their rapid filling of contrast, which equals that of the adjacent arteries **(Fig. 9.6)**. Depending on the location of the pseudoaneurysm and the clinical status of the patient, either transcatheter embolization or surgical intervention is indicated. **Hemorrhage** is best depicted on noncontrast CT as high attenuation within the pancreas, adjacent to the pancreas, or within preexisting fluid collections **(Fig. 9.7)**. Hemorrhage due to leakage from a pseudoaneurysm is associated with a mortality rate that approaches 50 percent. Thrombosis of the splenic vein or SMV represents another vascular complication of pancreatitis.

- **Fluid collections** are seen on CT in up to 50 percent of patients with acute pancreatitis. The majority of these collections resolve spontaneously, but up to 15 percent will organize and form **pancreatic pseudocysts.** These walled-off collections of pancreatic secretions require about 6 weeks to mature and are enclosed by a fibrous rim of granulation tissue. Many pseudocysts maintain communication with the pancreatic duct. Symptoms are dependent on size and location and include persistent abdominal pain, nausea and vomiting from duodenal or gastric outlet obstruction, and jaundice from biliary obstruction. Other complications of pseudocysts include spontaneous rupture into the retroperitoneum or peritoneal cavity and erosion into peripancreatic vessels. Pseudocysts are typically peripancreatic in location, although they can also dissect along fascial planes into adjacent organs, such as the liver, spleen, kidney, stomach, and more distant sites, such as the mediastinum **(Fig. 9.8)**.

CT is the diagnostic study of choice for the detection of pancreatic pseudocysts. An uncomplicated pseudocyst will demonstrate near water attenuation and a well-defined capsule. Increased density or inhomogeneity suggests complicating hemorrhage or infection. Unsuspected pseudocysts detected in patients without a proven history of pancreatitis can be mistaken for a cystic neoplasm **(see Section 9.4)**.

Management of pseudocysts depends on size and the presence of symptoms. Infected collections always require drainage, which can often be accomplished percutaneously with image guidance. Other indications for drainage include a size greater than 5 cm, increasing size, and new or worsening symptoms. Uninfected pseudocysts that are less than 4 or 5 cm in size often resolve spontaneously and can be followed with serial CT examination. The preferred surgical approach for an uncomplicated pseudocyst is internal drainage into the gastrointestinal tract. Endoscopic drainage procedures into the stomach or duodenum can also be accomplished by stenting or creating a fistula. Image-guided percutaneous drainage has been shown to be safe and effective. Pseudocyst hemorrhage can often be managed with angiographic embolization.

- **Chronic pancreatitis** represents progressive and irreversible destruction of pancreatic tissue. This disease process is clinically distinct from acute pancreatitis, which only rarely leads to chronic pancreatitis. Most cases are secondary to alcohol abuse, but additional causes include hyperlipidemia, hypercalcemia, and hereditary forms. Chronic pancreatitis presents clinically as epigastric pain in up to 95 percent of patients. Weight loss is a common associated finding. Malabsorption with steatorrhea occurs if more than 90 percent of the secretory capacity of the exocrine pancreas has been destroyed. Diabetes from endocrine dysfunction occurs in approximately 50 percent of patients, while abnormal glucose tolerance is seen in about 70 percent.

- **CT** demonstrates parenchymal atrophy, irregular dilatation and beading of the pancreatic duct, and coarse calcifications in the majority of patients with chronic pancreatitis **(Fig. 9.9)**. Other causes of pancreatic calcification are presented in **Differential 9.2.** Pseudocysts are relatively common in patients with chronic pancreatitis.

When parenchymal atrophy and ductal dilatation are present in the pancreatic body and tail on CT, the entire gland should be scrutinized to exclude a proximal obstructing tumor, which can have a similar appearance. Other complications of chronic pancreatitis include biliary ductal obstruction, duodenal obstruction, fistula formation, venous thrombosis, and pseudoaneurysm formation.

Biliary obstruction occurs in approximately 10 percent of patients with chronic pancreatitis and is due to stricture of the distal common bile duct within the pancreatic head. Alkaline phosphatase

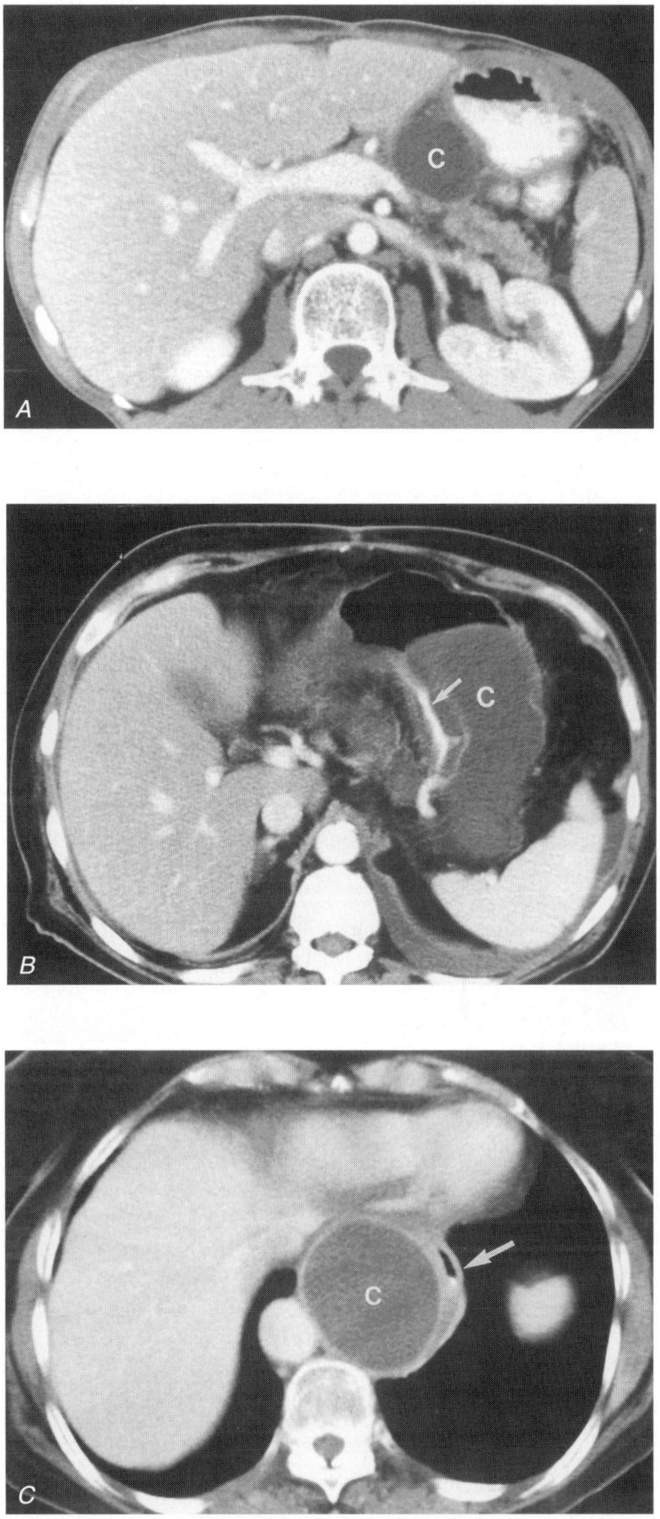

FIGURE 9.8 Pancreatic pseudocysts. *A*. Contrast-enhanced CT shows a rounded, well-defined fluid collection (C) anterior to the body of the pancreas. *B*. Contrast-enhanced CT shows a large fluid collection (C) within the wall of the stomach, compressing the air- and contrast-filled lumen *(arrow)*. *C*. Contrast-enhanced CT shows a pancreatic pseudocyst (C) that has dissected through the esophageal hiatus into the middle mediastinum. Note displacement of the esophagus *(arrow)*.

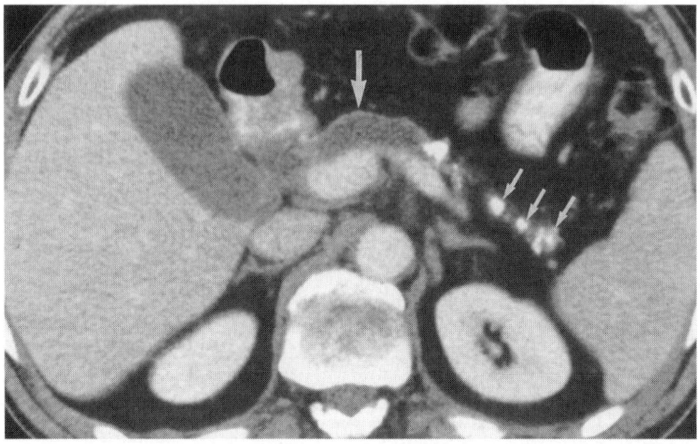

FIGURE 9.9 Chronic pancreatitis. Contrast-enhanced CT shows severe pancreatic atrophy with dilatation of the pancreatic duct *(large arrow)* and coarse calcifications in the pancreatic tail *(small arrows)*.

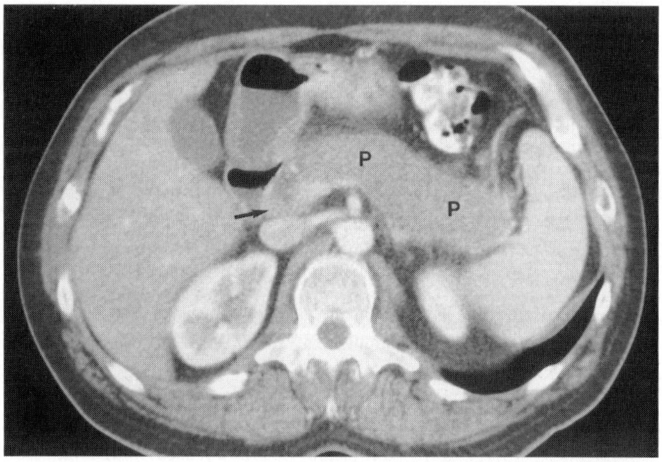

FIGURE 9.10 Idiopathic fibrosing pancreatitis. Contrast-enhanced CT in a 45-year-old man shows prominent enlargement and decreased enhancement of the pancreas (P), which spares only a portion of the head *(arrow)*. Multiple biopsies revealed interstitial fibrosis without evidence of malignancy.

and serum bilirubin are commonly elevated in these patients. CT depicts proximal ductal dilatation and absence of an obstructing tumor, but ERCP can better characterize the biliary duct morphology. Surgery may be necessary in patients with significant pain, jaundice, or cholangitis. Choledochoduodenostomy or Roux-en-Y choledochojejunostomy are preferred methods of biliary bypass. Pancreatic carcinoma should always be excluded in this setting.

Duodenal obstruction is an uncommon complication of chronic pancreatitis. CT demonstrates gastric and duodenal distention to the level of obstruction. These patients can be treated with a gastrojejunostomy.

Pancreatic fistulas can present as ascites or a pleural effusion that has an elevated amylase level. Repeated paracentesis or thoracentesis is often necessary. If conservative therapy is unsuccessful after 3 weeks, ERCP is performed to localize the leak. If the leak is located in the pancreatic tail, a distal pancreatectomy can be curative, whereas centrally located leaks can be drained into a Roux-en-Y jejunal loop. These procedures have a success rate over 80 percent. A pancreaticoenteric fistula represents drainage into an adjacent loop of bowel, often the transverse colon or splenic flexure, and usually requires operative intervention.

Splenic vein thrombosis can complicate acute or chronic pancreatitis. Isolated gastric varices may form along the greater curvature of the stomach in these patients **(see Fig. 6.9)**. Management of patients with bleeding gastric varices often includes splenectomy, which has a 90 percent success rate. As previously discussed, **pseudoaneurysms** can result from erosion into peripancreatic arteries **(see Fig. 9.6)**.

- **Treatment** of chronic pancreatitis includes abstaining from alcohol. Pancreatic enzymes and insulin are administered as needed. Intractable pain may require celiac nerve block. Endoscopic and surgical interventions for complications related to chronic pancreatitis were discussed above.
- **Idiopathic fibrosing pancreatitis** is a rare and unusual form of chronic pancreatitis characterized histologically by interstitial fibrosis that spares the acini. The typical CT findings of calcification, parenchymal atrophy, and pseudoaneurysm formation are absent in this form of pancreatitis. Instead, focal or diffuse pancreatic enlargement with decreased enhancement is depicted on CT and can mimic pancreatic adenocarcinoma **(Fig. 9.10)**. Patients may present with biliary obstruction if the pancreatic head is involved.

9.4 CYSTIC LESIONS

- **Pancreatic lesions** can be cystic, solid, or complex in nature. Pancreatic pseudocysts, discussed in **Section 9.3,** account for up to 90 percent of cystic lesions. Other cystic pancreatic masses include true epithelial cysts and cystic neoplasms, which include a spectrum of benign and malignant tumors **(Differential 9.3)**.
- True **epithelial pancreatic cysts** are rare and, when multiple, are usually associated with underlying conditions such as von Hippel-Lindau disease, autosomal dominant polycystic kidney disease, and cystic fibrosis. **Von Hippel-Lindau disease** is a neurocutaneous syndrome with autosomal dominant inheritance. Up to 70 percent of these patients have pancreatic cysts **(Fig. 9.11)**. Other associated findings include intracranial and spinal hemangioblastomas, retinal angiomas, renal cysts and renal cell carcinomas, pheochromocytomas, epididymal and broad ligament cystadenomas, and microcystic adenomas of the pancreas. Less than 5 percent of patients with **autosomal dominant polycystic disease** have pancreatic

9.2 PANCREATIC CALCIFICATION

Chronic pancreatitis—alcohol, hereditary, or biliary
Vascular calcifications
Tumors
- Adenocarcinoma—2%
- Islet cell tumor—20%
- Microcystic cystadenoma—40%, calcification of central scar
- Mucinous cystic neoplasm—10 to 15%, septal calcification
- Metastases—mucinous gastrointestinal primaries
- Cystic teratoma—fat and calcium
- Hemangioma—phleboliths

Chronic pseudocyst—calcification rare
Prior hematoma—trauma, coagulopathy

9.3

CYSTIC PANCREATIC LESION

Pseudocyst—develops in about 15% of pancreatitis
Microcystic adenoma—glycogen-rich fluid, small cysts
Mucinous cystic neoplasms—malignant evolution, mucin-rich fluid, large cysts
Solid and papillary epithelial neoplasm—low-grade malignancy of young women
Epithelial cyst
  Von Hippel-Lindau disease—about 70%
  Autosomal dominant polycystic kidney disease—less than 5%
  Cystic fibrosis
Hemangioma
Lymphangioma
Cystic teratoma
Cystic islet cell tumor
Parasitic cysts—echinococcal

cysts, whereas approximately 40 percent have hepatic cysts and virtually all have renal cysts. Patients with **cystic fibrosis** typically have diffuse fatty replacement of the gland but can also have multiple pancreatic cysts, which are usually only a few millimeters in size. Regardless of etiology, simple epithelial pancreatic cysts have the characteristic signature seen in other organs; namely, they are of water attenuation, lack enhancement and significant septations or calcifications, and have an imperceptible wall.

- Primary **cystic neoplasms** account for approximately 10 to 15 percent of pancreatic cystic lesions in published surgical series. The two major categories are the microcystic adenomas and the mucinous cystic neoplasms.
- **Microcystic adenomas** (also referred to as serous cystadenomas) most commonly affect older women, with 80 percent of cases occurring in patients over 60 years of age. These are benign tumors with no malignant potential. Therefore, recognition of microcystic adenomas on cross-sectional imaging is important primarily to avoid unnecessary intervention. Patients are often asymptomatic, but they may present with nonspecific symptoms or a palpable mass. Pathologically, microcystic adenomas contain numerous small cysts, most measuring less than 2 cm, although larger cysts are occasionally seen. The cytoplasm of the cells lining the cysts and the cyst fluid are glycogen-rich. A stellate central scar is characteristic of serous cystadenomas. These tend to be relatively large tumors, averaging over 5 cm in size, and have an equal distribution throughout the pancreas.

  On **CT,** microcystic adenomas are low-attenuation lobulated masses. The appearance following IV contrast will depend on the size of the tumor cysts. Most commonly, a multicystic appearance is seen, with a lacy or reticular pattern of enhancing septa **(Fig. 9.12)**. A stellate central scar, often with areas of dystrophic calcification, is characteristic of this benign tumor. The presence of central calcification is more common with microcystic adenomas than with any other pancreatic tumor **(Fig. 9.12)**.

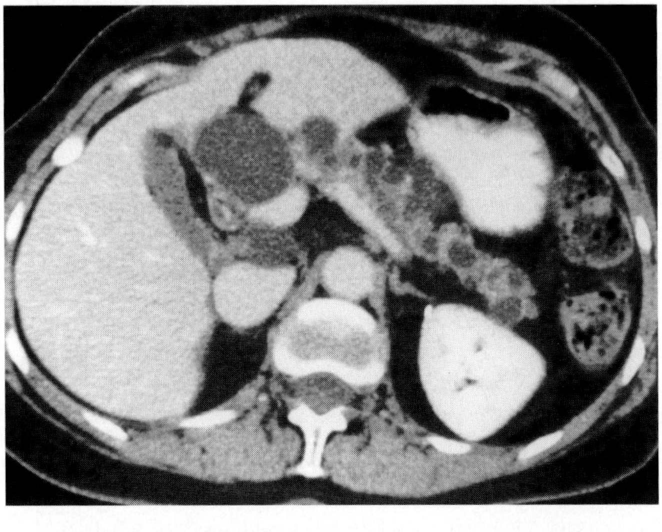

FIGURE 9.11 Pancreatic cysts. Contrast-enhanced CT in a 52-year-old woman with von Hippel-Lindau syndrome shows innumerable pancreatic cysts. Renal cysts and broad ligament cystadenomas were present on caudal images (not shown).

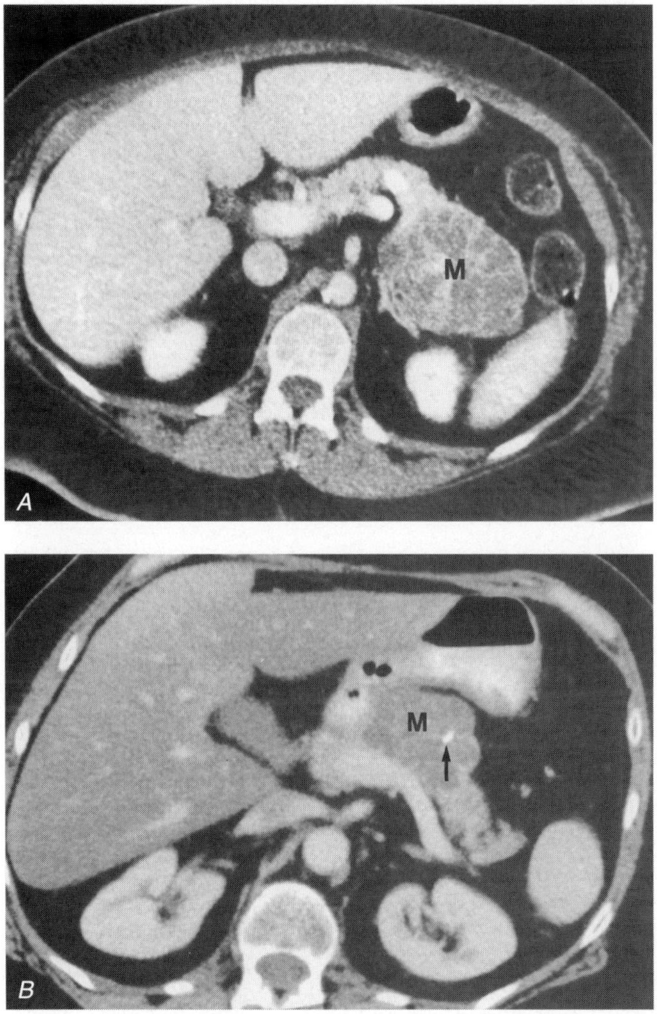

FIGURE 9.12 Microcystic adenoma. *A*. Contrast-enhanced CT in a 70-year-old woman shows a large low-attenuation mass (M) extending off the pancreatic tail. Multiple septations give rise to a lacy or reticular pattern of enhancement. *B*. Contrast-enhanced CT in a 65-year-old woman shows a large low-attenuation mass (M) in the body of the pancreas with central calcification *(arrow)*. Thin internal septations were better appreciated at other levels.

- **Mucinous cystic neoplasms** include both macrocystic cystadenoma and macrocystic cystadenocarcinoma, although all such tumors should be considered at least potentially malignant. These neoplasms are much more common among women, typically occurring in patients between 40 and 60 years of age. Approximately 85 percent are located within the pancreatic tail or distal body, where they can present as a palpable mass. Mucinous cystic neoplasms are typically quite large, with a mean diameter of 12 cm. The tumors contain single or multiple large mucin-containing macrocysts. Mucinous cystic neoplasms should be excised because of their tendency toward malignant progression. Even when malignant, they have a favorable prognosis compared with duct-cell adenocarcinoma once they have been completely excised.

  On **CT,** mucinous cystic neoplasms are large, well-defined unilocular or multilocular lesions located in the distal body or tail **(Fig. 9.13)**. The individual cysts generally measure over 2 cm in size and have thick walls. Curvilinear septal calcifications are present in 15 to 20 percent of cases. Like ovarian mucinous cystadenocarcinoma, cysts can contain mural nodules and solid excrescences. Unilocular tumors, however, can mimic the appearance of a pseudocyst. The tumor is predominantly hypovascular, but enhancement of the septa or solid components can be apparent. These tumors can spread locally or hematogenously to the liver, where metastases are often cystic in appearance.

  Duct-ectatic mucinous tumor is an uncommon variant of mucinous cystic neoplasms. Also referred to as intraductal papillary mucinous tumor or mucin-hypersecreting tumor, it consists of a papillary neoplasm of the main pancreatic duct or side branches and ranges from benign to frankly malignant in behavior. These tumors present at a similar age as the other mucinous cystic neoplasms, but the duct-ectatic variant occurs more frequently among men. When focal, the process is typically located in the uncinate portion of the pancreatic head, manifesting as localized ductal dilatation. In more advanced cases, the entire ductal system may be dilated. Duct-ectatic mucinous tumors have a relatively good prognosis, since parenchymal and extrapancreatic extension occur late in the disease course.

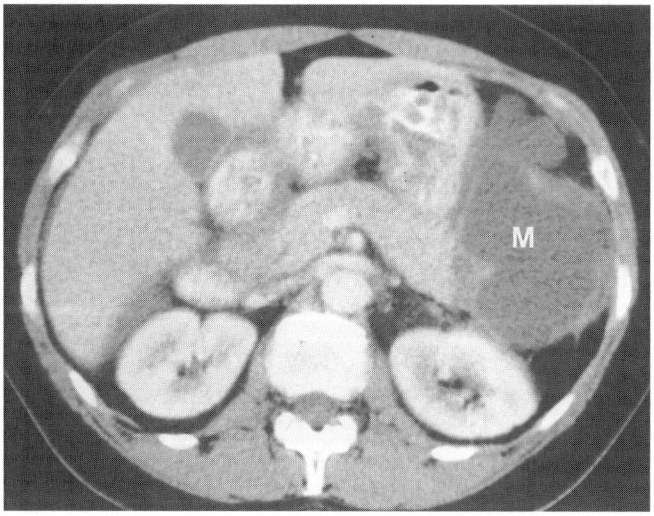

FIGURE 9.13 Mucinous cystic neoplasm (macrocystic cystadenocarcinoma). Contrast-enhanced CT in a 51-year-old woman shows a large, lobulated cystic mass (M) extending off the pancreatic tail. The tumor was composed of thick-walled macrocysts measuring over 2 cm in size.

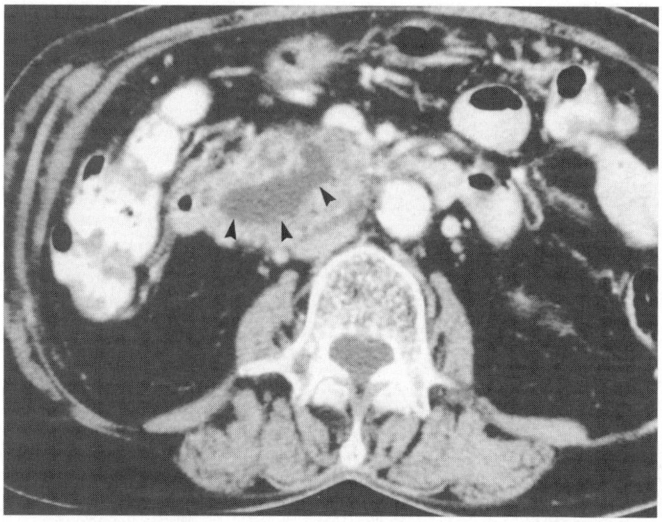

FIGURE 9.14 Duct-ectatic mucinous tumor. Contrast-enhanced CT in an 81-year-old woman shows prominent ductal dilatation involving the uncinate *(arrowheads)*. The entire ductal system was ectatic and of slightly higher attenuation than the fluid in the common bile duct.

  On **CT,** the primary feature of mucin-hypersecreting tumors is prominent cystic dilation of the involved portion of the pancreatic ductal system **(Fig. 9.14)**. The uncinate region is usually involved. ERCP is the preferred method of diagnosis, where abundant mucus production and outpouring at the papilla is evident and intraductal filling defects can be demonstrated.

- **Solid and papillary epithelial neoplasm (SPEN)** is a rare, low-grade pancreatic malignancy that typically affects young women, with a disproportionately higher rate among African Americans. It is treated with surgical excision and the prognosis is generally excellent. Solid and papillary epithelial neoplasms are usually located within the pancreatic tail and are large, encapsulated tumors with variable amounts of cystic and solid elements. Consequently, they are depicted on **CT** as complex cystic and solid lesions. Thick-walled cysts with mural nodules are characteristic **(Fig. 9.15)**. The mean tumor diameter is about 10 cm. A fluid-debris level from previous hemorrhage and cystic degeneration can be seen. Dystrophic calcification may be present in a minority of cases.

- **Cystic teratomas** only rarely occur within the pancreas and are benign. On CT, they are depicted as well-defined masses with a variable amount of fat and calcium and may contain fat-fluid levels.

9.5 SOLID TUMORS

- **Ductal adenocarcinoma** accounts for 95 percent of all pancreatic cancers and represents the fourth leading cause of cancer death in the United States **(Differential 9.4).** Ductal adenocarcinoma usually affects older adults beyond the sixth decade of life, and the overall incidence continues to rise. Despite advances in tumor detection and treatment, the prognosis remains dismal. Purported risk factors include diabetes mellitus, cigarette smoking, and chronic pancreatitis.

  The clinical presentation of pancreatic ductal adenocarcinoma is often nonspecific. Jaundice, with or without pain, is the presenting complaint in up to one-half of patients with tumors of the pancre-

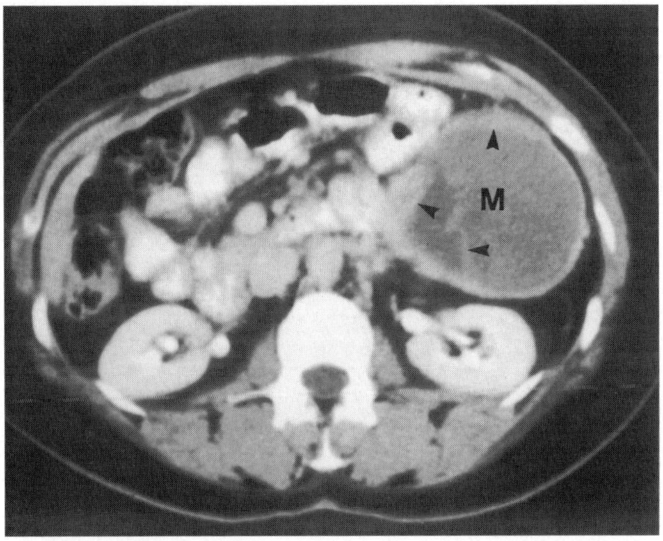

FIGURE 9.15 Solid and papillary epithelial neoplasm. Contrast-enhanced CT in a young woman shows a complex cystic and solid mass (M) extending off the pancreatic tail. Note thickened wall and septation *(arrowheads)*. The cystic components demonstrate varying degrees of attenuation. (Case courtesy of Dr. Arthur Bishop, Peoria, IL.)

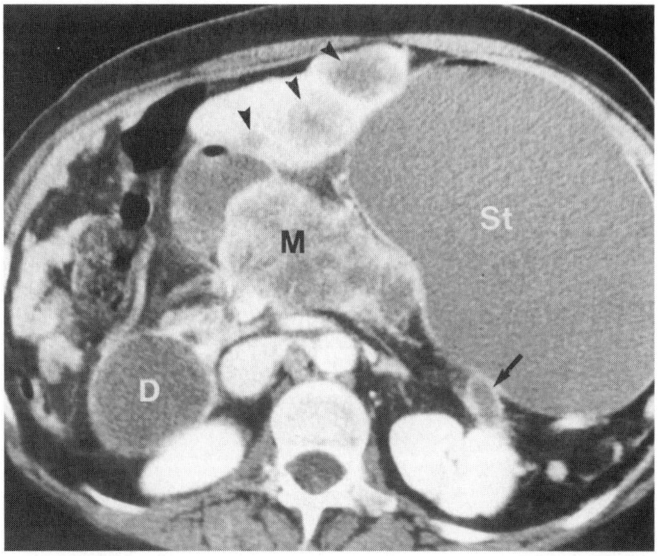

FIGURE 9.16 Pancreatic ductal adenocarcinoma. Contrast-enhanced CT in a 69-year-old woman shows a large hypoattenuating mass (M) centered in the pancreas. Dilatation of the stomach (St) and duodenum (D) is due to obstruction of the third portion of the duodenum by tumor. Note atrophy and ductal dilatation of the pancreatic tail *(arrow)* and liver metastases *(arrowheads)*.

atic head. Pain is the most common symptom in patients with tumors of the body and tail. Other symptoms include weight loss, fatigue, nausea and vomiting, diabetes, and depression. On physical exam, an enlarged, palpable, nontender gallbladder (Courvoisier sign) may be detected. Patients can also present with spontaneous migratory venous thrombosis (Trousseau sign). CA 19-9, a serum tumor marker, is elevated in up to 90 percent of patients with ductal adenocarcinoma but is not specific for cancer. The tumor is characteristically dense and fibrous with an infiltrative pattern of growth. Up to 70 percent of tumors arise within the pancreatic head, with the remainder involving the body and tail.

CT is the method of choice for the diagnosis and preoperative staging of pancreatic cancer, with a detection rate of approximately 99 percent. The tumor is typically depicted on CT as an area of focal low attenuation following contrast administration **(Fig. 9.16)**. Lesion conspicuity tends to be greatest during the early portal venous or "pancreatic" phase, occurring 40 to 70 s after injection.

9.4

SOLID PANCREATIC MASS

Ductal adenocarcinoma
Islet-cell tumor—insulinoma, gastrinoma, nonfunctioning, glucagonoma, somatostatinoma, VIPoma*
Lymphoma
Metastases—melanoma, renal cell, breast, lung, stomach
Solid and papillary epithelial neoplasm—cystic component
Mimics—peripancreatic adenopathy, adrenal mass, splenule
Focal pancreatitis
Idiopathic fibrosing pancreatitis
Pancreaticoblastoma—children
Acinar cell carcinoma

*Vasoactive intestinal peptide tumor.

Focal enlargement or deformity of the gland's contour by the tumor is usually present but may be absent with smaller lesions. Tumors of the pancreatic head often cause ductal obstruction, resulting in biliary and pancreatic ductal dilatation **(Fig. 9.17)**. Isolated pancreatic ductal dilatation and parenchymal atrophy in the body or tail should raise the concern for an obstructing cancer. Changes of pancreatitis and pseudocyst formation can be seen with obstructing tumors, resulting in significant overlap in the CT appearances of adenocarcinoma and focal pancreatitis. Apparent focal sparing of age-related fatty atrophy of the pancreas is also suspicious for adenocarcinoma **(Fig. 9.18)**. Tumor calcification is rare, seen in less than 2 percent of cases. In about one-half of cases, tumor extends into the retropancreatic space, obliterating the fat plane adjacent to the celiac axis or SMA and invading the lymphatics, rendering the tumor unresectable **(Fig. 9.19)**. Duodenal obstruction from direct tumor invasion is sometimes apparent **(Fig. 9.16)**. Metastases most commonly involve the liver and regional lymph nodes **(Figs. 9.16 and 9.17)**. Peritoneal, pleural, pulmonary, and skeletal metastases are less common. Direct ligamentous extension to adjacent retroperitoneal and peritoneal structures is occasionally seen.

Spiral CT has proved to be valuable in predicting tumor resectability. The degree of vascular involvement determines the feasibility of complete surgical resection, which remains the only hope for cure. If the tumor completely encircles the SMV and SMA on CT, the lesion is unresectable. Likewise, tumor sparing of the vasculature with preservation of the fat planes surrounding the arteries suggests resectability. Difficulty in prediction arises, however, when there is variable tumor contact without frank encasement of the mesenteric vessels on CT. Most patients with equivocal studies are offered the benefit of the doubt and undergo exploration. Overall, less than 20 percent of tumors confined to the pancreas are deemed resectable. Unfortunately, the tumor recurrence rate following "curative" surgery is high and 1-year survival after surgery is about 10 percent.

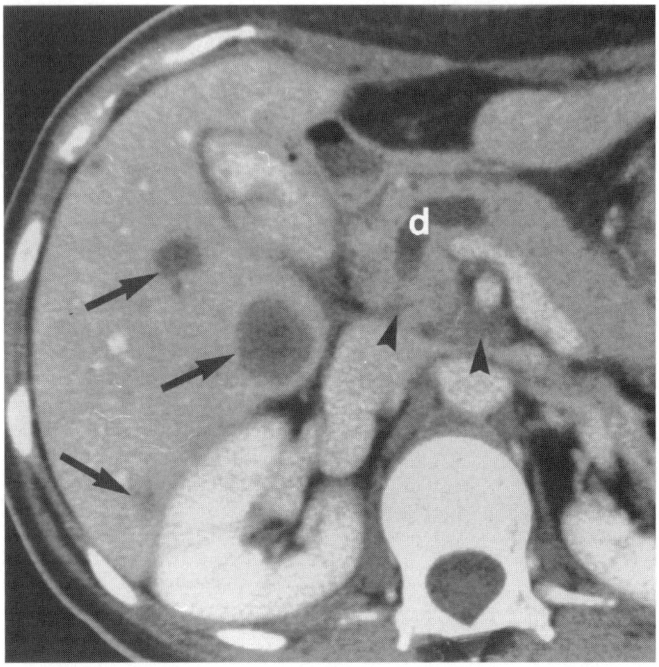

FIGURE 9.17 Pancreatic adenocarcinoma. Contrast-enhanced CT in a 39-year-old woman shows a subtle low-attenuation mass in the head of the pancreas *(arrowheads)* that contacts the superior mesenteric artery and obstructs the pancreatic duct (d). Note liver metastases *(arrows)*.

- **Unusual variants of adenocarcinoma** include pleomorphic giant-cell carcinoma, adenosquamous carcinoma, and anaplastic carcinoma. Rare nonepithelial and mesenchymal tumors include sarcomas and nerve sheath tumors. These can mimic the appearance of ductal adenocarcinoma on CT.
- **Islet cell tumors** of the pancreas are uncommon and arise from the specialized neuroendocrine cells that populate the pancreatic islets. These cells are derivatives of the APUD (amine precursor uptake and decarboxylation) line, similar in origin to pheochromocytoma, melanoma, carcinoid tumor, and medullary thyroid carcinoma. Islet cell tumors occur sporadically or are associated with multiple endocrine neoplasia type I **(MEN 1)**. MEN 1, also known as Werner syndrome, is also associated with adenomas of the pituitary and parathyroid.

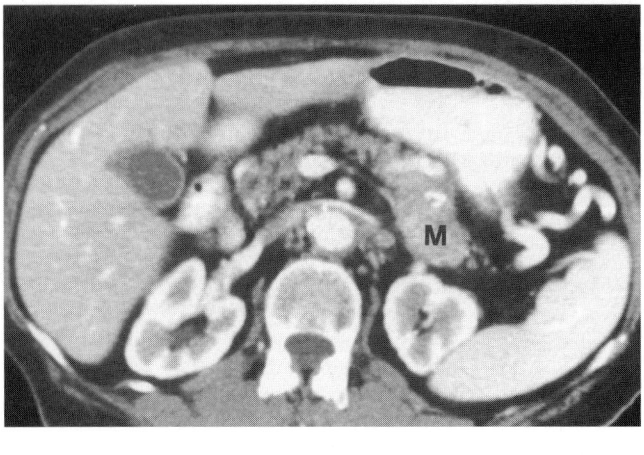

FIGURE 9.18 Pancreatic adenocarcinoma. Contrast-enhanced CT in a 66-year-old woman shows a solid mass (M) in the tail of the pancreas. The tumor is more conspicuous owing to the fatty involution involving the rest of the pancreas.

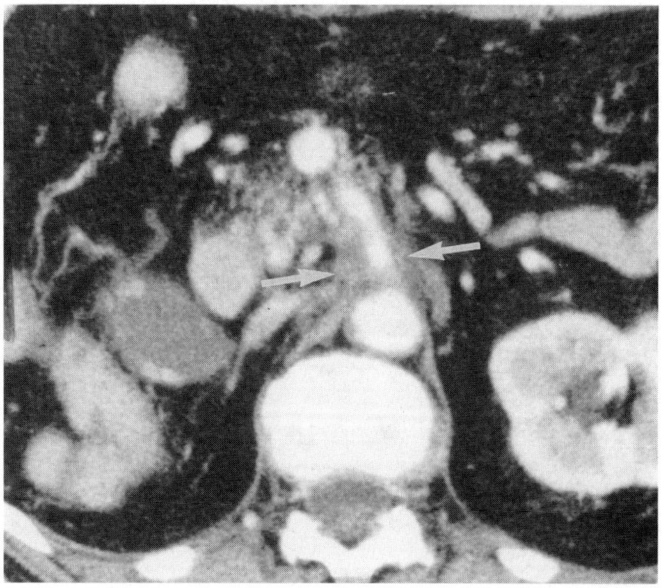

FIGURE 9.19 Encasement of the superior mesenteric artery (SMA) by adenocarcinoma. Contrast-enhanced CT in a 75-year-old man with pancreatic cancer shows tumor encasement of the SMA *(arrows)*, a characteristic pattern of spread for ductal adenocarcinoma.

Islet cell tumors are classified as **functional** (85 percent) if they secrete an active hormone and **nonfunctional** (15 percent) if they do not. Functional tumors are named according to their hormonal product, with insulinoma and gastrinoma representing the most common types. Less common islet cell tumors include glucagonoma, VIPoma (vasoactive intestinal peptide), and somatostatinoma. Not surprisingly, symptomatology depends on the tumor subtype. Patients with functional islet cell tumors tend to present earlier with small lesions and symptoms related to the endocrine effect of the hormone produced, whereas those with nonhyperfunctioning lesions present later with mass effect due to large tumor size. Differentiating a nonfunctional islet cell tumor from ductal adenocarcinoma is important, since these patients often respond favorably to surgery and chemotherapy and have a better overall prognosis.

On **CT,** most functional islet cell tumors are seen as small hypervascular pancreatic masses **(Differential 9.5)**. They are optimally imaged during the early arterial phase, performed with thin collimation. The tumor will enhance to a greater extent than the surrounding parenchyma, helping to differentiate an islet cell tumor from an adenocarcinoma **(Fig. 9.20)**. Additionally, islet cell tumors calcify in up to 20 percent of cases, whereas calcium is detectable on CT in less than 2 percent of ductal adenocarcinomas. Islet cell tumors demonstrate vascular encasement and central necrosis much less frequently than pancreatic adenocarcinomas. Cystic necrosis is occasionally seen with the large, nonhyperfunctioning lesions.

There is a wide variation in the rate of malignant transformation among islet cell tumors, depending on the subtype. For instance, less than 10 percent of insulinomas are considered malignant, but

9.5 HYPERVASCULAR PANCREATIC MASS

Islet cell tumor—insulinoma, gastrinoma, nonhyperfunctioning
Microcystic adenoma—serous fluid, generally small cysts
Metastases—renal cell, melanoma, carcinoid
Solid and papillary epithelial neoplasm (SPEN)
Pseudoaneurysm—following pancreatitis or trauma; hepatic, splenic, or gastroduodenal arteries

over 60 percent of gastrinomas are malignant. Malignancy is determined by the presence of local invasion or metastases rather than by histologic evaluation.

- **Insulinoma** is the most common functional islet cell tumor, usually affecting middle-aged adults in a sporadic fashion but also occurring as part of the MEN 1 syndrome. Patients present with symptoms caused by spontaneous hypoglycemia (< 50 mg/dL) during fasting or exercise. There is no site of predilection within the pancreas. Over 90 percent of insulinomas are benign.

  Insulinomas are often difficult to diagnose by **CT,** since the vast majority measure less than 2 cm and seldom deform the pancreatic contour. Most are hypervascular and require optimal CT technique with arterial-phase imaging to demonstrate the transient early tumor enhancement **(Fig. 9.20)**. Insulinomas are usually solitary lesions, but up to 10 percent are multiple. Calcification can occur and is suggestive of malignancy.
- **Gastrinoma** is the second most common islet cell tumor and is associated with MEN 1 in up to 40 percent of cases. Patients can present clinically with **Zollinger-Ellison syndrome,** consisting of recurrent peptic ulcer disease and diarrhea due to the hypergastrinemic state. Gastrinomas occur most frequently within the "gastrinoma triangle," a region that includes the pancreatic head (most common site), the second and third portions of the duodenum, the distal stomach, and peripancreatic nodes. Extrapancreatic tumors are often difficult to detect on any imaging modality. Compared with insulinoma, gastrinoma is more often multifocal and more often malignant.

  On **CT,** gastrinomas are hypervascular and average 3 to 4 cm in diameter. In over one-half of cases, multiple lesions are present. Thickened gastric and small bowel folds may be present from increased gastric acid secretion and malabsorption. Approximately 60 percent of patients have metastases at the time of diagnosis, most often to the liver and lymph nodes.
- **Nonfunctioning islet cell tumors** are the third most common type of islet cell tumors. The majority of these tumors actually do secrete detectable peptides, such as pancreatic polypeptide (PPomas), but they do not result in a discernible hormonal syndrome. Patients are usually asymptomatic, but some present with a palpable mass or with obstructive symptoms. Most nonhyperfunctioning islet cell tumors occur within the pancreatic head, but they can arise anywhere within the pancreas. They are typically large at the time of detection, often greater than 10 cm in size.

  On **CT,** these tumors are depicted as large, heterogeneous, enhancing masses, occasionally with areas of cystic necrosis **(Fig. 9.21)**. Approximately 25 percent contain coarse calcifications. Encasement of the celiac artery or superior mesenteric artery is rare. Metastases to regional lymph nodes or liver demonstrate pronounced enhancement. Because these patients lack a hormonal syndrome, the main differential consideration is ductal adenocarcinoma.
- Rare islet cell tumors include VIPoma, glucagonoma, and somatostatinoma. Patients with VIPoma can present with watery diarrhea, hypokalemia, and achlorhydria (WDHA syndrome), also known as Verner-Morrison syndrome. Multiple nondilated fluid-filled bowel loops due to the secretory diarrhea can be seen on CT **(Fig. 9.22)**. The tumor itself averages 5 to 10 cm in diameter and occurs most frequently in the pancreatic body and tail. VIPomas often contain solid and cystic components and are usually hypervascular. Approximately one-half undergo malignant transformation. The hallmark clinical manifestation of glucagonoma is a skin rash, called necrolytic migratory erythema. Patients can also present with diabetes, weight loss, and anemia. Glucagonomas are most common in the body or tail of the pancreas. The majority are malignant. **Somatostatinomas** present with a syndrome of diabetes, cholelithiasis, and steatorrhea. These tumors are hypervascular and most exceed 4 cm in size. The rate of malignant transformation is high.

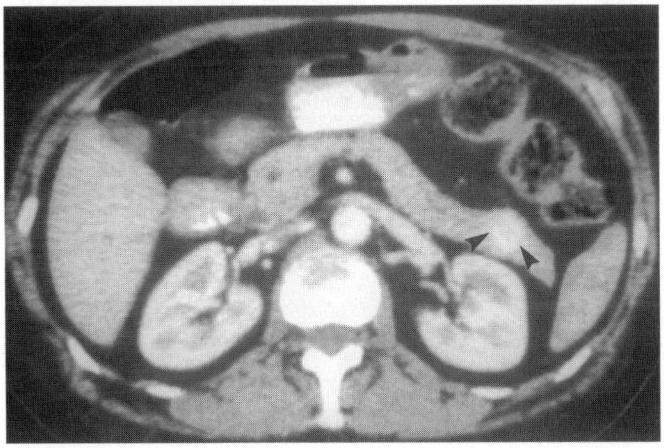

FIGURE 9.20 Islet cell tumor (insulinoma). Contrast-enhanced CT in a patient with symptoms and biochemical evidence of an insulinoma shows a subtle hypervascular mass *(arrowheads)* involving the pancreatic tail.

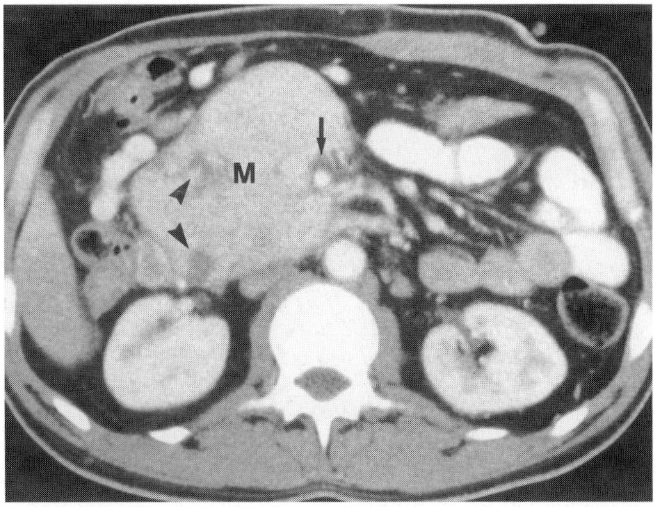

FIGURE 9.21 Nonfunctioning islet cell tumor. Contrast-enhanced CT in a 43-year-old woman shows a large enhancing mass (M) involving the pancreatic head. Areas of cystic necrosis are present *(arrowheads)*. Despite the large tumor size, the fat plane surrounding the superior mesenteric artery is preserved *(arrow)*. These features, along with the demonstrable enhancement, argue against adenocarcinoma.

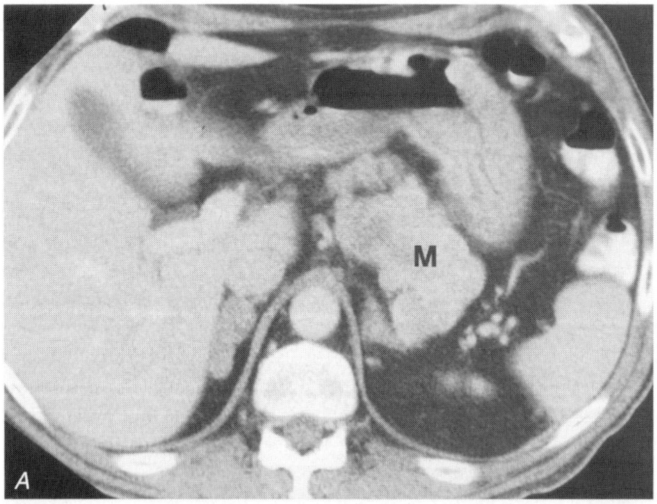

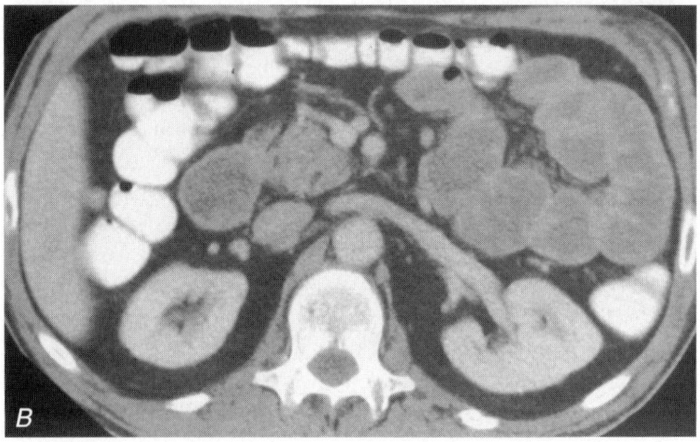

FIGURE 9.22 Vasoactive intestinal peptide tumor (VIPoma) with WDHA syndrome (watery diarrhea, hypokalemia, and achlorhydria). *A*. Contrast-enhanced CT in a 60-year-old man with profuse, watery diarrhea and weight loss shows a large lobulated pancreatic mass (M) involving the body and tail. VIPoma was diagnosed by pancreatic biopsy. *B*. Note multiple fluid-filled small bowel loops due to hypersecretion.

- **Pancreaticoblastoma** is rare but represents the most common pancreatic tumor in young children. Most of these tumors are located in the pancreatic head, arising from the ventral anlage, and present as large, palpable masses that measure between 5 and 15 cm in size. If detected early and completely excised, they have a favorable prognosis. However, patients with evidence of metastatic disease at presentation do poorly. On CT, pancreaticoblastomas are typically large, heterogeneous masses with areas of hemorrhage and necrosis **(Fig. 9.23)**.
- **Primary pancreatic lymphoma** is rare and almost always represents non-Hodgkin lymphoma. Multifocality and/or bulky masses favor lymphoma over pancreatic adenocarcinoma **(Fig. 9.24)**. Peripancreatic nodal lymphoma or secondary involvement of the pancreas by retroperitoneal nodal disease is much more common than primary pancreatic lymphoma; other sites of involvement will usually be apparent. In equivocal cases, biopsy can be performed to differentiate lymphoma from ductal adenocarcinoma, since the former is treated with chemotherapy and the latter with surgery. Extensive extranodal involvement with lymphoma is more common in the setting of immunocompromise, as in patients with AIDS. Diffuse infiltration and enlargement of the pancreas can rarely occur with lymphoma or leukemia. Areas of central necrosis can be seen with some high-grade lymphomas.

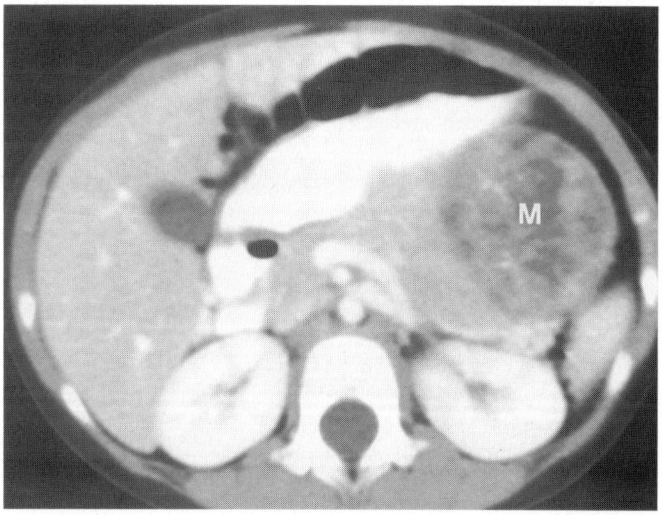

FIGURE 9.23 Pancreaticoblastoma. Contrast-enhanced CT in a 3-year-old girl shows a heterogeneous low-attenuation mass (M) extending off the pancreatic tail. (Case courtesy of Dr. Marilyn Siegel, St. Louis, MO.)

- **Metastases** to the pancreatic parenchyma are rarely of clinical concern. Involvement from direct tumor extension or peripancreatic nodal disease is more common than hematogenous spread. Melanoma, lung, breast, colon, renal, or osteosarcoma primaries have all been reported. Metastases from renal cell carcinoma appear to be the most common. These tumors can have an appearance similar to that of ductal adenocarcinoma on CT, although vascular encasement, biliary obstruction, and infiltration of the retropancreatic fat are less common with metastatic disease.

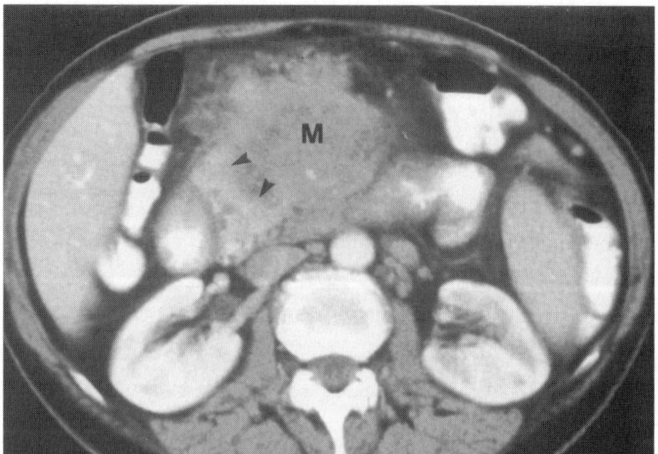

FIGURE 9.24 Pancreatic lymphoma. Contrast-enhanced CT in a 63-year-old woman shows a large, ill-defined pancreatic mass (M) that infiltrates into the peripancreatic fat. A portion of the pancreatic head is spared *(arrowheads)*.

TABLE 9.1

CLINICOPATHOLOGIC FEATURES OF PANCREATIC TUMORS						
Tumor	**Relative Incidence**	**Typical Patient**	**Typical Location**	**Morphology**	**Calcification**	**Behavior**
Adenocarcinoma	Common	Elderly, M > F	Head > body > tail	Solid mass	Rare	Malignant
Microcystic adenoma	Relatively common	Elderly, F > M	Variable	Small cysts	Central scar calcification	Benign
Mucinous cystic neoplasms	Relatively common	Middle-aged women	85% in body/tail	Large cysts	Septal calcification	Malignant evolution
Duct-ectatic mucinous tumor	Uncommon	Elderly, M > F	Uncinate process	Cystic expansion of duct	Uncommon	Malignant evolution
Islet cell	Uncommon	MEN 1*	Variable	Hypervascular mass	20%	Variable
Metastases	Uncommon	Oncologic history	Variable	Solid, often multifocal	Depends on primary	Malignant
Solid and papillary epithelial neoplasm	Rare	Young women	Tail	Areas of cystic degeneration	Dystrophic	Low-grade malignancy
Pancreaticoblastoma	Rare	Children	Head	Areas of hemorrhage and necrosis	Occasionally	Malignant potential
Primary lymphoma	Rare	Immune compromise	Variable	Solid, low attenuation	No	Malignant
Acinar cell	Very rare	Elderly	Body	Lobulated mass	No	Malignant

*Multiple endocrine neoplasia type 1.

- **Acinar cell carcinoma** is a rare exocrine pancreatic neoplasm that tends to occur in elderly patients. Occasionally, patients present with systemic fat necrosis from excess production of lipase by hyperfunctioning tumor cells. They typically present as large, lobulated masses in the body of the pancreas with areas of central necrosis. Prognosis is poor, with metastatic disease usually present at the time of diagnosis.
- An overview of the clinical, radiologic, and pathologic features of the various pancreatic tumors is provided in **Table 9.1.**

9.6 FATTY REPLACEMENT

- Fatty involution of the pancreas occurs normally with aging **(see Fig. 9.18)**. More dramatic **fatty replacement** of the pancreas is seen with obesity, diabetes mellitus, Cushing disease, and steroid administration (**Differential 9.6**). Pancreatic exocrine function is usually adequate in these conditions. Symptomatic total fatty replacement of the pancreas can be seen in cystic fibrosis, Schwachman-Diamond syndrome, Johanson-Blizzard syndrome, and malnutrition. **Cystic fibrosis** is a relatively common autosomal recessive disorder of exocrine gland function that typically affects white children. Common clinical manifestations of cystic fibrosis include chronic bronchopulmonary infections and pancreatic insufficiency. Complete fatty replacement of the pancreas is often depicted on CT **(Fig. 9.25)**. Patients with cystic fibrosis can also develop multiple pancreatic cysts, biliary cirrhosis, hepatic steatosis, and alterations within the bowel wall. Schwachman-Diamond syndrome is rare but represents the second most common cause, after cystic fibrosis, of pancreatic exocrine insufficiency in children. Similar fatty replacement is seen on CT. Recurrent infections and metaphyseal dysplasia are additional findings in this condition. Johanson-Blizzard syndrome consists of dwarfism, deafness, absence of permanent teeth, aplasia of the nasal alae, malabsorption, and pancreatic insufficiency. These patients have total fatty replacement of the pancreas, with both exocrine and endocrine insufficiency.

9.7 PANCREATIC SURGERY

- Pancreatic surgery is performed in certain cases of acute and chronic pancreatitis, for open drainage of pseudocysts, and for resection of pancreatic tumors. Surgical options in the setting of **acute pancreatitis** include cholecystectomy and intraoperative cholangiography for choledocholithiasis, debridement for necrotic pancreatic tissue, and drainage of infected fluid collections.

  Indications for surgery in the setting of **chronic pancreatitis** include intractable pain, obstruction of the common bile duct (CBD), and the possibility of tumor. A variety of surgical options exist for pancreatic ductal drainage or resection, including the Peustow proce-

9.6

PANCREATIC FATTY CHANGE

Aging—normal glandular atrophy
Cystic fibrosis
Obesity
Steroids or Cushing syndrome
Diabetes mellitus
Malnutrition
Chronic pancreatitis
Viral infection
Schwachman-Diamond syndrome
Johanson-Blizzard syndrome

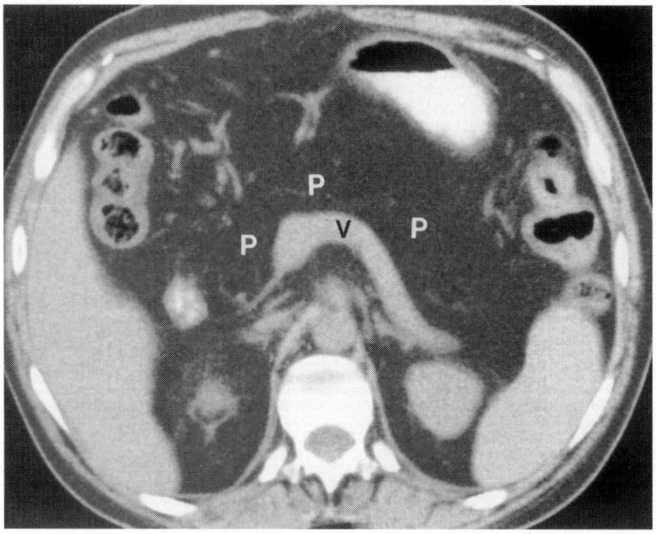

FIGURE 9.25 Cystic fibrosis. Noncontrast CT in a 36-year-old woman with cystic fibrosis shows total replacement of the pancreas (P) by fat, which increases the conspicuity of the splenic vein (V).

dure, distal pancreatic resection, Whipple procedure, total or subtotal pancreatectomy, and resection with end-to-side Roux pancreaticojejunostomy (Duval procedure). Operative mortality can be as high as 10 percent. Pain is relieved in up to 75 percent of patients.

The goals of pancreatic surgery for neoplasia include diagnosis, palliation, and cure. Surgical options include laparoscopy, biopsy, bypass, cholecystojejunostomy, choledochojejunostomy, partial resection, enucleation (for some islet cell tumors), and pancreatectomy. The operative mortality ranges from 2 to 10 percent.

- **Total pancreatectomy** for multifocal or diffuse disease is rarely performed. The pancreas is excised and an extensive lymphadenectomy is performed, with all patients developing insulin-dependent diabetes postoperatively. During the late 1960s, total pancreatectomy was advocated for patients with pancreatic cancer. Subsequent studies have shown better results following the Whipple procedure.
- The **Whipple procedure** (pancreaticoduodenectomy) is performed for pancreatic carcinoma or pancreatitis localized to the pancreatic head. Classically, it consists of resection of the pancreatic head, neck, and uncinate process and resection of the duodenum, gastric antrum, gallbladder, and distal CBD. Anastomoses include the pancreas to the small intestine (pancreaticojejunostomy), the remaining CBD to the jejunum (choledochojejunostomy), and the remaining stomach and duodenum to the small intestine (duodenojejunostomy). A pylorus-sparing Whipple procedure is now performed when feasible. Overall, there is a lower incidence of postoperative diabetes mellitus compared with total pancreatectomy. A 5 percent mortality rate is associated with this procedure.
- The **Peustow procedure,** a lateral pancreaticojejunostomy, is a ductal drainage procedure performed for chronic pancreatitis in which the pancreas is opened transversely and a side-to-side pancreaticojejunostomy is performed. The pancreaticojejunal anastomosis can be identified immediately anterior to the pancreatic body on CT in 75 percent of cases and the Roux-en-Y loop is demonstrable in 70 percent. The Roux-en-Y loop can mimic the appearance of a pancreatic or parapancreatic abscess on CT. Complications include fluid collections, abscess, pseudocyst, hematoma, and Roux-en-Y obstruction.
- **Distal pancreatectomy** is performed for chronic pancreatitis and distal pancreatic tumors. It includes resection of up to 75 percent of the distal gland as well as splenic resection.
- **Pancreatic transplantation** is usually performed in combination with renal transplantation. In early transplants, pancreatic drainage was peritoneal or enteric via a Roux-en-Y pancreaticojejunostomy. Subsequently, pancreatic drainage into the urinary bladder was accomplished with anastomosis of a short duodenal segment containing the ampulla of Vater directly to the bladder. Vascular supply is usually via the common iliac vessels. Complications include rejection (35 percent), pancreatitis (35 percent), peripancreatic hemorrhage (35 percent), abscess (35 percent), and vascular thrombosis (20 percent).

  CT is helpful in identifying adjacent fluid collections or anastomotic leaks in transplant patients with abdominal pain and fever. Complete bowel opacification with oral contrast is critical for adequate evaluation, as is an understanding of the surgical technique employed. CT is not useful in evaluating for transplant rejection.

Bibliography

Balthazar EJ, Freeny PC, vanSonnenberg E. Imaging and intervention in acute pancreatitis. *Radiology* 1994;193:297–306.

Bluemke DA, Cameron JL, Hruban RH, Pitt HA, Siegelman SS, Soyer P, Fishman EK. Potentially resectable pancreatic adenocarcinoma: Spiral CT assessment with surgical and pathologic correlation. *Radiology* 1995;197:381–385.

Buetow PC, Buck JL, Pantongrag-Brown L, Beck KG, Ros PR, Adair CF. Solid and papillary epithelial neoplasm of the pancreas: Imaging-pathologic correlation in 56 cases. *Radiology* 1996;199:707–711.

Buetow PC, Rao P, Thompson LDR. Mucinous cystic neoplasms of the pancreas: Radiologic-pathologic correlation. *Radiographics* 1998;18:433–449.

Diehl SJ, Lehmann KJ, Sadick M, Lachmann R, Georgi M. Pancreatic cancer: Value of dual-phase helical CT in assessing resectability. *Radiology* 1998;206:373–378.

Freed KS, Paulson EK, Frederick MG, Keogan MT, Pappas TN. Abdomen after a Puestow procedure: Postoperative CT appearance, complications, and potential pitfalls. *Radiology* 1997;203:790–794.

Gazelle GC, Saini S, Mueller PR, eds. *Hepatobiliary and Pancreatic Radiology: Imaging and Intervention.* New York: Thieme; 1998:630–676.

Hough DM, Stephens DH, Johnson CD, Binkovitz LA. Pancreatic lesions in von Hippel-Lindau disease: Prevalence, clinical significance, and CT findings. *AJR* 1994;162:1091–1094.

Katz DS, Hines J, Math KR, Nardi PM, Mindelzun RE, Lane MJ. Using CT to reveal fat-containing abnormalities of the pancreas. *AJR* 1999;172:393–396.

Procacci C, Graziani R, Bicego E, Bergamo-Andreis IA, Mainardi P, Zamboni G, Pederzoli P, Cavallini G, Valdo M, Pistolesi GF. Intraductal mucin-producing tumors of the pancreas: Imaging findings. *Radiology* 1996;198:249–257.

Ros PR, Hamrick-Turner JE, Chiechi MV, Ros LH, Gallego P, Burton SS. Cystic masses of the pancreas. *Radiographics* 1992;12:673–686.

Slone RM, Fisher AJ. *Pocket Guide to Body CT Differential Diagnosis.* New York: McGraw-Hill, 1999.

Stanley RJ, Semelka RC. Pancreas. In: Lee JKT, Sagel SS, Stanley RJ, Heiken JP, eds. *Computed Body Tomography with MRI Correlation,* 3rd ed. Philadelphia: Lippincott-Raven; 1998:873–959.

Vaughn DD, Jabra AA, Fishnan EK. Pancreatic diease in children and young adults: Evaluation with CT. *Radiographics* 1998;18:1171–1187.

Chapter 10

PERITONEUM AND RETROPERITONEUM

Perry J. Pickhardt

10.1 Anatomy and Technique
10.2 Ascites
10.3 Pneumoperitoneum
10.4 Peritoneal Inflammation and Abscess
10.5 Cystic Peritoneal Lesions
10.6 Solid Peritoneal Masses
10.7 Retroperitoneal Hemorrhage
10.8 Retroperitoneal Fibrosis
10.9 Retroperitoneal Masses
10.10 Lymphadenopathy
10.11 Lymphoma

10.1 ANATOMY AND TECHNIQUE

- Diseases of the peritoneal cavity and retroperitoneum represent a significant diagnostic challenge for clinicians because of their nonspecific symptoms and the difficulties in the physical examination of these areas. Consequently, clinicians have increasingly relied on **computed tomography** (**CT**) for the detection of peritoneal and retroperitoneal diseases. This chapter focuses on pathologic conditions primarily affecting these spaces; disease processes involving the abdominal solid organs and hollow viscera are covered in their respective chapters. Although separate consideration of peritoneal and retroperitoneal disease processes has been a traditional and worthwhile approach, it should be recognized that there is continuity between these compartments which allows for the bidirectional spread of pathologic processes.
- The **peritoneal cavity** is partitioned into communicating compartments by various ligaments that support the intraperitoneal organs **(Fig. 10.1).** The **transverse mesocolon** divides the peritoneum into supramesocolic and inframesocolic compartments. The more complex **supramesocolic compartment** contains derivatives of the embryologic ventral mesentery: the **falciform ligament,** which divides the right and left subphrenic spaces anterior to the liver, and the **lesser omentum,** which comprises the **gastrohepatic ligament** and the **hepatoduodenal ligament.** The **right subphrenic space** extends from the falciform ligament along the broad hepatic surface that abuts the right hemidiaphragm; it communicates posteriorly with the **right subhepatic space,** often referred to as **Morison's pouch.** The **left anterior subphrenic space** communicates with the **left anterior** and **posterior perihepatic spaces** and with the left posterior subphrenic space or **perisplenic space.** The left posterior perihepatic space (or **gastrohepatic recess**) is immediately anterior to the gastrohepatic ligament (see **Fig. 10.13**).

  The **lesser sac** is relatively isolated from the greater peritoneal cavity, communicating only through the epiploic **foramen of Winslow,** identified on CT between the inferior vena cava (IVC) and portal vein (see **Fig. 6.18**). The borders of the lesser sac include the stomach, gastrohepatic ligament, proximal duodenum, and hepatoduodenal ligament anteriorly; the splenorenal ligament, spleen, and gastrosplenic ligament laterally; the pancreas and parietal peritoneum posteriorly; and the transverse mesocolon and gastrocolic ligament inferiorly. During early development, the gastrosplenic ligament billows out inferiorly and forms the gastrocolic ligament, greater omentum, and superior layer of the transverse mesocolon **(Fig. 10.2).** Incomplete fusion of the greater omental leaves accounts for the occasional presence of a prominent omental bursa. The **superior recess** is located behind the gastrohepatic ligament and surrounds the caudate lobe of the liver.

  The **inframesocolic space** is divided by the broad, fan-shaped **small bowel mesentery** into the right and left infracolic spaces. The larger **left infracolic space** communicates freely with the intraperitoneal pelvis and has access to the right paracolic gutter **(Fig. 10.1).** The **right infracolic space** is more restricted inferiorly by the ileocecal mesentery. The **right paracolic gutter** freely communicates superiorly with the right subhepatic and perihepatic spaces, whereas the **left paracolic gutter** is restricted superiorly by the **phrenicocolic ligament,** a small peritoneal fold that extends laterally from the transverse mesocolon. Like the small bowel mesentery, the **sigmoid mesentery** presents a relative boundary for intraperitoneal spread of fluid or cells. The **pelvic cul-de-sac** is a peritoneal reflection that represents the most inferior portion of the peritoneal cavity.
- The **retroperitoneum** is bounded anteriorly by the parietal peritoneum, posteriorly by transversalis fascia, and superiorly by the diaphragm. Inferiorly, the retroperitoneum communicates with the extraperitoneal pelvis. The retroperitoneum contains portions of the colon and duodenum as well as the pancreas, kidneys, adrenal glands, aorta, IVC, and major lymph node groups. Retroperitoneal fat surrounds most organs on CT. The retroperitoneum is classically divided into three compartments by the **perirenal fascia** and

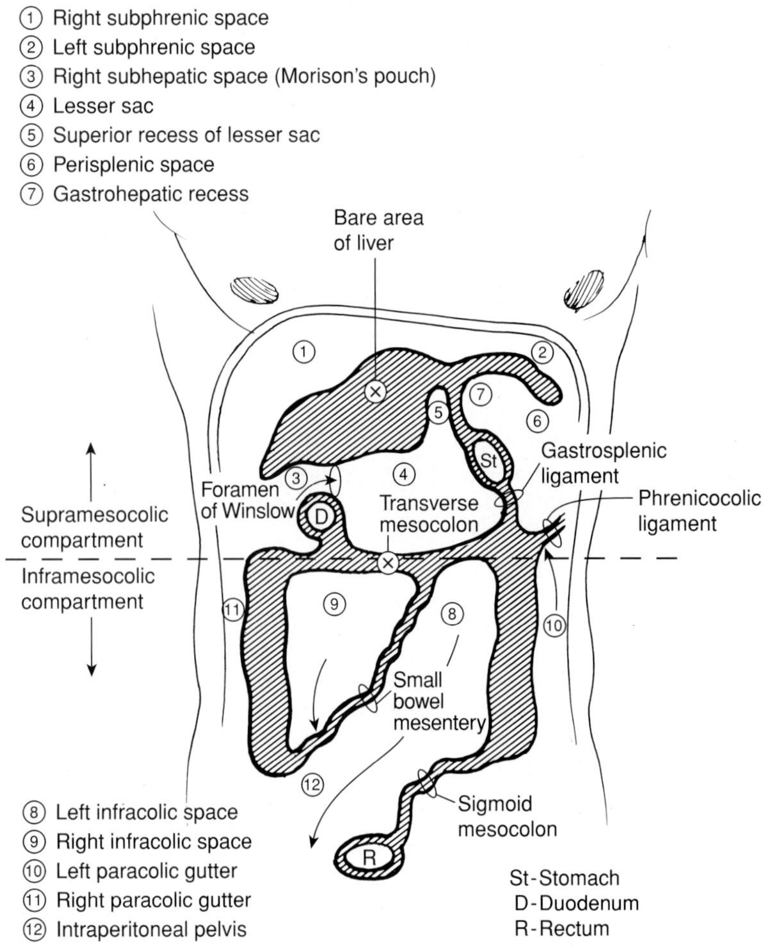

FIGURE 10.1 Peritoneal anatomy. Diagram of the posterior peritoneal reflections, which give rise to the major peritoneal spaces. The transverse mesocolon divides the peritoneum into supramesocolic and inframesocolic compartments.

lateroconal fascia: the perirenal, anterior pararenal, and posterior pararenal spaces **(Fig. 10.3).**

The borders of the **anterior pararenal space** include the anterior renal fascia posteriorly, the posterior parietal peritoneum anteriorly, and the lateroconal fascia laterally. The ascending and descending colon, pancreas, and retroperitoneal duodenum are contained within this space. The boundaries of the **perirenal space** are formed by the anterior and posterior perirenal fascia. This space contains the kidneys, adrenal glands, renal vessels, and proximal collecting system. Fibrous **bridging septa** span the perinephric space. The **posterior pararenal space** is bounded by the posterior perirenal fascia anteriorly and by the transversalis fascia posteriorly. The posterior pararenal space contains only fat but is a potential compartment for pathologic collections. Recent work has shown that the perirenal and lateroconal fascia are more complex than single membranes but actually represent fusion planes that are potential spaces and conduits for the spread of retroperitoneal disease. These fusion planes have been termed the ***retromesenteric plane, retrorenal plane,*** and ***lateroconal plane*** **(Fig. 10.3).** The anterior and posterior perirenal fascia, or **Gerota's fascia,** form a cone by fusing inferiorly. The fused layers continue into the extraperitoneal pelvis and form a potential pathway that extends into the presacral and perirectal regions. Pathologic fluid collections can communicate between the extraperitoneal pelvis and retroperitoneum, or vice versa, along these fascial planes.

- Normal **abdominal lymph nodes** are routinely seen on CT scans. Their common names reflect their anatomic location. The major **retroperitoneal lymph nodes** have a perivascular distribution alongside the aorta and IVC and include the paraaortic, aortocaval, and paracaval chains. Lymph nodes are also present in the renal hilum and the **retrocrural** space, which bridges the posterior mediastinum and retroperitoneum. **Peritoneal lymph nodes** are present in the porta hepatis, the gastrohepatic ligament, and the perisplenic, celiac, superior mesenteric, mesenteric, and peripancreatic regions. Major **pelvic lymph nodes** accompany large vessels and include the common, internal, and external iliac groups. **Obturator lymph nodes** are part of the external iliac chain and are often the first to be involved by pelvic malignancies. More superficially, the **inguinal lymph nodes** reside in the superior portion of the femoral triangle. Additional pelvic lymph nodes include the sacral and gluteal groups.
- **CT technique** for imaging of the peritoneum, retroperitoneum, and lymph nodes consists of standard 5- to 10-mm collimation. Examination with spiral technique allows single-breath-hold imaging over a large region and reduces spatial misregistration. Both oral and intravenous IV contrast should be routinely administered unless contraindicated. One exception occurs in the setting of suspected retroperitoneal hemorrhage, where emergency examination can be performed without oral or IV contrast. Practically speaking, CT has replaced lymphangiography for the evaluation of lymph node pathology. Although lymphangiography provides evaluation of internal nodal architecture, it is a tedious, difficult, and somewhat invasive study compared with CT. Another advantage of CT is its ability to evaluate the celiac, mesenteric, retrocrural, and periportal nodes, which are not opacified by lymphangiography.

10.2 ASCITES

- **Ascites** is simply fluid in the peritoneal cavity and is a common abnormal finding on CT **(Differential 10.1).**Transudative etiologies include cirrhosis, congestive heart failure, hypoproteinemia, renal failure, venous occlusion, and constrictive pericarditis. Exudative ascites results from inflammatory and neoplastic processes. Inflammatory etiologies include peritonitis from any cause and inflammation centered in the gut or other organs. Neoplastic

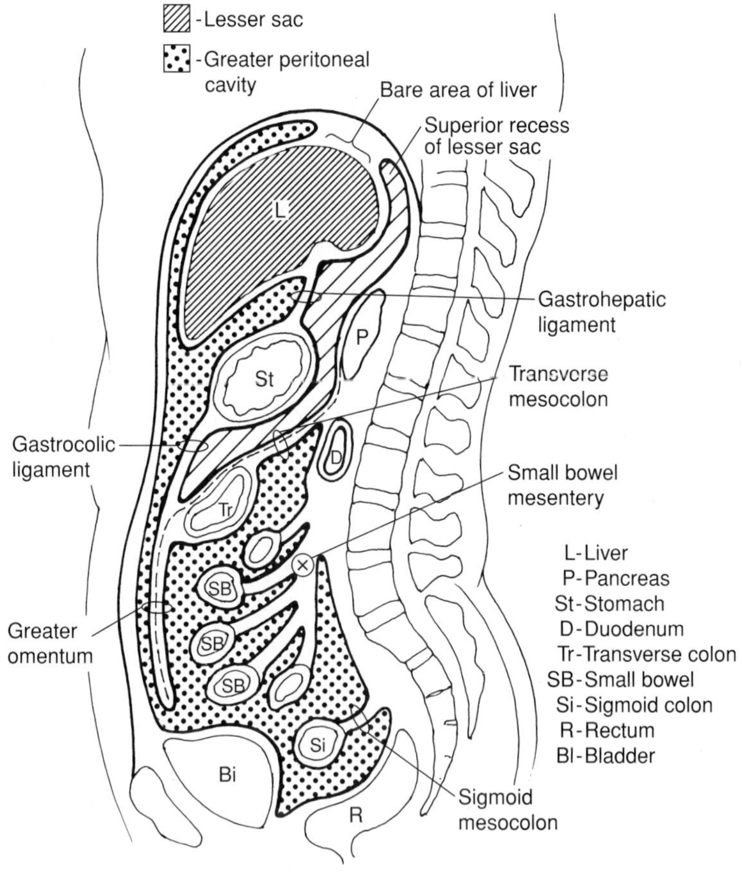

FIGURE 10.2 Peritoneal anatomy. Diagram of left parasagittal section to demonstrate the relationship of the mesenteries with the greater and lesser peritoneal sacs. Note the continuity between the intraperitoneal and extraperitoneal portions of the subperitoneal space. The dashed lines represent fusion planes.

involvement of the peritoneum leading to ascites can be seen with intraperitoneal seeding from ovarian or gastrointestinal (GI) malignancies, lymphoma, and, rarely, primary peritoneal tumors. In the setting of acute trauma, hemoperitoneum is commonly seen. Chylous ascites can result from lymphatic injury or obstruction. Urine ascites and bile peritonitis can be seen with laceration of the urinary system and biliary tree, respectively.

Even small amounts of peritoneal fluid can be detected on CT, with common locations including the pelvic cul-de-sac, perihepatic spaces, and Morison's pouch. With larger collections, bowel loops are often displaced centrally by fluid filling the paracolic gutters **(Fig. 10.4);** fluid can extend between leaves of the small bowel mesentery. Loculated ascites represents confinement of a peritoneal fluid collection and often appears rounded, sometimes exerting mass effect on adjacent structures. The appearance can simulate an abscess or cystic neoplasm. Loculated collections of fluid may be due to postoperative, inflammatory, or neoplastic adhesions. CT findings associated with bacterial or chemical **peritonitis** include focal or diffuse peritoneal thickening and enhancement associated with loculated ascites **(Fig. 10.5)**. Asymmetric accumulation, as within the lesser sac, should suggest a localized disease process or, alternatively, malignant ascites.

Coexisting findings on abdominal CT will often divulge the cause of ascites. Specific examples include a nodular liver and portal hypertension in cirrhosis **(Fig. 10.4);** cardiac enlargement, dilated hepatic veins, and hepatic congestion in congestive heart failure; and peritoneal soft tissue implants from metastatic involvement **(Fig. 10.15).** Although exudative causes of ascites may exhibit increased attenuation on CT, this finding is nonspecific. Likewise, traumatic hemoperitoneum often demonstrates attenuation values greater than 30 HU, but a lower value should not be assumed to represent preexisting ascites. Conversely, delayed enhancement of uncomplicated ascites can be seen in up to one-half of patients undergoing CT examination.

Pseudomyxoma peritonei is a rare condition due to rupture of a mucinous cystadenocarcinoma of the appendix, causing intraperitoneal accumulation of gelatinous material, tenacious ascites with septated locules displacing intra-abdominal organs, and scalloping of the liver margin and other organs **(Fig. 10.6).** Septal calcification is often seen in more chronic cases.

10.3 PNEUMOPERITONEUM

- **Pneumoperitoneum,** free air within the peritoneal cavity, is an important finding **(Differential 10.2).** The most common cause is perforation of a viscus due to ulceration, instrumentation, inflammation, ischemia, or trauma. Free intraperitoneal air soon after abdominal surgery is a normal finding but should resolve within 7 to 10 days. Procedures such as paracentesis, peritoneal dialysis, or biopsies may introduce air into the peritoneal cavity; this is generally of no clinical consequence. Rupture of a subserosal air cyst in a patient with benign pneumatosis cystoides intestinalis is an uncommon cause of free air **(Fig. 10.7).** Finally, a pneumothorax may rarely give rise to pneumoperitoneum via pleuroperitoneal communication. Care must be taken not to miss subtle extraluminal gas over the liver or adjacent to bowel loops on CT. Review of CT images with lung window settings can aid in the detection of small amounts of peritoneal air.

CT is also sensitive for detecting **pneumoretroperitoneum,** or air dissecting along retroperitoneal planes. The most common cause is perforation of the retroperitoneal duodenum or colon **(Fig. 10.8).** Other causes include retroperitoneal surgery and emphysematous pyelonephritis.

10.4 PERITONEAL INFLAMMATION AND ABSCESS

- CT is the favored imaging modality for detecting an intra-abdominal **abscess,** a finding that significantly affects clinical management. An abscess represents a localized collection of purulent ma-

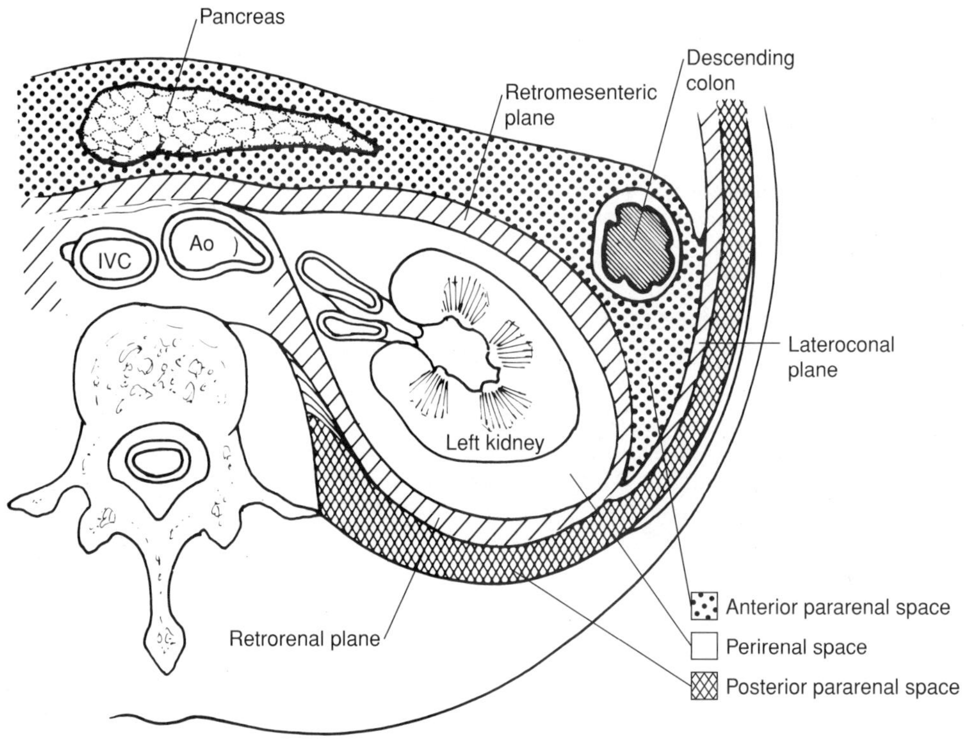

FIGURE 10.3 Retroperitoneal anatomy. Diagram of retroperitoneal anatomy. The classic anterior pararenal, perirenal, and posterior pararenal spaces are separated by fascial fusion planes (retromesenteric, retrorenal, and lateroconal) that represent potential pathways for the spread of pathologic processes. *Key:* IVC, inferior vena cava; Ao, aorta.

terial usually requiring percutaneous or open drainage. The clinical presentation commonly includes fever, leukocytosis, and abdominal pain. In patients receiving corticosteroids or who are otherwise immunocompromised, however, few clinical signs or symptoms may be present. The causes of abscess formation are myriad **(Differential 10.3).** The postoperative period, bowel perforation, pancreatitis, and pelvic inflammatory disease are common settings that can be complicated by abscess formation. Perforated bowel can occur with appendicitis, diverticulitis, Crohn disease, trauma, perforated cancer, foreign-body ingestion, and ischemia.

10.1

ASCITES

Cirrhosis
Carcinomatosis
CHF
Inflammation
  Pancreatitis, appendicitis, diverticulitis, peritonitis, tuberculosis
Trauma—hemoperitoneum
Renal failure
Hypoproteinemia—nephrotic syndrome, malabsorption
Constrictive pericarditis
Inferior vena cava or portal vein obstruction
Lymphoma
Disrupted or obstructed lymphatics
Primary peritoneal tumor

The classic **CT findings** of abscess consist of a focal fluid collection with an enhancing rim **(Fig. 10.9).** Most abdominal abscesses are rounded, but their appearance can be modified by their location **(Fig. 10.10).** Abscesses are commonly septate and

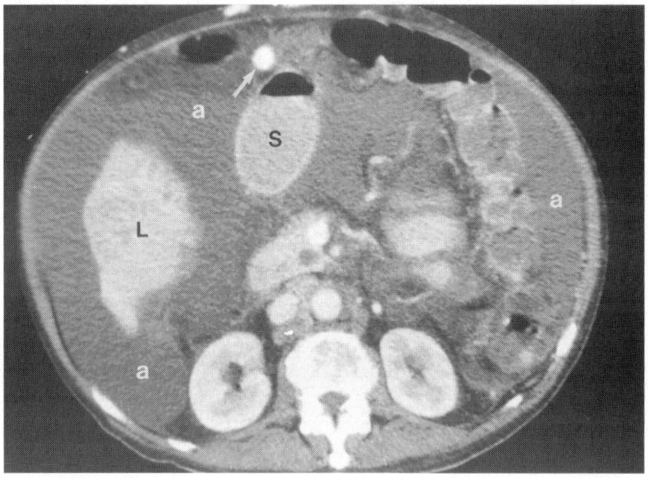

FIGURE 10.4 Ascites. Contrast-enhanced CT in a 72-year-old man with alcoholic cirrhosis shows massive ascites (a) displacing and separating the intraperitoneal structures. Note the nodular and heterogeneous appearance of the liver (L) and the enhancing paraumbilical portosystemic collateral vein *(arrow).* S, stomach.

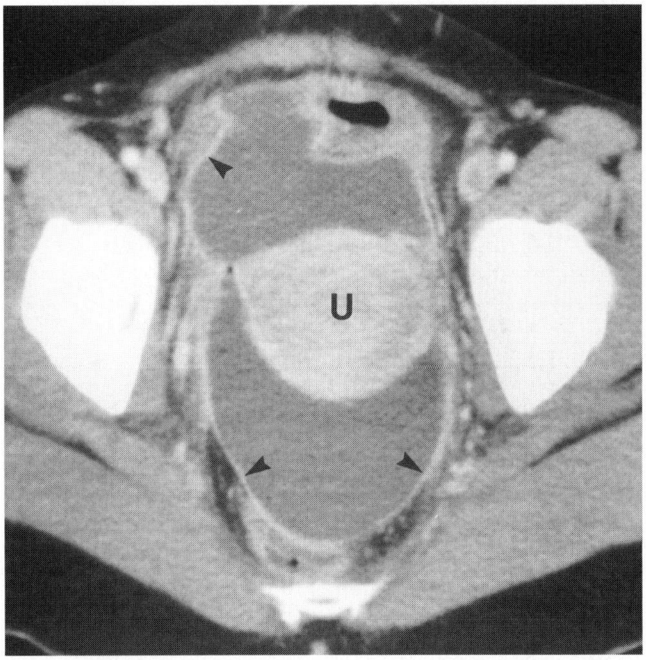

FIGURE 10.5 Peritonitis. Contrast-enhanced CT in a 42-year-old woman with a ruptured appendix shows fluid distending the peritoneal spaces that surround the uterus (U) and uniform thickening and enhancement of the parietal peritoneum *(arrowheads).*

thick-walled. Gas bubbles or an air-fluid level within an abscess is present in approximately one-third of cases. Surrounding inflammatory changes such as fat stranding, fascial thickening, and ascites are supportive findings. The pelvic cavity and subphrenic, subhe-

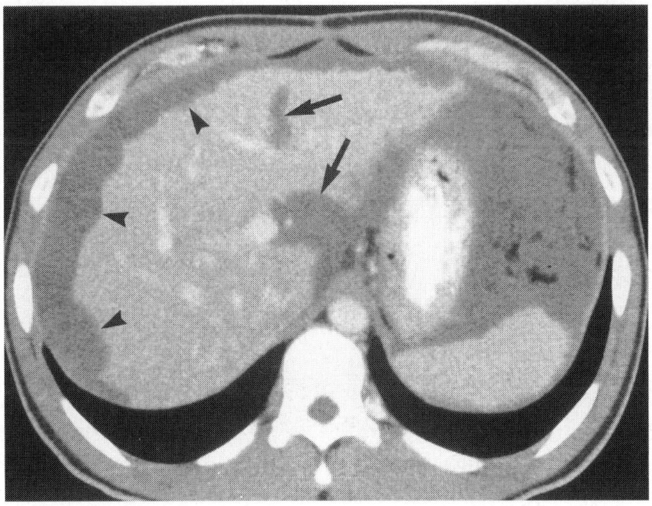

FIGURE 10.6 Pseudomyxoma peritonei. Contrast-enhanced CT in a 26-year-old man with pseudomyxoma peritonei shows fluid-attenuation gelatinous material surrounding the liver and filling the gastrosplenic region. Note scalloping of the liver margin *(arrowheads)* and widening of the fissures *(arrows).*

10.2

PNEUMOPERITONEUM

Perforated viscus—appendicitis, diverticulitis, ulcer, obstruction, trauma, ischemia, cancer, endoscopy
Recent surgery
Paracentesis
Peritoneal dialysis
Pneumatosis cystoides intestinalis—cyst rupture
Pneumothorax—pleuroperitoneal communication
Transvaginal introduction

patic, and perihepatic spaces are common locations for intraperitoneal abscesses. The location of retroperitoneal abscesses commonly reflects the underlying etiology. For example, abscess of the anterior pararenal space is often due to pancreatitis, duodenal perforation, or colonic disease; perinephric abscess usually reflects renal pathology; and psoas abscess may be due to spinal osteomyelitis and discitis. Interloop abscesses are often elongated, contain an air-fluid level, and may be mistaken for a dilated bowel loop. Diagnosis of a suspected abscess can often be confirmed with CT- or ultrasound-guided fine-needle aspiration.

Difficulties in diagnosis arise when imaging is performed during the earliest stages of infection, before liquefactive necrosis has occurred. In these cases, CT imaging demonstrates an irregular area of soft tissue density that represents an enhancing inflammatory mass or **phlegmon,** without a focal fluid collection. Attempted drainage is not fruitful in these cases and repeat imaging may be useful to follow maturation of the process. Because CT is not specific for the presence of infection, other lesions can mimic the appearance of an abscess, including pancreatic pseudocysts, mesenteric cysts, loculated ascites, duplication cysts, lymphoceles, bilomas, urinomas, chronic hematomas, large diverticula, and

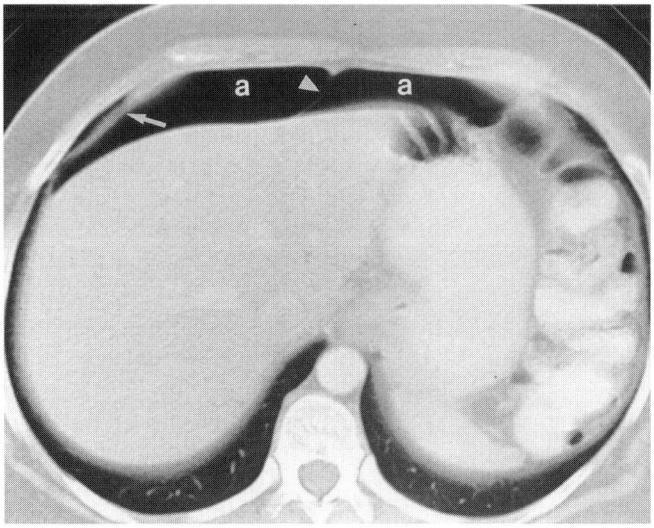

FIGURE 10.7 Pneumoperitoneum. CT with lung window shows free intraperitoneal air (a) anterior to the liver, beneath the diaphragm *(arrow),* and outlining the falciform ligament *(arrowhead).* The cause of pneumoperitoneum was spontaneous rupture of a subserosal cyst in this 46-year-old woman with benign pneumatosis coli (see **Fig. 6.39**).

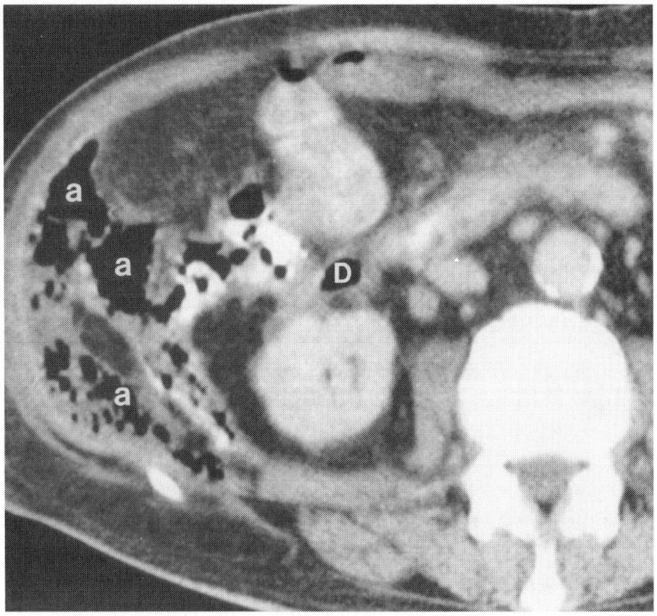

FIGURE 10.8 Pneumoretroperitoneum. Contrast-enhanced CT in a 73-year-old man demonstrates retroperitoneal contrast and air (a) in contiguity with the duodenum (D) and extending along the right pararenal space. A large perforated duodenal ulcer was confirmed at surgery.

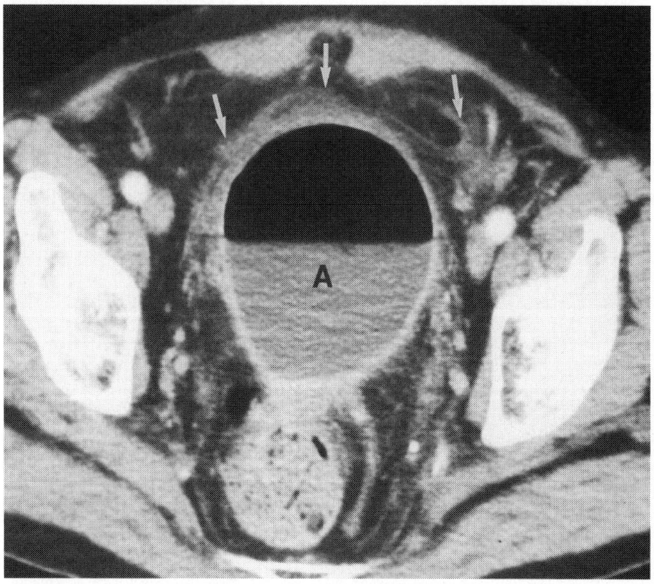

FIGURE 10.9 Abscess. Contrast-enhanced CT in a 64-year-old man with a 1-week history of left-lower-quadrant pain shows a rounded pelvic collection containing air and fluid (A) with an enhancing rim and inflammatory stranding of the adjacent fat *(arrows)*. Findings of sigmoid diverticulitis adjacent to this peridiverticular abscess were present on other levels. The urinary bladder was displaced caudally by the abscess.

necrotic tumors. Unopacified fluid-filled bowel loops and even the urine-filled bladder can also simulate the appearance of an abscess; delayed imaging may be necessary in some situations to ensure contrast opacification of these structures.

- CT can help distinguish among several unusual peritoneal inflammatory conditions that can clinically simulate more common diseases. **Mesenteric adenitis** results from benign inflammation of mesenteric lymph nodes, usually in the right lower quadrant, and is often clinically indistinguishable from acute appendicitis. In one large series, mesenteric adenitis accounted for about 8 percent of patients admitted for suspected appendicitis. CT findings consist of a cluster of three or more lymph nodes in the right lower quadrant measuring at least 5 mm in the short axis and a normal-appearing appendix. **Mesenteric panniculitis,** also known as *retractile mesenteritis* and *mesenteric lipodystrophy,* is an idiopathic inflammatory process characterized by fibrofatty thickening of the mesentery. CT findings vary from soft tissue infiltration of the mesentery to irregular mesenteric mass lesions **(Fig. 10.11). Segmental omen-**

10.3 ABDOMINAL ABSCESS

Postoperative
Bowel perforation—diverticulitis, appendicitis, Crohn disease, ischemia, perforated cancer, ingested foreign body, trauma, perforated ulcer
Pancreatitis
Tubo-ovarian
Trauma
Tuberculosis
Pyelonephritis
Mimics—loculated ascites, unopacified bowel, true cyst, pseudocyst, hematoma, lymphocele, biloma, urinoma, necrotic tumor

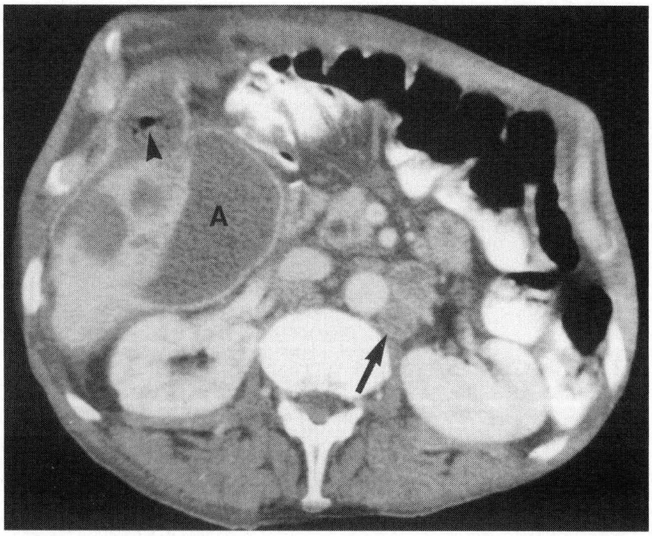

FIGURE 10.10 Perihepatic abscess. Contrast-enhanced CT in a 64-year-old man with weight loss and jaundice shows a crescentic fluid collection (A) with an enhancing rim surrounding the liver tip. Gas bubbles are present within the collection *(arrowhead)*. Liver lesions and retroperitoneal lymphadenopathy are also present *(arrow)*. Ultrasound-guided fine-needle aspiration biopsy of the fluid collection and liver yielded frank pus and poorly differentiated carcinoma, respectively.

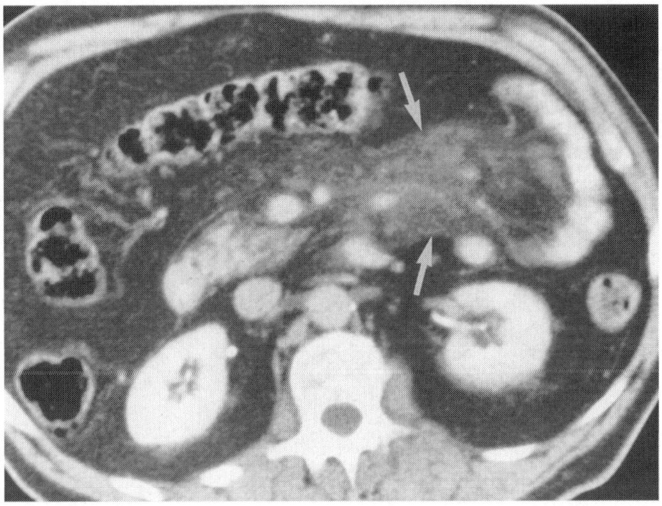

FIGURE 10.11 Mesenteric panniculitis. Contrast-enhanced CT in a 72-year-old man shows hazy soft tissue infiltration confined to a portion of the small bowel mesentery *(arrows)*.

tal infarction is a rare entity that may be related to adhesions, torsion, or a fragile blood supply to the omentum. Patients present with acute abdominal pain. Right-sided omental infarction often mimics acute appendicitis clinically. On CT, focal hazy soft tissue infiltration involving a portion of the omentum is characteristic. If this is recognized on imaging, patients can be spared unnecessary surgery, as treatment is conservative. **Epiploic appendagitis** results from torsion and infarction of a fatty appendage projecting off the colonic serosa. The clinical presentation consists of nonspecific acute abdominal pain. CT can suggest this diagnosis and prevent unnecessary surgery.

10.5 CYSTIC PERITONEAL LESIONS

- Cystic lesions of the peritoneum, mesentery, and omentum may result from a variety of neoplastic and nonneoplastic causes **(Differential 10.4)**. **Mesenteric cysts** are well-defined fluid attenuation lesions that most often arise in the small bowel mesentery **(Fig. 10.12)**. **Lymphangiomas** are closely related to mesenteric cysts but are typically multilocular and insinuate themselves between bowel loops. Lymphangiomas sometimes demonstrate an attenuation lower than that of water, reflecting a chylous component. Neither mesenteric cysts nor lymphangiomas demonstrate a malignant potential, but symptoms occasionally arise from mass effect on adjacent structures.

Duplication cysts are congenital and typically unilocular. They may occur anywhere along the GI tract and rarely communicate with the true lumen. **Mesothelial cysts** result from the incomplete fusion or delayed separation of the leaves of the greater omentum and are also characteristically unilocular. **Peritoneal pseudocysts** commonly result from pancreatitis and are often in or near the lesser sac, but they may occasionally dissect into the splenic hilum, porta hepatis, small bowel mesentery, transverse mesocolon, or mediastinum. Peritoneal pseudocysts are less commonly due to ovarian fluid that is subsequently trapped by peritoneal adhesions. Such inclusion cysts are usually located within the pelvis.

10.4 CYSTIC PERITONEAL LESION

Peritoneal carcinomatosis
Abscess
Loculated ascites
Postoperative seroma
Duplication cyst
Mesenteric cyst
Lymphangioma
Pancreatic pseudocyst
Peritoneal inclusion cyst
Lymphocele
Biloma
Peritonitis
Tuberculosis
Endometriosis
Pseudomyxoma peritonei
Cystic mesothelioma
Mesenteric teratoma
Chronic hematoma
Necrotic tumor
Echinococcal cyst

Involvement of the peritoneal cavity by **endometriosis** is usually not detectable on CT, although macroscopic solid and cystic lesions (endometriomas) are occasionally present (see **Fig. 13.16**). These lesions may demonstrate increased attenuation or fluid-fluid levels from prior hemorrhage. **Bilomas** are intraperitoneal collections of bile due to biliary leak from spontaneous rupture, trauma, instrumentation, or surgery. Intraperitoneal bile is usually walled off in a subhepatic or perihepatic location but otherwise has a nonspecific appearance **(Fig. 10.13)**. **Lymphocele** represents focal accumulation of lymphatic fluid caused by prior retroperitoneal or pelvic surgery. Lymphoceles are less commonly intraperitoneal because lymphatic leakage in such cases usually results in chylous ascites.

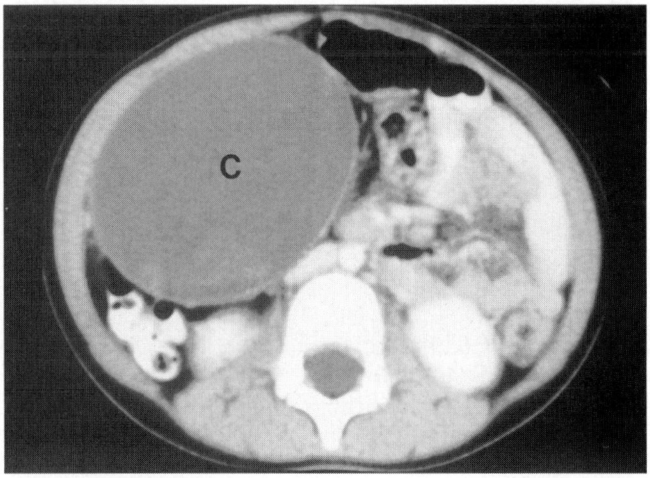

FIGURE 10.12 Mesenteric cyst. Contrast-enhanced CT in a 6-year-old girl demonstrates a large unilocular cyst (C) located within the small bowel mesentery.

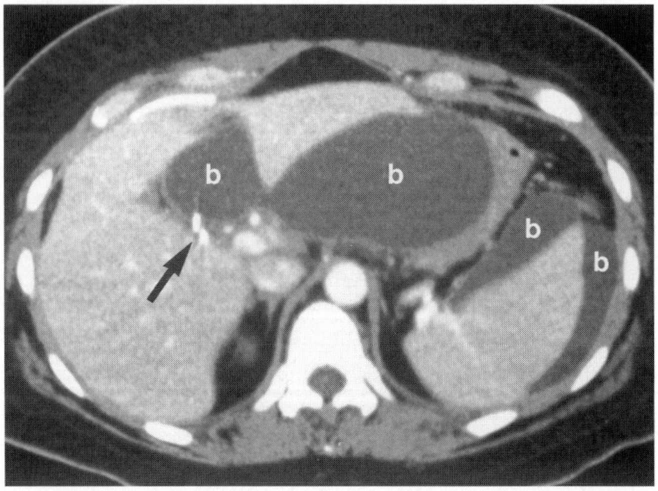

FIGURE 10.13 Biloma. Contrast-enhanced CT in a 46-year-old woman with persistent abdominal pain following laparoscopic cholecystectomy shows several loculated peritoneal fluid collections (b). The largest collection extends from the gallbladder fossa, where surgical clips are present *(arrow),* into the gastrohepatic recess. A biliary leak was confirmed by hepatobiliary scintigraphy prior to repair.

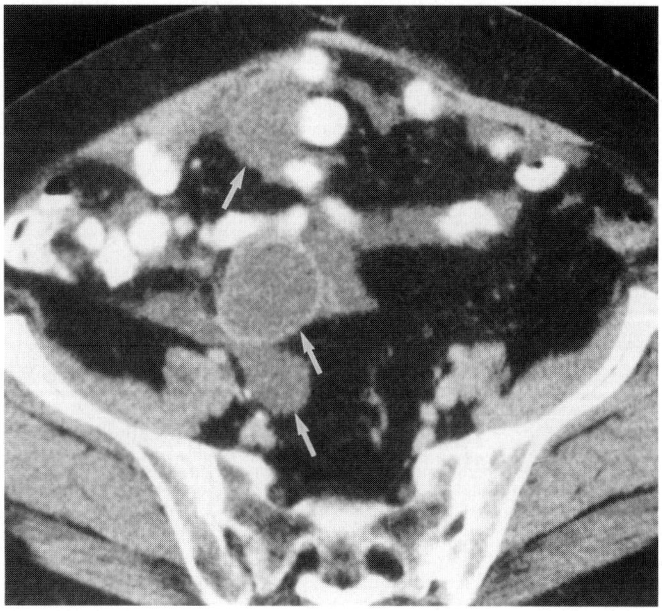

FIGURE 10.14 Cystic mesothelioma. Contrast-enhanced CT in a 62-year-old woman demonstrates multiple cystic lesions *(arrows)* involving the omentum and mesentery. The patient has been followed by CT for over 10 years and has had several recurrences in that period of time.

- **Cystic neoplasms** of the peritoneal cavity include the mature cystic teratoma and cystic mesothelioma. **Mesenteric teratomas** are predominately tumors of infancy. Although they are predominantly cystic, CT demonstration of mature fat, calcification or bone, and soft tissue elements is characteristic. Determining the anatomic site of origin of large tumors is difficult in young patients (see **Fig. 10.26**). **Cystic mesothelioma** of the peritoneum is generally benign and not related to asbestos exposure or malignant mesothelioma, although local recurrence after resection is common. On CT, multifocal cystic involvement of the mesentery and omentum is typical **(Fig. 10.14).** Pseudomyxoma peritonei results from rupture of a mucinous cystadenocarcinoma and has already been discussed (see **Fig. 10.6**). Peritoneal carcinomatosis has a multilocular cystic appearance from adhesions and malignant ascites; this entity is covered further in the next section. Peritoneum-based masses, whether primary or secondary, can occasionally appear cystic on CT if extensive necrosis is present.

10.6 SOLID PERITONEAL MASSES

- The differential diagnosis for solid peritoneal masses is broad and includes various neoplastic, inflammatory, and miscellaneous processes **(Differential 10.5).** Patient age, gender, symptoms, and history of a known primary malignancy will narrow the differential possibilities considerably. Associated CT findings—such as an organ-based primary tumor, ascites, or surrounding inflammatory changes—provide additional clues to the diagnosis.

  Metastatic carcinoma is the most common malignant process involving the peritoneum. Diffuse intraperitoneal seeding from ovarian carcinoma or GI malignancies such as pancreatic, gastric, or colon cancer is referred to as **peritoneal carcinomatosis.** Common areas for metastatic serosal implants reflect the preferred pathways of intraperitoneal flow of fluid and cells; these are determined by both gravitational effects and sites of mesenteric attachment (see **Fig. 10.1**). Therefore, the dependent pelvic cul-de-sac, the sigmoid mesocolon, and the ileocecal mesentery represent frequent sites of metastatic seeding. Perihepatic spread and omental involvement are also common.

  CT is somewhat limited in the detection of peritoneal metastatic disease, since individual implants are often less than 1 cm in size and difficult to distinguish from adjacent bowel or other structures.

10.5
SOLID PERITONEAL LESION

Tumor
- **Peritoneal carcinomatosis**
- **Lymphoma**
- **Lymphadenopathy**
- **Carcinoid**
- Desmoid (fibromatosis)
- Malignant mesothelioma
- Melanoma
- Sarcoma—MFH, leiomyosarcoma
- Benign stromal tumor—neurofibroma, hemangioma
- Desmoplastic small round cell tumor
- *Primary papillary serous carcinoma*

Infection—tuberculosis, actinomycosis, MAI, Whipple disease
Hematoma—trauma, surgery, coagulopathy
Mesenteric panniculitis (retractile mesenteritis)
Splenosis
Castleman disease
Extramedullary hematopoiesis
Leiomyomatosis peritonealis disseminata

Key: MAI, *Mycobacterium avium-intracellulare;* MFH, malignant fibrous histiocytoma.

Although nonspecific, ascites may be the only obvious finding of peritoneal involvement on CT, and its presence warrants a careful search for peritoneal implants. Despite its limitations, CT remains the primary imaging modality for the detection of peritoneal disease. When metastatic peritoneal deposits are detected on CT, they appear as well-defined nodules or masses, infiltrative or stellate lesions, or as diffuse peritoneal thickening **(Fig. 10.15).** Perihepatic serosal metastases often scallop the liver margin **(Fig. 13.21).** Prominent soft tissue infiltration and thickening of the omentum is referred to as **omental caking.**

Extranodal involvement of the omentum and mesentery with non-Hodgkin lymphoma (NHL) can appear as well-defined masses or as an infiltrative process that, when extensive, is referred to as **peritoneal lymphomatosis (Fig. 10.16).** Malignant melanoma may exhibit large peritoneal soft tissue masses **(Fig. 10.17).** Mesenteric involvement from a small bowel carcinoid tumor manifests on CT as a stellate, retractile, and often calcified mass that tethers thickened small bowel loops (see **Fig. 6.15).** Other primary malignancies—such as renal cell carcinoma, endometrial carcinoma, and transitional cell carcinoma—can rarely metastasize by intraperitoneal seeding.

Cancers can also involve the peritoneum by extending along peritoneal ligaments and mesenteries. Common examples include the spread of colon and pancreatic cancer along the transverse mesocolon, spread of colon and stomach cancer along the gastrocolic ligament, and spread of stomach and gallbladder cancer along the gastrohepatic ligament.

- **Primary peritoneal neoplasms** are rare compared with metastatic involvement. **Peritoneal mesothelioma** can be a solitary process or may occur in combination with pleural mesothelioma. As in the case of its pleural counterpart, there is an association between this entity and asbestos exposure and a prolonged latency period. CT findings include nodular or infiltrative peritoneal, mesenteric, and omental soft tissue thickening and a variable amount of ascites **(Fig. 10.18).** In isolation, these CT findings may be indistinguishable from peritoneal carcinomatosis, peritoneal lymphomatosis, tuberculous peritonitis, and pseudomyxoma peritonei.

  Intra-abdominal **desmoid tumors** (mesenteric fibromatosis) are a common complication of **Gardner syndrome** and are especially likely to be found in patients who have undergone prior abdominal surgery. Other manifestations of this autosomal dominant disorder include multiple adenomatous polyps of the colon and stomach, periampullary tumors, and multiple osteomas. On CT, desmoid tumors appear as soft tissue masses with either a well-defined or spiculated margin that frequently enhance following contrast administration.

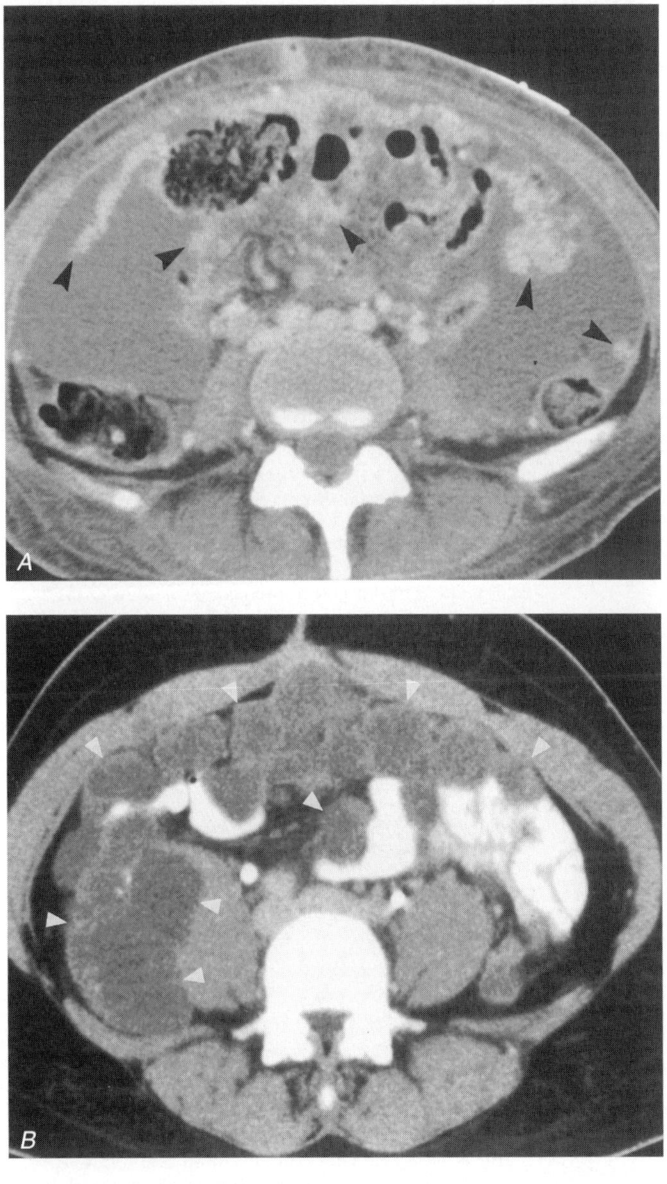

FIGURE 10.15 Peritoneal carcinomatosis. *A.* Contrast-enhanced CT in a 45-year-old woman with metastatic breast cancer shows diffuse nodular thickening of the omentum, mesentery, and parietal peritoneum *(arrowheads). B.* Contrast-enhanced CT in a 35-year-old woman with metastatic colon cancer shows multiple rounded peritoneal soft tissue masses *(arrowheads)* without ascites.

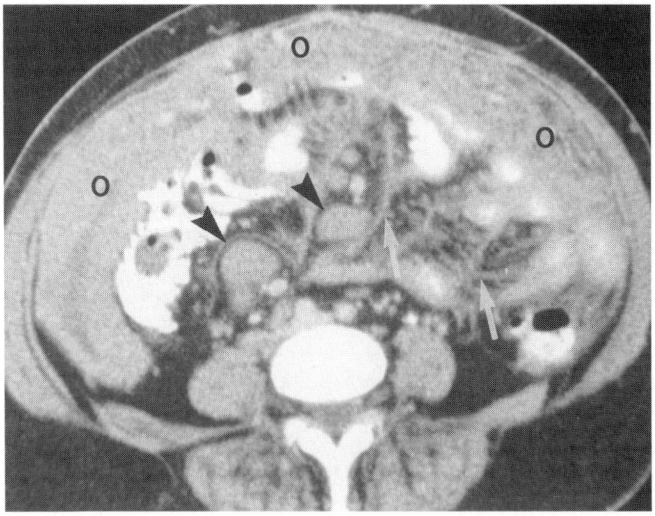

FIGURE 10.16 Peritoneal lymphomatosis. Contrast-enhanced CT in a 63-year-old woman with non-Hodgkin lymphoma demonstrates soft tissue caking of the omentum (O) and diffuse soft tissue thickening of the mesentery *(arrows).* Discrete mesenteric lymphadenopathy is also present *(arrowheads).*

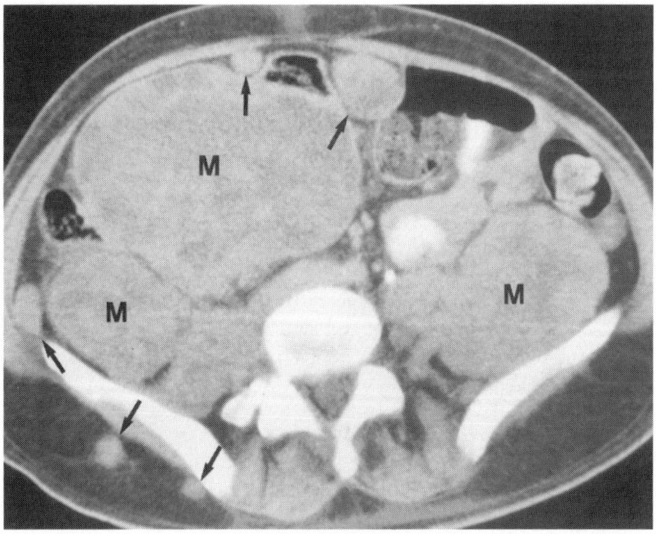

FIGURE 10.17 Melanoma. Contrast-enhanced CT in a 44-year-old woman with melanoma shows multiple large, peritoneal-based soft tissue masses (M). Smaller peritoneal and subcutaneous nodules are also present *(arrows)*.

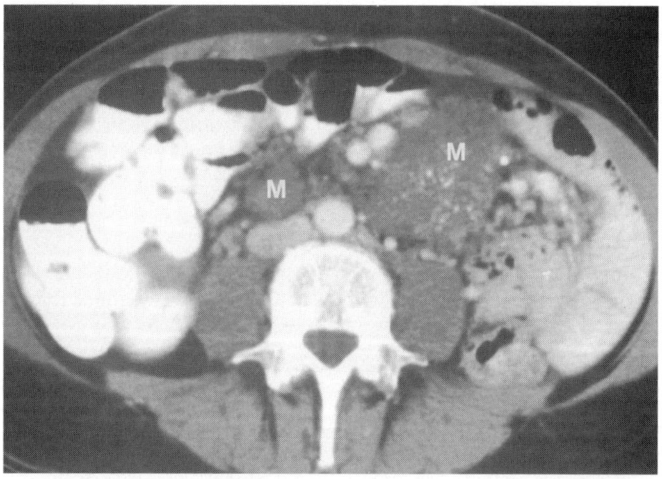

FIGURE 10.19 Mesenteric hemangioma. Contrast-enhanced CT in a 49-year-old woman with abdominal pain demonstrates ill-defined mesenteric soft tissue masses (M). The diagnosis of hemangioma was suggested by the presence of multiple punctate calcifications in the larger mass; these represent phleboliths. The patient also had multiple liver hemangiomas. (Case courtesy of Dr. Jeffrey Friedland, Denver, CO.)

Hemangiomas may arise in the peritoneum and are usually clinically silent. Punctate calcifications representing phleboliths are a distinguishing feature **(Fig. 10.19). Malignant fibrous histiocytoma (MFH)** is the most common soft tissue sarcoma to arise in the peritoneal cavity and is depicted on CT as a nonspecific soft tissue mass. **Desmoplastic small round cell tumor (DSRCT)** is an aggressive malignancy that tends to occur in adolescents and young adults. Typical CT findings include multiple peritoneal-based soft tissue masses with evidence of necrosis and hemorrhage **(Fig. 10.20).** Hematogenous or serosal liver metastases can be seen but no organ-based primary site is found. **Primary peritoneal papillary serous carcinoma** is a rare tumor that closely resembles

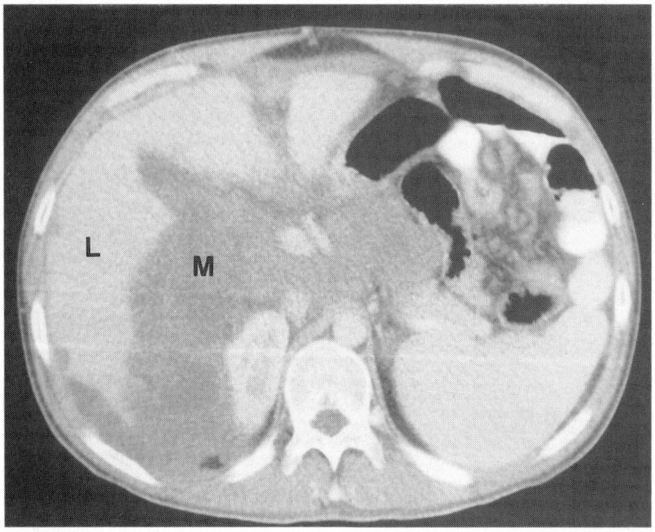

FIGURE 10.18 Peritoneal mesothelioma. Contrast-enhanced CT in a 29-year-old man with primary peritoneal mesothelioma demonstrates a confluent peritoneal-based soft tissue mass (M) that scallops the liver (L). Note similarity in CT appearance with pseudomyxoma peritonei **(Fig. 10.6)** and peritoneal carcinomatosis **(Fig. 13.21).**

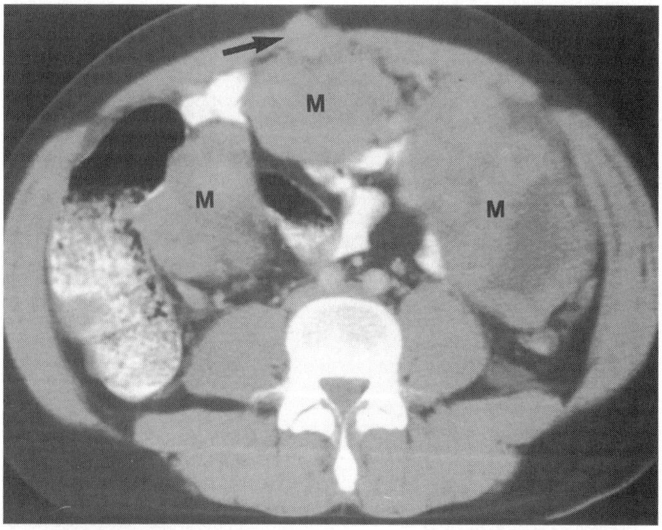

FIGURE 10.20 Desmoplastic small round cell tumor. Contrast-enhanced CT in a 35-year-old man with increasing abdominal girth shows multiple large peritoneal-based masses (M). A Sister Mary Joseph node is present at the umbilicus *(arrow)*. No organ-based primary site was found. (From Pickhardt PJ, Fisher AJ, Balfe DM, Dehner LP, Huettner PC. Desmoplastic small round cell tumor of the abdomen: Radiologic-histopathologic correlation. *Radiology* 1999;210:633–638. With permission.)

serous ovarian papillary carcinoma. Elderly women are most commonly affected. CT characteristics include multiple peritoneal and omental soft tissue masses with extensive calcification and normal-appearing ovaries.

Atypical infections may also result in solid-appearing peritoneal lesions that can simulate neoplasms. **Tuberculous peritonitis** is unusual but can demonstrate a variety of appearances on CT, including low-attenuation mesenteric masses or adenopathy, nodular peritoneal thickening, and high-attenuation ascites. **Actinomycosis** has a tendency to violate normal anatomic boundaries and may extend into the peritoneal cavity, appearing as an infiltrative soft tissue mass on CT.

Peritoneal involvement with systemic **amyloidosis** usually manifests itself on CT with soft tissue infiltration of the mesentery and encasement of mesenteric vessels. Intra-abdominal **splenosis** can also simulate tumor, exhibiting multiple intraperitoneal soft tissue lesions; a history of prior splenectomy or splenic trauma can suggest this possibility. Mesenteric **hemorrhage** can appear mass-like and mimic peritoneal carcinomatosis. **Castleman disease** (angiofollicular lymph node hyperplasia) most commonly involves the mediastinum but rarely can manifest as single or multiple peritoneal masses that demonstrate prominent enhancement on CT. Extramedullary hematopoiesis can rarely involve the mesentary.

10.7 RETROPERITONEAL HEMORRHAGE

- CT is an accurate and noninvasive method for confirming the diagnosis of retroperitoneal hemorrhage when it is suspected on clinical grounds **(Differential 10.6).** Common clinical findings include abdominal or back pain, abdominal fullness or mass, and a decrease in hematocrit; however, many times the diagnosis is not clinically obvious. When there is high clinical suspicion for retroperitoneal hemorrhage, CT may be performed urgently without oral or IV contrast administration.

Acute onset of severe back or abdominal pain in a patient with a known abdominal aortic aneurysm (AAA) is one such setting. CT is indicated for the evaluation of suspected **AAA leak or rupture** only in patients who are hemodynamically stable. Aneurysm rupture is usually obvious on CT, with varying amounts of mixed-attenuation periaortic blood infiltrating along retroperitoneal fascial planes **(Fig. 10.21).** In such instances, these studies should be promptly terminated to facilitate emergent surgery. AAA rupture carries a high mortality, ranging from 50 to 90 percent. Occasionally, aneurysm leaks are fairly subtle, with minimal soft tissue infiltration of the periaortic region **(Fig. 10.22).**

Iatrogenic causes of retroperitoneal hemorrhage include complications of recent surgery, percutaneous biopsy, and percutaneous nephrostomy. Another cause includes recent femoral arterial puncture for angiography. **Spontaneous** retroperitoneal hemorrhage may occur in patients receiving anticoagulation therapy or in those with an underlying bleeding diathesis. Retroperitoneal hemorrhage is a common finding following blunt abdominal **trauma. Retroperitoneal tumors** may present with hemorrhage; common examples include benign neoplasms such as renal angiomyolipomas and adrenal myelolipomas **(Fig. 10.23)** or malignant tumors such as renal cell carcinoma.

The **CT appearance** of acute retroperitoneal hemorrhage consists of soft tissue infiltration of the retroperitoneal spaces and interfascial planes, often with areas of increased attenuation that re-

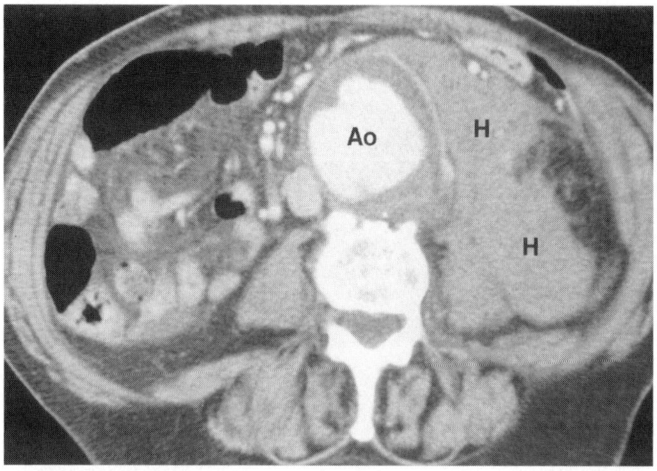

FIGURE 10.21 Ruptured abdominal aortic aneurysm (AAA). Contrast-enhanced CT in a 79-year-old man with abdominal pain demonstrates high-attenuation retroperitoneal hemorrhage (H) associated with an aortic aneurysm (Ao). If AAA leak or rupture had been suspected prior to CT, noncontrast images would have been sufficient.

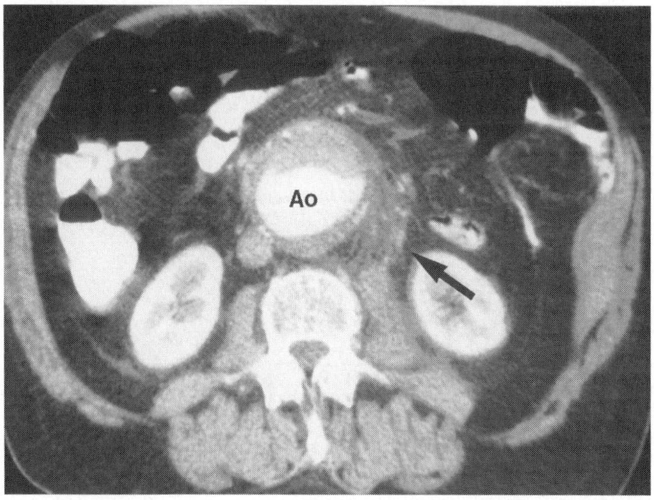

FIGURE 10.22 AAA leak. Contrast-enhanced CT in a 76-year-old man with a 5-day history of worsening abdominal pain shows soft tissue stranding *(arrow)* adjacent to an aortic aneurysm (Ao). No frank retroperitoneal hemorrhage was present. The patient was immediately taken to surgery and a leaking AAA was confirmed and repaired.

10.6 RETROPERITONEAL HEMORRHAGE

AAA leak or rupture
Trauma
Anticoagulation therapy
Postoperative
Femoral arterial puncture
Bleeding diathesis
Percutaneous biopsy/nephrostomy
Tumor

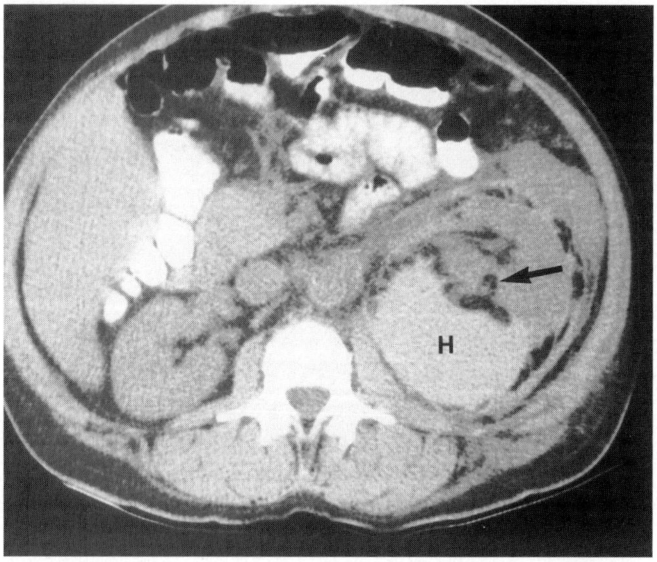

FIGURE 10.23 Retroperitoneal hemorrhage due to tumor. Noncontrast CT in a 56-year-old man presenting with acute left abdominal pain demonstrates high-attenuation blood (H) displacing the left kidney anteriorly. A small renal angiomyolipoma *(arrow)* was the cause of spontaneous hemorrhage.

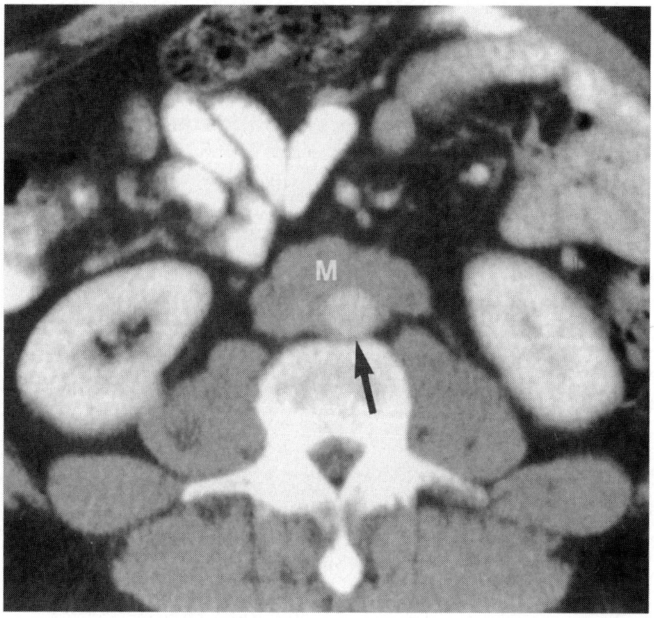

FIGURE 10.24 Retroperitoneal fibrosis. Contrast-enhanced CT in a 58-year-old man with idiopathic retroperitoneal fibrosis shows a soft tissue mass (M) anterior to the spine partially surrounding the aorta *(arrow)* and compressing the IVC, which is no longer visible.

flect acute hemorrhage. Significant mass effect on retroperitoneal structures is usually present. Bidirectional communication along the retroperitoneal and pelvic extraperitoneal planes is often appreciated with blood extending along these planes.

10.8 RETROPERITONEAL FIBROSIS

- **Retroperitoneal fibrosis** describes the end result of a variety of inflammatory and reactive conditions that incite the proliferation of fibrous tissue around the aorta, IVC, and ureters **(Differential 10.7).** The clinical presentation is usually related to IVC compression or ureteral obstruction. Up to one-half of these cases are **idiopathic.** Recognized causes of retroperitoneal fibrosis include certain drugs (methysergide), inflammatory AAA, metastases, retroperitoneal surgery, and granulomatous infection.

A mantle of perianeurysmal fibrosis seen in some patients with AAA has led to the term ***inflammatory AAA*** and is possibly related to an immune-mediated response to a component within the aneurysm wall. Desmoplastic retroperitoneal metastatic disease leading to fibrosis is most typical of breast cancer but can rarely be seen with other malignancies. Prior surgery for aortic aneurysm repair or prior retroperitoneal hemorrhage may also lead to fibrosis. Granulomatous infections such as tuberculosis or histoplasmosis can induce a process analogous to fibrosing mediastinitis. In approximately 15 percent of idiopathic cases, other fibrosing processes are present, such as sclerosing cholangitis, Riedel thyroiditis, orbital pseudotumor, or fibrosing mediastinitis.

CT findings usually consist of varying degrees of confluent soft tissue encasing the aorta and IVC, usually without significant displacement of these structures **(Fig. 10.24).** Encasement of the ureter is also common. Renal compromise may develop, even without hydronephrosis. With an inflammatory AAA, fibrosis is perianeurysmal and forms a circumferential cuff of soft tissue around the dilated aorta **(Fig. 10.25).**

CT cannot reliably distinguish between benign and malignant causes of retroperitoneal fibrosis. Furthermore, a CT-guided biopsy that yields only fibrosis does not completely exclude the possibility of malignancy. The main differential diagnostic considerations on CT include lymphoma, metastatic lymphadenopathy, and hemorrhage. Anterior displacement of the aorta and IVC from the spine by soft tissue favors tumor over fibrosis. Prognosis of retroperitoneal fibrosis depends on the underlying etiology, with benign causes generally having a more favorable outcome. Corticosteroid therapy may be beneficial in some cases.

10.7 RETROPERITONEAL FIBROSIS

Idiopathic
Inflammatory aneurysm—perianeurysmal fibrosis
Medications—particularly methysergide
Granulomatous infection—tuberculosis, histoplasmosis
Metastases—breast, colon cancer
Postoperative
Hemorrhage
Radiation
Lymphoma
Inflammation—pancreatitis, Crohn disease

10.9 RETROPERITONEAL MASSES

- Tumors of the retroperitoneum can be benign or malignant and can represent primary or metastatic disease **(Differential 10.8). Benign**

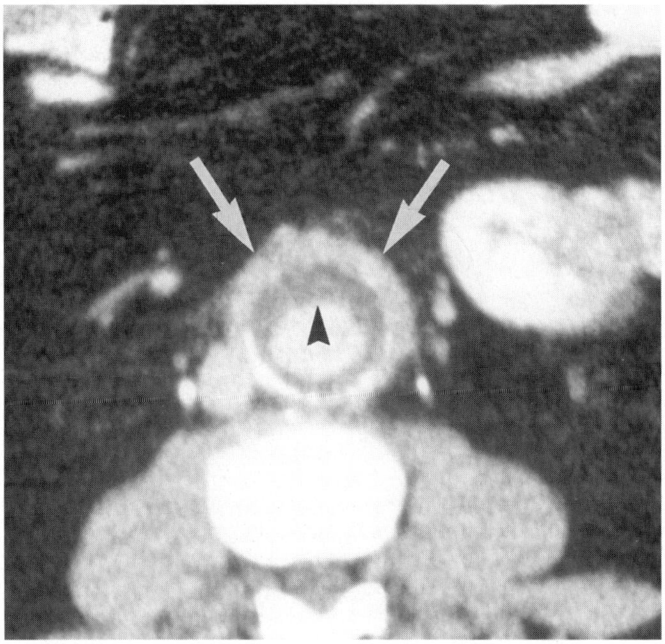

FIGURE 10.25 Inflammatory AAA. Contrast-enhanced CT in a 58-year-old man with AAA shows a rim of perianeurysmal soft tissue *(arrows)*. Intimal calcification and low-attenuation thrombus *(arrowhead)* are also present.

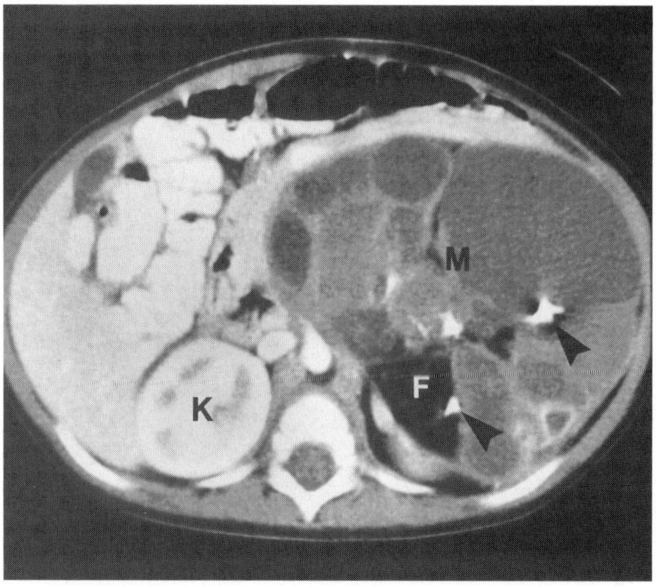

FIGURE 10.26 Retroperitoneal teratoma. Contrast-enhanced CT in a 1-year-old infant demonstrates a multilocular cystic mass (M) that also contains coarse calcification *(arrowheads)* and macroscopic fat (F). The kidney was displaced inferiorly. The lesion was identified incidentally on chest radiography because of the calcification. K, right kidney.

tumors of the retroperitoneum are rare. The CT appearance combined with the patient's clinical history can suggest the diagnosis in some instances. Retroperitoneal **lipomas** have a characteristic appearance on CT, with homogeneous fat density. Very rarely, a well-differentiated liposarcoma may be mistaken for a lipoma, but most liposarcomas have a discernible soft tissue component that argues against the diagnosis of a simple lipoma. **Lymphangiomas** are usually found in children and also demonstrate negative attenuation values because of their chylous composition. **Mature teratomas** often contain areas of macroscopic fat, calcification or ossification, and soft tissue, which combine to give a unique appearance on CT **(Fig. 10.26).** Fat-fluid levels are occasionally seen within teratomas and are diagnostic.

10.8

RETROPERITONEAL MASS

Lymphoma
Hematoma—see Differential 10.6
Lymphadenopathy—testicular, cervical, breast, other
Fibrosis—see Differential 10.7
Primary malignancy
  Liposarcoma—most common primary
  Malignant fibrous histiocytoma
  Leiomyosarcoma
Benign tumors—lipoma, lymphangioma, hemangioma, teratoma, neurofibroma, paraganglioma
Cystic lesions—abscess, pseudocyst, true cyst, lymphocele, urinoma

Retroperitoneal **nerve sheath tumors** occur predominantly in patients with neurofibromatosis and are often extensive, enveloping nearby retroperitoneal vessels. In patients with neurofibromatosis type I, these tumors are usually of a density near that of water and mimic low-attenuation retroperitoneal lymphadenopathy **(Fig. 10.27). Paragangliomas** are extra-adrenal pheochromocytomas and can arise anywhere along the sympathetic chain that runs along the abdominal aorta. A classic retroperitoneal location is at or near the level of the aortic bifurcation, a region termed the organ of Zuckerkandl **(Fig. 10.28).** Paragangliomas often demonstrate prominent enhancement on CT. **Hemangiomas** arising in the retroperitoneum are usually an incidental finding that can be suggested by the presence of phleboliths.

- **Primary malignant tumors** of the retroperitoneum are imaged more often than benign tumors but are nonetheless uncommon lesions. The majority of retroperitoneal malignancies are of mesenchymal or neurogenic origin and tend to be very large (>10 cm) at presentation. In addition, these lesions are heterogeneous because of necrosis, hemorrhage, and cystic degeneration. Liposarcoma, MFH, and leiomyosarcoma are the most common primaries, with the relative frequency among these three tumors depending on the series cited.

With retroperitoneal **liposarcoma,** a specific diagnosis is often possible on CT provided that the tumor is relatively well differentiated and contains at least some recognizable fat **(Fig. 10.29).** In actuality, even the more poorly differentiated and pleomorphic variants of liposarcoma usually have a detectable fatty component on CT. Compared with those having other retroperitoneal malignancies, patients with liposarcoma have a prolonged survival but may need to undergo multiple debulking operations for slowly advancing tumor recurrence.

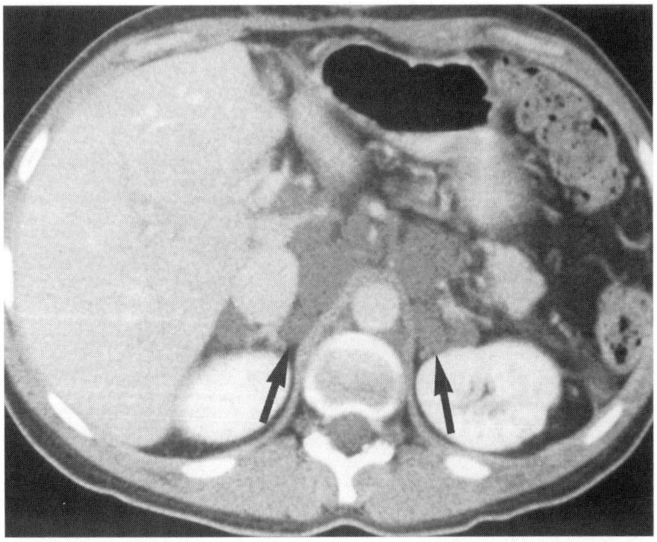

FIGURE 10.27 Retroperitoneal neurofibromas. Contrast-enhanced CT in a 24-year-old woman with neurofibromatosis type I demonstrates multiple retroperitoneal neurofibromas *(arrows)*. The appearance mimics low-attenuation lymphadenopathy.

MFH is more common than liposarcoma according to some series. On CT, the lone distinguishing feature of MFH is the presence of dystrophic calcification, which is seen in approximately 25 percent of cases. Such calcification is unusual in other retroperitoneal malignancies. **Leiomyosarcoma** may arise from the IVC or elsewhere in the retroperitoneum **(Fig. 10.30).** An intimate association with the IVC can suggest the diagnosis, but other large tumors, such as adrenocortical carcinoma, can often mimic this appearance. Regardless of the site of origin, leiomyosarcomas are typically heterogeneous, with large areas of central low attenuation.

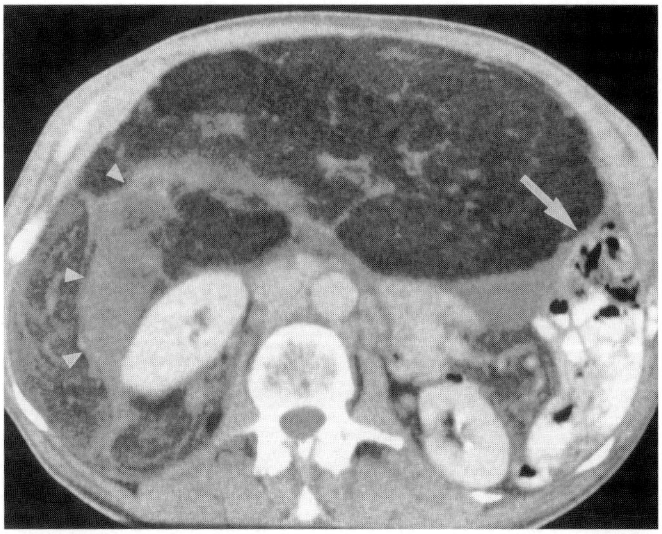

FIGURE 10.29 Retroperitoneal liposarcoma. Contrast-enhanced CT in a 77-year-old man with slowly increasing abdominal girth demonstrates a predominately fatty mass that occupies the majority of the abdomen. Soft tissue elements are present *(arrowheads)*. A retroperitoneal origin can be inferred from displacement of the right colon *(arrow)* and pararenal involvement.

Other rare primary retroperitoneal malignancies include fibrosarcoma, malignant germ-cell tumors, hemangiopericytoma, and rhabdomyosarcoma **(Fig. 10.31).** Hemangiopericytomas tend to be more vascular than the other tumors and therefore may demonstrate intense enhancement on CT. Retroperitoneal lymphadenopathy from non-Hodgkin lymphoma (NHL) and metastatic disease from a variety of malignancies occur much more

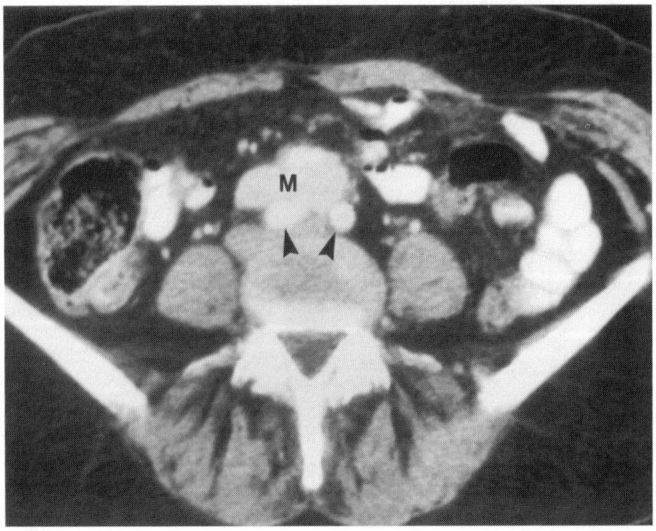

FIGURE 10.28 Paraganglioma. Contrast-enhanced CT in a 63-year-old woman shows a brightly enhancing mass (M) anterior to the common iliac arteries *(arrowheads)* near the bifurcation. A paraganglioma in this region arises from the so-called organ of Zuckerkandl.

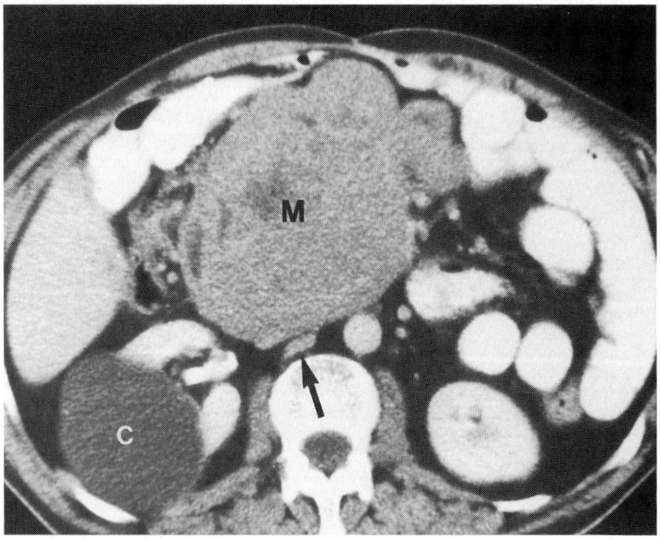

FIGURE 10.30 Leiomyosarcoma of IVC. Contrast-enhanced CT in a 73-year-old shows a heterogeneous mass (M) involving the IVC, which displaces contrast-filled bowel loops. Note the right diaphragmatic crus *(arrow)* and simple cyst involving the right kidney (C).

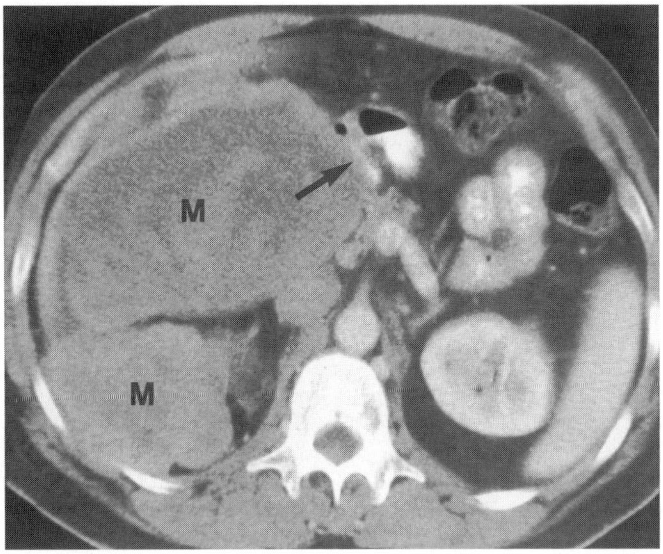

FIGURE 10.31 Retroperitoneal rhabdomyosarcoma. Contrast-enhanced CT in a 42-year-old man with a heterogeneous lobulated mass (M) arising from the retroperitoneum. Note the displacement of the right colon *(arrow)*.

frequently than primary retroperitoneal tumors; these topics are expanded upon in the upcoming sections.

10.10 LYMPHADENOPATHY

- CT is the primary imaging modality for the detection of intra-abdominal **lymphadenopathy.** The major CT criterion for diagnosing metastatic involvement of a lymph node is based on abnormal enlargement. This has inherent weaknesses, since normal-sized nodes can be involved with tumor and enlarged nodes are sometimes reactive and do not contain metastases. Despite this, CT offers rapid, noninvasive, and reasonably accurate evaluation of abdominal and pelvic lymph nodes for both initial diagnosis and follow-up after therapy.

  Abnormal **lymph node enlargement** is usually determined by a short-axis measurement on CT; the specific size criteria vary for different nodal groups. Retrocrural lymph nodes measuring >6 mm should be considered abnormal; gastrohepatic nodes measuring >8 mm are likely abnormal; retroperitoneal, celiac, and mesenteric nodes measuring >10 mm are abnormal; and porta hepatis nodes over 15 mm are considered abnormal. An isolated foramen of Winslow lymph node measuring over 15 mm in the short axis is a normal finding. Pelvic nodes measuring greater than 10 mm are considered abnormal by most radiologists, although some authors advocate a 15-mm threshold. In addition to size criteria, an abnormal number of normal-sized nodes can be an indication of disease and should be viewed with suspicion. Although certain CT features—such as lymph node size, morphology, density, and degree of enhancement—may suggest a specific cause, CT cannot reliably distinguish benign from malignant etiologies. Furthermore, other entities can mimic the appearance of lymphadenopathy on CT **(Differential 10.9). Benign causes** of lymphadenopathy include infectious etiologies such as mycobacterial and fungal agents and Whipple disease **(Fig. 10.32),** and noninfectious etiologies such as reactive hyperplasia, sarcoidosis, amyloidosis, and Castleman disease. **Castleman disease** involves abdominal and pelvic nodes in approximately 20 percent of cases and characteristically demonstrates prominent enhancement after IV contrast administration **(Fig. 10.33).**

10.9
MIMICS OF LYMPHADENOPATHY

Unopacified bowel loops
Diaphragmatic crus
Splenule(s)
Fibrosis
Large collateral vessels
Papillary process of caudate lobe
Hematoma
Lymphocele
Seroma
Abscess
Neurofibromatosis type I—nerve sheath tumors

- **Malignant lymphadenopathy** can exhibit a variety of appearances on CT, including discrete lymph node enlargement, conglomeration of multiple matted nodes, or a coalescent mass with obscuration of individual nodal borders. The majority of lymph nodes measuring over 15 mm harbor metastases in patients with a known primary malignancy; however, because of the significant overlap in appearance with benign causes, biopsy is usually indicated for confirmation. CT is commonly performed for staging and follow-up examinations in patients with lymphoma (see **Section 10.11**). CT is also useful for evaluating patients with abdominal and extra-abdominal primary malignancies and allows for assessment of nodal and extranodal involvement.

  Testicular neoplasms deserve special mention since the primary route of spread is via lymphatic pathways. Testicular tumors are the most common malignancy affecting men in their third decade of life. The vast majority (>85 percent) are of germ-cell

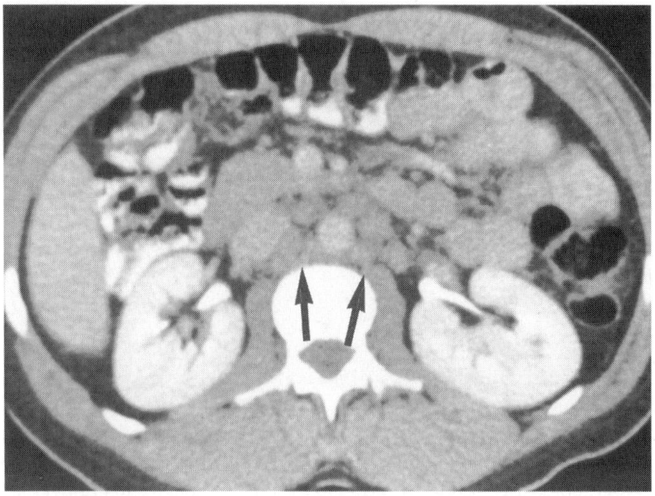

FIGURE 10.32 Histoplasmosis. Contrast-enhanced CT in a 33-year-old HIV-positive man with persistent fever demonstrates multiple, slightly enlarged retroperitoneal lymph nodes in the paraaortic and paracaval regions *(arrows)*. CT-guided biopsy was positive for *Histoplasma capsulatum*.

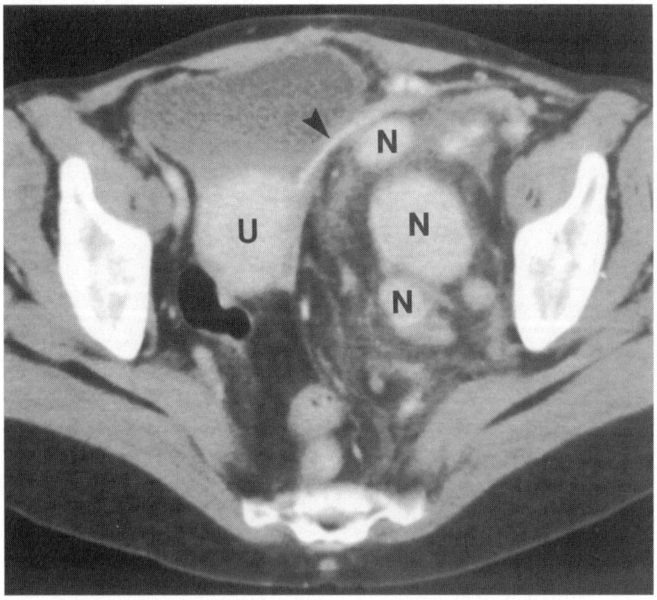

FIGURE 10.33 Castleman disease. Contrast-enhanced CT in a 58-year-old woman shows multiple brightly enhancing left iliac lymph nodes (N) displacing the uterus (U) and round ligament *(arrowhead).* Infiltration and expansion of the fat surrounding the involved nodes is present. Nodal biopsy revealed the plasma cell type of Castleman disease. The appearance remained unchanged on CT over a 5-year period.

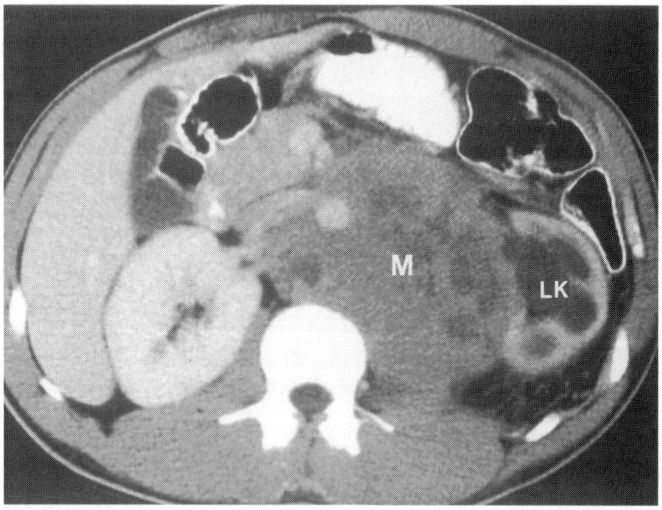

FIGURE 10.34 Testicular cancer. Contrast-enhanced CT in a 27-year-old man with a testicular nonseminomatous germ-cell tumor shows massive necrotic retroperitoneal lymphadenopathy (M) centered at the left renal hilum. The mass has obstructed the left kidney (LK).

origin and approximately 40 percent of these are seminomas. Seminomas are radiosensitive tumors that have a good prognosis, with a reported 10-year survival of 90 percent. Nonseminomatous germ-cell tumors—including embryonal cell carcinoma, choriocarcinoma, teratocarcinoma, yolk sac tumors, and mixed types—have a worse prognosis. Lymph node metastases reflect the normal lymphatic drainage pattern of the testes, which follows the course of the gonadal veins. Therefore, nodal metastases appear to "skip" the pelvis and first involve the renal hilar region on the left and paracaval region on the right. On CT, bulky retroperitoneal lymphadenopathy, often with large areas of central low attenuation, is a common finding **(Fig. 10.34).** CT monitoring and serum tumor-marker assays are employed for detecting recurrent disease. Posttherapy fibrosis can be difficult to distinguish from true recurrence on a single CT examination.

- Lymphadenopathy is a common finding on CT in patients with the **acquired immunodeficiency syndrome (AIDS).** Even before developing clinical AIDS, HIV-positive patients may present with a "lymph node syndrome" that represents a benign reactive process. An increased number of normal-sized lymph nodes is the most common finding on CT. Lymphadenopathy from disseminated Kaposi sarcoma is characteristically higher in attenuation than that due to other causes. AIDS-related B-cell lymphoma is very aggressive; CT demonstrates extranodal disease in over 80 percent of patients with abdominal disease. Mycobacterial infection commonly presents with lymphadenopathy. Both tuberculosis and *Mycobacterium avium-intracellulare* (MAI) can give rise to low-attenuation lymphadenopathy **(Fig. 10.35),** although it is somewhat more common with the former. Fungal infection can also result in lymphadenopathy **(Fig. 10.32).** Prophylaxis for *Pneumocystis carinii* with aerosolized pentamidine has led to an increased incidence of extrapulmonary disease. The presence of small, punctate calcifications involving the liver, spleen, and abdominal lymph nodes is a characteristic finding of prior disseminated infection.

- **Low-attenuation lymphadenopathy** on CT can result from various infections, neoplasms, and miscellaneous causes **(Differential 10.10).** Mycobacterial disease has already been discussed. Whipple

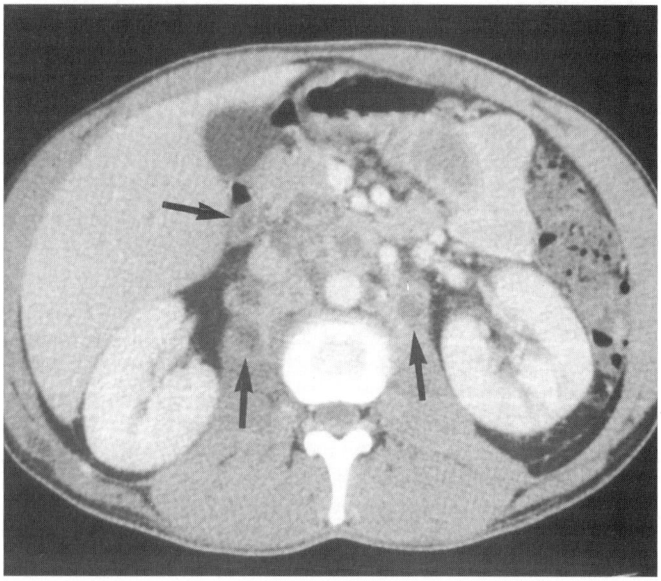

FIGURE 10.35 MAI. Contrast-enhanced CT in a 37-year-old HIV-positive man with persistent fever demonstrates multiple enlarged retroperitoneal lymph nodes with central low attenuation *(arrows).*

10.10

LOW-ATTENUATION LYMPHADENOPATHY

Infection—mycobacterial (TB, MAI), Whipple disease
Metastases—testicular, ovarian, necrotic squamous cell cancer
Lymphoma—especially posttherapy
Lymphangioleiomyomatosis (LAM) —mediastinal most common
Mimics—neurofibromatosis type I, lymphocele, cyst

10.11

CALCIFIED LYMPH NODES

Old granulomatous disease—histoplasmosis, tuberculosis
Lymphoma—particularly treated
Lymphangiographic contrast (mimic)
Disseminated *P. carinii*—AIDS patients
Metastatic cancer—mucinous adenocarcinoma, osteosarcoma
Amyloidosis—may be very dense
Thorotrast

disease can appear identical to MAI infection on CT, with diffuse bowel wall thickening and low-attenuation lymph nodes. These findings result from the accumulation of bacterial glycoprotein within macrophages. Arthralgias and central nervous system symptoms are also common. Metastatic lymph nodes with central necrosis are more common with squamous cell cancer and testicular tumors. Low-attenuation adenopathy in patients with lymphoma can be seen after therapy or in untreated patients with aggressive subtypes. **Lymphangioleiomyomatosis (LAM)** is a rare disorder that affects women of reproductive age and results from the benign proliferation of smooth muscle along the lymphatic system. Thoracic manifestations predominate, but low-attenuation abdominal adenopathy can be seen and may be associated with chylous ascites **(Fig. 10.36).** Retroperitoneal nerve sheath tumors in patients with neurofibromatosis type I are typically of near-water attenuation and can simulate low-attenuation adenopathy (see **Fig. 10.27**).

Lymph node calcification is less common in the abdomen **(Differential 10.11)** compared with the thorax but is usually due to old, healed granulomatous disease from histoplasmosis or tuberculosis. Punctate nodal calcification from disseminated *P. carinii* infection in AIDS patients has already been discussed. Other causes include treated lymphoma, metastatic disease from mucinous primaries or osteosarcoma, and amyloidosis.

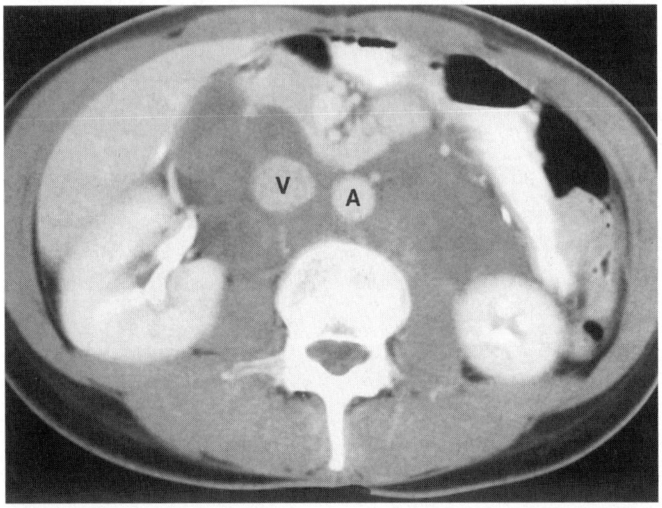

FIGURE 10.36 Lymphangioleiomyomatosis (LAM). Contrast-enhanced CT in a 41-year-old woman with worsening dyspnea shows confluent low-attenuation retroperitoneal lymphadenopathy that encases the aorta (A) and IVC (V). LAM was diagnosed by CT-guided retroperitoneal lymph node biopsy. The patient eventually went on to lung transplantation. (From Pickhardt PJ, Kazerooni EA, Flint A. Diagnosis of lymphangioleiomyomatosis by CT-guided retroperitoneal biopsy. *Clin Radiol* 2000 (in press). With permission.)

- **Hypervascular lymph nodes** on CT **(Differential 10.12)** are most commonly the result of metastatic disease from a hypervascular primary, such as renal cell, thyroid, melanoma, Kaposi sarcoma, and neuroendocrine tumors. Lymphoma frequently demonstrates at least moderate enhancement with dynamic imaging. Castleman disease is a benign cause of hypervascular adenopathy **(Fig. 10.33).**
- **CT-guided lymph node biopsy** is a safe and accurate diagnostic procedure. Commonly used methods include fine-needle aspiration with a 20- or 22-gauge needle and core biopsy with a spring-loaded "biopsy gun." A coaxial technique allows for multiple passes without repositioning of the outer needle. The particular method employed depends on several factors, including the anatomic location of the lesion, expertise of the cytopathologist, and specific clinical questions to be addressed. In cases of suspected lymphoma, core biopsy is generally preferred, since it preserves the histologic architecture of the specimen and provides more tissue for flow cytometry **(Fig. 10.37).**

10.11 LYMPHOMA

- **Hodgkin disease (HD)** usually affects adults in the third to fifth decades of life. Diagnosis requires cytologic detection of the Reed-Sternberg cell. There are four recognized histopathologic subtypes. The **nodular sclerosing** variant accounts for approximately 65 percent of cases and is most frequent among young women, who often present with mediastinal lymphadenopathy. The **mixed cellularity type** represents 25 percent of HD and more commonly involves paraaortic lymph nodes and the spleen. The **lymphocytic-predominant** and **lymphocytic-depleted** forms are unusual. The Ann Arbor staging classification is predictive of clinical outcome and describes involvement of a single nodal region (stage I), involvement of two or more nodal regions on one side of the diaphragm (stage II), involvement of both sides of the diaphragm (stage III), and diffuse involvement of at least one extralymphatic organ (stage IV).

  HD is typically radiosensitive and the overall 10-year survival is approximately 90 percent. HD has a predictable pattern of spread

10.12

HYPERVASCULAR LYMPH NODES

Metastases—renal cell, melanoma, thyroid, Kaposi sarcoma (AIDS), neuroendocrine tumors
Castleman disease
Lymphoma—occasionally demonstrates prominent enhancement
HIV lymph node syndrome

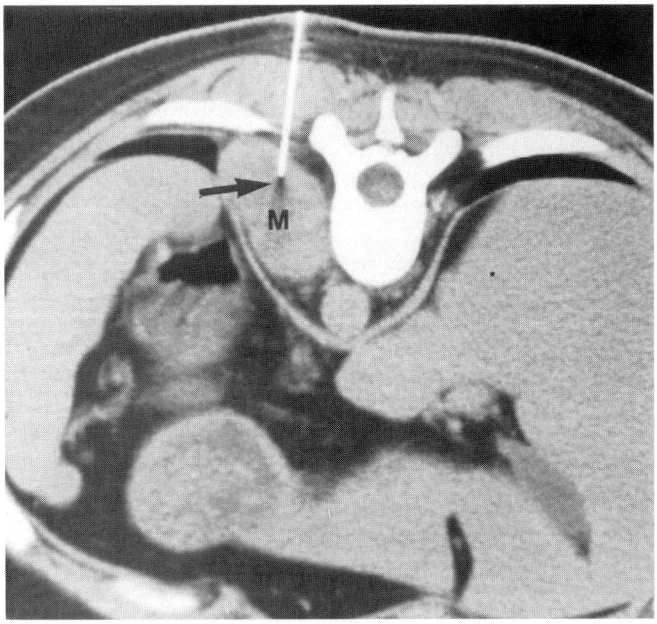

FIGURE 10.37 CT-guided lymph node biopsy. Prone CT image from percutaneous needle biopsy in a 26-year-old woman with an enlarged retrocrural lymph node (M) shows shadowing artifact *(arrow)* confirming the position of the needle tip within the mass. Core biopsy was performed for suspected lymphoma but pathologic examination revealed Castleman disease.

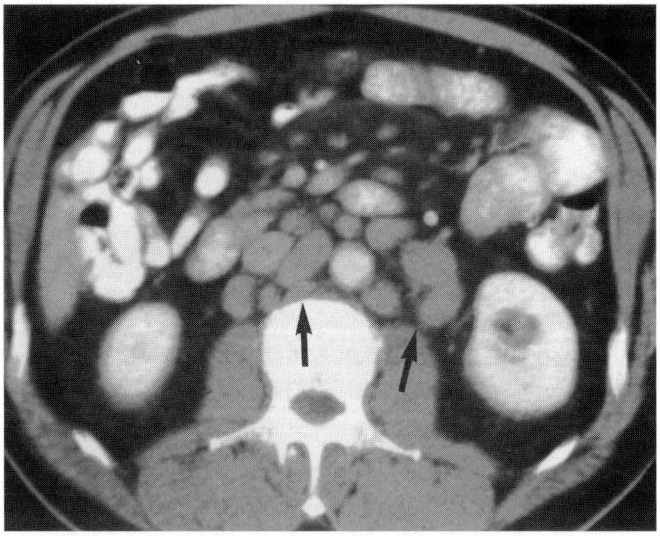

FIGURE 10.38 Non-Hodgkin lymphoma (NHL). Contrast-enhanced CT in a 60-year-old man with NHL shows multiple enlarged paraaortic and aortocaval lymph nodes *(arrows)*.

with extension to contiguous nodal groups. Extranodal disease beyond the spleen and abdominal involvement are less common than in NHL. Accurate staging is critical for patient management. Although CT is noninvasive and has a 70 to 90 percent accuracy in HD, lymphangiography is still performed at some centers for detection of disease in normal-sized retroperitoneal and peritoneal nodes, especially when lymph node enlargement is absent on CT. CT diagnosis of abdominal and pelvic lymphadenopathy is based on pathologic enlargement, but biopsy is necessary to confirm the diagnosis.

- **Non-Hodgkin lymphoma (NHL)** encompasses a diverse group of neoplasms and consequently demonstrates less predictable clinical behavior. Various classification systems have been employed in the past, with the "Working Formulation" representing the one most frequently used. This system broadly divides NHL into low-, intermediate-, and high-grade groups. Although the higher-grade tumors demonstrate more aggressive clinical behavior, the possibility for cure is better for this than for lower-grade disease. The Ann Arbor staging classification has also been applied to NHL. Overall, NHL involves the abdomen more frequently than HD, with mesenteric lymphadenopathy present in over one-half of all cases. In addition, extranodal involvement beyond the spleen is more common and is seen in approximately 25 percent of cases. Patients with congenital or acquired immunodeficiency are at significantly increased risk for developing a B-cell NHL and exhibit a higher frequency of extranodal disease (80 percent).

CT is the primary imaging modality for diagnosis and for evaluating response to therapy in patients with NHL. Bulky paraaortic and mesenteric lymphadenopathy is common; this can appear as discrete lymph node enlargement or as a coalescent mass **(Fig. 10.38).** Confluent lymphadenopathy with envelopment of mesenteric vessels on CT is called the **sandwich sign (Fig. 10.39).** Involved nodes are typically seen as homogeneous soft tissue attenuation on CT, although nodal calcification and central low attenuation are occasionally seen, especially following treatment. Moderate nodal enhancement is commonly seen after IV contrast administration. Diffuse peritoneal involvement can result in omental caking that resembles carcinomatosis (see **Fig. 10.16**).

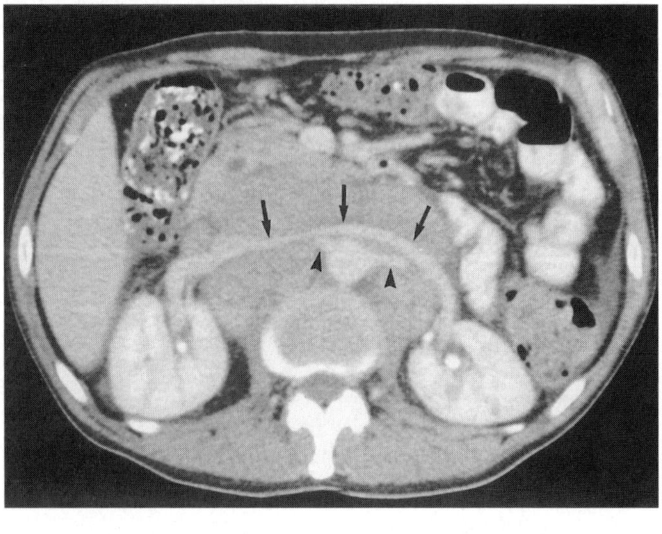

FIGURE 10.39 Sandwich sign in lymphoma. Contrast-enhanced CT in a 67-year-old man with NHL demonstrates confluent lymphadenopathy encasing but not occluding the left renal vein *(arrows)* and renal arteries *(arrowheads)*.

Bibliography

Cohan RH, Dunnick NR. The retroperitoneum. In: Haaga JR, ed. *Computed Tomography and Magnetic Resonance Imaging of the Whole Body,* 3rd ed. St Louis: Mosby-Yearbook; 1994:1292–1326.

Cooper C, Silverman PM, Davros WJ, Zeman RK. Delayed contrast enhancement of ascitic fluid on CT: Frequency and significance. *AJR* 1993; 161:787–790.

Einstein DM, Singer AA, Chilcote WA, Desai RK. Abdominal lymphadenopathy: Spectrum of CT findings. *Radiographics* 1991;11:457–472.

Fujiyoshi F, Ichinari N, Kajiya Y, Nishida H, Shimura T, Nakajo M, Matsunaga Y, Furoi A, Imaguma M. Retractile mesenteritis: Small-bowel radiography, CT, and MR imaging. *AJR* 1997;169:791–793.

Heiken JP, Winn SS. Abdominal wall and peritoneal cavity. In: Lee JKT, Sagel SS, Stanley RJ, Heiken JP, eds. *Computed Body Tomography with MRI Correlation,* 3rd ed. Philadelphia: Lippincott-Raven; 1998:971–1022.

Lee JKT, Hiken JN, Semelka RC. Retroperitoneum. In: Lee JKT, Sagel SS, Stanley RJ, Heiken JP, eds. *Computed Body Tomography with MRI Correlation,* 3rd ed. Philadelphia: Lippincott-Raven; 1998: 1023–1085.

Molmenti EP, Balfe DM, Kanterman RY, Bennett HF. Anatomy of the retroperitoneum: Observations of the distribution of pathologic fluid collection. *Radiology* 1996;200:95–103.

North LB, Wallace S, Lindell MM Jr, Jing B-S, Fuller LM, Allen PK. Lymphography or staging lymphomas: Is it still a useful procedure? *AJR* 1993;161:867–869.

Oliphant M, Berne AS, Meyers MA. The subperitoneal space of the abdomen and pelvis: Planes of continuity. *AJR* 1996;167:1433–1439.

Pickhardt PJ, Fisher AJ, Balfe DM, Dehner LP, Huettner PC. Desmoplastic small round cell tumor of the abdomen: Radiologic-histopathologic correlation. *Radiology* 1999;210:633–638.

Puylaert JBCM. Right-sided segmental infarction of the omentum: Clinical, US, and CT findings. *Radiology* 1992;185:169–172.

Rao PM, Rhea JT, Novelline RA. CT diagnosis of mesenteric adenitis. *Radiology* 1997;202:145–149.

Rao PM, Wittenberg J, Lawrason JN. Primary epiploic appendagitis: Evolutionary changes in CT appearance. *Radiology* 1997;204:713–717.

Stafford-Johnson DB, Bree RL, Francis IR, Korobkin M. CT appearance of primary papillary serous carcinoma of the peritoneum. *AJR* 1998;171:687–689.

Walensky RP, Venbrux AC, Prescott CA, Osterman FA Jr. Pseudomyxoma peritonei. *AJR* 1996;167:471–474.

Chapter 11

ADRENAL GLANDS

Andrew J. Fisher

11.1 Anatomy, Physiology, and Technique
11.2 Congenital Abnormalities
11.3 Hyperplasia, Infection, and Hemorrhage
11.4 Endocrine Abnormalities
11.5 Adrenal Adenomas
11.6 Other Benign Masses
11.7 Metastases
11.8 Other Malignant Masses

11.1 ANATOMY, PHYSIOLOGY, AND TECHNIQUE

- The **adrenal glands** lie along the anterosuperior renal margin, adjacent to the diaphragmatic crura. They are encompassed by the perinephric fat and contained within Gerota's fascia. The three morphologic components are the medial limb, lateral limb, and body.

  The adrenal glands coalesce from two distinct entities. The cortex develops from coelomic epithelium at the lower thoracic level. The adrenal medulla is formed by neural crest cells that migrate into the gland during embryogenesis. The kidneys ascend from the pelvis and abut the adrenals at 8 weeks of gestation, thus altering their appearance.

- The **adrenal cortex** has three layers: the zona glomerulosa, which produces aldosterone; the zona fasciculata, which synthesizes cortisol; and the zona reticulosa, which makes androgens, primarily testosterone. The **adrenal medulla** synthesizes catecholamines, namely epinephrine and norepinephrine. There is analogous tissue in the paravertebral sympathetic chain. Consequently, tumors that arise from the adrenal medulla occur in this distribution as well.

  Arterial supply is via the superior adrenal artery, arising from the inferior phrenic artery; the middle adrenal artery, arising from the aorta; and the inferior adrenal artery, arising from the renal artery. Venous drainage is usually via a single central vein that drains to the inferior vena cava (IVC).

- On **computed tomography (CT), normal adrenal glands** appear as thin, inverted Y- or V-shaped soft tissue structures with smooth medial and lateral limbs **(Fig. 11.1)**. These limbs should be roughly as thin as the adjacent diaphragmatic crus, approximately 4 mm in axial thickness. Adrenal margins should be flat or concave without significant nodularity. The normal adrenal gland has a 2- to 4-cm cephalocaudal span; the right is usually slightly more cephalad than the left. The gland is normally of uniform soft tissue attenuation, similar to the hepatic parenchyma.

  The right gland is superomedial to the kidney, posterior to the IVC, medial to the right hepatic lobe, and lateral to the right diaphragmatic crus. The left adrenal gland is more anterior in relation to the kidney than the right. It is bordered by the pancreatic body and tail and the stomach anterolaterally, the left diaphragmatic crus medially, and the kidney inferoposteriorly.

- On routine 5- to 8-mm thick **abdominal CT images,** the adrenal glands are usually well demonstrated, but they can be better characterized with dedicated adrenal technique. This generally involves 2- to 3-mm-thick contiguous sections through the adrenal fossae using a small field of view (FOV). It should be noted, however, that most adrenal lesions are identified on routine CT imaging, and dedicated thinner slices generally do not further contribute to lesion characterization. Helical CT can help in detecting small lesions by acquiring the target volume during a single breath-hold, thus avoiding respiratory misregistration. Also, multiplanar reconstructions can aid in determining the organ of origin in selected cases. Complete assessment involves evaluating the size, shape, contour, density, and symmetry of the glands.

- **Intravenous (IV) contrast** optimally demonstrates the relationship of an adrenal mass to adjacent vessels and parenchymal organs but is not necessary when specifically searching for or characterizing an adrenal lesion. In fact, noncontrast images are more valuable in distinguishing the most common benign lesion, the adenoma, from other adrenal masses. Enhancement patterns generally do not aid in differential diagnosis, although recent investigations suggest that enhancement patterns and contrast washout may help in distinguishing adrenal adenomas from metastatic disease **(Section 11.7).** Of note, IV contrast is often mistakenly withheld in cases of suspected pheochromocytoma owing to the largely historical potential for inciting a hypertensive crisis **(Section 11.6).**

11.2 CONGENITAL ABNORMALITIES

- Congenital absence of the adrenal gland is rare. Absence of both the adrenal gland and kidney is usually a result of prior surgery, as the adrenal glands are present in approximately 90 percent of cases of **renal agenesis** or other **congenital anomalies,** such as crossed ectopy. The adrenal's shape, however, is altered in these conditions, often demonstrating an elongated, discoid morphology **(Fig. 11.2).** This discoid morphology is also a relatively common normal variation, occurring (usually in the right adrenal gland) in patients with

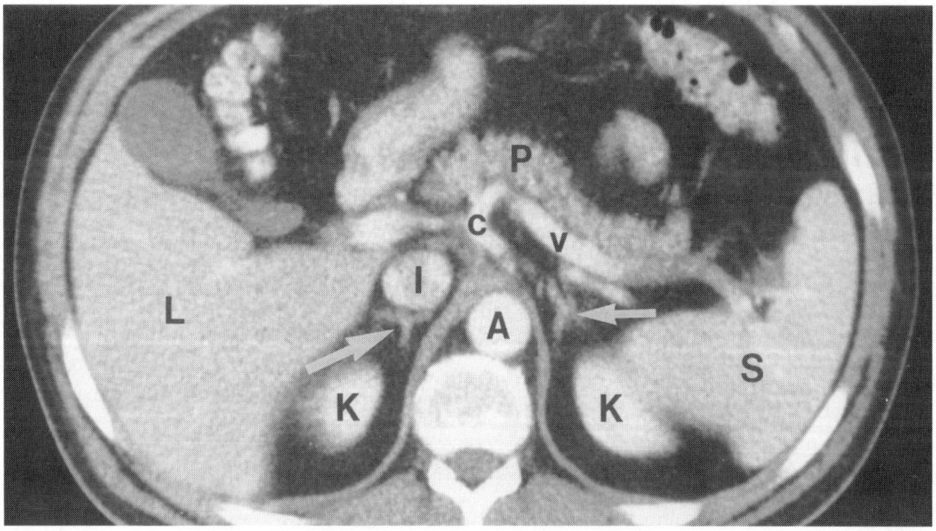

FIGURE 11.1 Normal adrenal glands. The normal adrenal glands *(arrows)* have an "inverted Y" shape and are only as thick as the adjacent diaphragmatic crura. L, liver; K, kidney; I, IVC; P, pancreas; c, celiax axis; A, aorta; v, splenic vein; S, spleen.

normal kidneys. Conversely, patients who have undergone nephrectomy with adrenal sparing will have normal adrenal morphology.

- **Congenital lesions** of the adrenal glands include hyperplasia, hemorrhage, and neuroblastoma. Congenital adrenal hemorrhage is the most common. Its presence sometimes signals an underlying congenital neuroblastoma; therefore, adrenal hemorrhages should be followed to resolution. It should be noted that patients with congenital neuroblastoma have a better prognosis than those who develop the tumor during childhood. These entities are more completely discussed in following sections.

11.3 HYPERPLASIA, INFECTION, AND HEMORRHAGE

- **Adrenal hyperplasia** is generally a bilateral process of adrenal enlargement, with increased cortisol secretion producing **Cushing syndrome.** In up to 85 percent of these patients, an adrenocorticotropic hormone (ACTH)-producing pituitary adenoma is the cause; however, exogenous steroids and paraneoplastic syndromes, especially from small cell carcinoma of the lung, can also produce this clinical condition.

  The adrenal glands may appear normal or smoothly thickened in the setting of hyperplasia **(Fig. 11.3).** Less commonly, they may demonstrate asymmetrical nodular thickening and may even appear as a dominant nodule simulating an adenoma. The most striking enlargement occurs in conjunction with ectopic ACTH production.
- **Macronodular hyperplasia** occasionally occurs. This process, often seen in long-standing hyperplasia, is generally ACTH-dependent; however, one or more nodules may be autonomous.

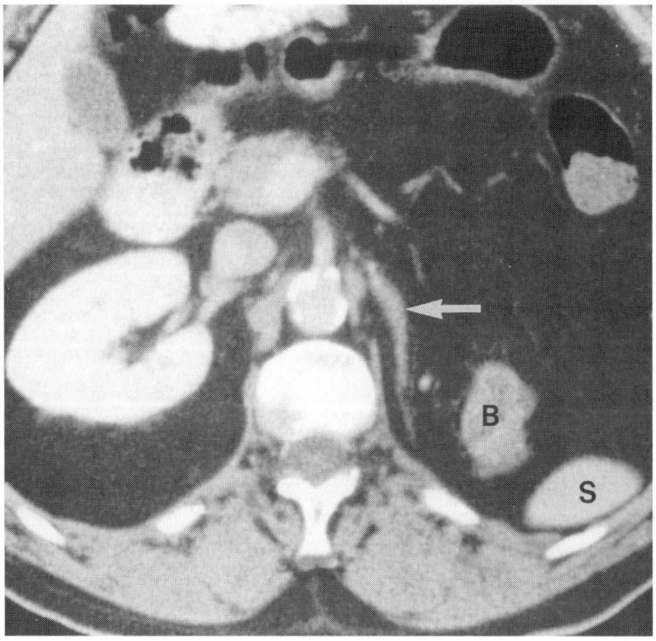

FIGURE 11.2 Renal agenesis. A disk-shaped left adrenal gland *(arrow)* is noted in this 72-year-old man with renal agenesis. A bowel loop (B) and the spleen (S) partially fill the renal fossa.

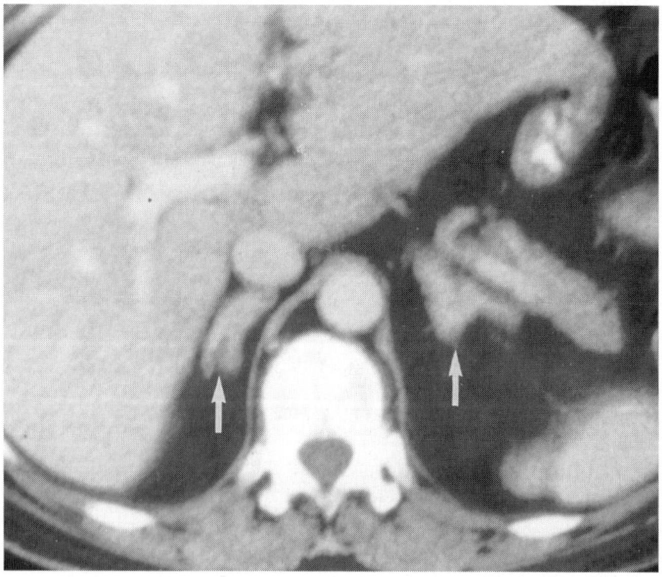

FIGURE 11.3 Adrenal hyperplasia. Bilateral adrenal thickening *(arrows)* due to an ACTH-secreting tumor in a 68-year-old woman. [From Slone RM, Gutierrez FR, Fisher AJ (eds.) *Thoracic Imaging: A Practical Approach.* New York: McGraw-Hill; 1999. With permission.]

Bilateral adrenalectomy may be necessary for definitive treatment. CT demonstrates diffusely thickened glands with one or more superimposed nodules.

- **Granulomatous disease,** generally histoplasmosis or tuberculosis, can involve the adrenal glands. Tuberculosis is a frequent cause of adrenal insufficiency (Addison disease), accounting for up to 30 percent of cases. Nearly half of all patients with disseminated histoplasmosis will develop Addison disease.

  During the acute phases of granulomatous infection, the adrenal glands enlarge and may become nodular in appearance. Central decreased attenuation and rim enhancement can be seen, and definitive diagnosis may require percutaneous biopsy. Over time, the adrenal glands may calcify diffusely **(Fig. 11.4).** This appearance is indistinguishable from prior hemorrhage or idiopathic adrenal calcification **(Differential 11.1).**

  Other infections are rare. These may be primary infections or superimposed upon existing abnormalities such as adrenal hematomas. Imaging may demonstrate only glandular enlargement; when a discrete mass occurs, it probably indicates development of an abscess.

- **Adrenal hemorrhage** may appear as a mass lesion. It is often precipitated by sepsis, birth trauma, or hypoxia in neonates and children. Another cause in children and adolescents is meningococcal sepsis leading to adrenal insufficiency **(Waterhouse-Friderichsen syndrome).** Adult adrenal hemorrhage is usually the result of blunt trauma, coagulopathy, or recent surgery. Only 2 percent of patients with severe abdominal trauma have radiologically evident findings of adrenal hemorrhage, although autopsy may reveal adrenal injury in up to 28 percent of this population. The overwhelming majority, approximately 90 percent, of adrenal hematomas related to blunt trauma occur on the right side.

  Acute hemorrhage is typically manifest as a round or oval adrenal mass with increased attenuation (50 to 90 HU) on noncontrast images **(Fig. 11.5).** Diffuse glandular enlargement is less common. There is often stranding and hemorrhage in the adjacent perinephric fat. Diagnosis is made by the combination of appropriate clinical history and decrease in size or attenuation of the adrenal mass on short-interval follow-up CT examination. Calcification and cyst formation are common as late sequelae.

- **Wolman disease** is a rare familial xanthomatosis. It is clinically manifest by failure to thrive, diarrhea, and malabsorption. The disease is usually fatal by 6 months of age. CT shows the results of lipid ester accumulation within abdominal organs, including bilateral adrenal enlargement with calcification and often hepatosplenomegaly. The adrenal attenuation is lower than normal due to increased lipid content. The adrenal calcifications may also be evident on plain films and sonography.

11.1

ADRENAL CALCIFICATION

Prior hemorrhage—coagulopathy, trauma, sepsis, dehydration
Tumor
  Neuroblastoma
  Adrenocortical carcinoma
  Metastases—mucinous primaries, posthemorrhage
  Adenoma
  Pheochromocytoma—"eggshell" calcification
  Ganglioneuroma
Idiopathic
Prior infection—granulomatous
Waterhouse-Friderichsen syndrome
Wolman disease

11.4 ENDOCRINE ABNORMALITIES

- Adrenal disease may result from intrinsic endocrinopathy, since the gland has significant hormonal function. Overproduction states,

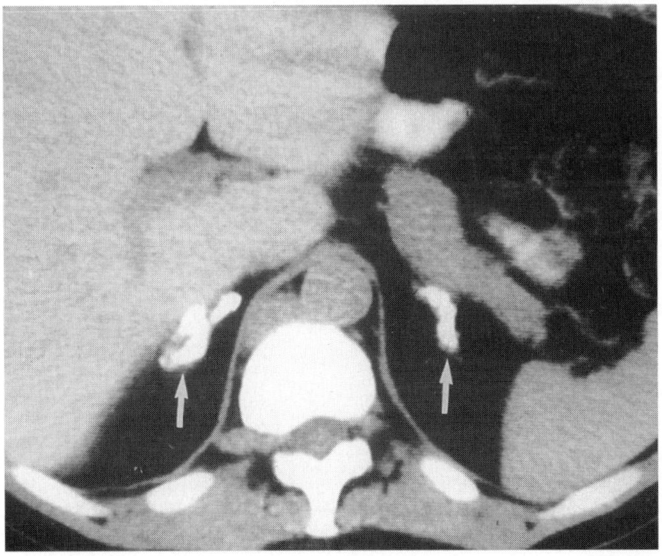

FIGURE 11.4 Adrenal calcification. The adrenal glands are diffusely calcified *(arrows)* in this patient, presumably from prior granulomatous disease. (Case courtesy of Dr. Jeffrey Brown, St. Louis, MO.)

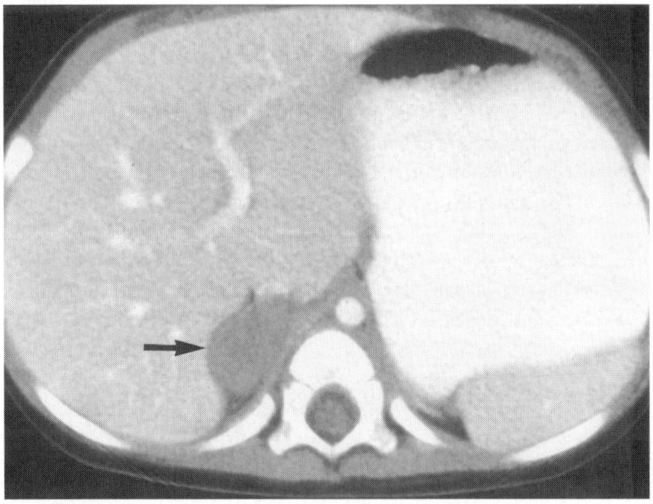

FIGURE 11.5 Adrenal hemorrhage. This 1-year-old girl had sustained a minor fall. There is a well-circumscribed low-attenuation right adrenal mass *(arrow)*. This resolved on follow-up imaging and is diagnostic of an adrenal hemorrhage. No other injury to a parenchymal organ was demonstrated. (Case courtesy of Dr. Jeffrey Friedland, Denver, CO.)

typically from adenomas and, less commonly, from adrenocortical carcinomas, include Cushing syndrome, Conn syndrome, and masculinization. Pheochromocytomas are often symptomatic from catecholamine secretion.

- **Cushing syndrome** results from excess serum cortisol. It is more common in women than in men (4:1), often presenting in the fourth decade. Manifestations include hypertension, "buffalo hump" fat deposition, abdominal striae, acne, amenorrhea, osteoporosis, and glucose intolerance. Laboratory evaluation reveals increased plasma cortisol and urinary 17-hydroxy catecholamine levels.

  Only 10 to 20 percent of **Cushing syndrome** patients have adrenal cortisol-producing adenomas. Of the remainder, 70 percent are attributable to pituitary adenomas or ectopic ACTH secretion resulting in adrenal hyperplasia. The final 10 percent are due to functional adrenocortical carcinomas or exogenous sources.

- **Conn syndrome** of hypokalemia, hypernatremia, and hypertension is a relatively uncommon entity. In contrast to Cushing syndrome, Conn syndrome is due to primary aldosterone-producing adenomas in the zona glomerulosa in almost 80 percent of cases. The remaining 20 percent are due to bilateral adrenal hyperplasia; adrenocortical carcinomas only rarely excrete aldosterone.

- Adenomas rarely produce the **androgenital syndrome.** Congenital androgenital syndrome results from an enzymatic deficiency in steroid synthesis, most commonly of 21-hydroxylase and 11-β-hydroxylase. The congenital form manifests as adrenal hyperplasia. Acquired androgenital syndrome is usually attributable to an adenoma of the zona reticularis and results in precocious puberty in boys and masculinization in women. Some 20 percent of cases are secondary to adrenocortical carcinoma.

- **Addison disease** is due to adrenal insufficiency. Symptoms develop insidiously and include fatigue, weakness, anorexia, nausea and emesis, and hypotension. Patients may have both mucosal and cutaneous pigmentation. Laboratory diagnosis centers around decreased serum cortisol levels.

  The acute and subacute forms of Addison disease are usually attributable to active adrenalitis or bilateral adrenal hemorrhage. Adrenalitis is most commonly the result of tuberculosis or fungal infections, while adrenal hemorrhage may be the result of shock, sepsis, coagulopathy, or trauma. Chronic Addison disease, present for 2 years or longer, is more commonly due to idiopathic adrenal atrophy and is usually autoimmune in nature. Previous granulomatous disease is another common cause of chronic Addison disease.

  CT imaging is clinically more helpful in acute cases, occasionally demonstrating bilateral adrenal hemorrhage, hematomas, or active adrenalitis. Imaging in chronic Addison disease is less helpful, as it is impossible to distinguish idiopathic adrenal atrophy from previous granulomatous disease. Both typically demonstrate small, calcified glands.

11.5 ADRENAL ADENOMAS

Adrenal adenomas are the most common benign tumors of the adrenal gland **(Differential 11.2).** They produce variable amounts of glucocorticoids, androgens, or mineralocorticoids. Clinical presentation depends on the type and amount of hormone production; the vast majority are identified as incidental lesions, and represent nonhyperfunctioning adenomas. An adrenal lesion may be seen on up to 4 percent of all abdominal CTs with over one-third of these lesions incidentally identified. Well over half of these adrenal lesions represent adenomas, with many occurring in oncologic patients.

11.2

ADRENAL MASS

Benign tumor
- **Adenoma**
- Myelolipoma
- Pheochromocytoma
- Ganglioneuroma

Malignant tumor
- **Metastases**—lung, breast, renal cell, melanoma
- **Neuroblastoma**
- Adrenocortical carcinoma
- Lymphoma—non-Hodgkin

Hyperplasia—bilateral
Hematoma—coagulopathy, severe stress, trauma, sepsis
Granulomatous disease—tuberculosis, histoplasmosis
Cyst
Mimic—pancreatic tail, fluid-filled bowel, renal apex, gastric diverticulum, collateral vessels, IVC, renal vein

Key: IVC, inferior vena cava.

- On **CT,** adenomas appear as nodules of varying size and attenuation. Generally, they are round or ovoid soft tissue masses. Adenomas that give rise to Cushing syndrome are often 2 cm or greater in size, while those in Conn syndrome are frequently smaller, typically 1 cm or less in size. Thus, thin-section images are necessary to properly evaluate patients with suspected adenomas. CT has a sensitivity of almost 100 percent for adenomas producing Cushing syndrome but only 90 percent for those producing Conn syndrome **(Fig. 11.6).**

  Adrenal adenomas imaged by noncontrast CT have **low attenuation** due to intracellular lipid deposition from steroid synthesis **(Fig. 11.7).** Various noncontrast attenuation levels have been proposed for diagnosing adenomas. An attenuation of less than 10 HU on noncontrast CT is considered diagnostic. Although

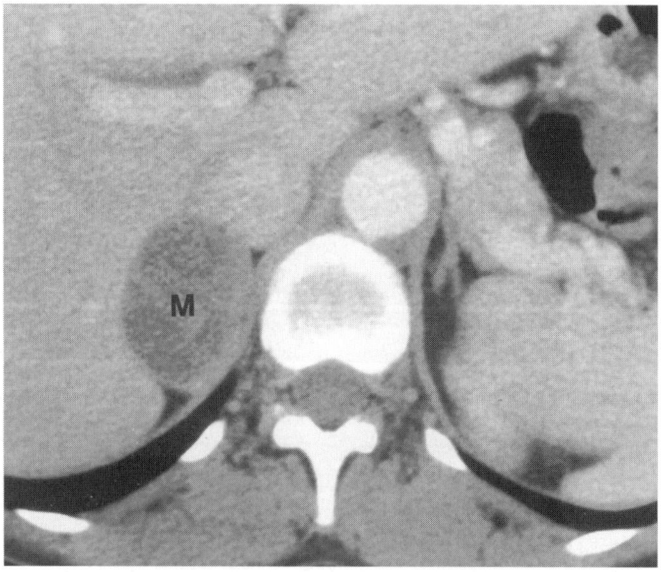

FIGURE 11.6 Hyperaldosteronoma. A 37-year-old woman with hypertension and hypokalemia. There is a low-attenuation (22 HU) right adrenal mass (M) that is likely an adrenal adenoma. This is in keeping with Conn syndrome.

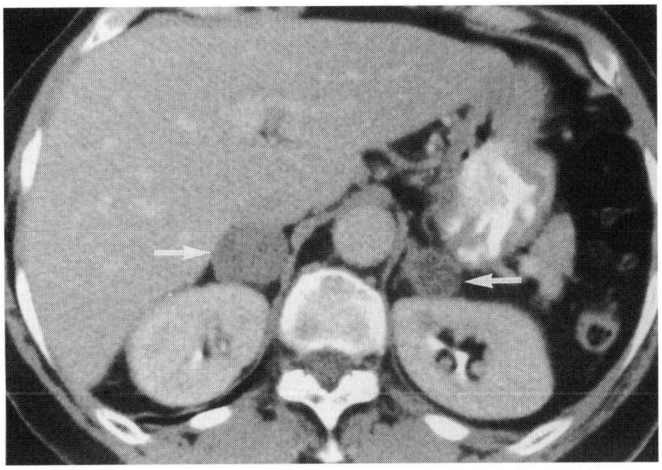

FIGURE 11.7 Bilateral adrenal adenomas. A 67-year-old woman with symmetrical, near-water-attenuation adrenal masses *(arrows)* even following administration of IV contrast.

adenomas may demonstrate prominent enhancement similar to that of metastases, they will usually have lower HU values on delayed images due to more rapid washout of contrast. One proposed cutoff is an attenuation value less than 24 HU at 15 minutes. More recent work with contrast washout curves has shown that a 15-minute postcontrast attenuation of 37 HU has a 96 percent sensitivity and specificity for adenoma, with a similar value at 30 minutes giving a 93 percent sensitivity and 100 percent specificity.

- **Magnetic resonance imaging** (MRI) can usually confirm an adrenal adenoma if attenuation values on noncontrast CT are equivocal. In-phase and opposed-phase imaging capitalizes on the differences in precessional frequencies of fat and water protons. This results in intravoxel cancellation of microscopic fat and water present in adenomas. Consequently, signal dropout on opposed-phase imaging is highly specific for adenomas, confirming the diagnosis **(Fig. 11.8).** Adrenal biopsy may be necessary in indeterminate cases or when histologic sampling is required prior to therapy.

11.6 OTHER BENIGN MASSES

- **Pheochromocytomas,** or adrenal paragangliomas, are neuroendocrine tumors of chromaffin-cell origin arising from the adrenal medulla. Their production of catecholamines can lead to episodic symptoms of headaches, flushing, hypertension, and palpitations. Urinary catecholamines and vanillylmandelic acid (VMA) are elevated and serve as clinical clues to the diagnosis.

  Approximately 90 percent of pheochromocytomas are unilateral and arise within the adrenal gland. Extra-adrenal pheochromocytomas may occur anywhere along the sympathetic chain, including the organ of Zuckerkandl, a site located between the origin of the inferior mesenteric artery and the aortic bifurcation.

  There is inheritance of pheochromocytomas in 10 percent of cases. **Multiple endocrine neoplasia (MEN) syndrome type IIA** (Sipple syndrome) is the combination of pheochromocytoma, medullary carcinoma of the thyroid, and parathyroid adenoma. **MEN IIB** (mucosal neuroma syndrome) is the combination of pheochromocytoma, medullary carcinoma of the thyroid, and mucosal neuromas. In these conditions, the patient typically has

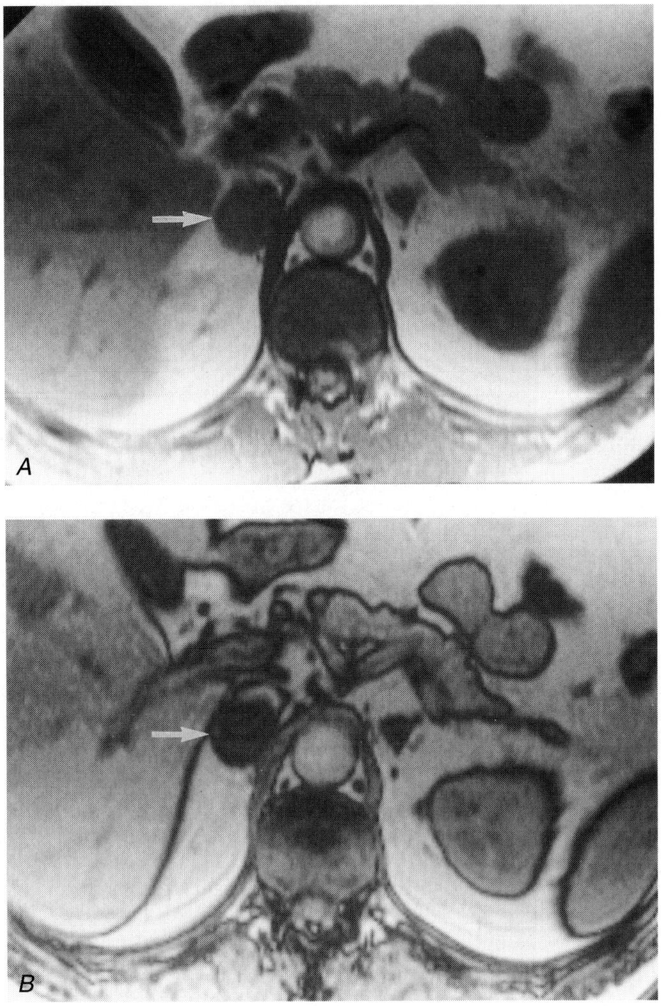

FIGURE 11.8 Adrenal adenoma. A 51-year-old man being evaluated for renal artery stenosis with an adrenal lesion. In-phase MR image *(A)* demonstrates a 1-cm right adrenal lesion *(arrow)* that is isointense to the hepatic parenchyma. Out-of-phase MR image *(B)* shows lower intensity in the lesion than in the liver owing to intravoxel cancellation of water and fat (signal dropout), diagnostic of an adrenal adenoma.

smaller and often bilateral pheochromocytomas. Other inherited conditions associated with pheochromocytomas include the neurocutaneous syndromes of von Hippel-Lindau, tuberous sclerosis, and neurofibromatosis. A familial form of isolated pheochromocytomas also exists.

- On **CT,** pheochromocytomas appear as soft tissue adrenal lesions that densely enhance following IV contrast administration. Hemorrhagic central necrosis may be present in this hypervascular tumor, particularly with increasing tumor size **(Fig. 11.9).** Calcifications are present in 10 percent of cases and generally are thin and peripheral.

  Limited noncontrast thin sections through the adrenal fossa can be obtained if a pheochromocytoma is clinically suspected. This is done both to avoid IV contrast administration and to identify the lesion in the appropriate clinical setting. IV contrast is often withheld owing to concern for precipitating a hypertensive crisis, although recent reports suggest that nonionic contrast is safe in these patients. Alpha-adrenergic blockade by phentolamine can be

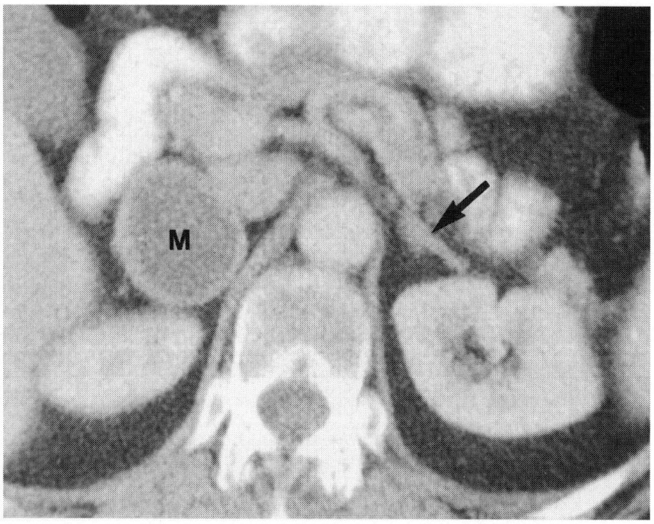

FIGURE 11.9 Pheochromocytoma. A 59-year-old woman with hypertension. A right adrenal mass (M) is present, with central necrosis and peripheral enhancement. The left adrenal gland *(arrow)* is normal.

employed to reduce the likelihood of precipitating a symptomatic hypertensive episode.

Pheochromocytomas are characteristically of low signal intensity on T1-weighted MRI and "light bulb bright" on T2-weighted images. Reported sensitivity in lesion detection approaches 100 percent.

- **Paragangliomas** are extra-adrenal pheochromocytomas. As mentioned, they can occur anywhere along the sympathetic chain from the mediastinum through the retroperitoneum and pelvis. Paragangliomas have a slightly greater malignant potential than adrenal pheochromocytomas.

  This tumor can be solitary or multiple and its imaging characteristics are nonspecific **(Fig. 11.10).** They are enhancing soft tissue paraspinal masses sometimes demonstrating low-attenuation central necrosis. On CT, malignant paragangliomas are difficult to distinguish from other retroperitoneal malignancies. Ectopic lesions can be localized with indium-111 octreotide or iodine-131 methyliodobenzylguanidine (MIBG) scintigraphy.

- **Ganglioneuromas** are benign neural crest tumors that can arise anywhere along the sympathetic chain, but approximately 40 percent occur in the adrenal gland. Although they are less common than the malignant neuroblastoma **(Section 11.7),** ganglioneuromas may result from the spontaneous differentiation of a neuroblastoma. This is most frequently seen in patients under 2 years of age. A ganglioneuroblastoma **(Fig. 11.11).** is an intermediate lesion with malignant potential.

  On **CT imaging,** ganglioneuromas are often indistinguishable from their malignant counterpart, usually having an infiltrative appearance and containing calcifications. Ganglioneuromas may, however, demonstrate a more benign appearance with margination, homogeneous low attenuation, and enhancement following IV contrast administration. Demonstrable lack of growth over time or excision is required to assure benignity or confirm the diagnosis.

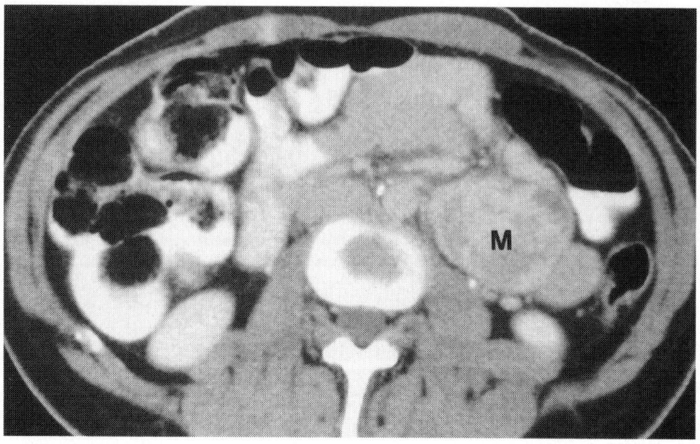

FIGURE 11.10 Left paraganglioma. IV contrast–enhanced CT demonstrates a heterogeneous, partially necrotic paravertebral mass (M) in this 41-year-old woman with hypertension.

- **Myelolipomas** are uncommon, benign adrenal tumors containing bone marrow and soft tissue elements. They do not produce hormones and consequently are detected in asymptomatic patients unless they hemorrhage or compress adjacent structures.

  CT demonstrates macroscopic fat (-30 to -110 HU), obviating the need for biopsy **(Fig. 11.12).** These attenuation values are markedly lower than expected for cortical adenomas. Soft tissue myeloid elements may predominate and can demonstrate enhancement following IV contrast administration. Dystrophic calcification is seen in about 20 percent. No treatment is required unless the pa-

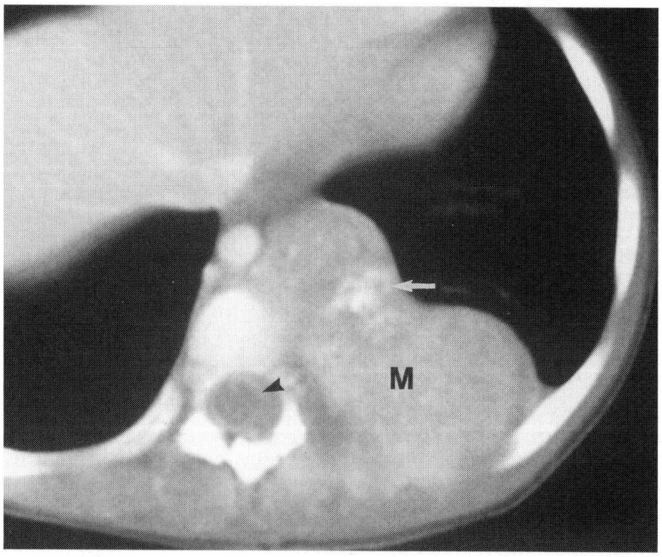

FIGURE 11.11 Ganglioneuroblastoma. A young boy with neurologic symptoms. CT after IV contrast demonstrates an enhancing left paravertebral mass (M) with regions of calcification *(arrow).* The eccentric position of the thecal sac *(arrowhead)* confirms tumor extension into the spinal canal, which was demonstrated to better advantage on subsequent MR imaging. (Case courtesy of Dr. Jeffrey Friedland, Denver, CO.)

tient is symptomatic. Rarely, the tumor occurs in an extra-adrenal location and can be mistaken for a liposarcoma, necessitating biopsy or excision.

On **MRI,** portions of the lesion will follow fat signal on all sequences. This macroscopic fat will not show signal dropout with opposed-phase imaging since there are no water protons to cancel the fat protons; however, decreased signal can be seen with radiofrequency (RF) fat saturation, confirming the diagnosis. Variable soft tissue components will demonstrate low to intermediate signal intensity on T1-weighted MRI and higher signal intensity on T2-weighted images.

- **Adrenal cysts** are rare and typically asymptomatic. They may produce pain from mass effect, following hemorrhage, or due to superimposed infection. Adrenal cysts are either true epithelial cysts, pseudocysts, or parasitic cysts. Pseudocysts lack a cellular lining and result from prior hemorrhage; they constitute almost 40 percent of adrenal cysts. Parasitic adrenal cysts are distinctly rare and typically associated with echinococcal disease. Hemorrhagic adrenal cysts may be seen following trauma or in conjunction with Beckwith-Wiedemann syndrome (macroglossia, gigantism, organomegaly, omphalocele, exophthalmos).

  On **CT** images, adrenal cysts possess imaging characteristics similar to those of simple cysts anywhere in the body. Pseudocysts or parasitic cysts are more likely to contain foci of mural calcifications than true adrenal cysts. Cysts may be indistinguishable from adenomas on noncontrast CT because of their comparable attenuation. Lack of IV contrast enhancement demonstrates their true cystic nature. Adrenal cysts may demonstrate increased attenuation subsequent to hemorrhage or infection.

- **Adrenal pseudotumors** are simulated masses in the expected location of the gland itself. Etiologies vary depending on the anatomic site. On the left, etiologies include splenules, unopacified small bowel loops, gastric diverticulae **(Fig. 11.13),** renal masses, and tortuous splenic or renal vessels. Right-sided adrenal pseudotumors may be attributable to tortuous renal vessels, the IVC, the duodenum, or renal pathology. Examination of contiguous slices is essential, and thin collimation may be necessary to identity the true nature of these "lesions." Helical CT with multiplanar reconstructions or MRI may demonstrate the organ of origin to greater advantage in difficult cases.

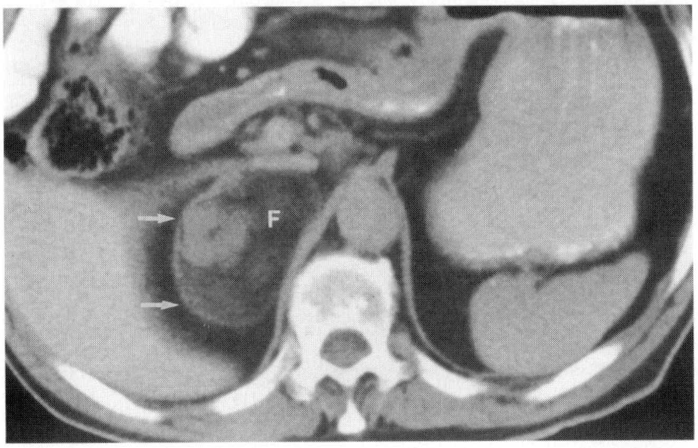

FIGURE 11.12 Myelolipoma. Contrast-enhanced CT demonstrates a heterogeneous mass in the right adrenal gland *(arrows)* with macroscopic fat (F) confirming a myelolipoma.

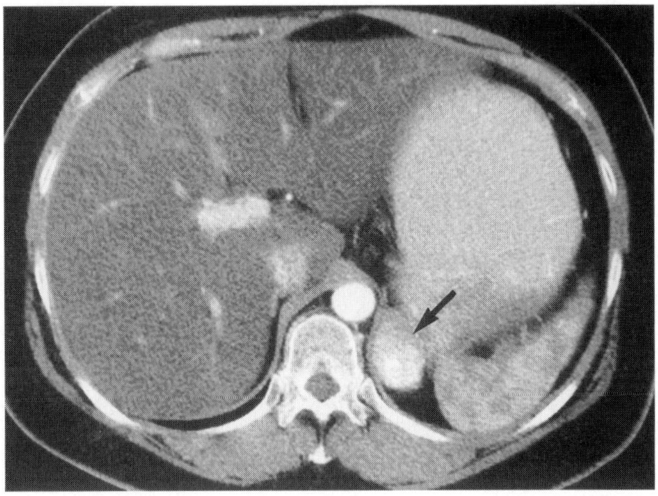

FIGURE 11.13 Adrenal pseudotumor. There is a high-attenuation mass *(arrow)* in the expected location of the left adrenal gland. This is a gastric diverticulum, with the increased attenuation resulting from pooling of oral contrast. A normal left adrenal gland was identified more inferiorly. The liver had diffuse fatty infiltration.

11.7 METASTASES

- Chest CTs traditionally extend through the adrenal glands to exclude **metastatic disease** in patients with known or suspected malignancy. Metastases commonly occur in the adrenal gland; up to one-quarter of patients with a known malignancy have adrenal metastases at autopsy. Adrenal metastases, however, rarely occur in the absence of a known or suspected primary neoplasm. Less than 10 percent of incidentally discovered adrenal masses are malignant.

  The most frequent primary malignancies include bronchogenic, renal cell, breast, melanoma, and gastrointestinal malignancies. Adrenal metastases may be found on CT in up to 24 percent of patients with known bronchogenic carcinoma; however, adenomas still account for at least two-thirds of adrenal masses in this population. Some adrenal metastases may hemorrhage spontaneously and produce acute flank pain.

- The **CT imaging** characteristics of metastatic deposits are variable and rarely permit a definitive diagnosis. Typically, an adrenal metastasis appears as a nodule of variable size that enhances following IV contrast administration **(Fig. 11.14).** Metastases in general are larger and less well defined than adenomas. Of course, there is significant overlap; many metastatic deposits measure less than 3 cm and, conversely, larger lesions can prove to be benign.

  Adrenal metastases may be heterogeneous in attenuation and demonstrate an enhancing rim. Unless noncontrast CT images demonstrate an attenuation of less than 10 HU, characteristic of benign adenomas, the lesion should be considered indeterminate. Recent work suggests that delayed CT (1 hour after IV contrast administration) shows adenomas to have a mean attenuation of 11 HU and metastases to have a mean attenuation of 49 HU. Consequently, below a 30-HU cutoff, sensitivity was 95 percent and specificity was 100 percent for adenomas. The presence of metastatic lesions elsewhere, particularly in the liver, serves as a clue to the correct diagnosis. Hemorrhagic metastases will demonstrate lesion irregularity and heterogeneity, often with stranding in the adjacent perinephric fat **(Fig. 11.15).**

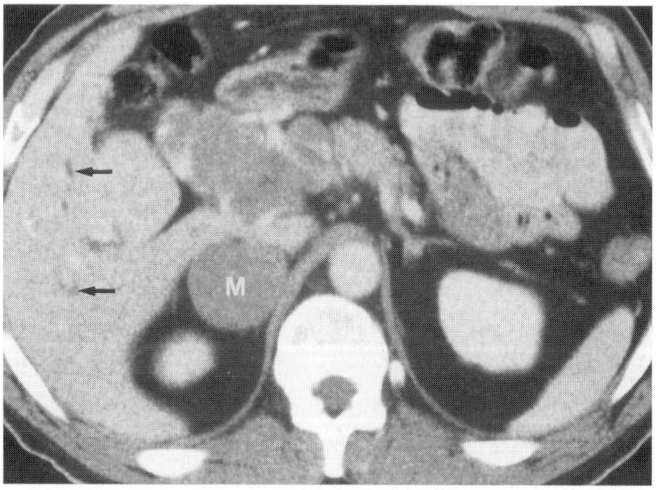

FIGURE 11.14 Adrenal metastasis. There is a circumscribed, hypoenhancing right adrenal metastasis (M) that replaces the gland in this man with known metastatic melanoma. This lesion is greater than 20 HU. Biliary dilatation *(arrows)* was secondary to a mass of the pancreatic head. [From Slone RM, Gutierrez FR, Fisher AJ (eds.) *Thoracic Imaging: A Practical Approach.* New York: McGraw-Hill; 1999. With permission.]

MRI can confirm that an adrenal lesion is an adenoma if there is signal dropout on opposed-phase imaging, but the lack of signal dropout does not entirely exclude an adenoma. Therefore, such a lesion should be considered indeterminate, possibly representing a metastatic focus. The multiplanar capabilities of MRI are beneficial in determining the organ of origin. Definitive diagnosis requires biopsy using either CT or sonographic guidance.

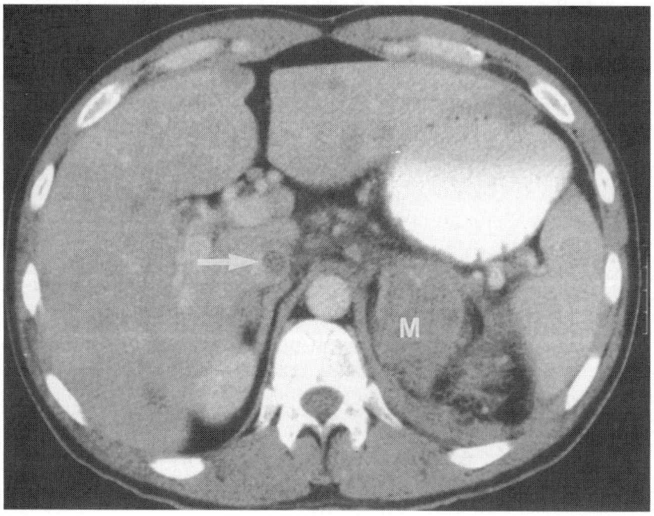

FIGURE 11.15 Hemorrhagic adrenal metastasis. A 38-year-old man with testicular cancer and acute left flank pain. There is a heterogeneous left adrenal mass (M) with low-attenuation regions and adjacent soft tissue stranding. Thrombus is present within the IVC *(arrow)* and there are multiple hepatic metastases.

Adrenal biopsy may be required in indeterminate cases or for histologic evaluation prior to commencing cancer therapy. CT generally is the guidance modality of choice, although larger lesions may be readily demonstrable on sonography. A posterior approach is taken, with attention paid to the posterior pleural reflections. A coaxial system with an 18-gauge outer guide needle allows for multiple samples to be obtained using a smaller biopsy needle without repositioning **(Fig. 11.16).**

11.8 OTHER MALIGNANT MASSES

- **Adrenocortical carcinomas** are rare malignancies. They occur in patients around 40 years of age and demonstrate no gender predilection. Adrenocortical carcinomas are functional in about 50 percent of cases, with Cushing syndrome the most common hormonal presentation. This may be seen in conjunction with virilization. The remainder are discovered incidentally or in a patient complaining of abdominal fullness or tenderness. Prognosis is generally poor and, to date, chemotherapy has been ineffective.

  On **CT imaging,** adrenocortical carcinomas are typically large (>5 cm), heterogeneous, and partially necrotic tumors that arise from the adrenal cortex **(Fig. 11.17).** Bilateral tumors are present in fewer than 10 percent of cases. They enhance heterogeneously and calcify in up to 30 percent of cases. Adrenocortical carcinomas spread by local extension to involve the kidney, liver, or IVC; hematogenous dissemination to the pulmonary parenchyma and regional lymph nodes also occurs.

- **Lymphoma** of the adrenal gland is uncommon but may be evident in up to 4 percent of patients diagnosed with lymphoma. Non-Hodgkin lymphoma is most common, with the adrenal glands usually secondarily involved. Up to one-third of such patients will have bilateral adrenal involvement and may clinically present with Addison disease. Primary adrenal involvement with lymphoma is distinctly rare. Leukemia involving the adrenal glands will have a similar appearance.

  CT demonstrates soft tissue masses enlarging or replacing the gland. Contrast enhancement is similar to that seen with retroperitoneal adenopathy. Adrenal disease is often difficult to separate

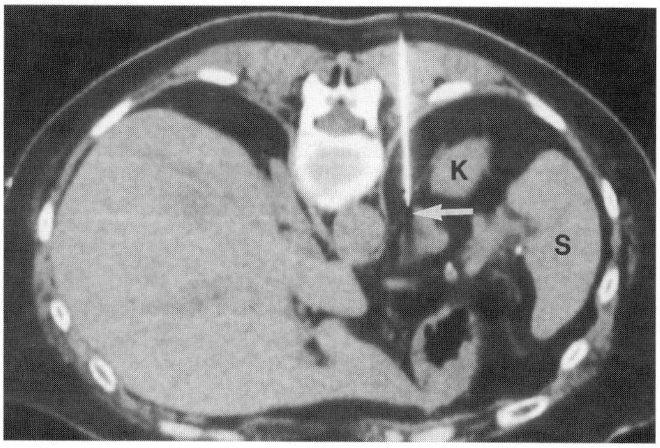

FIGURE 11.16 Adrenal biopsy. CT guidance is used to place the guide and biopsy needles in a coaxial fashion. The black streak artifact *(arrow)* localizes the needle tip. S, spleen; K, left kidney.

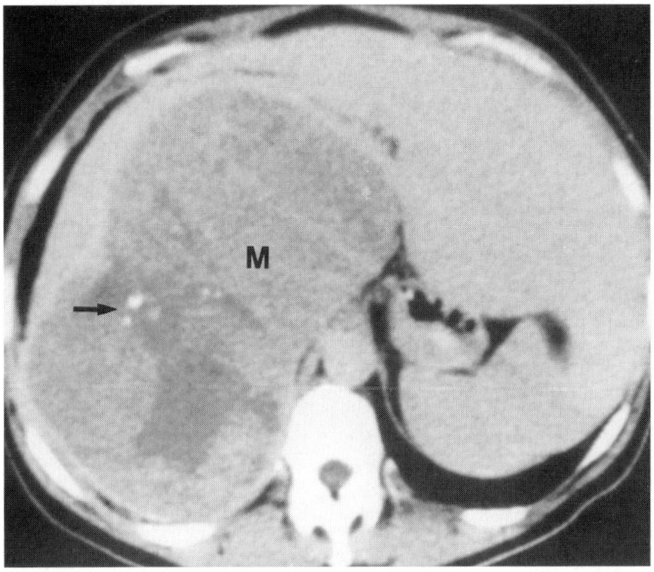

FIGURE 11.17 Adrenocortical carcinoma. This CT shows a large suprarenal mass (M) displacing the liver to the left. The mass has necrosis and central calcifications *(arrow).* [From Slone RM, Gutierrez FR, Fisher AJ (eds.) *Thoracic Imaging: A Practical Approach.* New York: McGraw-Hill; 1999. With permission.]

from adjacent retroperitoneal nodal masses, and most patients have concomitant adenopathy **(Fig. 11.18).** Ipsilateral renal and contralateral adrenal involvement are occasionally seen.

- **Neuroblastoma** is a primary adrenal malignancy arising from neural crest cells. It is the most common solid abdominal mass in infancy and the most common extracranial malignancy in young children. In addition to abdominal pain and mass, paraneoplastic presentations can include diarrhea from vasoactive intestinal peptide (VIP) secretion, paroxysmal flushing from catecholamine production, and myoclonus or opsoclonus. Most patients have a positive marrow aspirate at the time of diagnosis. Early presentation (diagnosis at less than 1 year of age) has a better prognosis. Some 1 percent convert spontaneously to benign ganglioneuromas or resolve completely.

  Neuroblastoma can arise anywhere along the sympathetic chain. On **CT,** adrenal lesions are large, heterogeneous, and irregularly marginated soft tissue masses **(Fig. 11.19).** They frequently demonstrate areas of necrosis. The majority contain stippled calcifications that serve as a diagnostic clue. Regional spread is common, as are nodal, hepatic, osseous, and pulmonary metastases. Intraspinal spread is more frequently seen in neuroblastoma arising from the extra-adrenal sympathetic chain.

- **The staging of neuroblastoma** is as follows:

  Stage I—Confined to the organ of origin.
  Stage II—Local tumor extension that does not cross midline.
  Stage III—Continuous involvement crossing the midline, bilateral lymph node involvement.
  Stage IV—Disseminated neuroblastoma.
  Stage IV-S—Patients less than 1 year old with stage I–II primary tumor and metastases limited to the skin, liver, and bone marrow yet without radiologic evidence of osseous metastases. Stage IV-S confers a more favorable prognosis.

- **Eponymic neuroblastoma syndromes** include pepper, blueberry muffin, and Hutchinson types. Pepper syndrome includes metastatic disease causing severe hepatomegaly; blueberry muffin syndrome includes multiple skin metastases; and Hutchinson syndrome includes cranial metastases and proptosis.

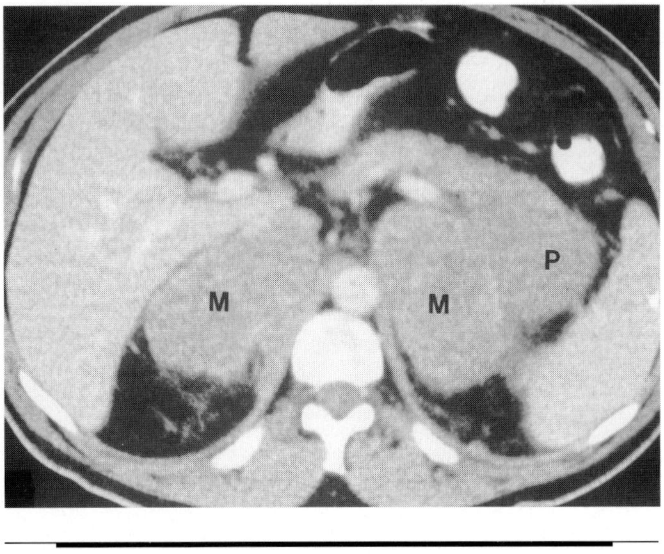

FIGURE 11.18 Adrenal lymphoma. A 52-year-old man with disseminated abdominal lymphoma has bilateral hypoenhancing masses (M) secondarily involving the adrenal glands. There is also a lymphomatous mass enlarging the pancreatic tail (P).

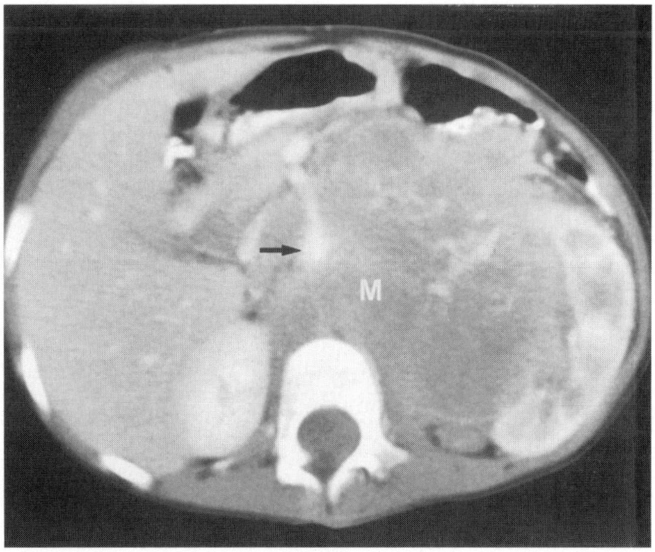

FIGURE 11.19 Neuroblastoma. CT after IV contrast demonstrates a large, infiltrating soft tissue mass (M) that extends across the midline, elevating the aorta *(arrow)* from the spine. The left kidney has a delayed nephrogram, indicating obstruction. (Case courtesy of Dr. Jeffrey Friedland, Denver, CO.)

Bibliography

Cirillo RL Jr, Bennett WF, Vitellas KM, Poulos AG, Bova JG. Pathology of the adrenal gland: Imaging features. *AJR* 1998;170:429–435.

Kawashima A, Sandler CM, Fishman EK, et al. Spectrum of CT findings in nonmalignant disease of the adrenal glands. *Radiographics* 1998;18:393–412.

Kenney PJ, Robbins GL, Ellis DA, Spirt BA. Adrenal glands in patients with congenital renal anomalies: CT appearance. *Radiology* 1985;155:181–182.

Korobkin M, Brodeur FJ, Francis IR, Quint LE, Dunnick NR, Londy F. Imaging of adrenal masses. *Urol Clin North Am* 1997;24:603–622.

Korobkin M, Brodeur FJ, Francis IR, et al. CT time-attenuation washout curves of adrenal adenomas and nonadenomas. *AJR* 1998;170:747–752.

Kenney PJ, Lee JKT: The adrenals. In: Lee JKT, Sagel SS, Stanley RJ, Heiken JP, eds. *Computed Body Tomography with MRI Correlation,* 3rd ed. Philadelphia: Lippincott-Raven; 1998:1171–1208.

Westra SJ, Zaninovic AC, Hall TR, Kangarloo H, Boechat MI. Imaging of the adrenal gland in children. *Radiographics* 1994;14:1323–1340.

Chapter 12

KIDNEYS

Andrew J. Fisher

12.1 Anatomy, Physiology, and Technique
12.2 Congenital Abnormalities
12.3 Nephrocalcinosis and Urolithiasis
12.4 Infectious, Inflammatory, and Vascular Conditions
12.5 Cystic Disease
12.6 Benign Masses
12.7 Malignant Masses
12.8 Surgery

12.1 ANATOMY, PHYSIOLOGY, AND TECHNIQUE

- The **kidneys** reside in the retroperitoneum, encompassed by perinephric fat and Gerota's fascia. Each kidney is encased within a fibrous renal capsule. Connective tissue septa extend outward from the capsular surface to Gerota's fascia. The kidneys' main purpose is to filter the blood and regulate arterial pressure. They also secrete erythropoietin. The renal cortex contains the glomeruli, while the medulla is predominantly composed of uriniferous tubules. Centrally, renal sinus fat surrounds the collecting system and the renal vessels. At the hilum of the kidney, the urine-containing calyces join, forming the renal pelvis. The pelvis transitions to the proximal ureter at the ureteropelvic junction.

  Embryologically, the kidney develops from two distinct parts of the mesoderm. Renal nephrons develop from the metanephric mesoderm, whereas the lower urinary tract—including the distal collecting tubules, calyces, renal pelvis, ureters, and bladder trigone—develops from the ureteral bud. Early in embryogenesis, the kidneys lie close together, positioned anterior to the sacrum with the hila directed anteriorly. As the fetus develops, differential growth causes the kidneys to migrate cephalad, away from the midline; at the same time, the hila rotate medially. The kidneys attain their adult position by the ninth gestational week.

  The kidneys are supplied by a main renal artery originating from the aorta, usually at the L2 level. Accessory renal arteries can be present and arise from the abdominal aorta or the common iliac arteries. There is usually a single main renal vein on each side that drains directly into the inferior vena cava (IVC). Although the left renal vein generally courses anterior to the abdominal aorta, it may travel posterior to the aorta (retrocaval left renal vein) or branch and encompass the aorta (circumaortic left renal vein).

- **The ureters** are paired structures that course from the renal hila to the bladder trigone. They take an oblique course from a medial, paravertebral position at their junction with the renal pelvis to cross over the iliac vasculature and then run adjacent to the pelvic sidewalls before deviating medially into the bladder. In its cephalad course, the ureter is lateral to the gonadal vein, but this relationship reverses near the level of the iliac crests. Because the ureter undergoes peristaltic contractions, the ureteral caliber varies significantly over its course.

  The ureter is composed of three histologic layers: the transitional epithelium of the mucosa with a supporting lamina propria; the double-layered muscularis; and the adventitia. The normal ureteral wall is less than 1 mm thick, but it can be demonstrated on CT imaging. The ureteral arterial supply is variable and poorly visualized on CT. Lymphatic drainage is shared proximally with that of the kidney and distally with that of the bladder. The lymphatic drainage of the midureter is variable.

  Conventional **computed tomography (CT) technique** using 5- to 10-mm collimation adequately demonstrates the kidneys in most cases. Helical CT is employed when there is clinical suspicion of subtle renal pathology, since it has the benefit of avoiding respiratory misregistration. Moreover, rapid acquisition enables dual-phase imaging and improved detection of transiently enhancing masses. Intravenous (IV) contrast is routinely used to allow differentiation of pathologic processes from the normal parenchyma. Corticomedullary differentiation is maximal on images obtained 30 seconds after the beginning of the contrast bolus; the nephrographic phase is best seen 70 to 100 seconds after the beginning of the bolus **(Fig. 12.1).**

  Helical CT is also used for the detection of acute urolithiasis. In this setting, neither oral nor IV contrast is administered. Consequently, focal high-attenuation regions are due to calcium-containing structures: vascular calcifications, pelvic phleboliths, or ureteral calculi. For this clinical indication, 5-mm collimation with a pitch of 1.4 to 1.6 is typically used. Additional imaging with IV contrast is helpful in confusing cases or in those where other etiologies for the acute presentation are identified and require further evaluation.

12.2 CONGENITAL ABNORMALITIES

- When there is an **empty renal fossa,** several entities should be considered. The kidney may have been atrophic or ectopic or it may have been surgically excised. Renal ectopia includes **horseshoe kidney,** where there is an isthmus of renal parenchyma or fibrous tissue joining low-lying kidneys that cross the midline **(Fig. 12.2).** Horseshoe kidneys are prone to vesicoureteral reflux, hydronephrosis, calculi, and trauma. In **crossed-fused ectopia,** the left kidney is

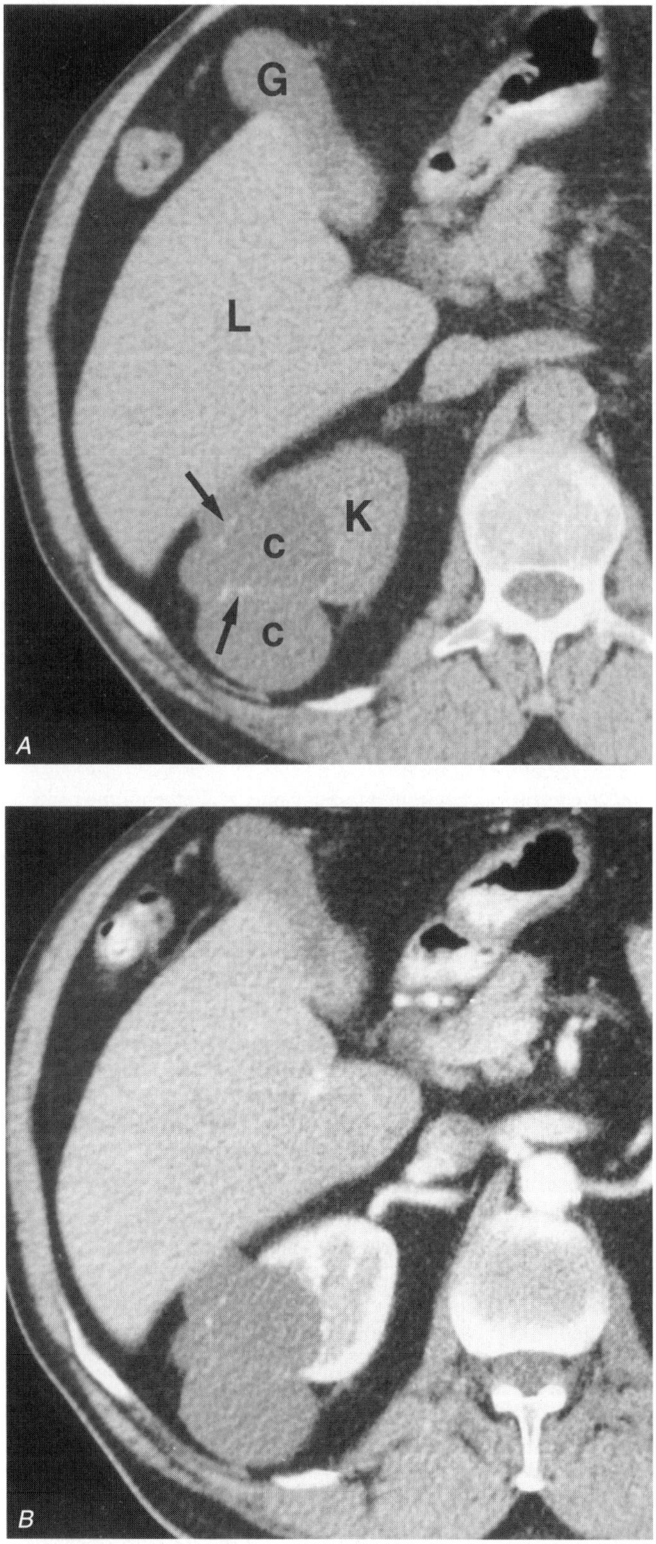

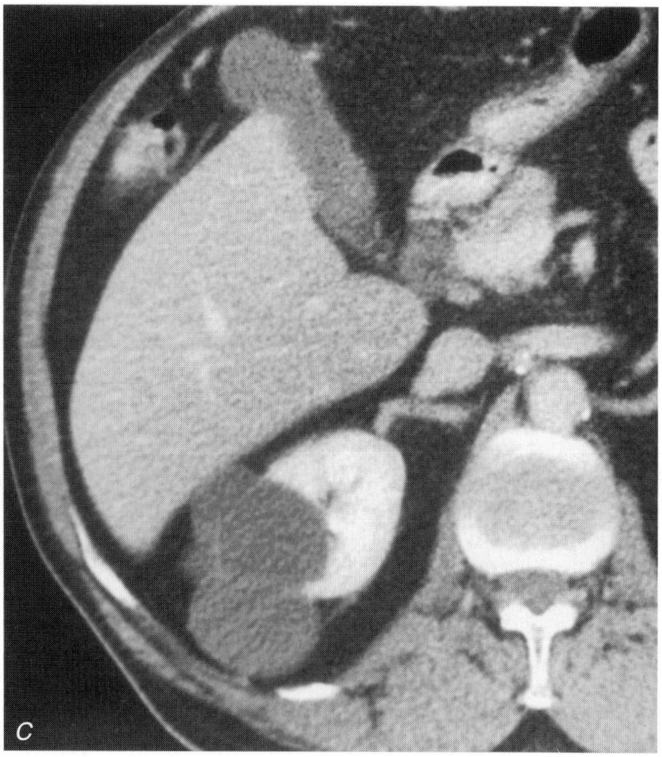

FIGURE 12.1 **Dual-phase renal CT.** Noncontrast *(A)*, corticomedullary *(B)*, and nephrographic *(C)* phase images in a 71-year-old man with hematuria. In the corticomedullary phase *(B)*, there is dense aortic and renal cortical enhancement, while in the nephrographic phase *(C)*, there is venous opacification and uniform renal enhancement. Additionally, there is a septated cyst (C) within the right kidney (K) containing several thin calcifications *(arrows)*. G, gallbladder; L, liver.

usually fused to the inferior pole of the right kidney. A **pelvic kidney** represents failed embryologic ascent of an otherwise normal kidney. Intrathoracic kidneys are a rare occurrence.

- There is significant variation in normal **renal size;** lengths range from 9 to 14 cm. A single small kidney suggests the differential of congenital hypoplasia; atrophy from previous obstruction, infection, or reflux; ischemia; or previous partial resection **(Differential 12.1).** Bilaterally small kidneys result from chronic glomerulonephritis, ischemia, chronic papillary necrosis or pyelonephritis, bilateral reflux nephropathy, or bilateral obstructive atrophy **(Differential 12.2).** A single large kidney is usually the result of compensatory hypertrophy following resection or failure of the contralateral kidney. Other causes of unilateral renal enlargement include obstruction, tumor, duplication, infection, acute renal vein thrombosis, or acute infarction **(Differential 12.3).** In cases of **collecting system duplication,** the upper-pole moiety inserts ectopically and tends to become obstructed, whereas the lower pole is affected by reflux disease (Weigert-Meyer rule). Bilateral renal enlargement is often due to diabetes, acute inflammation, bilateral masses, obstruction, or acute renal vein thrombosis **(Differential 12.4).**

  Renal development may also lead to focal renal variations. A **dromedary hump** represents a focal contour bulge of normal parenchyma along the lateral margin of the left kidney. **Fetal lobation** may persist throughout life. Prominent cortical parenchyma at the corticomedullary junction, referred to as a **column of Bertin,** can simulate a renal mass. This normal variation enhances in concert with the normal renal parenchyma. Prominent, hypertrophied parenchyma can be present adjacent to a renal scar.

- **Pelvicaliectasis** is dilatation of the renal collecting system, while **hydronephrosis** is dilatation with obstruction **(Fig. 12.3).**

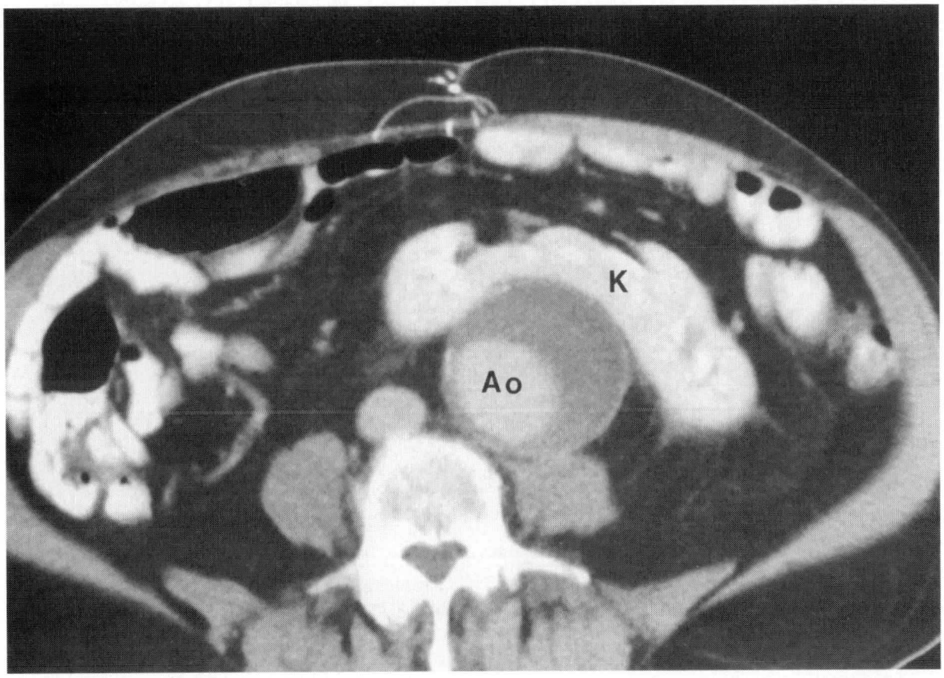

FIGURE 12.2 **Horseshoe kidney.** A 68-year-old man with an abdominal aortic aneurysm. The kidneys (K) are fused with a band of parenchyma passing anterior to the aorta (Ao). There is normal renal function and no hydronephrosis.

Hydronephrosis is most commonly caused by obstructing calculi, although it can be caused by transitional cell carcinoma, pelvic malignancies, sloughed papillae, blood clots, retroperitoneal fibrosis, aortic aneurysms, or reflux disease **(Differential 12.5).** Delayed contrast excretion or a delayed nephrogram can be evident. The reader should be able to readily connect dilated calyces with a distended renal pelvis, differentiating hydronephrosis from multiple renal or parapelvic cysts (see **Fig. 12.13).**

- **Obstruction of the ureteropelvic junction** resulting in hydronephrosis is the most common cause of an abdominal mass in a neonate. Abnormality of the proximal ureteral smooth muscle results in eventual fibrosis, although extrinsic compression from a crossing vessel can create a similar appearance. Patients may be asymptomatic or have flank pain, mass, hematuria, or fever.

  Many ureteropelvic junction obstructions are diagnosed on prenatal ultrasound. On CT, the finding of hydronephrosis with a decompressed ureter and lack of an obstructing mass should suggest the diagnosis. There may be decreased renal contrast excretion compared with the contralateral kidney.

- **Multicystic dysplastic kidney** results from obstruction of the ureter early in embryogenesis. The resulting kidney lacks functioning renal parenchyma and therefore fails to excrete contrast. Numerous renal cysts are present and are often separated by enhancing fibrous septa. The cysts do not communicate and should not be confused with dilated calyces of hydronephrosis **(Fig. 12.4).** This abnormality is often observed on prenatal ultrasound but can be incidentally discovered at any age. The majority involute over time. They are commonly associated with contralateral ureteropelvic junction obstruction.

12.3 NEPHROCALCINOSIS AND UROLITHIASIS

There are multiple sources of renal calcifications **(Differential 12.6).** These can occur within various renal masses, within the parenchyma (medulla or cortex), and within the collecting system.

- **Medullary nephrocalcinosis** describes calcific deposits within the medullary pyramids and is more common than cortical nephrocalcinosis **(Fig. 12.5).** It commonly results from hypercalcemic states (hyperparathyroidism), renal tubular acidosis (type 1, distal), and medullary sponge kidney. **Renal tubular acidosis** may be primary (from an inherited enzymatic defect) or secondary (Fanconi syndrome, Wilson disease, amphotericin B toxicity) to an acquired inability of the distal tubules to secrete hydrogen ions. Both processes result in an inability to acidify urine. Calcium ions are soluble in acid urine but much less soluble in alkaline urine, which permits precipitation of crystalline calcium salts.

  Medullary sponge kidney, also termed renal ***tubular ectasia,*** reflects dilatation of the collecting ducts of Bellini. Approximately 15 percent of these patients develop calcifications within the dilated

12.1 UNILATERAL SMALL KIDNEY (ATROPHY OR HYPOPLASIA)

Postobstructive atrophy
Congenital hypoplasia
Ischemia—atherosclerosis, FMD, trauma to vascular pedicle
Infarction
Reflux nephropathy
Partial resection
Postinfectious atrophy
Radiation nephritis
Hypoplastic form of multicystic dysplastic kidney

Key: FMD, fibromuscular dysplasia.

12.2 BILATERAL SMALL KIDNEY

Atherosclerosis with ischemia
Chronic glomerulonephritis
Chronic papillary necrosis—diabetes, sickle cell disease, analgesics
Bilateral obstructive atrophy
Chronic pyelonephritis
Reflux nephropathy
Chronic hypertension

12.3

UNILATERAL LARGE KIDNEY

Compensatory hypertrophy
Obstruction or hydronephrosis—stone, tumor, stricture
Primary tumor—renal cell carcinoma, Wilms tumor
Acute pyelonephritis
Idiopathic
Xanthogranulomatous pyelonephritis
Duplex system—20% bilateral
Cross-fused ectopia
Polycystic kidney disease—usually bilateral
Hematoma
Renal vein thrombosis—RCCA invasion, hypercoagulable state, sepsis, IVC clot extension
Acute infarction—trauma, thromboembolic disease, vasculitis
Multicystic dysplastic kidney
Multilocular cystic nephroma

Key: IVC, inferior vena cava; RCCA, renal cell carcinoma.

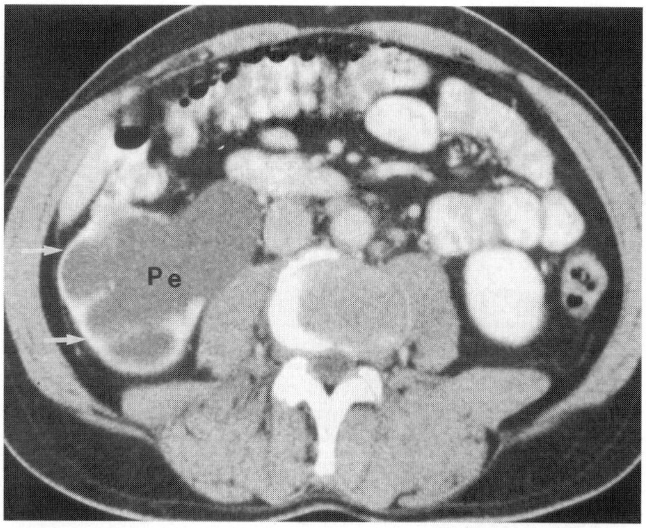

FIGURE 12.3 Hydronephrosis. There is dilatation of the renal pelvis (Pe) and calyces from an obstructing transitional cell carcinoma of the ureterovesical junction. A thin rim of enhancing renal parenchyma is present *(arrows)*.

tubules. Patients are usually asymptomatic, although hematuria and acute flank pain can result from passage of stones that form in the top of the papillae. Medullary sponge kidney can involve both kidneys, one kidney only, or even a single collecting system.

Hypercalcemia is most often due to hyperparathyroidism. Primary hyperparathyroidism results from a parathyroid adenoma; secondary hyperparathyroidism is most commonly due to renal disease. Excessive calcium ingestion (milk-alkali syndrome), sarcoidosis, vitamin D intoxication, and other entities can also result in medullary nephrocalcinosis.

- **Cortical nephrocalcinosis** is associated with chronic glomerulonephritis, oxalosis, acute cortical necrosis, and Alport syndrome. **Primary oxalosis** is a rare autosomal recessive abnormality that becomes clinically apparent as childhood urolithiasis and progresses to dense calcification of both the renal cortex and medulla. **Acute cortical necrosis** can occur in patients with shock, sepsis, ethylene glycol ingestion, or obstetric complications such as abruption or placenta previa. In the acute stage, diminished cortical enhancement is evident **(Fig. 12.6). Alport syndrome** is an autosomal dominant disorder characterized by nerve deafness and nephritis. Patients develop renal failure in midlife.

- **Renal calculi** are a common cause of emergency department visits. Almost 10 percent of the population develops a kidney stone by age 70. Initial presentation is often in the third or fourth decade of life, and there is a 4:1 male predominance. There is a well-established geographic distribution: renal calculi are much more prevalent in the southern United States than in the North.

  Over 75 percent of renal calculi consist of **calcium oxalate** either alone or in combination with calcium phosphate. Hypercalcemia is a common predisposing factor. Other causes of calcium

12.4

BILATERAL LARGE KIDNEY (>13 cm in length)

Diabetes mellitus
Inflammation
  Acute glomerulonephritis—streptococcal infection
  Pyelonephritis
  Acute interstitial nephritis—drug reaction, eosinophilia
  Acute tubular or cortical necrosis
  Wegener granulomatosis
  Goodpasture disease
  Lupus, polyarteritis nodosa
Masses
  Polycystic kidney disease
  Lymphoma or leukemia
  Metastases—lung, breast, lymphoma, contralateral RCCA
  Tuberous sclerosis—multiple AMLs or cysts
  Multiple myeloma
Normal variant
Acute papillary necrosis
Bilateral hydronephrosis—retroperitoneal fibrosis, pelvic tumor, radiation
Medullary sponge kidney
Renal vein thrombosis
Bilateral duplex system
Acute urate nephropathy
Amyloidosis

Key: AML, angiomyolipoma; RCCA, renal cell carcinoma.

12.5

HYDRONEPHROSIS

Ureteral obstruction—stone, tumor, extrinsic mass, retroperitoneal fibrosis
UPJ obstruction—congenital, crossing vessel
Reflux
Megacalicosis

Key: UPJ, ureteropelvic junction.

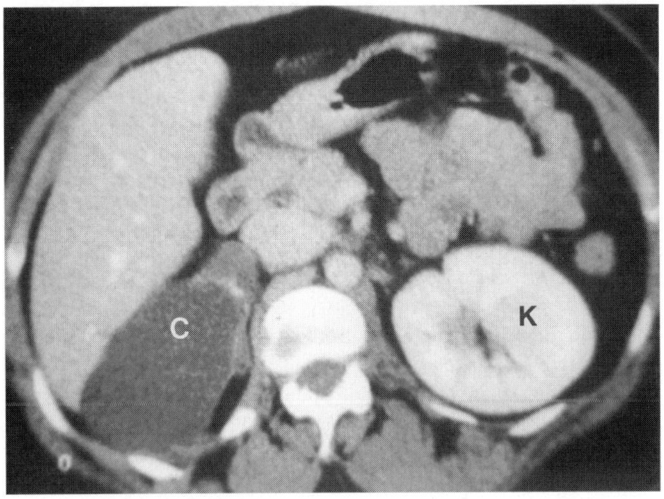

FIGURE 12.4 Multicystic dysplastic kidney. The right kidney is entirely replaced by a septated cystic mass (C). There is no residual renal parenchyma, and a normal left kidney (K) is present.

stones include hyperoxalosis, hyperuricosuria, and idiopathic hypercalciuria.

- **Stones of composition other than calcium oxalate** are less common and have their own predisposing factors. Pure **calcium phosphate stones** represent less than 10 percent of renal calculi and can be seen with hypercalciuria, renal tubular acidosis, and medications that alkalinize the urine (Diamox). **Struvite stones** are composed of magnesium ammonium phosphate and may be seen in conjunction with xanthogranulomatous pyelonephritis **(Section 12.4).** Struvite

12.6

RENAL CALCIFICATION

Atherosclerotic vessels
Nephrolithiasis
Medullary nephrocalcinosis
  Renal tubular acidosis
  Medullary sponge kidney
  Hypercalcemic states—**hyperparathyroidism**
  Paraneoplastic syndrome—secondary hypercalcemia
  Papillary necrosis—diabetes, sickle cell, phenacetin
Cortical nephrocalcinosis
  Chronic glomerulonephritis—poststreptococcal infection
  Oxalosis
  Acute cortical necrosis—shock, dehydration, abruption
  Chronic transplant rejection
  Alport syndrome—nephrocalcinosis and nerve deafness
Infection—tuberculosis, XPG, echinococcal cyst
Renal cyst
Tumor—renal cell, Wilms
Multicystic dysplastic kidney
Old hematoma
Furosemide therapy—children

Key: XPG, xanthogranulomatous pyelonephritis.

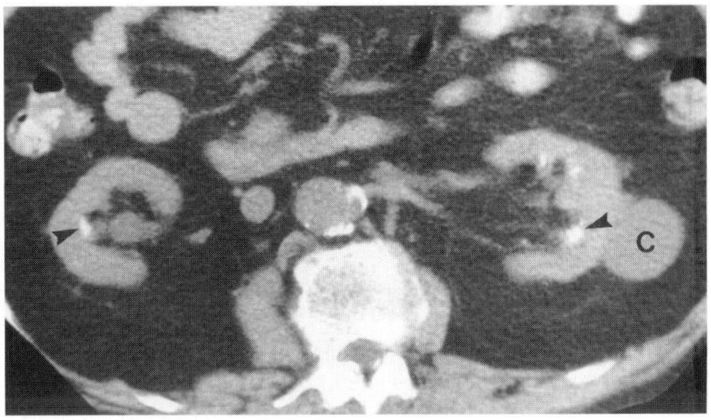

FIGURE 12.5 Medullary sponge kidney. Multiple medullary calcifications *(arrowheads)* are present within the renal papillae bilaterally. Incidental note is made of a left simple renal cyst (C).

stones are often found in the presence of urease-producing bacteria such as *Proteus mirabilis*. These stones can rapidly increase in size. **Uric acid stones** account for approximately 6 to 10 percent of all renal calculi and may be seen with acidic urine and hyperuricosuria from gout. Uric acid stones are radiolucent on conventional radiographs. Less common stone compositions include cysteine, xanthine, and matrix (coagulated mucoid material).

Essentially all renal and ureteral calculi have high attenuation on noncontrast CT; accordingly, this method has rapidly become the technique of choice in evaluating patients with suspected urolithiasis. CT has a sensitivity of 97 percent, a specificity of 96 percent, and an overall accuracy of 96 percent in detecting urolithiasis.

While only 85 percent of renal calculi are visible on plain films, all but matrix stones have a CT attenuation value of at least 100 HU, making them readily detectable **(Fig. 12.7).** Hydronephrosis

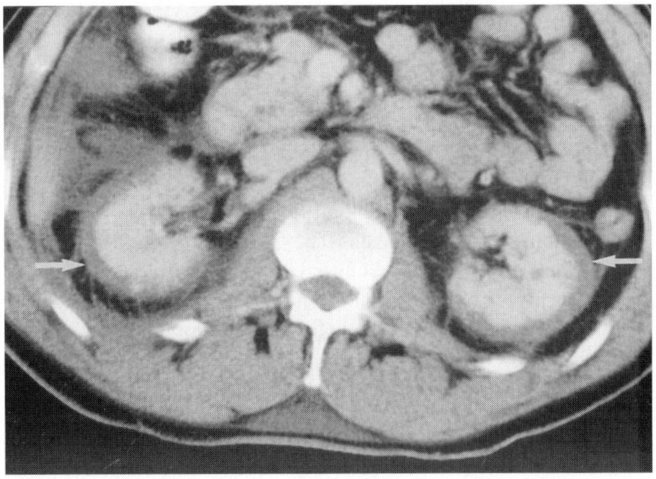

FIGURE 12.6 Acute cortical necrosis. IV contrast–enhanced CT in a 42-year-old postsurgical patient demonstrates peripheral soft tissue rimming both kidneys *(arrows)*. This is a region of ischemic cortex due to a recent episode of hypovolemia and shock. There is stranding in the perinephric space.

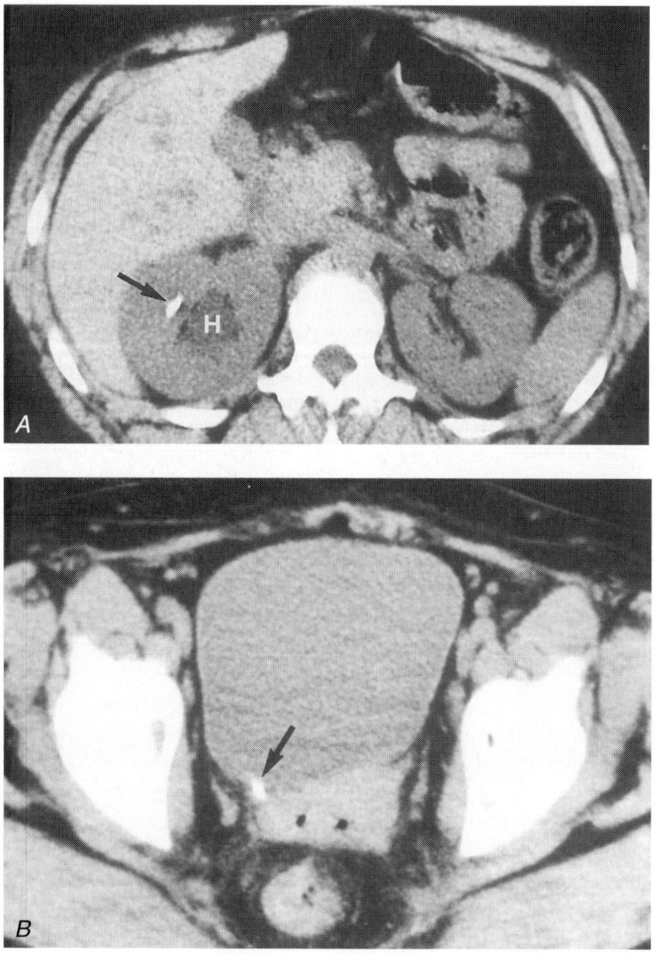

FIGURE 12.7 Urolithiasis. A 37-year-old woman with hematuria and right flank pain. *A*. There is right-sided hydronephrosis as well as an intrarenal calculus *(arrow)*. The right kidney is modestly enlarged. *B*. An obstructing calculus is present at the ureterovesical junction *(arrow)*.

and hydroureter are clearly demonstrated, as are other findings such as renal enlargement, perinephric stranding, and asymptomatic stones elsewhere. Significant obstruction can exist even when hydronephrosis is not present, since the collecting system can decompress via forniceal rupture. A soft tissue "rim sign" is often present surrounding a ureteral calculus but not a pelvic phlebolith, allowing the reader to differentiate the two. Ureteral dilatation can be present **(Differential 12.7),** although this has several other causes.

The most important **predictors of patient outcome** besides clinical symptoms are stone size and stone location, both of which are accurately and rapidly determined by CT. Future research should provide further insight to answer whether the findings on noncontrast CT can accurately predict the degree of functional obstruction. A final benefit of CT is that 10 percent of patients with clinically suspected urolithiasis have a different etiology for acute abdominal pain, and this alternative diagnosis can be made in a substantial fraction of patients undergoing CT.

12.4 INFECTIOUS, INFLAMMATORY, AND VASCULAR CONDITIONS

- **Pyelonephritis** is a common cause of flank pain, often associated with fever, pyuria, and leukocytosis. With the exceptions of tuberculosis and staphylococcal infection, bacterial pyelonephritis occurs by ascending infection from the bladder. Predisposing conditions include vesicoureteral reflux, neurogenic bladder, diabetes, prolonged catheterization, pregnancy, and immunocompromised states. Common offending organisms are *Escherichia coli, Proteus mirabilis,* and *Klebsiella.*

  Pyelonephritis is an infection of portions of the renal parenchyma, including the cortex, medulla, calyces, and pelvis. The medullary interstitium is the first site of involvement, and infection there quickly spreads to the cortex. Although there is often global renal involvement, a patchy distribution is also seen on occasion. Generally, focal nephritis will involve a medullary ray and therefore have a wedge-shaped distribution on CT imaging.

  On **CT,** the involved kidney can be focally or diffusely enlarged. The renal parenchyma can appear low in attenuation on precontrast images, and there are usually wedge-shaped regions of decreased enhancement following IV contrast administration **(Fig. 12.8).** These areas are well marginated by the renal lobule. Perinephric stranding or even perinephric abscesses can be present, and there is often thickening of Gerota's fascia and the bridging perinephric septa **(Fig. 12.9).** Pyonephrosis is often present, in which case layering debris can be detected within the collecting system.

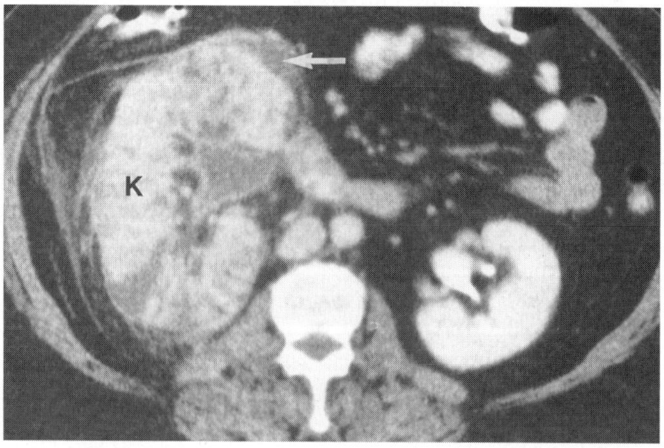

FIGURE 12.8 Pyelonephritis. A 59-year-old woman with abdominal pain and fever. There is severe right renal enlargement (K) with heterogeneous, striated contrast enhancement after IV contrast administration. Infiltration of the perinephric fat, thickening of Gerota's fascia, and a perinephric fluid collection *(arrow)* are also apparent. The left kidney is normal.

12.7 URETERAL DILATATION

Obstruction—stone, tumor/adjacent mass, inflammation, blood clot, fungus ball
Vesicoureteral reflux
Primary megaloureter

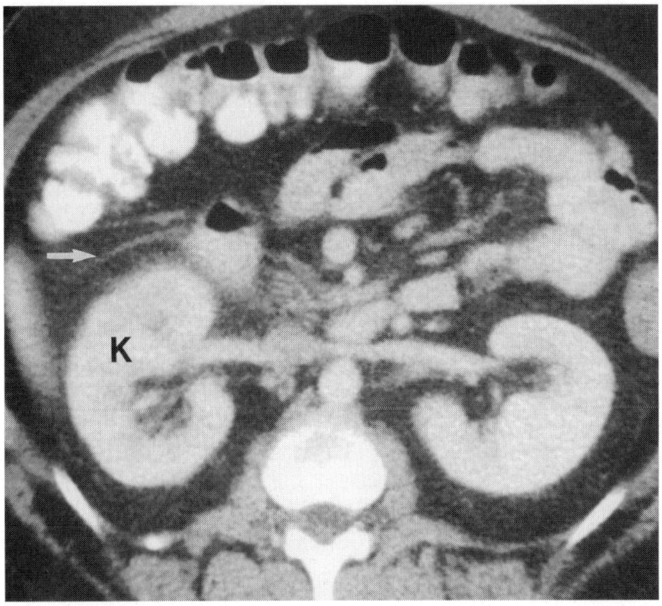

FIGURE 12.9 Pyelonephritis. A 40-year-old woman with fever, leukocytosis, pyuria, and right flank pain. IV contrast–enhanced CT shows mild right-sided renal enlargement (K), infiltration of the perinephric fat, indistinct renal margins, and fascial thickening *(arrow)*. The patient showed symptomatic resolution several days after beginning an antibiotic regimen.

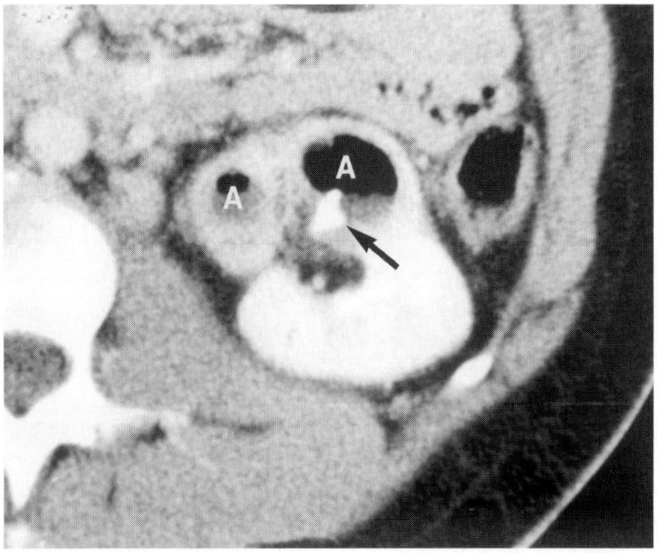

FIGURE 12.10 Renal abscess. A 31-year-old woman with left renal gas noted on abdominal sonography. There are two left renal midzone abscesses with air-fluid levels (A). These were secondary to the obstructing calculus *(arrow)*.

Adequately treated pyelonephritis usually causes no permanent damage, although papillary necrosis and cortical scarring can occur with incompletely treated or aggressive infections.

Focal pyelonephritis, previously termed ***acute focal bacterial nephritis,*** is a variant of bacterial renal infection. It is often due to staphylococcal infection or an ascending bacterial agent. Focal pyelonephritis primarily affects the renal cortex and reflects phlegmonous inflammation, which frequently progresses to form an abscess. On CT, focal pyelonephritis is depicted as a low-attenuation mass with heterogeneous enhancement. Its margins with surrounding normal kidney are usually indistinct; well-defined margins more likely represent a complicating parenchymal abscess.

- **Renal abscesses** are an uncommon complication of bacterial pyelonephritis. *Staphylococcus* and *Streptococcus* are usually the causative agents, although improved medical management has led to a shift toward gram-negative organisms. Renal abscesses are uncommon when adequate antibiotic treatment has been administered. Treatment may require percutaneous drainage if aggressive antibiotic therapy fails to clear the infection. Symptoms are similar to uncomplicated pyelonephritis and include fever, flank pain, and leukocytosis.

On **CT,** renal abscesses appear as solitary or multifocal areas of low attenuation within the renal parenchyma. These regions are usually rounded and well-marginated. Adjacent thickening of Gerota's fascia, perinephric stranding, and intralesional gas can also be demonstrated **(Fig. 12.10).** Hematogenous seeding may lead to bilateral renal parenchymal involvement as well as abscesses within the liver or spleen. Microabscesses, measuring only several millimeters in diameter, can also be demonstrated on CT; they commonly reflect infection by fungal agents, particularly *Candida albicans.*

- **Emphysematous pyelonephritis** is a more fulminant renal infection seen predominately in immunocompromised patients and diabetics, who account for over 90 percent of cases. It is postulated that the glucosuria in these patients provides a suitable environment for bacterial fermentation of glucose, producing carbon dioxide and hydrogen. *E. coli* is the causative agent in 70 percent of cases. Aggressive medical therapy and percutaneous drainage make up the minimum intervention, but nephrectomy is often warranted.

CT demonstrates gas within the renal parenchyma, collecting system, and sometimes the perinephric tissues. Other potential causes of renal gas include instrumentation, trauma, and fistulae from adjacent inflammatory processes. Viewing at lung window settings (W, 1800; L, −550) can improve the conspicuity of subtle foci of gas. There is associated renal enlargement, perinephric inflammation, and diminished or absent contrast excretion.

- **Xanthogranulomatous pyelonephritis (XGP)** is an uncommon cause of renal inflammation. There is parenchymal infiltration with lipid-laden macrophages associated with a staghorn calculus in 75 percent of cases. *Proteus mirabilis* is the usual causative organism, although *E. coli, Klebsiella,* and *Pseudomonas* can also produce this unusual immune response. Symptoms are nonspecific and often chronic; they include malaise, fever, flank pain, and leukocytosis. Patients are typically middle aged, and there is a female predominance (4:1).

CT in XGP may demonstrate the classic findings of a staghorn calculus, decreased excretion of contrast, and a low-attenuation renal mass. The affected kidney is often enlarged, and there may be associated obstruction of the ureteropelvic junction. Associated inflammatory changes can be extensive and involve the perinephric fat, retroperitoneum, and psoas and abdominal wall muscles, as well as more distant sites such as the pleural space **(Fig. 12.11).**

XGP diffusely involves the affected kidney in 85 percent of cases; the remaining 15 percent demonstrate local renal parenchymal infiltration (tumefactive XGP), which may be difficult to differentiate from primary neoplasm.

- **Renal vascular disease** is very common and usually related to atherosclerotic stenosis of the renal artery ostium. This often precipitates renovascular hypertension by decreasing transmural pressure in afferent renal arterioles, activating the renin-angiotensin-aldosterone system. Renovascular hypertension accounts for less than 5 percent of all patients with hypertension. CT can demonstrate calcific atherosclerotic plaques within the abdominal aorta and its branches. In the future, CT angiography may play a more significant role in demonstrating the arterial narrowing, although conventional angiography can directly measure pressure gradients across the stenosis and provide therapeutic intervention. Other causes of renovascular hypertension include fibromuscular dysplasia, Takayasu arteritis, and polyarteritis nodosa. **Polyarteritis nodosa** is a systemic necrotizing vasculitis of small and medium-sized vessels. The kidney is the most frequently affected organ, often demonstrating arterial stenoses, intrarenal and main renal artery aneurysms, and small cortical infarcts.
- **Renal infarcts** are often the result of embolic disease, atherosclerosis, or collagen vascular disease. Presenting symptoms are nonspecific and include flank pain or low-grade fever. CT demonstrates a well-marginated segment of renal parenchyma that fails to enhance after IV contrast; however, there may be a thin rim of peripheral enhancement due to preserved capsular flow **(Fig. 12.12).** Infarcts are often multiple and can result in scarring and a contour abnormality.

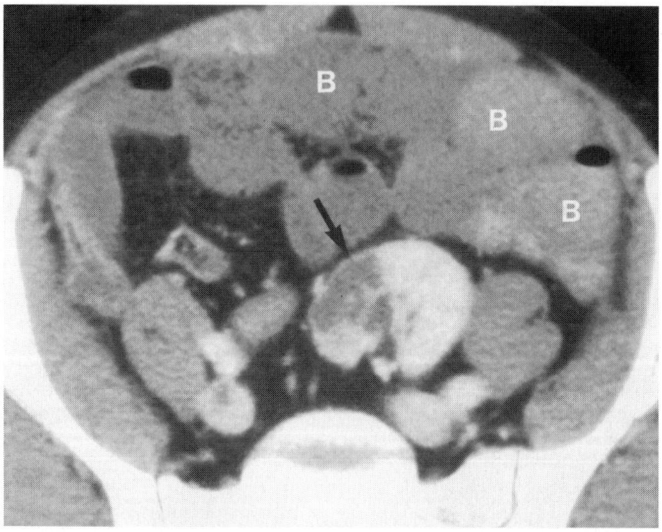

FIGURE 12.12 Renal infarct. This patient was undergoing high-dose estrogen therapy for gender reassignment and presented with acute abdominal pain. The pelvic kidney demonstrates a wedge-shaped region of absent enhancement representing a renal infarct. There is characteristic preserved capsular flow *(arrow)*. Dilated small bowel (B) is due to superior mesenteric artery thrombosis with bowel ischemia.

12.5 CYSTIC DISEASE

- **Renal cysts** are very common, and there are many causes **(Differential 12.8).** Simple cysts are seen in approximately one-half of patients over 50 years of age. Cysts do not cause symptoms unless they hemorrhage, become infected, or grow to a very large size. A simple renal cyst is a water-attenuation, nonenhancing mass with a smooth, imperceptible wall. It does not contain calcifications or septations. A slight elevation of the adjacent renal parenchyma

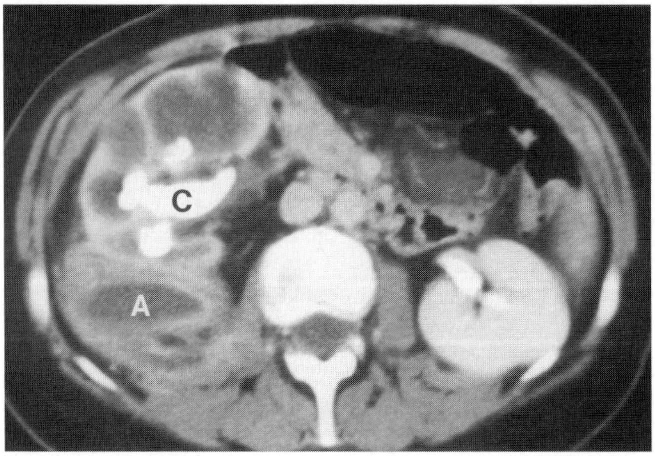

FIGURE 12.11 Xanthogranulomatous pyelonephritis. IV contrast–enhanced CT shows a staghorn calculus (C) within an infiltrated, low-attenuation kidney, displaced anteriorly by an associated abscess (A). [From Slone RM, Gutierrez FR, Fisher AJ (eds.) *Thoracic Imaging: A Practical Approach.* New York: McGraw-Hill; 1999. With permission.]

12.8

RENAL CYST

Cortical cyst (simple cyst)
Parapelvic cyst
Conditions associated with multiple cysts
  Autosomal dominant polycystic disease
  Autosomal recessive polycystic disease
  Acquired cystic disease
  Von Hippel-Lindau disease
  Medullary cystic disease
  Medullary sponge kidney
  Tuberous sclerosis
Cystic tumors
  Cystic renal cell carcinoma
  Multilocular cystic nephroma
  Multicystic dysplastic kidney
  Metastasis
Hydronephrosis
Calyceal diverticulum
Hematoma
Urinoma
Vascular—arteriovenous fistula, pseudoaneurysm
Hydatid

may be present (**beak sign**) (see **Fig. 7.31**). Cysts can be of increased attenuation if there has been prior hemorrhage or if the cyst contains high-attenuation material such as calcium or protein.

- **Bosniak** has divided cortical renal cysts into four categories based on their imaging features and the risk that the cyst is malignant:

Type I—Simple cyst.
Type II—Minimally complicated cysts (thin septations or calcifications, may be hyperdense, no enhancement). Hyperdense cysts should be less than 3 cm, have one-quarter of their circumference outside the kidney, be homogeneous, and not display enhancement after IV contrast. Type IIF cysts, slightly more complex type II lesions, are probably benign but require imaging follow-up.
Type III—Complex cysts (thick, irregular, multiple septations or calcifications, thick or nodular wall, no enhancement)
Type IV—Cystic neoplasm (irregular, thickened or enhancing wall or septa or a solid component).

Simple or minimally complicated cysts do not warrant follow-up; intermediate (IIF) lesions should be followed by CT after an interval of 3 to 6 months. Category III or IV cystic lesions should be excised, as they have a high likelihood of representing neoplasm. The Bosniak system is a useful guideline, but significant interobserver variability exists.

- **Parapelvic cysts** (renal sinus cysts) arise within the renal hilum. They are conjectured to be of lymphatic origin. Parapelvic cysts have the same imaging characteristics as cysts found within the parenchyma. They often deform the collecting system and are frequently bilateral **(Fig. 12.13).** They are higher in attenuation than sinus lipomatosis.

- **Autosomal dominant polycystic kidney disease (ADPCKD)** is a relatively common inherited disorder that progresses to renal insufficiency. Patients present in their twenties through forties with flank pain, hypertension, renal failure, a palpable abdominal mass, or hematuria. The flank pain is often the result of cyst hemorrhage, cyst enlargement with stretching of the renal capsule, or ureteral obstruction.

The CT features of ADPCKD are numerous bilateral simple renal cysts of varying sizes, resulting in moderate to severe renal enlargement. High-attenuation hemorrhagic cysts are present in the majority of patients **(Fig. 12.14).** There is no increased risk of renal cell carcinoma (RCCA) unless the patient is on prolonged dialysis. Associations include hepatic (>40 percent) and pancreatic (<10 percent) cysts and intracranial berry aneurysms (up to 40 percent).

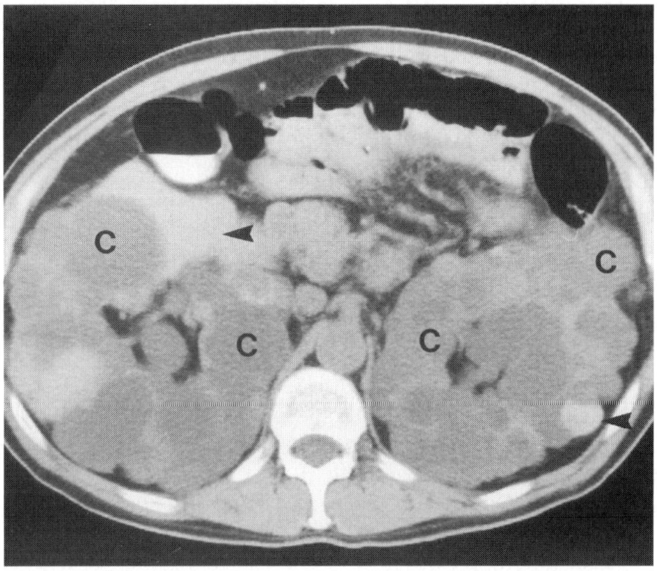

FIGURE 12.14 Autosomal dominant polycystic kidney disease. Innumerable cysts (C) essentially replace the normal renal parenchyma in this patient with known ADPCKD. Several hemorrhagic cysts *(arrowheads),* including a very large one in the right kidney anteriorly, are present.

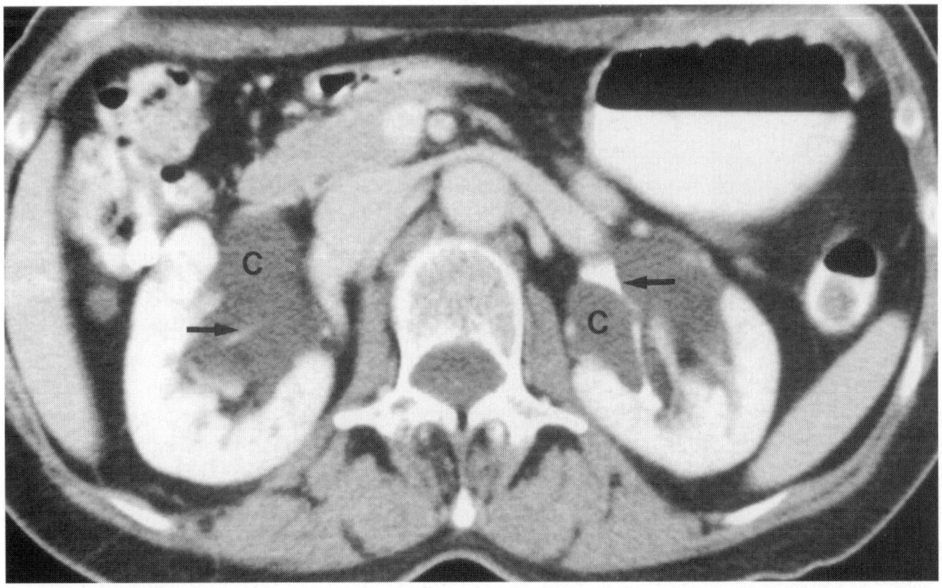

FIGURE 12.13 Parapelvic cysts. Hilar fluid-attenuation collections represent parapelvic cysts (C) with stretched collecting systems *(arrows)* opacified by contrast crossing this region.

- **Autosomal recessive polycystic kidney disease (ARPCKD)** is an inherited disease characterized by renal cyst formation (actually dilated tubules) and hepatic fibrosis. Infants may have renal failure at birth and minimal hepatic involvement. These patients succumb within the first weeks of life. When hepatic failure predominates, patients present later in childhood with marked hepatic fibrosis (often leading to portal hypertension) and tubular ectasia.

CT findings depend on the age of presentation. Infants have markedly enlarged kidneys that function poorly. Numerous tiny cystic spaces are often present. Those ARPCKD patients presenting in childhood have mildly enlarged kidneys with medullary ductal ectasia resulting in a striated nephrogram, numerous renal cysts, and CT findings of portal hypertension.

- **Acquired cystic disease** describes the development of numerous cysts within the native kidneys of patients on hemodialysis. After 3 years of dialysis, 40 percent of patients have renal cysts. Another, clinically more important, association is the development of oncocytomas and RCCA. Cysts frequently regress after renal transplantation. On CT, numerous, bilateral parenchymal cysts are present **(Fig. 12.15).** They are small but can contain hemorrhagic fluid or have mural calcification. The underlying kidney is atrophic and excretes IV contrast poorly.
- **Von Hippel-Lindau (VHL) disease** is an autosomal dominant inherited neurocutaneous syndrome. Extrarenal manifestations include intracranial and spinal hemangioblastomas, retinal angiomas, pheochromocytomas, pancreatic islet cell tumors, epididymal and broad ligament cystadenomas, and abdominal visceral cysts. Within the kidneys, 60 to 80 percent of these patients develop multiple, bilateral renal cysts, which may be indistinguishable from those of ADPCKD. Approximately 30 to 60 percent of VHL patients have pancreatic cysts and a small percentage have associated hepatic cysts; therefore, multiple renal cysts in conjunction with predominantly pancreatic cysts should favor VHL over ADPCKD **(Fig. 12.16).**

  Of greater concern is the 25 to 45 percent prevalence of RCCA in VHL patients. These tumors are present earlier than sporadic RCCA, and bilateral tumors are often discovered. Consequently, these patients undergo routine imaging evaluations, usually with CT, to exclude development of a RCCA. Nephron-sparing resection of small RCCAs is attempted in VHL patients to preserve as much normal parenchyma as possible.

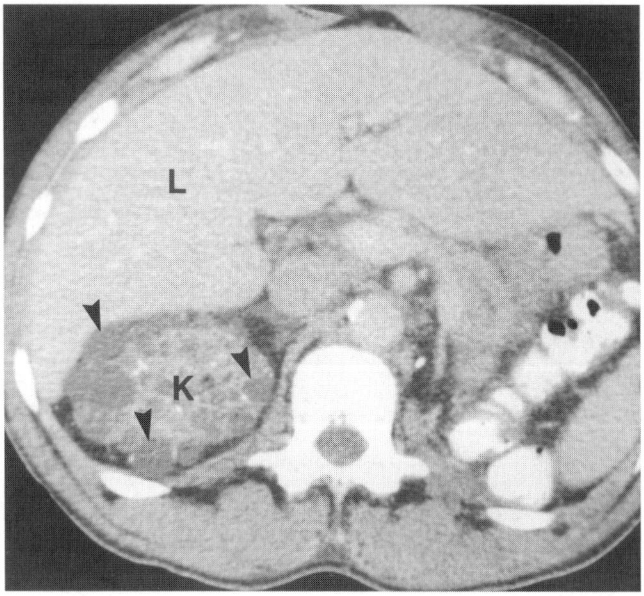

FIGURE 12.15 Acquired renal cystic disease. IV contrast–enhanced CT demonstrates a poorly functioning right kidney (K). There are numerous small simple renal cysts *(arrowheads)* representing acquired cystic disease. The more inferior left kidney demonstrated similar changes. L, liver.

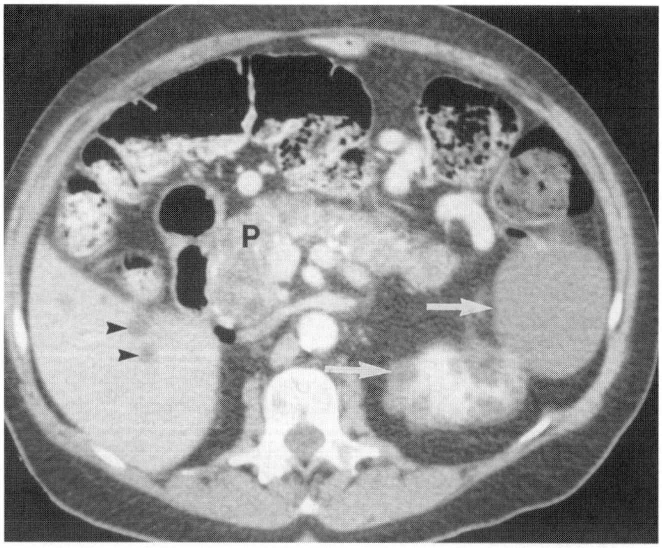

FIGURE 12.16 Von-Hippel Lindau disease. This patient has multiple simple cysts in the left kidney *(arrows)* and the liver *(arrowheads)*. There are numerous poorly resolved cysts throughout the pancreas (P).

- **Tuberous sclerosis (TS)** is another autosomal dominant neurocutaneous syndrome. It is characterized by facial angiofibromas and hamartomas of multiple organs. Some 80 percent of TS patients also have one or more renal angiomyolipomas. Renal cysts are often present and may be multiple and bilateral, simulating ADPCKD or VHL. Patients come to clinical attention because of mental retardation, seizures, or acute abdominal pain from hemorrhage of an angiomyolipoma.

12.6 BENIGN MASSES

- There are numerous causes of solid renal masses **(Differential 12.9).**
- **Angiomyolipomas (AMLs)** are benign, hamartomatous renal tumors. They are made up of varying amounts of vascular, fatty, and muscular elements. Typically, solitary AMLs are seen sporadically in the general population, while multiple AMLs are associated with tuberous sclerosis. These lesions are often resected or embolized owing to their potential for catastrophic hemorrhage.

  The **CT appearance** of AMLs can vary greatly. The CT finding of a solid renal mass containing macroscopic fat is essentially diagnostic of an AML **(Fig. 12.17);** RCCAs can very rarely show macroscopic fat, usually in areas of necrosis with osteoid metaplasia or from tumor encasement of perinephric fat **(Differential 12.10).** Other cellular elements within AMLs, particularly muscle, can predominate in some cases, making the diagnosis more difficult. Thin-collimation imaging may be necessary to identify small foci of fat. Additionally, lesions that have been complicated by spontaneous hemorrhage will have an altered CT appearance, with soft tissue stranding of the perinephric fat as well as heterogeneous high attenuation within the lesion itself **(Fig. 12.18).**
- **Oncocytomas** are uncommon renal tumors that are generally classified as benign, although their malignant potential is still unclear. They are usually large (>5 cm) at the time of diagnosis and often

12.9

RENAL MASS

Renal cyst
Normal variant—dromedary hump, column of Bertin
Malignant tumor
  Renal cell carcinoma
  Transitional cell carcinoma
  Wilms
  Lymphoma/leukemia
  Metastasis—lung, breast, gastrointestinal, melanoma
  Squamous cell carcinoma
  Clear cell sarcoma
  Rhabdoid tumor
  Sarcoma
Benign tumor—angiomyolipoma, multicystic dysplastic kidney, mesoblastic nephroma, multilocular cystic nephroma, oncocytoma, reninoma, *carcinoid, adenoma, mesenchymal tumor*
Abscess
Focal bacterial nephritis or infarct
Hematoma
Xanthogranulomatous pyelonephritis
Other childhood tumors—nephroblastomatosis (Wilms association)
Vascular—renal artery aneurysm, arteriovenous malformation
Tuberculoma

12.10

RENAL MASS WITH FAT

Angiomyolipoma
Xanthogranulomatous pyelonephritis—lipid-laden macrophage infiltration
Wilms tumor
Renal cell carcinoma
Liposarcoma/lipoma
Teratoma

detected in asymptomatic individuals. Oncocytomas appear on CT as homogeneous, nonencapsulated, low-density enhancing parenchymal masses. One-third of cases may have an identifiable central fibrous scar, which is suggestive of the diagnosis; however, these lesions are always excised, since RCCA cannot be excluded with certainty. If the diagnosis of oncocytoma is considered preoperatively, the surgeon can plan to perform wedge resection, thus preserving the remainder of the kidney.

- **Renal adenomas** are benign solid tumors that present in older patients. There is an increased prevalence in acquired cystic disease, trisomy 7, and trisomy 17. Renal adenomas have the nonspecific CT appearance of an enhancing soft tissue lesion. Although they are benign, renal adenomas are impossible to distinguish confidently from a RCCA; consequently, renal adenomas are excised.
- **Multilocular cystic nephromas (MLCNs)** are uncommon renal neoplasms. They have a bimodal demographic distribution, occurring in young boys and in women between 40 and 60 years of age. On CT, MLCNs appear as a complex cystic mass with multiple internal septations **(Fig. 12.19).** Calcifications can be present, particularly along the margins. Normal parenchyma should be present in the ipsilateral kidney. These lesions are managed surgically, as they can be difficult to confidently distinguish from cystic RCCAs and some have harbored Wilms tumors.
- **Mesoblastic nephroma** is a benign, hamartomatous tumor that is

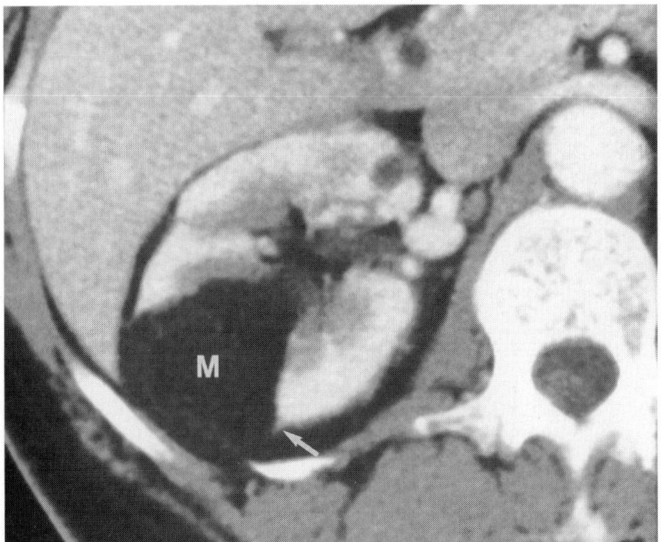

FIGURE 12.17 Angiomyolipoma. A 55-year-old woman being evaluated for colon cancer. There is a wedge-shaped 4-cm fat-attenuation mass (M) in the right renal midzone. A "beak" of normal renal parenchyma *(arrow)* is seen adjacent to the lesion, indicating its intrarenal nature. [From Slone RM, Gutierrez FR, Fisher AJ (eds.) *Thoracic Imaging: A Practical Approach.* New York: McGraw-Hill; 1999. With permission.]

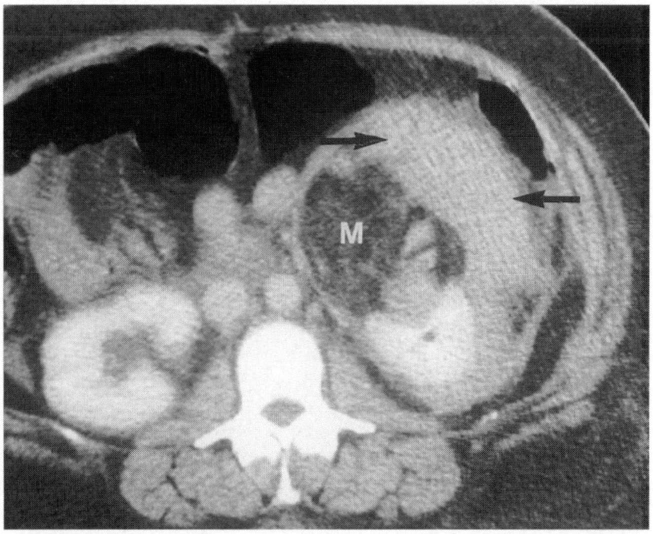

FIGURE 12.18 Hemorrhagic angiomyolipoma. IV contrast–enhanced CT in a 24-year-old woman with acute left flank pain. There is a fat-attenuation mass (M) indenting the anterior aspect of the left renal lower pole. Adjacent stranding and soft tissue attenuation represent acute hemorrhage *(arrows).* (Case courtesy of Dr. Jeffrey Friedland, Denver, CO.)

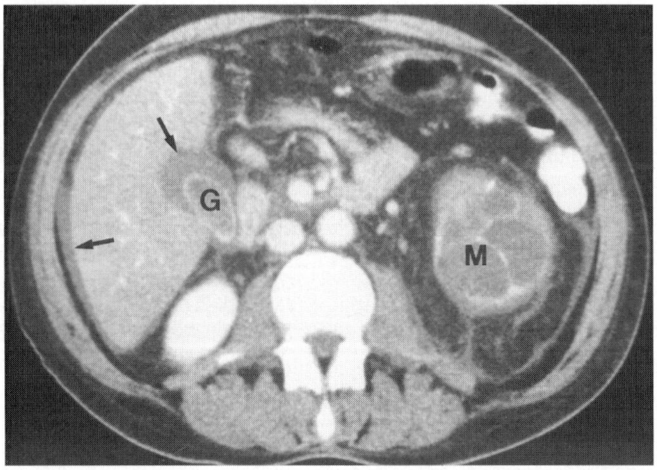

FIGURE 12.19 **Multilocular cystic nephroma.** This 49-year-old man presented with fever and right-upper-quadrant pain. There are findings of acute cholecystitis with pericholecystic and perihepatic fluid *(arrows)*. A complex cystic mass (M) arises from the left renal upper pole with surrounding parenchyma present. G, gallbladder.

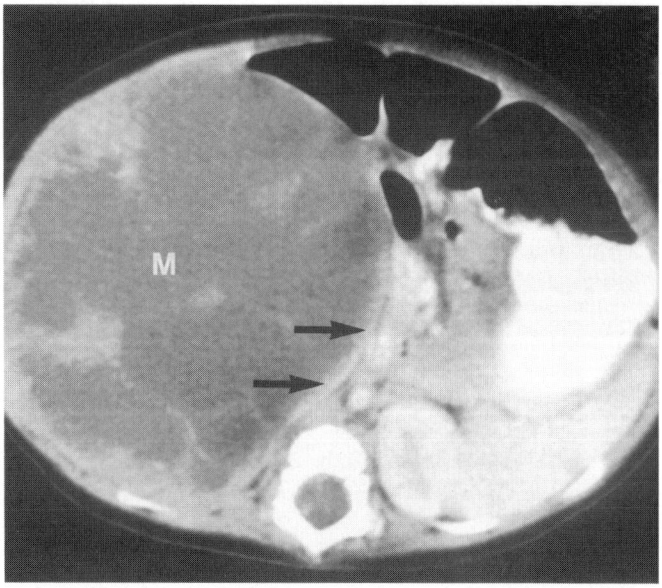

FIGURE 12.20 **Mesoblastic nephroma.** This infant has a palpable left abdominal mass. There is no recognizable normal left renal parenchyma; a thin rim of enhancing tissue is present peripherally *(arrows)*. A large, heterogeneous, and predominantly low-attenuation mass (M) is present in the left renal fossa. (Case courtesy of Dr. Jeffrey Friedland, Denver, CO.)

generally present at birth. It is clinically manifest as a nontender abdominal mass or may be identified on prenatal ultrasound. Rarely, the tumor can behave aggressively. Nephrectomy is curative. On CT, mesoblastic nephromas are large, nonencapsulated masses that show modest enhancement after IV contrast administration. Necrosis and hemorrhage are uncommon **(Fig. 12.20).**

12.7 MALIGNANT MASSES

- **Renal cell carcinoma (RCCA)** is the most common primary renal malignancy in adults. It accounts for approximately 85 percent of primary renal tumors. RCCA is also seen in association with von Hippel-Lindau syndrome and acquired cystic disease. Patients may present with fever, weight loss, hematuria, and anemia. Uncommonly, hepatic enzymes will be elevated without demonstrable liver parenchymal involvement, a condition referred to as ***Stauffer syndrome.***

  On **CT,** the tumor's appearance ranges from that of a complex renal cyst, which may have only a single demonstrable mural nodule **(Fig. 12.21),** to a large, heterogeneous, and densely enhancing solid mass. Lesions in excess of 3 cm often have central necrosis, as the tumor gradually outstrips its vascular supply **(Fig. 12.22).** RCCAs do not

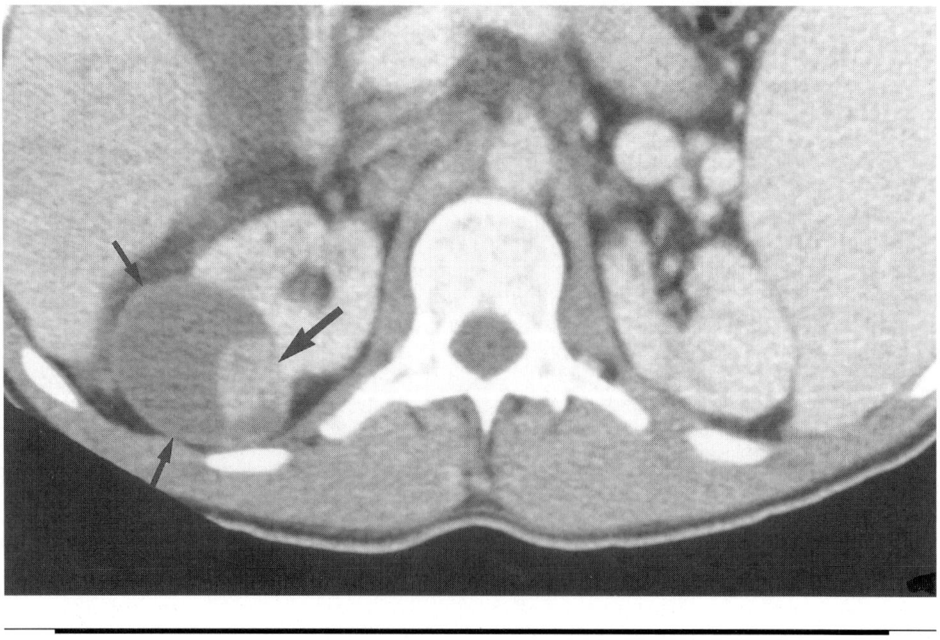

FIGURE 12.21 **Cystic renal cell carcinoma.** A cystic right renal mass with a thickened rim *(small arrows)* is seen, as well as a densely enhancing mural nodule *(large arrow)*. This is a Bosniak IV lesion and must be surgically resected.

contain fat unless they grow in an exophytic fashion to encompass a portion of the perinephric fat or develop osteoid metaplasia in an area of hemorrhage and necrosis (in which case coarse calcification

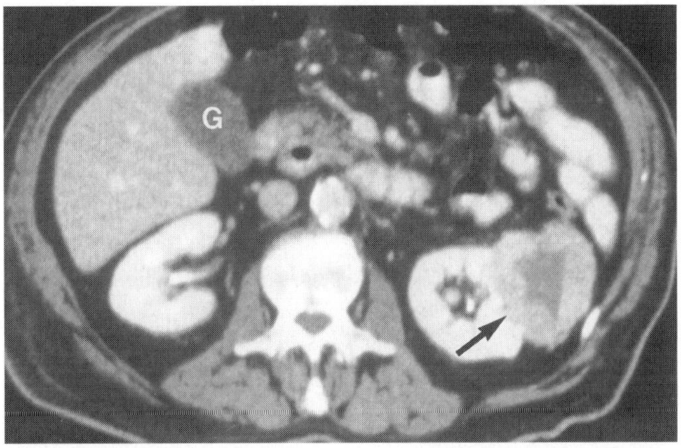

FIGURE 12.22 Renal cell carcinoma. IV contrast–enhanced CT showing a soft tissue mass *(arrow)* arising from the left renal midzone, with central area of low attenuation representing necrosis. G, gallbladder. [From Slone RM, Gutierrez FR, Fisher AJ (eds.) *Thoracic Imaging: A Practical Approach.* New York: McGraw-Hill; 1999. With permission.]

is also present). Calcifications are uncommonly present. RCCAs can invade the renal vein and IVC; on CT, an IVC tumor thrombus shows enhancement and expansion of the vascular lumen. As well, RCCAs can cause regional lymphoid or bilateral pulmonary hilar lymphadenopathy; lytic bone metastases; and adrenal, hepatic, pulmonary, and contralateral renal metastases.

Small, solid, enhancing parenchymal lesions should be presumed to represent RCCAs **(Fig. 12.23).** They can be surgically excised, although others have suggested monitoring with sequential short-interval follow-up exams. This approach can be beneficial in older patients or those who are poor surgical candidates. These small lesions have been shown to remain unchanged by CT follow-up for 2.5 years. Less than 6 percent of renal masses are indeterminate by CT imaging.

The Robson staging classification has been traditionally employed, although a TNM staging classification is now in place. RCCA stage is the best predictor of tumor behavior. The Robson staging system is as follows:

I—Tumor contained within the renal capsule. Treatment is with parenchyma-sparing local excision or nephrectomy.

II—Tumor contained within Gerota's fascia (can include ipsilateral adrenal metastases). Treatment is with nephrectomy.

III—A. Tumor with renal vein or IVC invasion. May be amenable to resection. Depending on the level of IVC or even left atrial involvement, a combined thoracoabdominal approach may be necessary.

B. Tumor with local lymphadenopathy.

C. Tumor with both vascular invasion and local lymphadenopathy.

IV—Tumor with distant metastases.

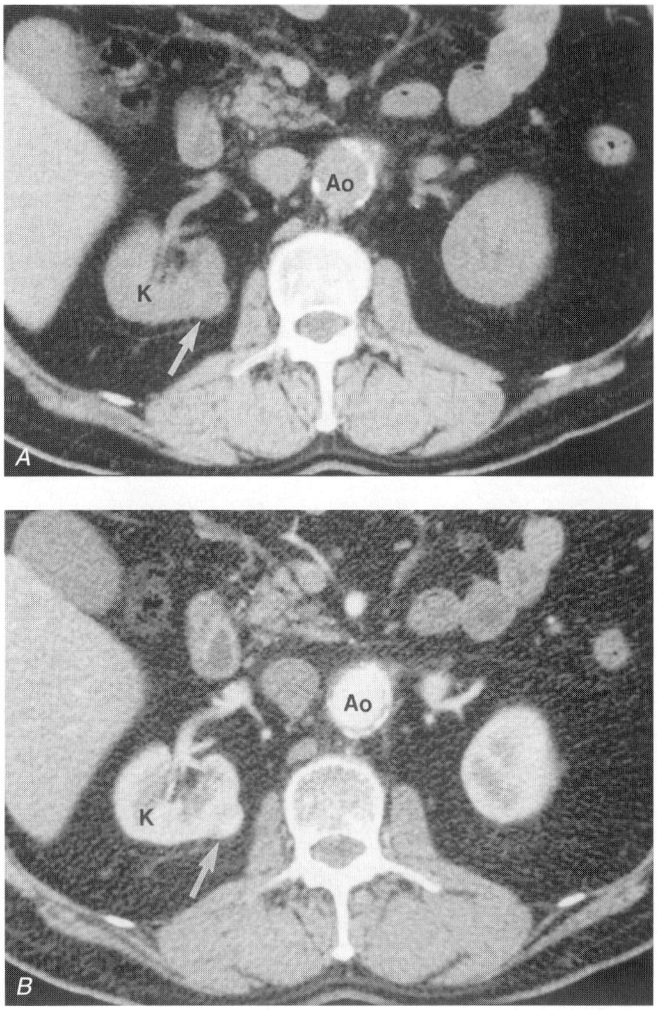

FIGURE 12.23 Small renal lesion. Noncontrast CT *(A)* demonstrates a less than 2-cm focal contour abnormality *(arrow)* along the medial aspect of the right kidney (K). Corticomedullary phase CT *(B)* shows that this mass *(arrow)* enhances like the aorta (Ao) and is highly suggestive of a renal neoplasm. Pathology revealed renal cell carcinoma.

- **Transitional cell carcinoma (TCCA)** arises from the urothelium and accounts for approximately 5 percent of primary renal malignancies. It can arise in the renal pelvis, although it is about 10 times more common in the bladder, and primary ureteral sites are even less frequently found. TCCA may be multifocal, since the entire urothelium is at risk. Consequently, surgical therapy consists of nephroureterectomy with excision of a cuff of bladder at the ureteral orifice.

  On **CT,** TCCA may be seen as a discrete mass arising in the renal hilum. It originates within the collecting system but can have indistinct margins with the surrounding parenchyma **(Fig. 12.24).** The tumor can be large and obstructing or give a "faceless" kidney, with absence of normal hilar morphology. The tumor is relatively hypovascular compared with both normal renal tissue and RCCAs. If it is infiltrative, the primary differential considerations are aggressive RCCA, lymphoma, metastases (often from a primary in the lung), pyelonephritis, and other, rarer renal malignancies.

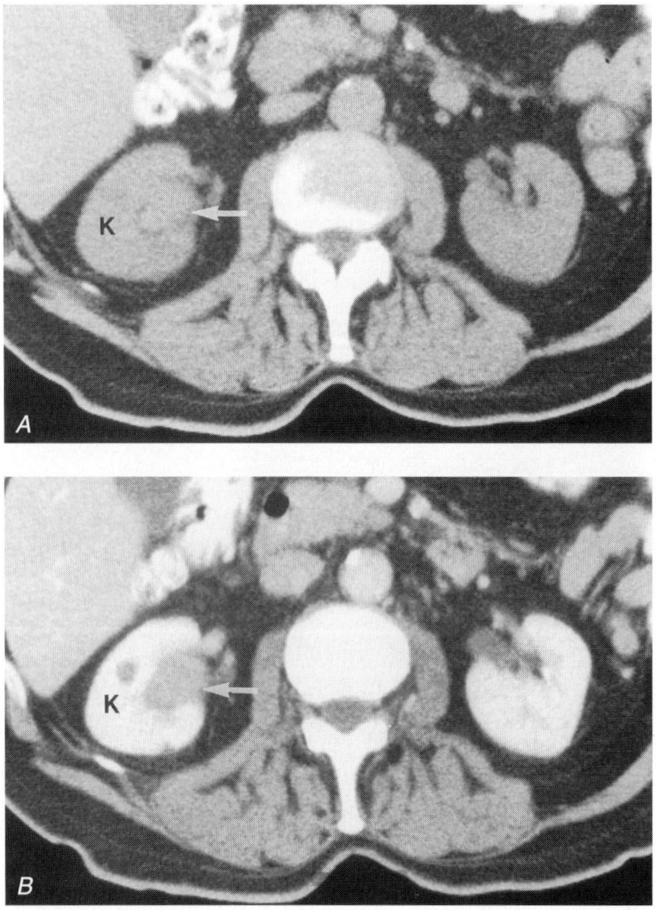

FIGURE 12.24 Transitional cell carcinoma of the renal pelvis. A 79-year-old man with hematuria. Noncontrast CT image *(A)* demonstrates soft tissue fullness *(arrow)* in the pelvis of the right kidney (K). After IV contrast *(B)*, the soft tissue mass *(arrow)* shows mild enhancement.

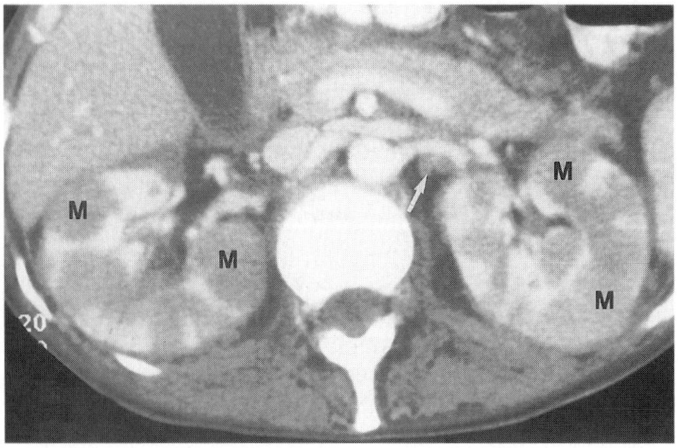

FIGURE 12.25 Renal lymphoma. IV contrast–enhanced CT demonstrates numerous low-attenuation renal parenchymal masses (M) bilaterally. Several small lymph nodes *(arrow)* are noted adjacent to the left renal artery.

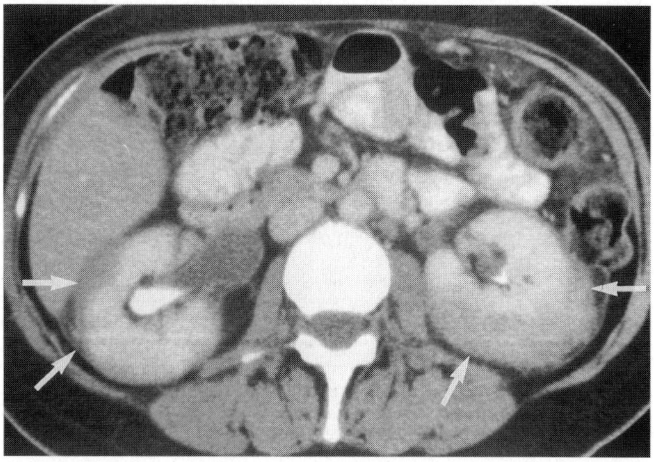

FIGURE 12.26 Renal leukemia. IV contrast–enhanced CT in a 38-year-old woman demonstrates bilateral subcapsular hypoenhancing soft tissue *(arrows)*. This infiltrative process has indistinct margins with the normal renal parenchyma.

- **Lymphoma** can arise within the kidney or result from direct extension of a large retroperitoneal mass. The cell type is usually of the non-Hodgkin variety. Renal involvement can be present in up to 5 percent of patients with lymphoma or up to 10 percent of those with AIDS-related disease.

The most common appearance of renal lymphoma after IV contrast administration is a single lesion or multiple rounded, low-attenuation parenchymal lesions that are hypoenhancing compared with the normal parenchyma. These masses can be distinguished from RCCA by their multifocality, relative hypovascularity, frequent associated retroperitoneal lymphadenopathy, and lack of central necrosis or intravascular tumor extension **(Fig. 12.25).** Renal lymphoma can enlarge the kidney diffusely when it preferentially involves the renal cortex. Renal leukemia can have a similar appearance **(Fig. 12.26).**

An additional presentation is **perinephric lymphoma,** depicted as a homogeneous soft tissue density arising within Gerota's fascia and at least partially encompassing the kidney **(Differential 12.11).** Invasion of the renal hilum or extension along the subcapsular space, where tissue planes offer limited resistance, is sometimes seen. More commonly, however, the kidney is involved secondarily from adjacent retroperitoneal lymphadenopathy. Lymphoma rarely causes ureteral obstruction or vascular compromise since it is a "soft" tumor **(Fig. 12.27).**

12.11

PERINEPHRIC LESION

Hematoma—trauma, tumor, anticoagulation, ESWL, AAA
Perinephric abscess—pyelonephritis, tuberculosis
Lymphoma—non-Hodgkin
Renal cell carcinoma
Adrenal mass
Urinoma
Pancreatitis
Sarcoma

Key: AAA, abdominal aortic aneurysm; ESWL, extracorporeal shock wave lithotripsy.

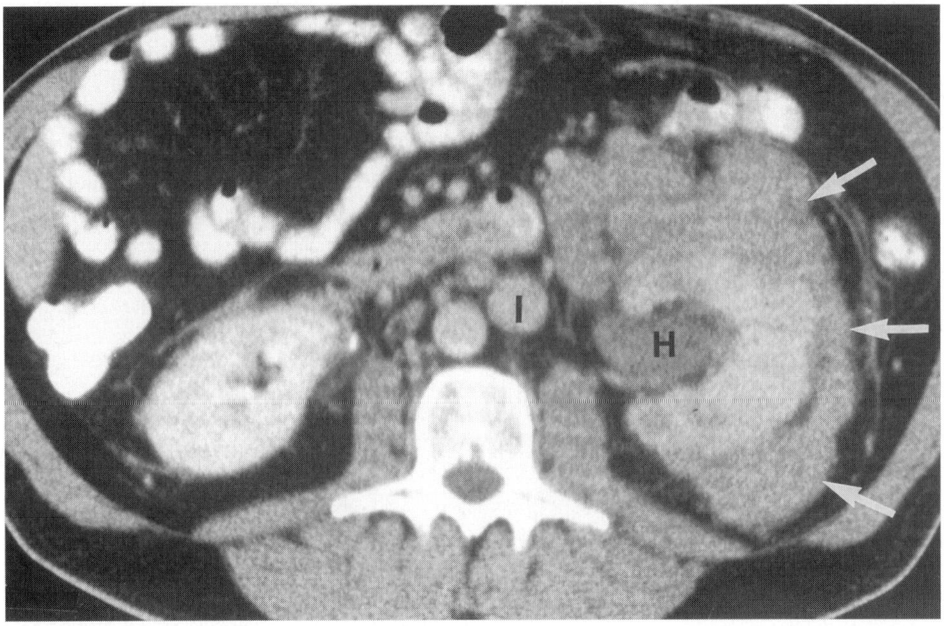

FIGURE 12.27 Perinephric lymphoma. This 52-year-old man left-lower quadrant pain and an abnormal intravenous pyelogram. There is a soft tissue mass *(arrows)* encompassing the left kidney. The delayed nephrogram is secondary to moderate proximal ureteral obstruction and hydronephrosis (H). Incidental note is made of a left-sided IVC (I).

- **Metastases** to the kidney are common at autopsy series, which report them in more than 10 percent of patients with disseminated carcinoma. Yet renal metastases are infrequently seen on imaging studies. When visible, they usually originate from primary sites in the adrenal gland, lung, or breast or from a melanoma.

  Renal metastases are generally small and multifocal, although a solitary mass can be present in either the cortex or medulla. Except for metastases from melanoma, metastases demonstrate relatively poor enhancement as compared with normal adjacent parenchyma. Occasionally, it can be difficult to distinguish metastases from a primary renal malignancy or renal inflammatory disease.

- **Wilms tumor** is the most common malignant renal tumor in children and adolescents. It is rarely seen in adults. Also termed ***nephroblastoma,*** a Wilms tumor contains embryonic blastema, epithelium, and stroma. There are associations with hemihypertrophy, sporadic aniridia, Beckwith-Wiedeman syndrome, and Drash (Wilms tumor, pseudohermaphroditism, and glomerulonephritis) syndrome. Presentation is usually due to a palpable mass, although fever, pain, hypertension, and anorexia are frequently present. Most pediatric cases are initially imaged with ultrasound. On CT, the lesions are typically over 10 cm in size and hypoenhancing; they occasionally invade the IVC **(Fig. 12.28).** Bilateral involvement is present in 5 to 10 percent of cases. Metastases most commonly occur to lung parenchyma. Adult Wilms tumors can appear as soft tissue masses with central necrosis, making distinction from RCCA impossible.

- **Nephroblastomatosis** represents persistence of multiple rests of embryologic metanephric blastoma. There is a close association with Wilms tumor, and nephroblastomatosis shares similar associations. Malignant transformation occurs in less than 1 percent of young children with nephrogenic rests. Because of the potential complicating Wilms tumor, careful imaging follow-up in these patients is warranted as a minimum; some authors advocate chemotherapy.

  Nephrogenic rests may be solitary, multifocal, or diffuse and bilateral. They are typically subcapsular in distribution. Nephroblastomatosis enhances less markedly than the renal-parenchyma; rapid growth and increasing lesion complexity suggest malignant disease.

- **Other pediatric renal malignancies** include clear cell sarcoma and rhabdoid tumor of the kidney. They are not believed to represent variants of Wilms tumor. **Clear cell sarcoma of the kidney** possesses the same age distribution and site of origin as Wilms tumor but has a significantly worse prognosis. Skeletal and pulmonary metastases are particularly common. **Rhabdoid tumor of the kidney** occurs in infants and very young children. Brain and lung metastases are frequent and the prognosis is grave **(Fig. 12.29).**

- **Renal sarcomas** other than sarcomatous RCCA are distinctly rare. They arise from the renal capsule and typically invade and displace the kidney. The most common is a capsular leiomyosarcoma, although other histologies—including liposarcomas, fibrosarcomas, and hemangiopericytomas—can be found. Most appear on CT as masses of soft

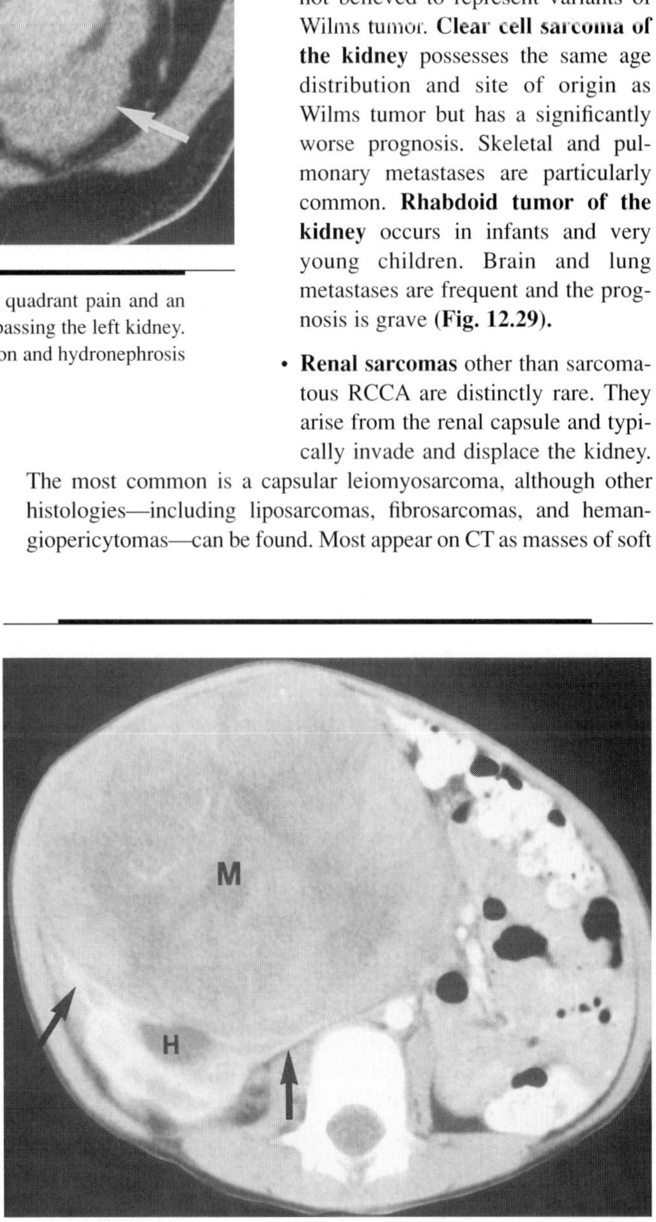

FIGURE 12.28 Wilms tumor. This 4-year-old boy has a visible deformity of the right abdominal wall. There is a large, heterogeneous, enhancing mass (M) in the right midabdomen. The beak of encompassing renal parenchyma *(arrows)* belies its renal origin. The tumor is causing hydronephrosis (H), and hepatic invasion was seen on other images.

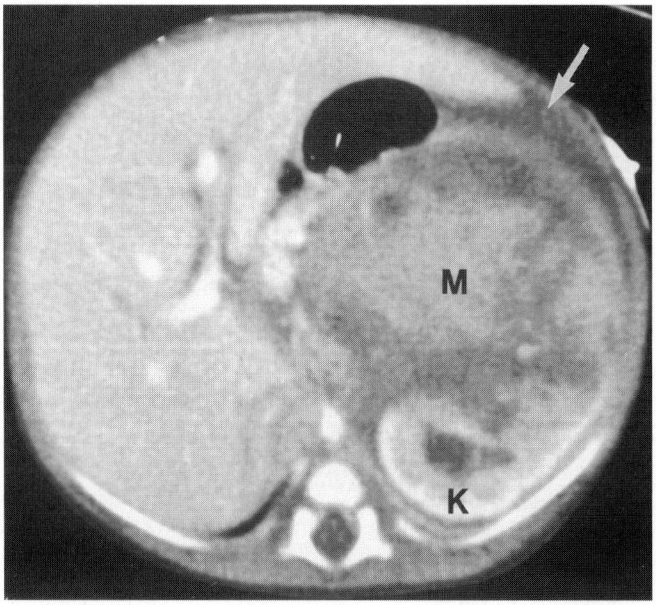

FIGURE 12.29 Malignant rhabdoid tumor. There is a large, partially enhancing mass (M) arising from the midzone of the left kidney (K) in this 1-day-old infant. The remaining abdominal contents are displaced. Areas of low density represent necrosis, and there is free fluid *(arrow)* within the abdomen.

tissue density with variable enhancement, which is most pronounced in hemangiopericytomas. Macroscopic fat suggests an AML or liposarcoma. Nephrectomy and wide excision are warranted.

- **Renal medullary carcinoma** is an uncommon malignancy occurring with higher frequency in patients with sickle cell anemia. Patients usually present in the second or third decade of life. Renal medullary carcinoma is an aggressive tumor appearing as an infiltrative, heterogeneously enhancing central renal mass.

There are numerous **less common renal tumors,** including juxtaglomerular, neuroendocrine, and stromal tumors; collecting duct and squamous cell cancers; and tumor-like conditions such as XGP and malakoplakia.

12.8 SURGERY

Total nephrectomy is often performed for renal neoplasms and less commonly for infectious or inflammatory processes. In this procedure, the contents of the perinephric space are excised, including the adrenal gland as well as the kidney itself. CT consequently demonstrates an empty renal fossa, which is often occupied by displaced structures such as small bowel or the spleen. CT readily demonstrates postoperative complications such as hematomas and abscesses as well as local tumor recurrence.

A **partial nephrectomy** is performed in an attempt to maximize preservation of renal function. This is performed for small tumors, for lesions that are considered likely benign by preoperative imaging, or in patients with a solitary kidney. A focal parenchymal defect is seen by CT. Laparoscopic resection can be performed through a posterior retroperitoneal approach. Complications include postoperative fluid collections and hernias along the trocar track.

Bibliography

Bechtold RB, Chen MY, Dyer RB, Zagoria RJ. CT of the ureteral wall. *AJR* 1998;170:1283–1289.

Bosniak MA, Birnbaum BA, Krinsky GA, Waisman J. Small renal parenchymal neoplasms: Further observations on growth. *Radiology* 1995;197:589–597.

Buckley JA, Urban BA, Soyer P, Scherrer A, Fishman EK. Transitional cell carcinoma of the renal pelvis: A retrospective look at CT staging with pathologic correlation. *Radiology* 1996;201:194–198.

Choyke PL, Glenn GM, Walther MM, Patronas NJ, Linehan WM, Zbar B. Von Hippel-Lindau disease: Genetic, clinical, and imaging features. *Radiology* 1995;194:629–642.

Dunnick NR, Newhouse JH, Sandler CM, Amis ES, (eds.): *Textbook of Uroradiology,* 2nd ed. Baltimore: William & Wilkins; 1997.

Dyer RB, Chen MYM, Zagoria RJ. Abnormal calcifications of the urinary tract. *Radiographics* 1998;18:1405–1424.

Kawashima A, Sandler CM, Goldman SM, Raval BK, Fishman EK. CT of renal inflammatory disease. *Radiographics* 1997;17:851–866.

Kenney PJ, Lee JKT: The adrenals. In: JKT Lee, Sagel SS, Stanley RJ, Heiken JP, eds. *Computed Body Tomography with MRI Correlation,* 3rd ed. Philadelphia: Lippincott-Raven, 1998:1171–1208.

Lonergan GJ, Martinez-Leon MI, Agrons GA, Montemarano H. Nephrogenic rests, nephroblastomatosis, and associated lesions of the kidney. *Radiographics* 1998;18:947–968.

Miller FH, Parikh S, Gore RM, Nemcek AA Jr, Fitzgerald SW, Vogelzang RL. Renal manifestations of AIDS. *Radiographics* 1993;13:587–596.

Scher HI, Leibel SA, Lange P, Raghavan D, (eds.): *Principles and Practice of Genitourinary Oncology.* Philadelphia: Lippincott-Raven, 1997.

Sheeran SR, Sussman SK. Renal lymphoma: Spectrum of CT findings and potential mimics. *AJR* 1998;171:1067–1072.

Slone RM, Fisher AJ. *Pocket Guide to Body CT Differential Diagnosis.* New York: McGraw-Hill, 1999.

Smith RC, Verga M, McCarthy S, Rosenfield AT. Diagnosis of acute flank pain: Value of unenhanced helical CT. *AJR* 1996;166:97–101.

Chapter 13

PELVIS

Perry J. Pickhardt

13.1 Anatomy and Technique
13.2 Bladder
13.3 Uterus
13.4 Ovaries
13.5 Prostate
13.6 Inflammatory Diseases of the Pelvis
13.7 Pelvic Masses

13.1 ANATOMY AND TECHNIQUE

- Evaluation of the pelvis is made clinically challenging by the diversity of potential pathologic processes that may affect it. Genitourinary (GU), gastrointestinal (GI), musculoskeletal, and neurovascular structures all coexist within the confined pelvic space. In addition, disease processes that originate in the upper abdomen may also involve the pelvis by direct peritoneal or extraperitoneal extension. Consequently, diagnostic imaging plays an important role in patients with suspected pelvic disease. **Computed tomography (CT),** ultrasound, and magnetic resonance imaging (MRI) are complementary techniques, and each has its own particular advantages and indications within the pelvis. This chapter focuses on the CT evaluation of pelvic disease.

  In general, CT is not relied upon for precise staging of most GU neoplasms, but it is nonetheless helpful in treatment planning. Therefore, the various staging classifications are not addressed in detail, but important features on CT that can affect patient management are emphasized. The utility of CT lies more in the evaluation of advanced stages of cancer, where it surpasses clinical examination in accuracy.

- A thorough understanding of normal **pelvic anatomy** is essential for accurate CT interpretation. In common practice, the pelvis on CT may be arbitrarily defined as extending from the superior margin of the iliac crests to below the public symphysis. In more anatomic terms, the false pelvis lies superior to the true pelvis and is separated from it by an oblique plane subtended by the sacral promontory and symphysis pubis. Unlike in the upper abdomen, gender consideration is of paramount importance in the pelvis, given the disparate anatomic features that exist between men and women **(Fig. 13.1).** Pelvic features that are common to both sexes include the major vessels, bladder, rectum, and major musculoskeletal structures. The pelvic skeletal anatomy consists of an osseous ring formed by the innominate bones and sacrum. The major muscles of the pelvis include the iliacus, psoas, obturator internus, piriformis, and pelvic diaphragm.

  The pelvis is made up of three major anatomic compartments: the peritoneal pelvis, the extraperitoneal pelvis, and the perineum. The **peritoneal pelvis** includes the space above the reflection of parietal peritoneum that overlies the superior aspect of the bladder, the proximal one-third of the rectum, and, in women, the uterus and adnexa. The dependent portions formed by peritoneal reflections include the rectouterine **pouch of Douglas** and vesicouterine recess in females and the rectovesical recess in males **(Fig. 13.1).** The peritoneal pelvis is largely occupied by small bowel loops, colon, and appendix.

  The **extraperitoneal pelvis** is continuous with the retroperitoneal space, allowing for bidirectional spread of pathologic processes. Major components of the extraperitoneal pelvis include the presacral space, the perirectal space, and the retropubic **space of Retzius,** all of which potentially intercommunicate **(Fig. 13.1).** The extraperitoneal pelvis contains the major GU organs and the distal two-thirds of the rectum.

  The **perineum** is separated from the extraperitoneal pelvis by the muscular pelvic floor or diaphragm, which is formed by the levator ani and coccygeus muscles. The **ischiorectal fossa** is the largest component of the perineum and forms a pyramidal space that is bounded by the levator ani and external sphincter muscles medially and the obturator internus muscle laterally **(Fig. 13.2).**

  The **urinary bladder** is a distensible reservoir and its CT appearance will depend upon the degree of luminal filling. When the bladder is urine- or contrast-filled, its wall thickness should not exceed 5 mm. Opacified urine usually lies dependent to unopacified urine. This relationship, however, can be reversed in patients with significant glycosuria. The distal ureters lie immediately posterior to the parietal peritoneum and cross the common iliac vessels at the pelvic brim. The ureterovesical junction is located at the bladder trigone near the posterior base. The ureters are readily identified on CT when dilated or opacified with excreted contrast material.

- The intrapelvic portions of the **female genital tract** are significantly more complex than those of the male **(Fig. 13.1).** The appearance of the **uterus** will vary depending on the patient's age, hormonal status, uterine position, and presence of fibroids. The uterus normally appears as a homogeneous, ovoid structure on axial CT images. The endometrium and myometrium demonstrate prominent contrast enhancement on CT compared with the pelvic wall musculature (see **Fig. 13.15**). The endometrial cavity is usually identified as a central low-attenuation stripe within the uterus.

  The uterine **cervix** is usually depicted on CT as a rounded or donut-shaped structure at the inferior aspect of the uterus. The **vagina** typically has a flattened or elongated transverse orientation and lies between the bladder and rectum **(Fig. 13.3).** The **fallopian**

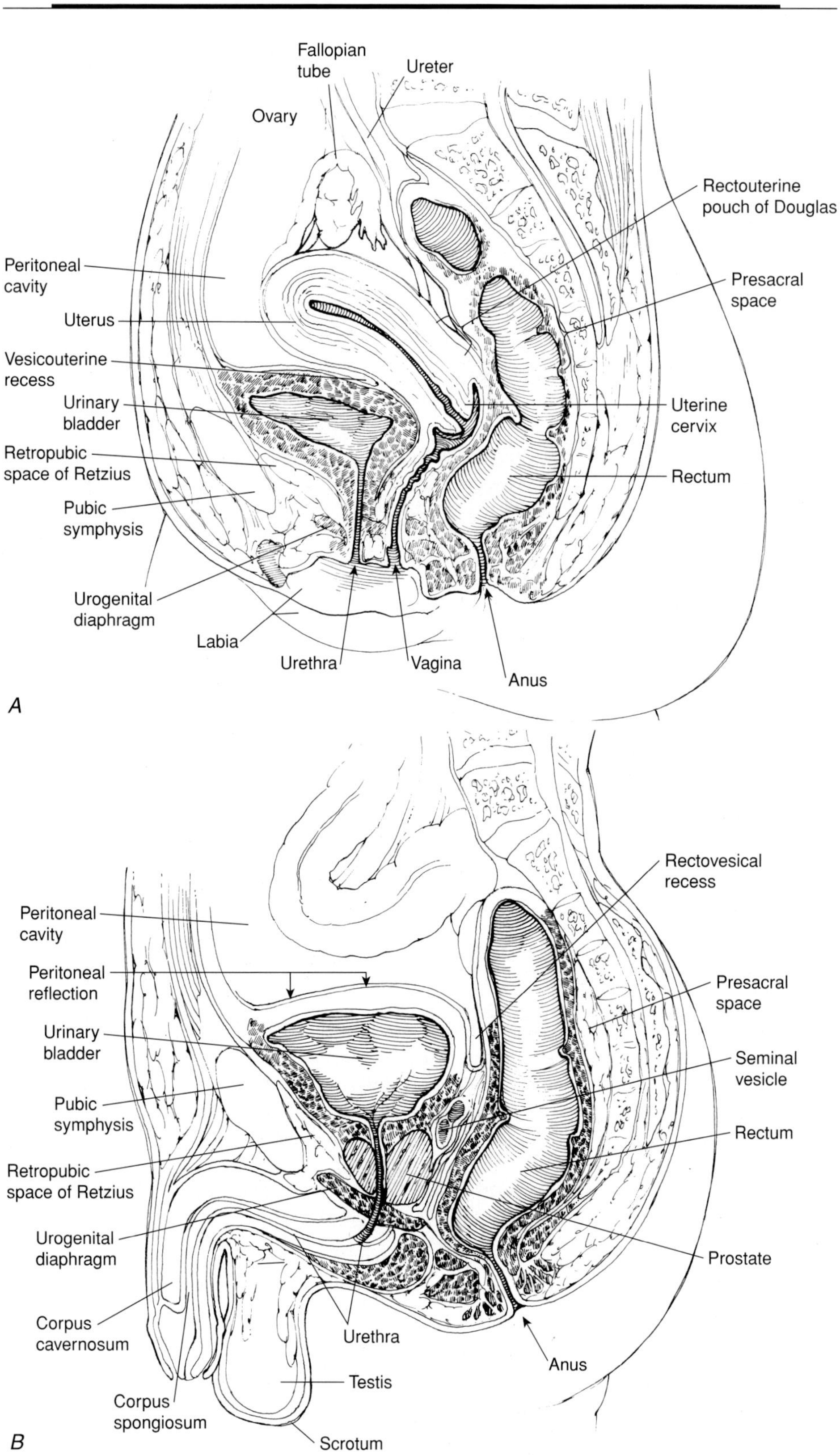

FIGURE 13.1 Pelvic anatomy. Diagram of sagittal sections of the female *(A)* and male *(B)* pelvis.

tubes extend laterally from the uterine cornua and drape over the ovaries laterally (see **Fig. 13.17**). The fallopian tubes form the free edge of a fold of peritoneum called the **broad ligament.** It contains the parametrial vessels, which often show prominent enhancement on CT in premenopausal women. The base of the broad ligament is formed by the cardinal ligament, which extends from the cervix to the lateral pelvic wall. The ureters are seen just anterior to the triangular cardinal ligaments.

The **ovaries** also demonstrate many different normal appearances and positions on CT. Occasionally, normal ovaries are difficult to define clearly and separate from adjacent structures, especially in postmenopausal women. Identification of multiple cystic follicles can be helpful in finding the ovaries on CT. The **round ligaments** are usually identifiable on CT and extend from the uterine fundus to the labia majora via the inguinal canal (see **Fig. 10.33**).

- On CT, the **prostate gland** in male patients is depicted as a walnut-sized homogeneous soft tissue structure beneath the bladder base. The normal gland should not exceed 4 cm in diameter. The **seminal vesicles** occupy the posterior niche between the bladder and prostate gland and are easily identified on CT **(Fig. 13.4).** The **spermatic cords** are composed of vessels, nerves, lymphatics, and the vas deferens and can usually be traced along their course through the inguinal canal and into the scrotum. When the entire scrotum is imaged on CT, the normal **testes** are identified as homogeneous ovoid structures.

- Standard **CT technique** for imaging the abdomen will generally apply to the pelvis as well. In fact, images of both the abdomen and pelvis are routinely obtained as a single study. The artifact that is introduced from respiratory motion is less of a problem in the pelvis than in the chest and abdomen. Adequate contrast opacification and distention of the GI tract is imperative, since unopacified bowel loops can often simulate true pelvic pathology. Intravenous (IV) contrast should be administered unless contraindicated. In selected cases, delayed postcontrast imaging allows for confirmation of unopacified bowel or further evaluation of a nondistended bladder. Additional CT techniques within the pelvis include CT cystography in the setting of pelvic trauma (see **Chapter 15**) or fistula formation with adjacent structures. When filling defects are identified in the bladder,

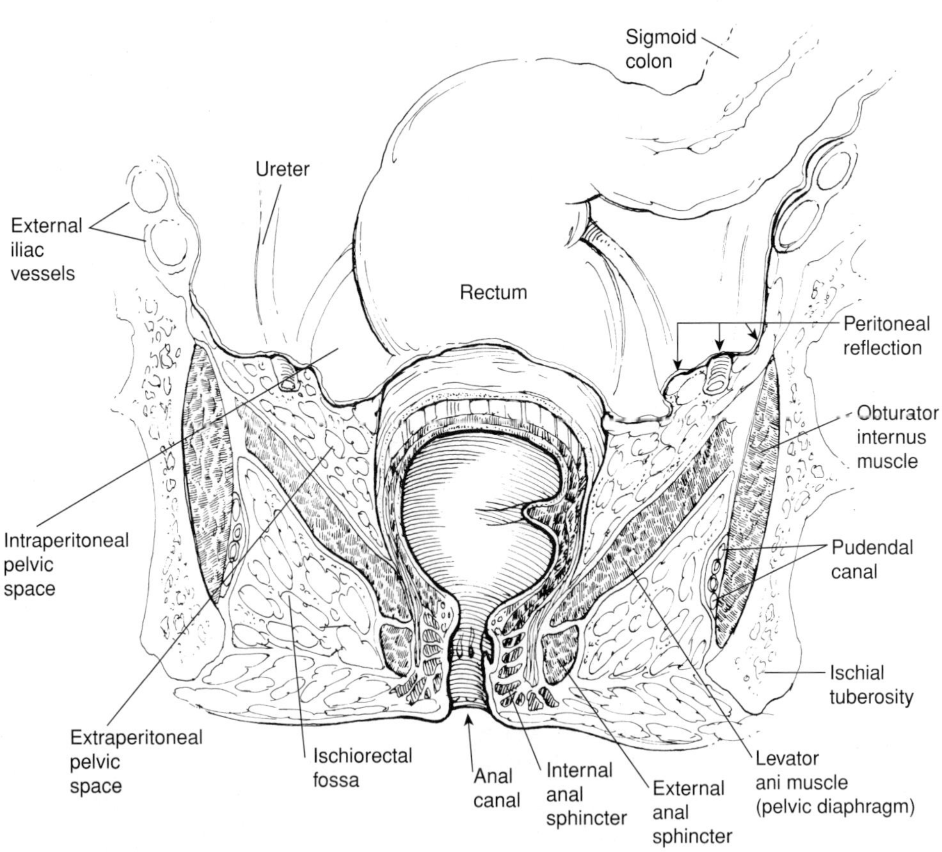

FIGURE 13.2 Pelvic anatomy. Diagram of a coronal section through the posterior pelvis shows the relationship of the intraperitoneal pelvis, extraperitoneal pelvis, and perineum.

decubitus positioning can be performed to determine whether they are mobile. Rectal contrast can also be given in selected cases. A vaginal tampon is placed prior to scanning at some centers to clearly mark the position of the vagina.

13.2 BLADDER

- Confident diagnosis of **bladder wall thickening** on CT requires adequate luminal distention. CT allows for characterization of bladder lesions, distinguishes between focal and diffuse disease, and evaluates for perivesical involvement.

  Focal thickening of the bladder wall must be differentiated from mobile intraluminal filling defects **(Differential 13.1).** Causes of localized wall thickening include tumors and inflammatory conditions. Prostatic enlargement is a common cause of a filling defect of the bladder base in older men. **Mobile filling defects** can be confirmed on CT by demonstrating movement of the lesion on prone imaging. Intraluminal blood clots can result from GU trauma, tumors, or calculi. Acute hemorrhage will usually result in attenuation values greater than 40 HU. Foreign bodies within the bladder may have been inserted by the patient or may result from iatrogenic causes, with a Foley-type balloon catheter being by far the most common entity (see **Fig. 13.26**). Calculi are most commonly seen in patients with bladder outlet obstruction or chronic infection. Fungal balls are an uncommon cause of a bladder filling defect and are usually seen in diabetic patients.

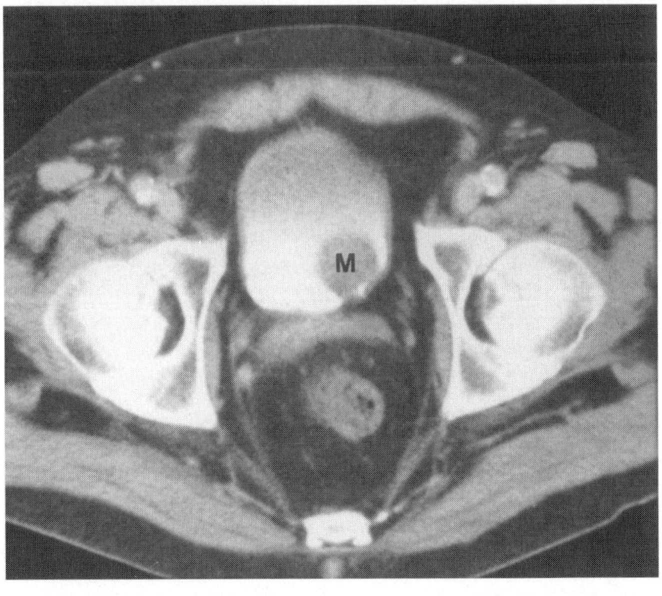

FIGURE 13.3 Bladder transitional cell carcinoma (TCC). Contrast-enhanced CT in a 65-year-old woman shows a rounded soft tissue mass (M) within the bladder near the left ureteral orifice. The position of the lesion did not change after repeat imaging in the prone position.

- **Transitional cell carcinoma (TCC)** accounts for over 90 percent of urothelial bladder tumors and occurs most commonly in elderly patients. Hematuria is the usual clinical presentation. Known or reported risk factors for developing TCC include smoking, exposure to aniline or azo dyes, cyclophosphamide therapy, analgesic abuse, Balkan nephropathy, chronic infection, and urinary stasis. Approximately 80 percent of bladder TCCs at diagnosis are superficial papillary tumors, whereas 20 percent are invasive. Multifocal involvement is seen in about one-third of papillary tumors. Synchronous upper tract tumors are found in less than 3 percent of cases, but patients with bladder TCC remain at risk for development of upper tract disease. Up to 40 percent of patients with upper tract TCC eventually develop TCC of the bladder.

  Bladder TCC is seen on CT as focal wall thickening or as an endophytic mass **(Fig. 13.3).** The lateral bladder wall is the most common site of involvement, followed by the trigone and dome. Tumor staging reflects the degree of mural infiltration or perivesical extension. CT is useful for demonstrating extravesical extension, lymphadenopathy, and ureteral obstruction, but it cannot reliably assess the degree of bladder wall invasion. Superficial lesions are typically fulgurated, tumors involving the bladder wall muscu-

13.1

FOCAL BLADDER LESION OR FILLING DEFECT

Enlarged prostate
Foreign body—particularly Foley catheter
Blood clot—trauma, tumor, stone, intervention
Urothelial tumor—90% transitional, 5% squamous, 2% adenocarcinoma, embryonal rhabdomyosarcoma, paraganglioma
Calculus
Perivesical inflammation—diverticulitis, PID, UVJ stone
Urethral diverticulum—"female prostate"
Cystitis cystica/glandularis
Schistosomiasis
Ureterocele
Fungus ball
Malakoplakia
Endometriosis
Amyloidois

Key: PID, pelvic inflammatory disease; UVJ, ureterovesical junction.

lature require cystectomy, and patients with inoperable tumors receive chemotherapy or palliation.

A slightly higher incidence of TCC has been reported to occur within bladder diverticula, probably because of urinary stasis. Extravesical spread of such tumors can occur earlier, since diverticula lack a muscular barrier **(Fig. 13.4).** CT is also useful for detecting disease recurrence following radical cystectomy, which involves pelvic lymph nodes in approximately two-thirds and the cystectomy bed in one-third of cases.

- **Squamous cell carcinoma** accounts for approximately 5 percent of bladder malignancies. Most patients will have a history of chronic or recurrent bladder infection, often with associated calculi. Infestation with *Schistosoma haematobium* also predisposes to squamous cell carcinoma. Differentiation of squamous cell carcinoma from TCC is not possible on CT. **Adenocarcinoma** of the bladder accounts for only 1 to 2 percent of malignancy. These tumors are associated with bladder extrophy, cystitis glandularis, and urachal remnants. The majority of **urachal carcinomas** are mucinous adenocarcinomas. On CT, these lesions involve the bladder dome and often extend superiorly along the course of the urachus **(Fig. 13.5).** Calcification is present in up to 70 percent of cases. In children, **embryonal rhabdomyosarcoma** of the bladder represents an aggressive malignancy with a poor prognosis.

- **Benign bladder tumors** are rare. Leiomyoma is the most common benign tumor and is typically seen in adult women. The tumor may project into the bladder lumen or grow in an extravesical manner, where it can become rather large before causing any symptoms. Paragangliomas of the bladder are rare and usually occur near the trigone. The classic presentation of these tumors includes sweating, headache, and palpitations on micturition in a hypertensive patient. Other benign tumors include fibroepithelial polyps, nephrogenic adenomas, neurofibromas, and hamartomas.

- **Nonneoplastic causes** of focal bladder wall thickening primarily consist of infection-related and extrinsic processes. Perivesical inflammation from diverticulitis, appendicitis, Crohn disease, or pelvic inflammatory disease is a common cause of focal bladder wall thickening (see **Fig. 6.28**). Cystitis cystica is related to recurrent urinary tract infections and is histologically characterized as benign submucosal nests of epithelial cells that are typically located at the bladder base. Cystitis glandularis is a related condition that represents further metaplasia of the submucosal nests and is considered premalignant. Malakoplakia is also related to chronic infection and is characterized by soft plaques that project into the

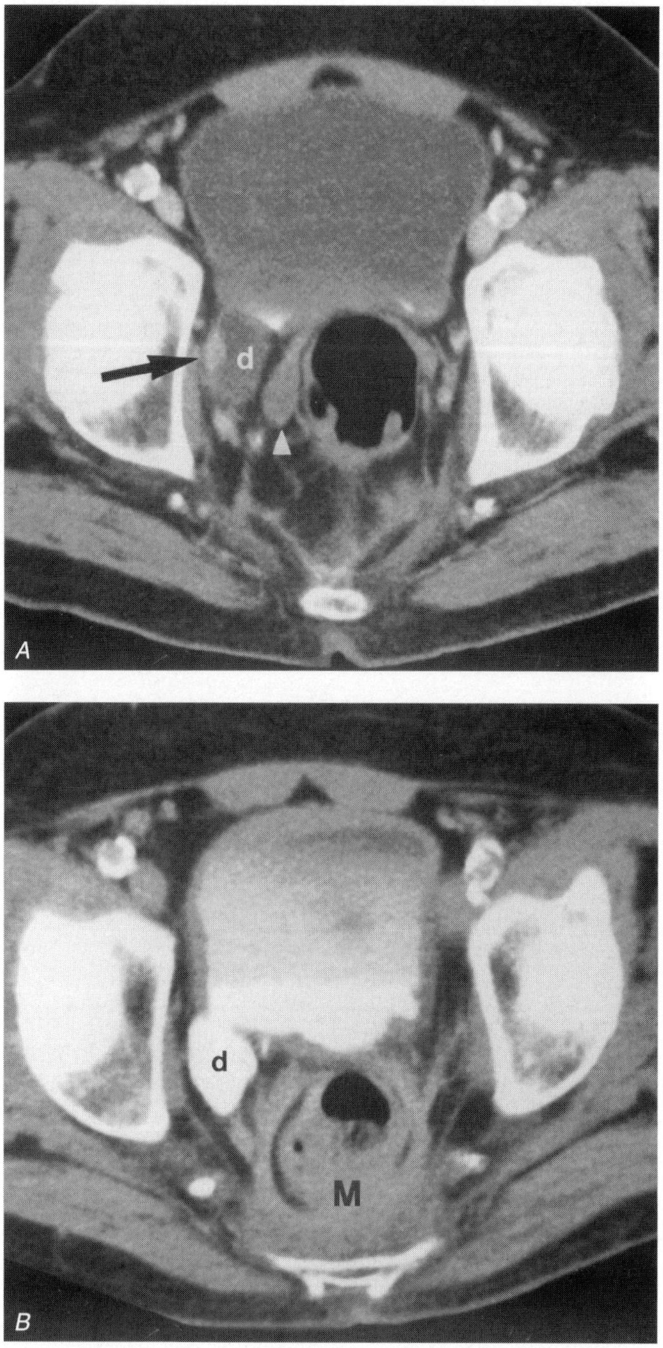

FIGURE 13.4 TCC within bladder diverticulum. *A.* Contrast-enhanced CT in an 81-year-old man shows a diverticulum (d) extending from the right posterior bladder. The small soft tissue nodule in the lateral aspect of the diverticulum *(arrow)* was found to be TCC at cystoscopy and was fulgurated. Right seminal vesical *(arrowhead)*. *B.* Follow-up study 6 months later shows new perirectal and presacral soft tissue (M). Extension of TCC was proven on biopsy. The patient had not received radiation therapy.

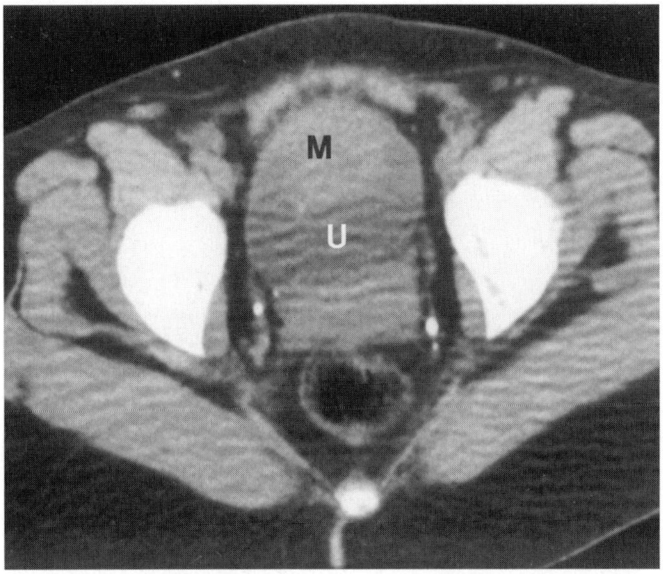

FIGURE 13.5 Urachal adenocarcinoma. Contrast-enhanced CT in a 40-year-old man shows a soft tissue mass (M) involving the anterior bladder dome surrounded by unopacified urine (U). The mass extended superiorly from the bladder on other images. This proved to be an adenocarcinoma arising within a urachal remnant.

bladder lumen. Histologic examination shows intracellular collections of phagocytized bacteria (Michaelis-Gutmann bodies) within histiocytes. Amyloidosis and endometriosis may also rarely involve the bladder.

- **Diffuse thickening of the bladder wall** is most often secondary to inflammation, bladder outlet obstruction, or neurogenic causes **(Differential 13.2).** The underlying cause is usually apparent from the clinical history and associated findings on CT. Incomplete bladder distention simulates diffuse bladder wall thickening on CT. In cases of bladder outlet obstruction, as with benign prostatic hypertrophy, or neurogenic bladder from detrusor hyperreflexia, a corrugated contour from trabeculation may be apparent.
- **Bladder infection** may be caused by bacterial, fungal, viral, or parasitic pathogens. Cystitis from any organism can result in diffuse wall thickening **(Fig. 13.6).** Acute bacterial cystitis is extremely common and is most often due to coliform bacteria such as *Escherichia coli.*
- **Emphysematous cystitis** is typically seen in diabetic patients and is most often due to *E. coli* infection. The presence of intramural gas is readily detected on CT **(Fig. 13.7).** A mucosal breach results in intraluminal gas. If air is seen only within the bladder lumen and not within the bladder wall, causes such as catheterization, candidiasis, or fistula formation with bowel should be considered (see **Fig. 6.28) (Differential 13.3).**

13.2 DIFFUSE BLADDER WALL THICKENING

Nondistended bladder
Cystitis
Infection—bacterial, fungal, parasitic, viral
Radiation, *eosinophilic, interstitial*
Outlet obstruction—prostatic enlargement most common
Neurogenic bladder

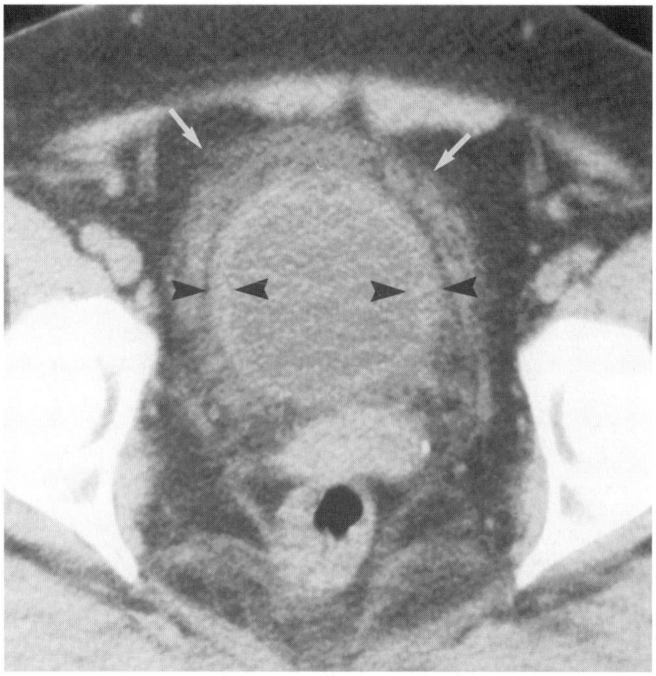

FIGURE 13.6 Cystitis. Contrast-enhanced CT in a 48-year-old woman with abdominal pain and urinary frequency shows diffuse bladder wall thickening *(arrowheads)* and soft tissue infiltration of the perivesical fat *(arrows)* from bacterial cystitis.

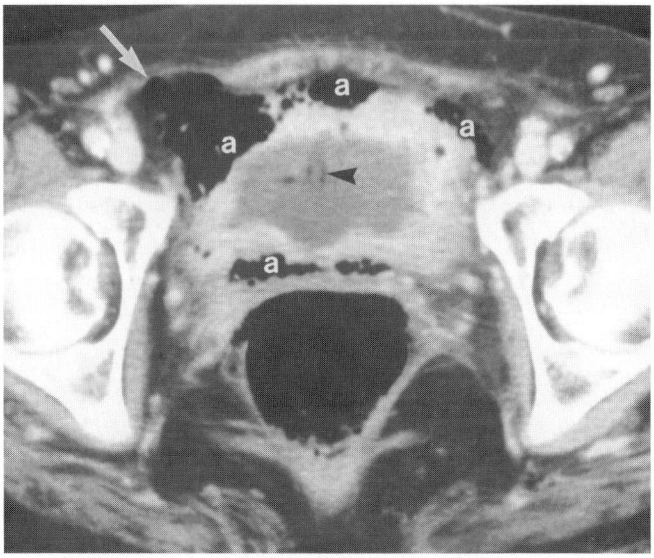

FIGURE 13.7 Emphysematous cystitis. Contrast-enhanced CT in a 72-year-old diabetic woman with *E. coli* cystitis shows air bubbles (a) throughout the thickened bladder wall. Air appears to extend beyond the confines of the bladder wall anteriorly *(arrow).* A Foley catheter is in place *(arrowhead).*

13.3 AIR IN BLADDER WALL OR LUMEN

Instrumentation—catheterization, cystoscopy, ureteroscopy
Fistula with colon, small bowel, or vagina—radiation, cancer, Crohn disease, diverticulitis, surgery
Trauma
Emphysematous cystitis—bacterial, diabetics, air initially in wall
Candidiasis—diabetics, air in lumen

Tuberculous cystitis results from a descending infection of the upper tract and occasionally causes bladder wall calcification. Bladder infection with *Schistosoma haematobium,* which is common in parts of northern Africa, results in inflammation and fibrosis of the bladder wall. Long-standing disease often results in calcification and predisposes to squamous cell carcinoma. Other causes of bladder wall calcification are less common and include radiation cystitis, cyclophosphamide therapy, amyloidosis, and bladder tumors. Calcification from TCC is seen in less than 1 percent of untreated patients.

- Bladder wall thickening and irregularity from **radiation cystitis** is due to edema and hemorrhage in the acute phase and from fibrosis in the chronic phase. Prominent bladder wall edema and hemorrhage are also associated with cyclophosphamide therapy. Other forms of cystitis include eosinophilic and interstitial types.
- A contour deformity of the bladder from extrinsic compression is a nonspecific finding on conventional urography, but the cause is usually apparent on CT. Normal structures such as the uterus and bowel commonly indent the bladder. Causes of a vertical orientation or "pear-shaped" bladder include pelvic hematoma, lymphadenopathy, prominent iliopsoas muscles, and pelvic lipomatosis **(Fig. 13.8).**

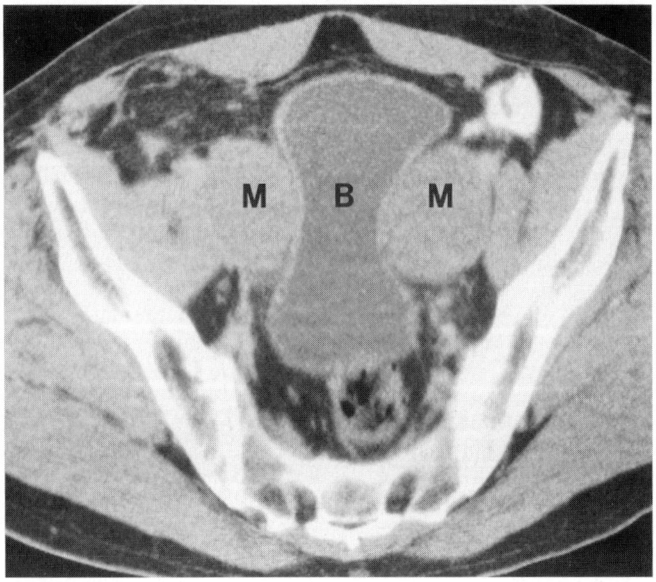

FIGURE 13.8 Extrinsic mass effect on bladder. Contrast-enhanced CT in a 60-year-old man with metastatic prostate cancer shows bulky iliac lymphadenopathy (M) that deforms the bladder contour (B).

13.3 UTERUS

- **Leiomyoma** of the uterus is a very common benign tumor of the myometrium, seen in 25 to 50 percent of women over 30 years of age. Commonly referred to as "fibroids," these tumors vary widely in size and are frequently multiple. Leiomyomas are classified as submucosal, intramural, or subserosal, depending on their relative location within the uterine corpus. Cervical fibroids are uncommon. Most of these tumors do not cause symptoms and are discovered incidentally on imaging. Occasionally, symptoms arise because of tumor size, location, torsion, or red degeneration. Rare and enigmatic variants of leiomyomas include the benign metastasizing leiomyoma and leiomyomatosis peritonealis disseminata.

  On **CT,** uterine leiomyomas demonstrate a variety of appearances and, along with pregnancy, are the most common causes of uterine enlargement **(Differential 13.4).** Generally, the tumors are rounded, they distort the uterine contour, and they often contain areas of low attenuation **(Fig. 13.9).** The presence of coarse calcifications supports the diagnosis. A uterine origin is sometimes difficult to appreciate with subserosal fibroids, and these lesions can extend into the broad ligament and simulate other adnexal lesions. MRI provides a more complete evaluation due to improved soft tissue contrast and multiplanar display.
- Endometrial thickening can result from polyps, hyperplasia, or malignancy. Although endometrial abnormalities can be detected on CT, ultrasound (especially hysterosonography) is the preferred imaging modality for the evaluation of endometrial thickening. **Endometrial carcinoma** is the most common invasive malignancy of the female genital tract. Postmenopausal bleeding is the typical presentation. Staging of endometrial carcinoma is surgical and determined by the degree of uterine invasion, cervical involvement, extrauterine extension, lymph node spread, bladder or bowel involvement, and distant metastases.

  On **CT,** endometrial carcinoma is usually depicted as a heterogeneous mass that fills and expands the uterine cavity **(Fig. 13.10).** Expansion can be due in part to hydrometros or hematometros from cervical obstruction by tumor. Myometrial or extrauterine extension may be apparent on CT but is better assessed by MRI. CT is more useful for the detection of advanced stages of disease, as seen with lymphadenopathy, bowel or bladder invasion, and distant metastases. CT is also valuable in assessing for disease recurrence.
- **Cervical cancer** affects premenopausal women more frequently than does endometrial or ovarian cancer and is usually detected early by cervical Pap smear. The great majority of cervical cancers are squamous cell carcinomas. Direct parametrial extension is the primary mode of spread, followed by pelvic lymph node dissemi-

13.4 ENLARGED UTERUS

Fibroids—25 to 50% of women, multiple, may calcify
Pregnancy
Obstruction—cervical stenosis, cervical carcinoma, polyps
Endometrial cancer—>90% adenocarcinoma
Adenomyosis—endometrial invasion of myometrium
Endometrial hyperplasia—unopposed estrogen
Endometrial polyps—20% multiple, <4% malignant
Gestational trophoblastic disease (GTD)
Pyometra
Uterine sarcoma

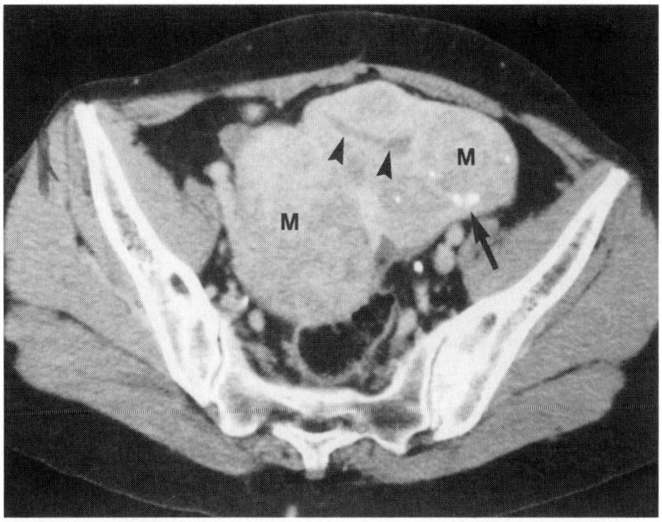

FIGURE 13.9 Uterine leiomyomas. Contrast-enhanced CT in a 79-year-old woman shows lobulated enlargement of the uterus by heterogeneous masses (M) that distort the uterine contour. Coarse calcifications are present *(arrow)*. Note the eccentric position of the endometrial stripe *(arrowheads)*.

nation. Distant metastases occur late in the disease course. Tumors without obvious parametrial spread are generally treated surgically, whereas radiation therapy is indicated in patients with locally advanced disease.

On **CT,** the primary tumor is usually depicted as a low-attenuation mass that enlarges the cervix. The tumor may obstruct the endocervical canal, resulting in fluid accumulation that enlarges the uterine cavity **(Fig. 13.11).** CT is most helpful in advanced stages of disease and can demonstrate unresectability in cases with prominent parametrial or pelvic side-wall involvement, lymphadenopathy, hydronephrosis from ureteral obstruction, or distant metastases. Unfortunately, both false-positive and false-negative CT interpretations for local extension are relatively common in less advanced stages of disease. MRI more accurately stages local extension of cervical cancer. CT is frequently employed in patients with suspected tumor recurrence. CT findings of recurrent disease usually consist of new soft tissue within the pelvis, but differentiation from radiation or postsurgical fibrosis often requires biopsy.

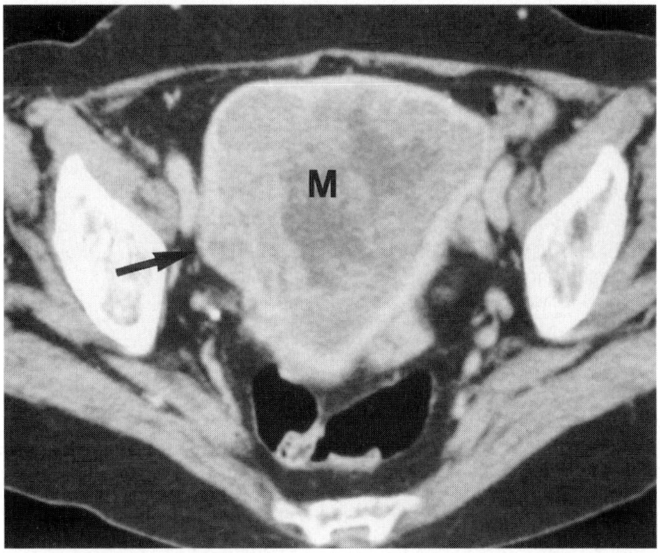

FIGURE 13.10 Endometrial cancer. Contrast-enhanced CT in a 72-year-old woman shows expansion of the endometrial cavity by an irregular soft tissue mass (M). Central low attenuation may represent necrosis, fluid from obstruction, or blood. The ill-defined tumor margin with the enhancing myometrium on the right represents local invasion *(arrow)*.

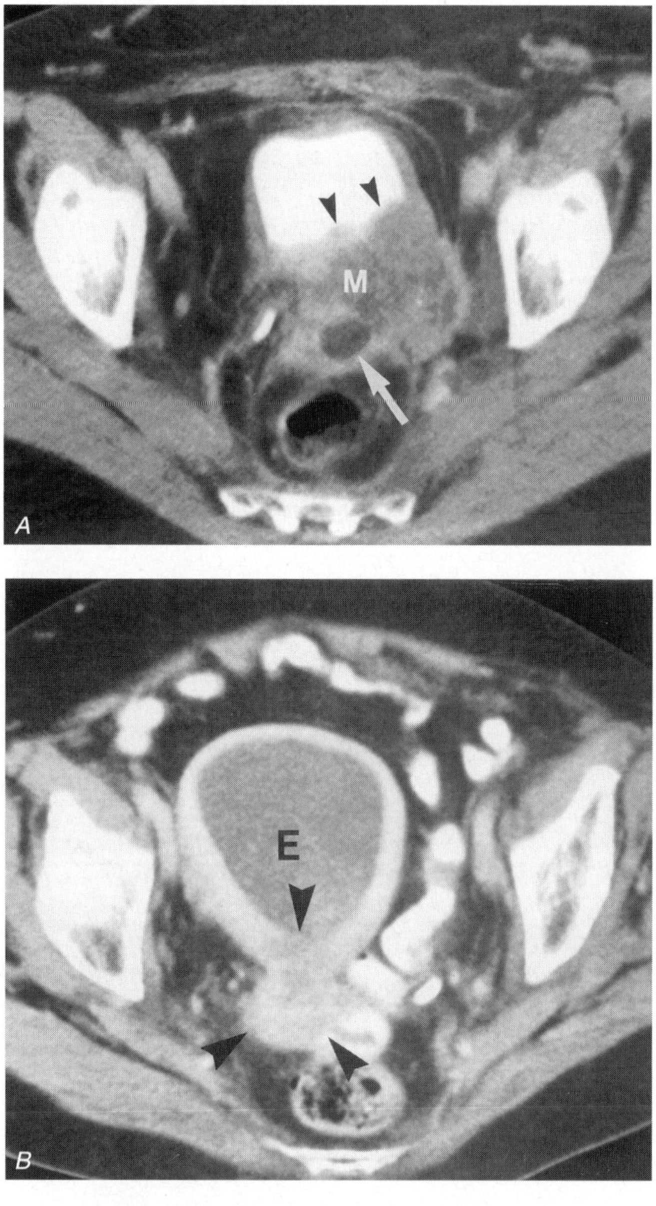

FIGURE 13.11 Cervical cancer. *A*. Contrast-enhanced CT in a 42-year-old woman shows a large cervical mass (M) with left parametrial extension, invasion of the urinary bladder *(arrowheads)*, and dilatation of the left ureter due to obstruction *(arrow)*. *B*. Contrast-enhanced CT in an 85-year-old woman shows hydrometros with homogeneous fluid expanding the endometrial cavity (E) due to obstruction from a cervical mass *(arrowheads)*.

- **Uterine sarcomas** may arise from the endometrium or myometrium. Malignant mixed müllerian tumors (MMMT) are derived from totipotential endometrial stromal cells and make up the majority of uterine sarcomas. Endometrial stromal sarcomas are less common than MMMT. Both sarcomas are clinically aggressive and, on CT, appear as large heterogeneous masses centered within the uterine cavity **(Fig. 13.12).** Leiomyosarcomas are derived from the myometrium but do not arise from preexisting leiomyomas. These tumors are also typically large and heterogeneous at presentation. Unfortunately, there are no imaging features that can reliably differentiate leiomyosarcomas from large leiomyomas.

- **Gestational trophoblastic disease (GTD)** represents a spectrum of abnormal trophoblastic proliferation that includes hydatidiform mole (partial or complete), invasive mole, and choriocarcinoma. The hydatidiform mole is the most common form of GTD and the typical presentation includes a uterus that is too large for dates and abnormal elevation of serum beta human chorionic gonadotropin (β-hCG) level. Approximately 15 percent of patients develop an **invasive mole** after evacuation of a hydatidiform mole, but invasive moles can also occur after normal pregnancy or abortion. Penetration of the myometrium by trophoblastic tissue defines invasion. **Choriocarcinoma** occurs in 5 percent of women with a previous mole, but approximately one-half of all cases follow abortion or pregnancy. This highly malignant tumor is characteristically hemorrhagic and frequently metastasizes.

  CT is not routinely performed for molar pregnancy, since ultrasound is adequate for imaging diagnosis of hydatidiform moles. CT and MRI are more valuable for the evaluation of invasive moles and choriocarcinoma. On CT, invasion of the myometrium by an ill-defined mixed-attenuation mass is characteristic **(Fig. 13.13).** Evidence of hemorrhage is more typical of choriocarcinoma, and hemorrhagic metastases may also be detected on cross-sectional imaging. Prominent cystic enlargement of the ovaries develops in up to 50 percent of patients with GTD and represents theca-lutein cysts from β-hCG stimulation.

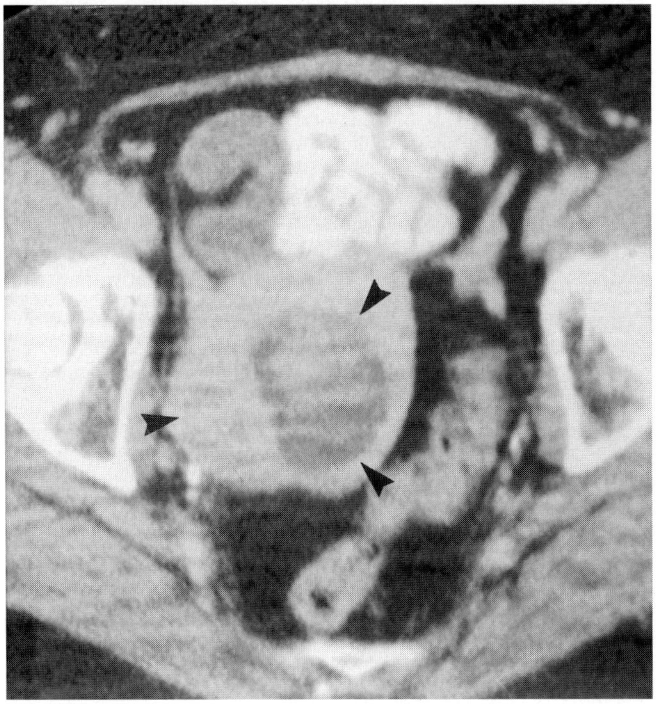

FIGURE 13.12 Uterine sarcoma. Contrast-enhanced CT in a 66-year-old woman shows a large heterogeneous mass within the uterus *(arrowheads)*, which proved to be a malignant mixed müllerian tumor (MMMT). Differentiating uterine sarcomas from other neoplasms, such as endometrial carcinoma or atypical leiomyoma, is often not possible on CT.

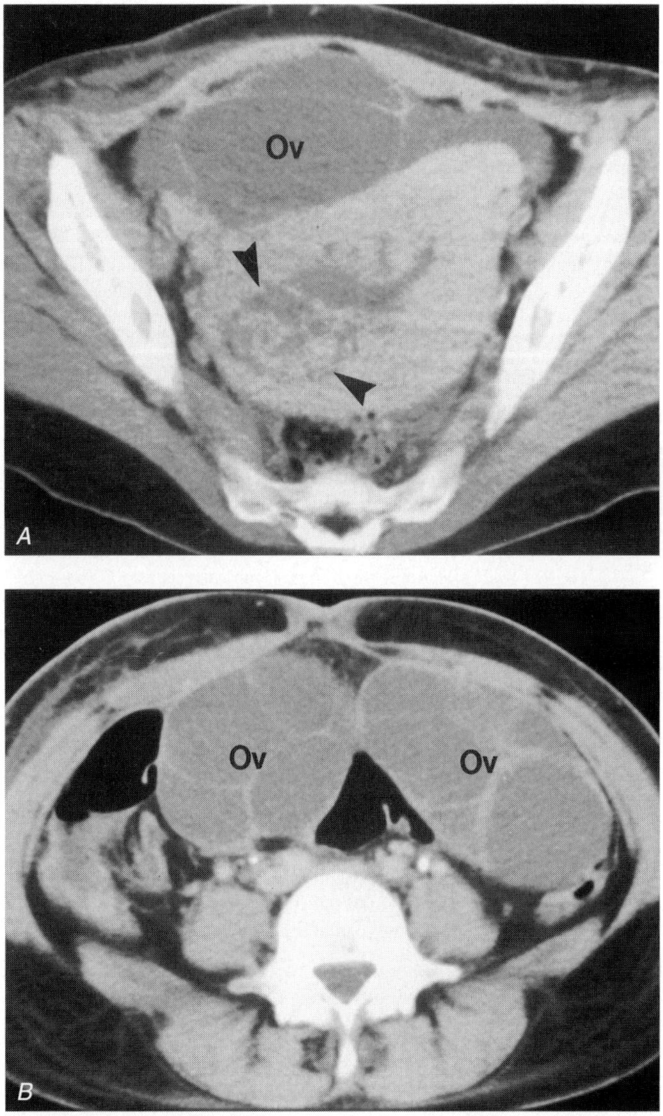

FIGURE 13.13 Gestational trophoblastic disease (invasive mole). Contrast-enhanced CT (*A* and *B*) in a 26-year-old woman who underwent evacuation of a molar pregnancy 3 weeks earlier shows invasion of myometrium by a heterogeneous mass lesion *(arrowheads)*. The uterus is enlarged. Massive bilateral cystic enlargement of the ovaries (Ov) represents multiple theca-lutein cysts.

- **Congenital uterine anomalies** may be detected on CT, although they are better evaluated on hysterosalpingography and MRI. These defects are often detected during evaluation for fertility problems, but other cases are found incidentally in asymptomatic women. Incomplete fusion, canalization, or development of the müllerian ducts can all result in anomalies. Failure of fusion results in duplication anomalies such as uterine didelphia. Canalization failures include a noncommunicating uterine horn and cervical agenesis. Unicornuate uterus and absent uterus are examples of nondevelopment. In utero exposure to diethylstilbestrol (DES) is responsible for a group of uterine malformations, a T-shaped uterus being the most widely recognized. These patients are at increased risk for developing clear cell adenocarcinoma of the vagina.

Bicornuate uterus can often be distinguished from septate uterus on cross-sectional imaging **(Fig. 13.14).** Hydrometrocolpos is seen with congenital vaginal obstruction or atresia. Because of concurrent development of the urinary system, renal anomalies commonly coexist with uterine anomalies. In males, ipsilateral renal agenesis is seen in approximately two-thirds of patients with congenital cysts of the seminal vesicles.

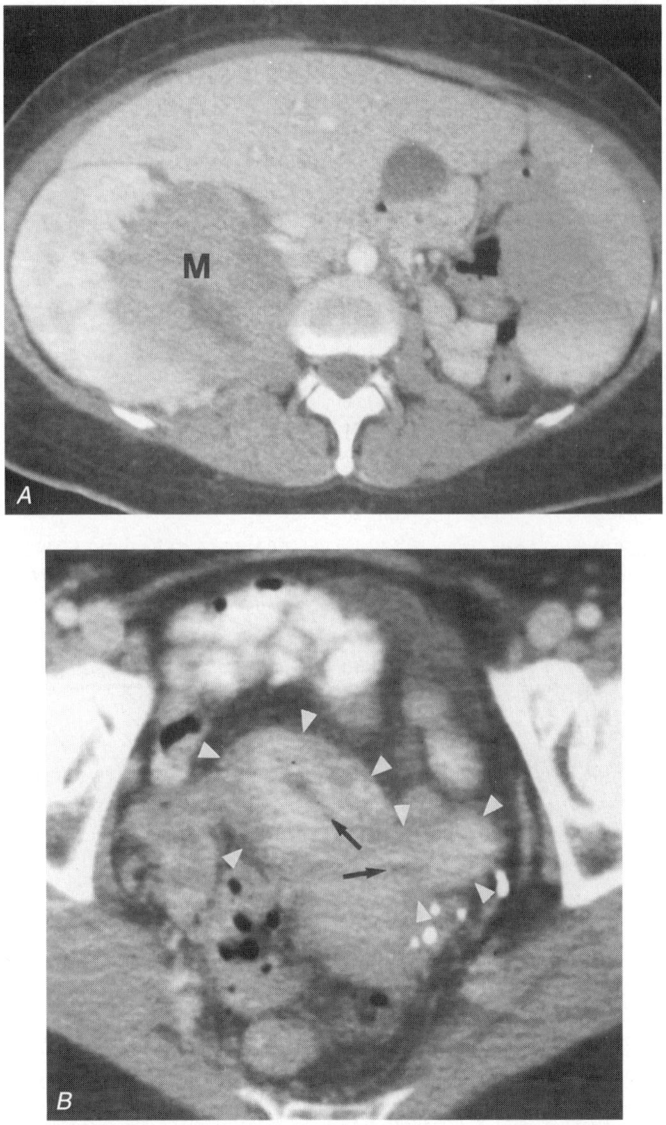

FIGURE 13.14 Uterine anomaly with associated renal agenesis. Contrast-enhanced CT (*A* and *B*) in a 57-year-old woman demonstrates a large infiltrating right renal mass (M), which proved to be a collecting duct carcinoma. Unsuspected agenesis of the left kidney was also found and congenital absence was supported by an associated bicornuate uterus *(arrowheads)*. Note separate endometrial stripes *(arrows)*. [From Pickhardt PJ. Collecting duct carcinoma arising in a solitary kidney. *Clin Imaging* 1999; 23:115–118. With permission.]

13.4 OVARIES

- Ultrasound is the primary imaging modality for ovarian pathology. In equivocal or indeterminate cases on ultrasound, MRI is now the next most appropriate imaging method of choice. Despite this, many ovarian lesions are first detected on CT, and an awareness of their appearance is important for their appropriate management.

- **Cystic adnexal lesions** are commonly seen on CT **(Differential 13.5).** Differential diagnostic considerations will be altered by the specific imaging appearance and clinical history. General categories of cystic lesions include nonneoplastic, benign neoplastic, and malignant. Tubo-ovarian abscess complicating pelvic inflammatory disease is discussed in **Section 13.6.**

- **Nonneoplastic cysts** are common in premenopausal women and are most often physiologic cysts **(Fig. 13.15).** When physiologic cysts become greater than 2.5 cm in size, they are termed ***functional cysts,*** with follicular and corpus luteum types being the most common. Functional cysts are usually simple and unilocular on CT. A follow-up ultrasound in 6 to 8 weeks is usually indicated for larger cysts in premenopausal women; most of these lesions represent functional cysts that typically resolve over time. **Theca-lutein cysts** are commonly seen in GTD and also with ovarian hyperstimulation in patients receiving fertility treatment (see **Fig. 13.13).** Theca-lutein cysts are usually multiple and bilateral; they can cause massive ovarian enlargement. **Serous inclusion cysts** are nonfunctional and are typically seen in postmenopausal women, where follow-up is necessary to exclude a cystic neoplasm. **Peritoneal pseudocysts** (mesenteric inclusion cysts) result from entrapment of peritoneal fluid released from the ovary during the normal cycle.

  Endometriosis usually consists of small, discrete endometrial implants on the peritoneal surface that cannot be resolved on imaging. If cyclic hemorrhage occurs, these lesions can grow into macroscopic cysts called ***endometriomas,*** which can be detected on CT. The ovaries and adnexal regions are most commonly involved. The appearance on CT will depend on the amount and timing of hemorrhage, with lesions ranging from fluid to soft tissue attenuation **(Fig. 13.16).**

- **Mature cystic teratoma (dermoid)** is the most common benign ovarian tumor in younger women. CT features of fat, calcification, and soft tissue within a well-defined adnexal mass are diagnostic of

13.5
PREDOMINATELY CYSTIC ADNEXAL LESION

Functional cysts—follicular, corpus luteum (>2.5 cm)
Tubo-ovarian abscess
Mature cystic teratoma
Cystadenoma > cystadenocarcinoma—over 50% of all neoplasms
Ectopic pregnancy
Hydrosalpinx
Endometrioma
Paraovarian cyst
Theca-lutein cysts—overstimulation, gestational trophoblastic disease
Metastases
Peritoneal pseudocyst
Mimics—loculated ascites, GI-related abscess, lymphocele

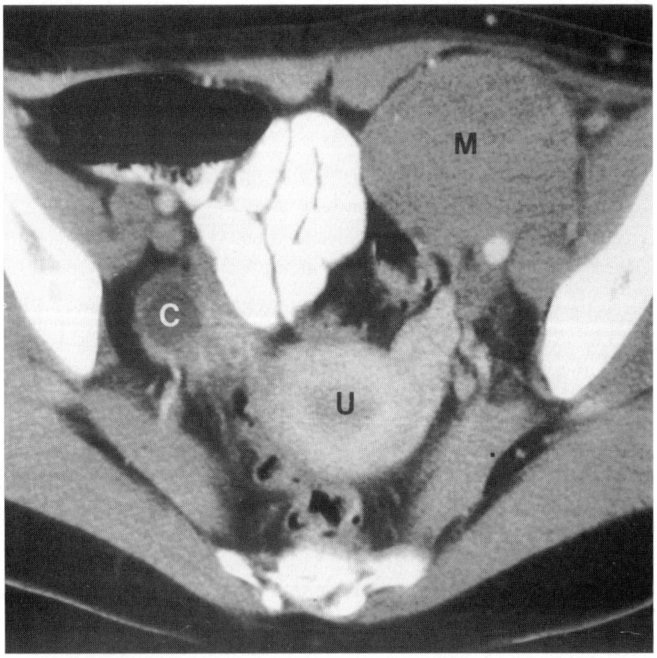

FIGURE 13.15 Physiologic ovarian cyst. Contrast-enhanced CT in a 16-year-old girl shows a 2-cm ovarian cyst (C). U, uterus. Left iliac nodal mass (M) represents a lymphoproliferative disorder occurring after heart transplantation. (From Pickhardt PJ, Siegel MJ. Abdominal manifestations of posttransplantation lymphoproliferative disorder. *AJR* 1998;171:1007–1013. With permission.)

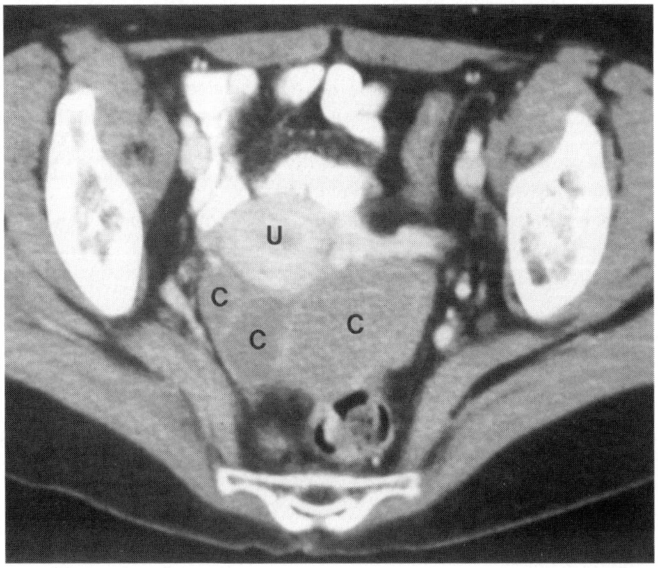

FIGURE 13.16 Endometriomas. Contrast-enhanced CT in a 51-year-old woman undergoing pretherapy evaluation for cervical carcinoma shows multiple cystic lesions (C) posterior to the uterus (U). The larger lesion on the left is slightly higher in attenuation than the other cysts. Endometriomas were found at radical hysterectomy for cervical cancer.

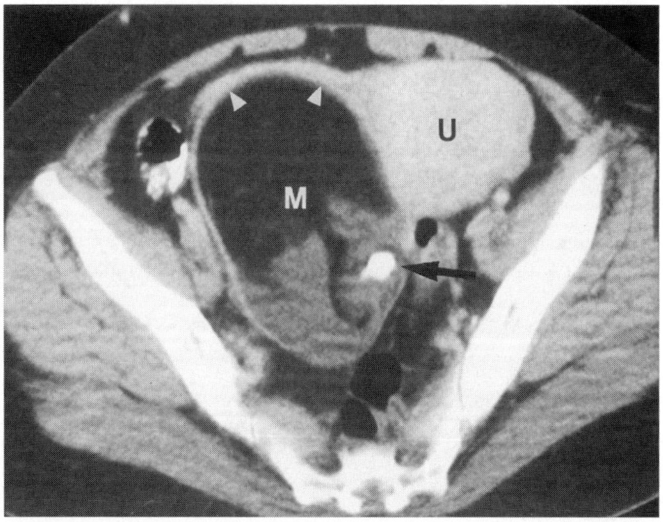

FIGURE 13.17 Mature ovarian teratoma. Contrast-enhanced CT in a 49-year-old woman shows a predominantly fatty mass (M), with areas of soft tissue attenuation and calcification *(arrow)*. Note right fallopian tube draping over lesion *(arrowheads)*.

a mature teratoma **(Fig. 13.17).** Fat-fluid levels and nodules of hair and tissue (dermoid plugs) are also characteristic findings. The fat attenuation within these lesions represents sebaceous material. Bilateral dermoids are seen in approximately 10 percent of cases **(Fig. 13.18).** Although benign, these tumors are removed because of their potential for torsion and rare malignant degeneration.

- Serous and mucinous **ovarian cystadenomas** are common benign epithelial tumors. Serous tumors account for 30 percent of all ovarian neoplasms, and 60 percent of these are benign. Most serous cys-

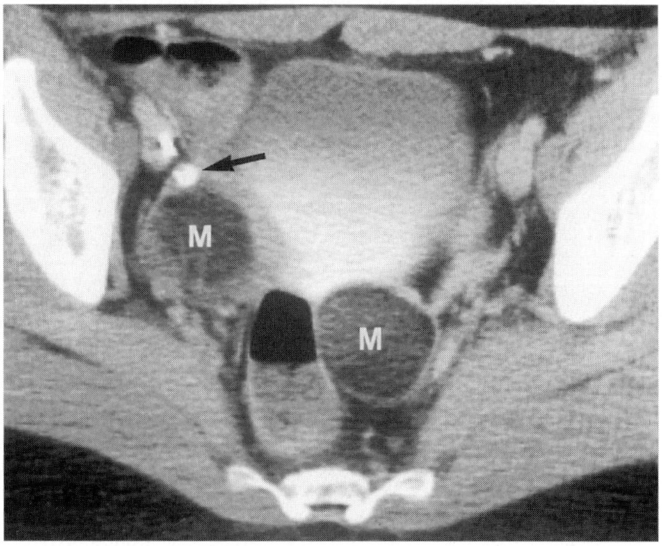

FIGURE 13.18 Bilateral ovarian dermoids. Contrast-enhanced CT in a 25-year-old woman shows bilateral fat-attenuation adnexal masses (M). Calcification is present on the right *(arrow)*. (Case courtesy of Dr. Matthew Fleishman, Denver, CO.)

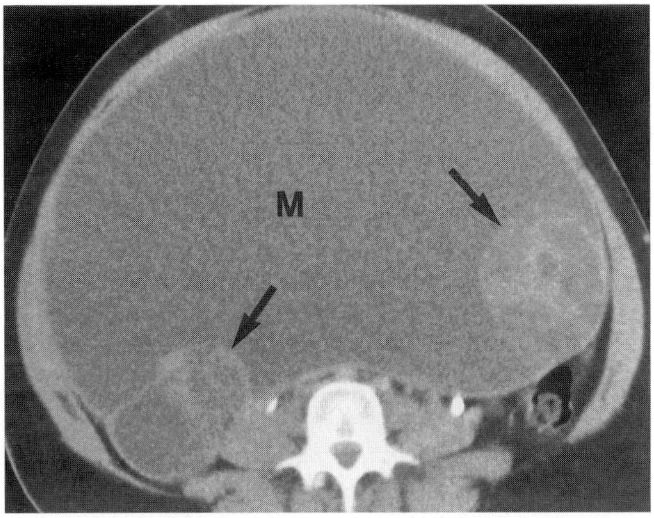

FIGURE 13.19 **Mucinous ovarian cystadenoma.** Contrast-enhanced CT in a 27-year-old woman shows a fluid-filled mass (M) that occupies nearly the entire abdomen. Smaller locules are present *(arrows)* in addition to the dominant cyst.

tadenomas are unilocular or contain a single septation. The tumors are usually 5 to 10 cm in size and are bilateral in about 10 percent of cases. Mucinous tumors represent 20 percent of all epithelial neoplasms, and 85 percent of these are benign. Mucinous cystadenomas tend to be larger than serous lesions (15 to 30 cm) and are typically multilocular in appearance **(Fig. 13.19).** Other types of epithelial tumors of the ovary include endometrioid, Brenner, and clear cell types.

- **Ovarian carcinoma** is not the most common gynecological malignancy but represents the most common cause of death since patients so often present with advanced disease. **Cystadenocarcinomas** account for 90 percent of all ovarian malignancies, of which approximately 40 percent are serous, 20 percent are endometrioid, and 10 percent are mucinous. Clear cell carcinoma is relatively rare. CT has been shown to be insensitive for the detection of small peritoneal implants, which limits its staging accuracy. However, despite only moderate accuracy in tumor staging, CT is an excellent predictor of tumor resectability. CT is also valuable in assessing for residual disease following therapy, since second-look laparotomies are no longer performed on a routine basis.

  On **CT,** features that favor malignancy in an adnexal mass include a size greater than 5 cm; solid tumor components; thick, enhancing septations; peritoneal implants; and ascites **(Fig. 13.20).** Cystadenocarcinomas are generally larger than their benign counterparts and involve both ovaries in 25 to 50 percent of cases. Although small peritoneal implants can be missed on CT, it remains the imaging method of choice for the detection of peritoneal spread. Omental caking, nodular peritoneal implants, scalloping of the liver margin, and ascites are all common findings **(Fig. 13.21).** Occasionally, calcification is identified within peritoneal implants on CT.

- **Metastases** to the ovary are most commonly derived from GI and breast primaries and represent about 10 percent of cancers involving the ovary. Spread of mucinous GI adenocarcinomas to the ovary typically results in bilateral solid and cystic masses often referred to as **Krukenberg tumors (Fig. 13.22).** Their discovery can precede that of the primary tumor. The imaging appearance is nonspecific and resembles that of primary neoplasms such as epithelial tumors, germ-cell tumors, and sex-cord stromal tumors.

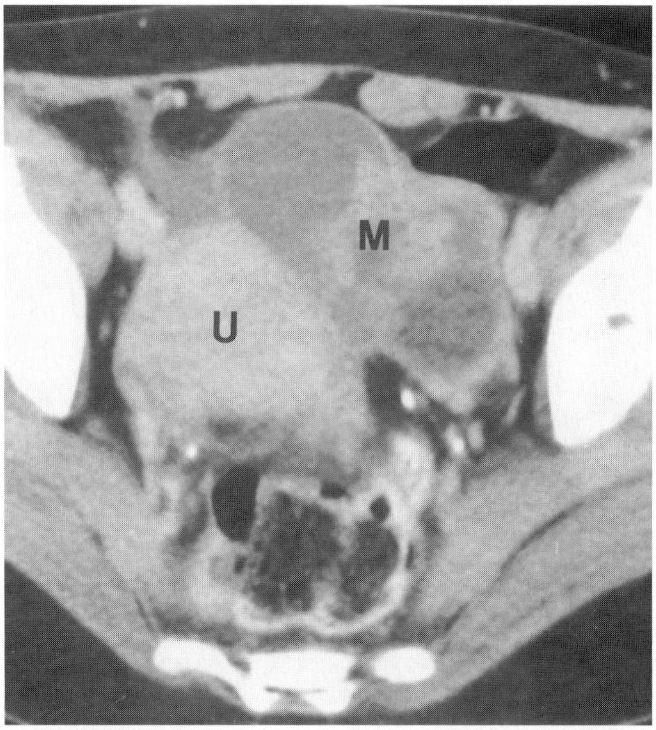

FIGURE 13.20 **Ovarian cystadenocarcinoma.** Contrast-enhanced CT in a 58-year-old woman shows a complex cystic and solid left adnexal mass (M). U, uterus. On pathologic examination, the tumor contained areas of papillary serous, clear cell, and endometrioid differentiation.

- The differential for predominantly **solid adnexal masses** overlaps significantly with that of the cystic lesions already discussed and also includes both neoplastic and nonneoplastic conditions **(Differential 13.6).** The solid component of ovarian cystadenocarcinomas is often less pronounced than their cystic component; however, because they represent over 90 percent of all malignancies, they still account for a significant percentage of predominantly solid tumors.

  Other, less common ovarian neoplasms are more characteristically solid in nature. **Sex-cord stromal tumors** include the lesions that commonly produce estrogen (granulosa cell tumors and thecomas) and tumors that can produce androgens (Sertoli-Leydig tumors). Ovarian fibromas and fibrothecomas are considered benign and can rarely be associated with ascites and right-sided pleural effusion **(Meig syndrome).** Granulosa cell tumors are usually considered malignant. On CT, sex-cord stromal tumors are typically depicted as solid adnexal masses **(Fig. 13.23).** Ovarian germ-cell tumors have a variety of appearances on CT but are often solid lesions. Dysgerminomas are analogous to testicular seminomas; endodermal sinus tumors are more common in children; and teratomas usually have a characteristic appearance, already discussed. Other tumors that can present as solid adnexal masses include subserosal leiomyomas in the broad ligament and ovarian metastases.

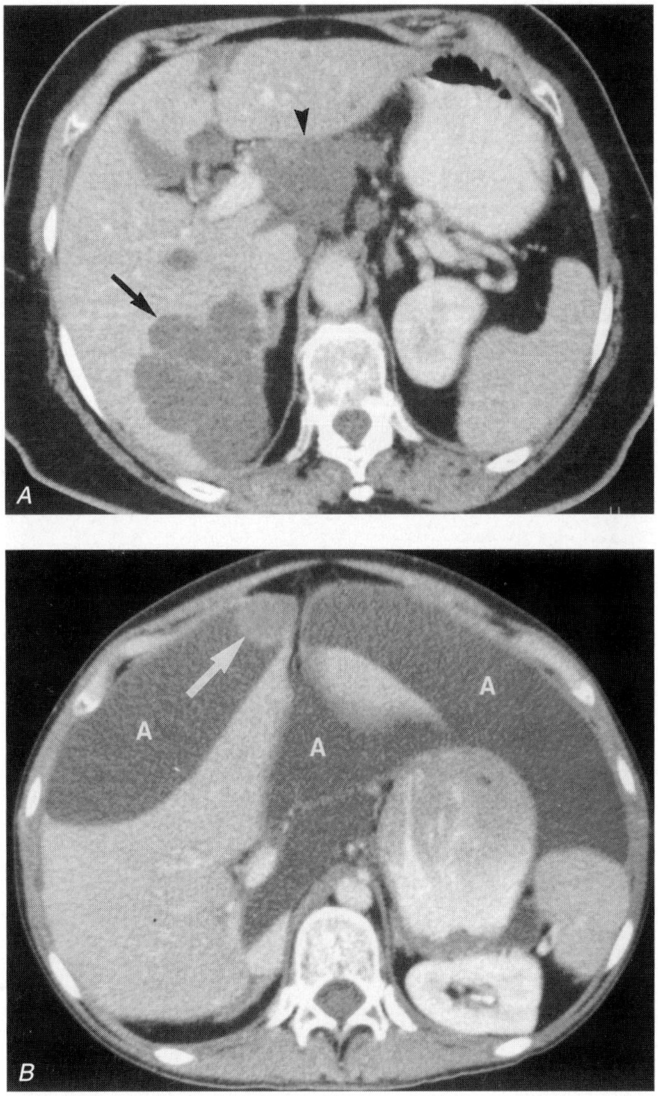

FIGURE 13.21 Peritoneal spread of ovarian cancer. *A.* Contrast-enhanced CT in a 76-year-old woman shows serosal implants that scallop the liver margin *(arrow)* and occupy the gastrohepatic region *(arrowhead)*. *B.* Contrast-enhanced CT in a 40-year-old woman shows loculated malignant ascites (A) that also scallops the liver contour. Note enhancing peritoneal soft tissue nodule *(arrow)*.

- **Ovarian torsion** usually presents with acute abdominal pain. Torsion can be related to an underlying adnexal tumor, most commonly from an ovarian dermoid, or can occur with an apparently normal ovary. Early diagnosis is important to avoid salpingo-oophorectomy. Affected patients are usually under 30 years of age. Findings on CT parallel the ultrasound findings of a complex solid mass, characteristically with multiple peripheral follicular-type cysts **(Fig. 13.24).** Adjacent pelvic fluid may be present as well.

13.5 PROSTATE

- The major diseases that affect the prostate gland include benign prostatic hypertrophy, prostatic cancer, and prostatitis. CT is not the primary modality for evaluating these, but—given the high prevalence of prostate disease among older men—such abnormalities are commonly depicted on CT. CT does play a limited role in patients with known prostatic cancer.

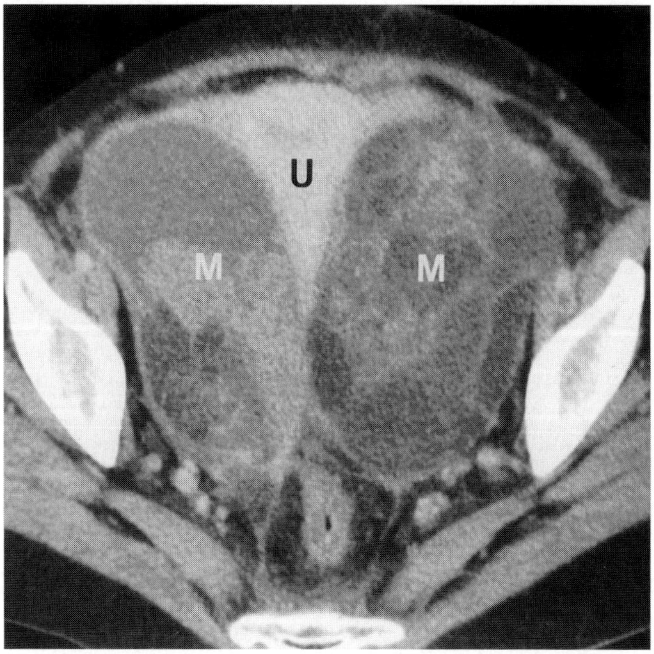

FIGURE 13.22 Krukenberg tumors. Contrast-enhanced CT in a 42-year-old woman shows large, bilateral cystic and solid adnexal masses (M) that flank the uterus (U). The masses represent ovarian metastases from colon carcinoma.

- **Benign prostatic hypertrophy (BPH)** describes hyperplastic changes of the periurethral gland and is an extremely common entity, affecting over one-half of men over the age of 50. Prostatic enlargement initially indents the bladder base but, with increasing size of the gland, may elevate it from the pelvic floor. The presence of

13.6 PREDOMINATELY SOLID ADNEXAL MASS

Epithelial tumors—90% of ovarian malignancies
  Cystadenocarcinoma
    Serous > endometrioid > mucinous > *clear cell*
Stromal tumors—<5% of ovarian malignancies
  Granulosa cell tumor—usually malignant
  Fibroma/fibrothecoma—usually benign
  Sertoli-Leydig tumor
Germ-cell tumors—<3% of ovarian malignancies
  Dermoid
  Dysgerminoma—young women
  Endodermal sinus tumor—children and young women
  Immature teratoma—malignant
Subserosal leiomyoma—broad ligament
Endometriosis
Metastases—Krukenberg tumors
Ovarian torsion—young women, peripheral cysts
Ovarian edema—usually due to intermittent torsion
Nongynecologic—hematoma, tumor
Sarcoma—fibrosarcoma

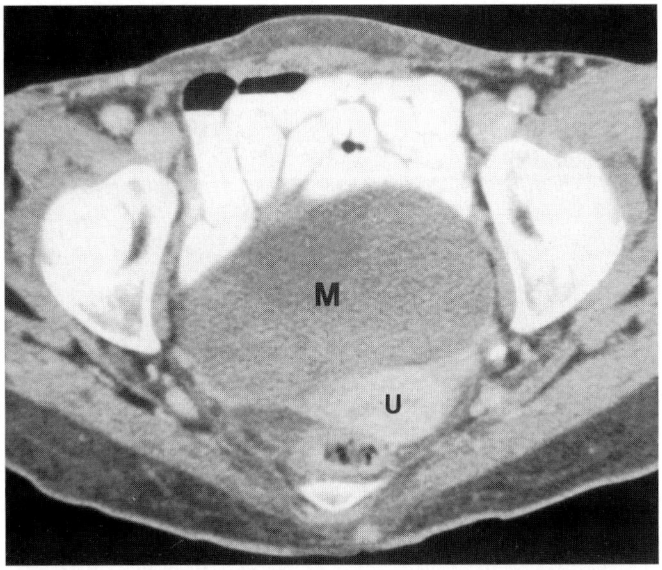

FIGURE 13.23 Ovarian fibroma. Contrast-enhanced CT in a 71-year-old woman shows a homogeneous solid mass (M) anterior to the uterus (U).

symptoms from bladder outlet obstruction correlates poorly with the overall size of the prostate. On CT, bladder wall thickening or trabeculation indicates an obstructive component; upper tract dilatation can be seen in severe cases. CT cannot exclude the possibility of coexisting carcinoma.

- **Prostatic carcinoma** is the most common cancer among men (excluding skin cancer). Over 95 percent of cases are adenocarcinoma and, unlike BPH, most often arise in the peripheral zone of the prostate gland. Early disease is being detected more frequently with routine screening for elevated levels of prostate-specific antigen (PSA) in conjunction with digital rectal examination. Tumor stage is affected by whether the lesion is palpable; presence of extracapsular extension; invasion of the seminal vesicles, bladder, rectum, or pelvic side wall; pelvic lymph node involvement; and distal metastatic disease.

  Controversy has surrounded the appropriateness of imaging evaluation for prostatic cancer. Skeletal scintigraphy for detecting osseous metastatic disease is probably not indicated when PSA levels are below 10 ng/ml. CT has been used for preoperative stag-

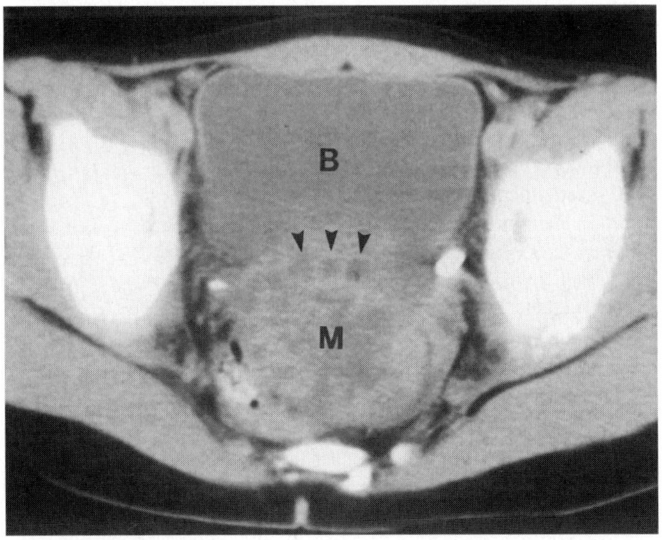

FIGURE 13.24 Ovarian torsion. Contrast-enhanced CT in an 8-year-old girl with severe pelvic pain of acute onset shows a large, complex pelvic mass (M), in the midline posterior to the bladder (B). The presence of peripheral cysts *(arrowheads)* is characteristic of ovarian torsion.

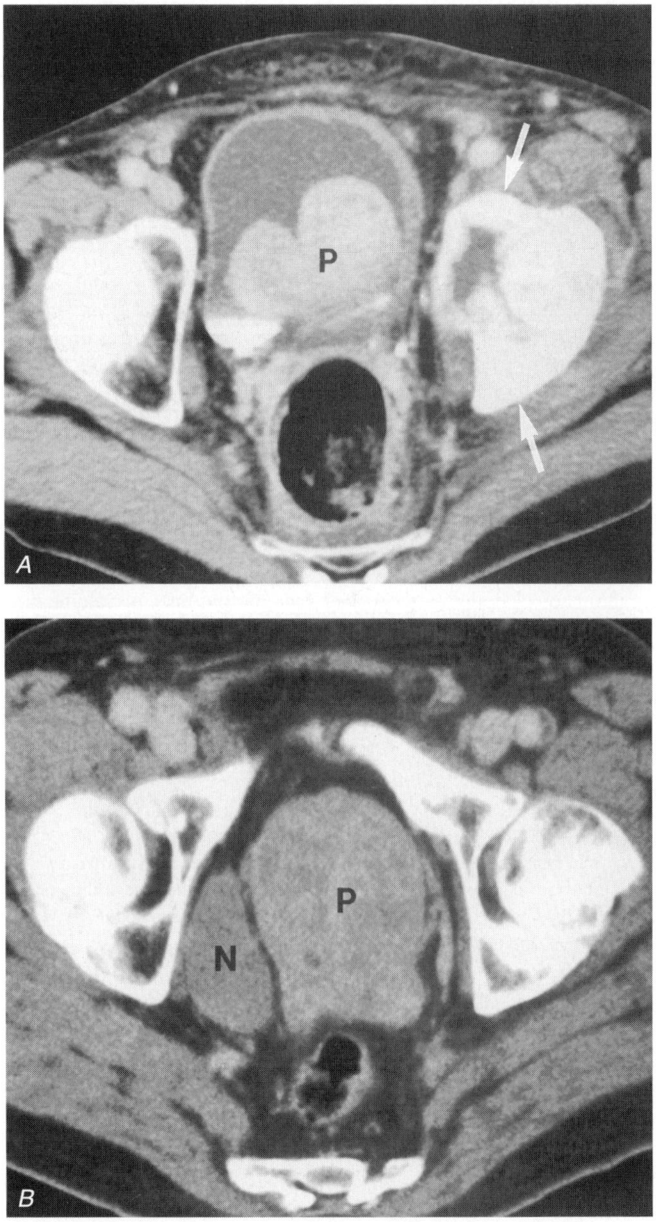

FIGURE 13.25 Metastatic prostate carcinoma. *A.* Contrast-enhanced CT in a 90-year-old man demonstrates prostatic enlargement (P) and a mixed lytic and sclerotic osseous pelvic metastasis *(arrows)*. *B.* Contrast-enhanced CT in a 78-year-old man shows prostatic enlargement (P) and right-sided obturator lymphadenopathy (N).

ing in the past but is inaccurate for assessing early extracapsular spread. It is, however, useful in more advanced disease and can demonstrate pelvic lymph node involvement and other distant metastases **(Fig. 13.25).** MRI with an endorectal coil has been touted for its ability to evaluate for local tumor extension but is not currently in widespread use for staging purposes.

- **Prostatitis,** or inflammation of the prostate gland, is usually due to a retrograde bacterial infection. *E. coli* is the most common organism. Granulomatous prostatitis from tuberculosis or fungal infection is less common. Imaging findings in prostatitis are nonspecific. **Prostatic abscess,** however, can be readily identified on CT as a focal area of low attenuation within an enlarged gland **(Fig. 13.26).**
- **Prostatic calcification** is most often inconsequential and idiopathic in nature, occurring predominantly in the peripheral zone. It can also occur with prostatic adenoma, prostatic carcinoma, and granulomatous prostatitis. Calcification of the seminal vesicles is usually due to diabetes mellitus but can be seen with granulomatous infection or may be idiopathic in nature.

13.6 INFLAMMATORY DISEASES OF THE PELVIS

- **Pelvic inflammatory disease (PID)** is typically an ascending infection that affects sexually active women. *Chlamydia trachomatis* is the single most common cause. Cross-sectional imaging is not necessary unless a complicating **tubo-ovarian abscess** is suspected. The typical CT findings of abscess are depicted and include a complex, septate adnexal fluid collection with an enhancing rim. Without clinical correlation, the imaging appearance is often indistinguishable from that of a cystic neoplasm **(Differential 13.5). Hydrosalpinx** or pyosalpinx will appear on CT as an enhancing fluid-filled tubular structure that can simulate an unopacified bowel loop **(Fig. 13.27).** Tuberculosis is a common cause of chronic granulomatous salpingitis worldwide, and the presence of calcification may suggest the diagnosis. Pelvic actinomycosis is associated with

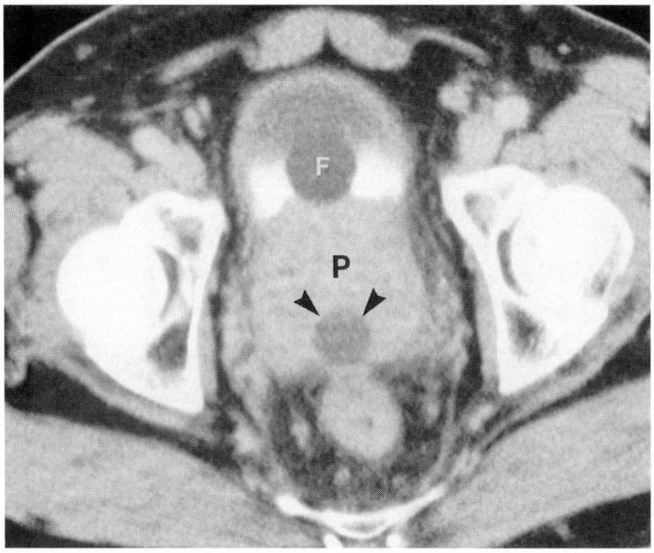

FIGURE 13.26 Prostatic abscess. Contrast-enhanced CT in a 69-year-old man with prostatitis shows a well-defined low-attenuation lesion *(arrowheads)* within a diffusely enlarged prostate. A Foley balloon catheter (F) is present in the bladder.

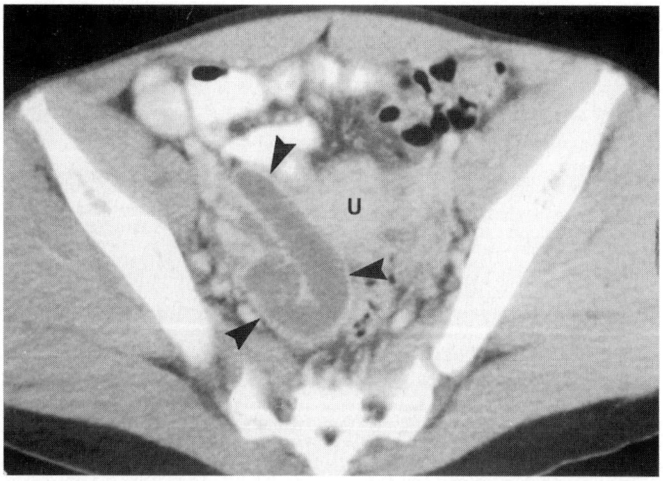

FIGURE 13.27 Hydrosalpinx. Contrast-enhanced CT in a 28-year-old woman with a history of pelvic inflammatory disease shows a fluid-filled tubular structure with an enhancing wall in the right adnexal region *(arrowheads).* U, uterus.

the use of an intrauterine device (IUD) and is depicted on CT as an ill-defined enhancing adnexal soft tissue mass, often with an associated cystic component **(Fig. 13.28).**

- Postpartum inflammatory conditions that can be visualized on CT include venous thrombosis, endometritis, and pyometra. **Ovarian vein thrombophlebitis** is most commonly due to postpartum endometritis. On CT, wall enhancement of ovarian veins that are

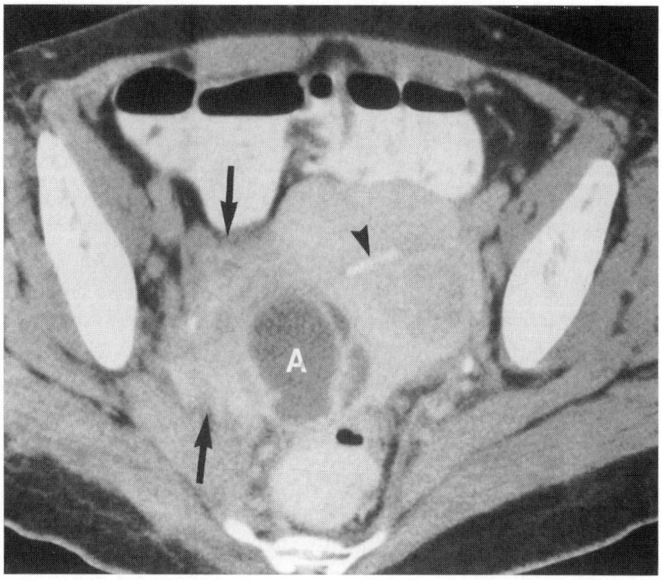

FIGURE 13.28 Tubo-ovarian abscess from actinomycosis. Contrast-enhanced CT in a 50-year-old woman undergoing evaluation for right-sided hydronephrosis shows a right-sided septate adnexal fluid collection with rim enhancement (A) as well as enhancing soft tissue *(arrows).* The presence of an intrauterine device *(arrowhead)* suggested the diagnosis of actinomycosis, but malignancy could not be excluded preoperatively.

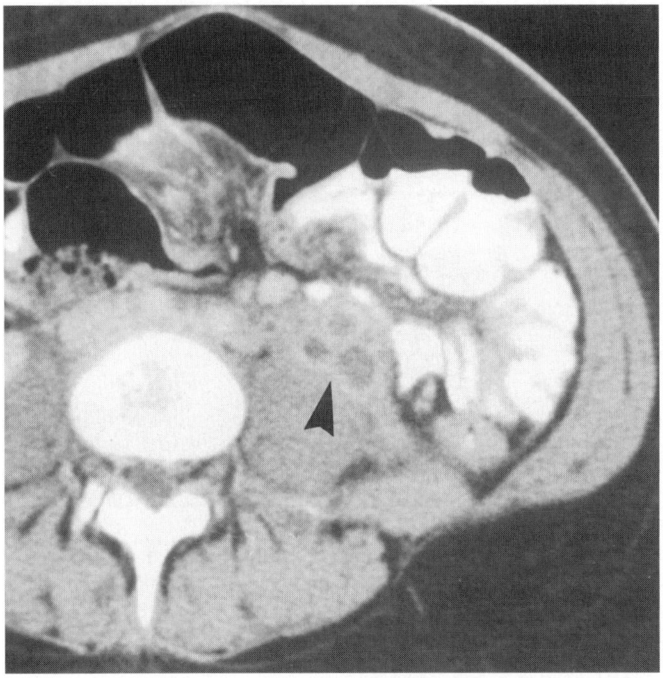

FIGURE 13.29 Ovarian vein thrombophlebitis. Contrast-enhanced CT in a 16-year-old woman with persistent abdominal pain, fever, and leukocytosis 7 days postpartum shows thrombosis and wall enhancement of dilated left ovarian veins *(arrowhead)*. Isolated left-sided involvement is atypical.

dilated by low-attenuation intraluminal thrombus is characteristic **(Fig. 13.29)**. The right side is involved in the majority of cases and isolated left-sided disease is seen in less than 10 percent. Ovarian vein thrombosis in patients who have undergone gynecologic cancer surgery is an incidental finding that usually requires no treatment. Endometritis is the most common cause of puerperal fever. In pyometra, marked distention of the endometrial cavity with pus may be difficult to distinguish from hematoma on CT.

- **Fournier gangrene** represents a fulminant necrotizing fasciitis involving the scrotum and perineum. Patients with diabetes mellitus are most often affected. Rapid diagnosis and treatment with appropriate antibiotics as well as prompt surgical debridement are critical for survival. Imaging is generally not indicated unless the diagnosis is uncertain or unsuspected. Subcutaneous emphysema and cellulitis are readily depicted on CT **(Fig. 13.30)**.
- **Lymphogranuloma venereum** is a sexually transmitted disease caused by *C. trachomatis*. Involvement of the rectum is relatively common and is usually due to lymphatic extension from the genital region, but it can also represent primary infection. Fibrosis of the rectal wall and stricture formation can be seen with long-standing disease **(Fig. 13.31)**.

13.7 PELVIC MASSES

- Masses involving the bladder, uterus, cervix, ovary, and prostate have been discussed in the preceding sections. Furthermore, the differentials for peritoneal and retroperitoneal masses covered in Chapter 10 largely apply to the intraperitoneal and extraperitoneal pelvis as well. Several additional entities are covered in the paragraphs that follow; these include the undescended testis, pelvic rhabdomyosarcoma, and presacral lesions.

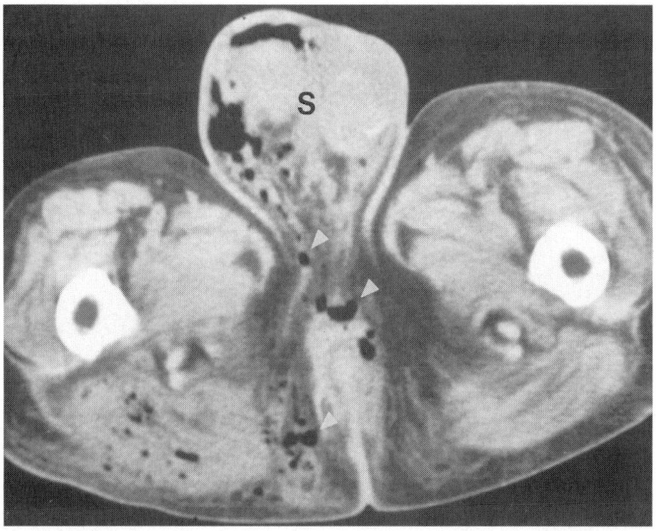

FIGURE 13.30 Fournier gangrene. Contrast-enhanced CT in a 45-year-old diabetic man who presented with scrotal swelling shows subcutaneous gas and soft tissue stranding within the scrotum (S) that extends into the perineum *(arrowheads)*. Extensive surgical debridement was required.

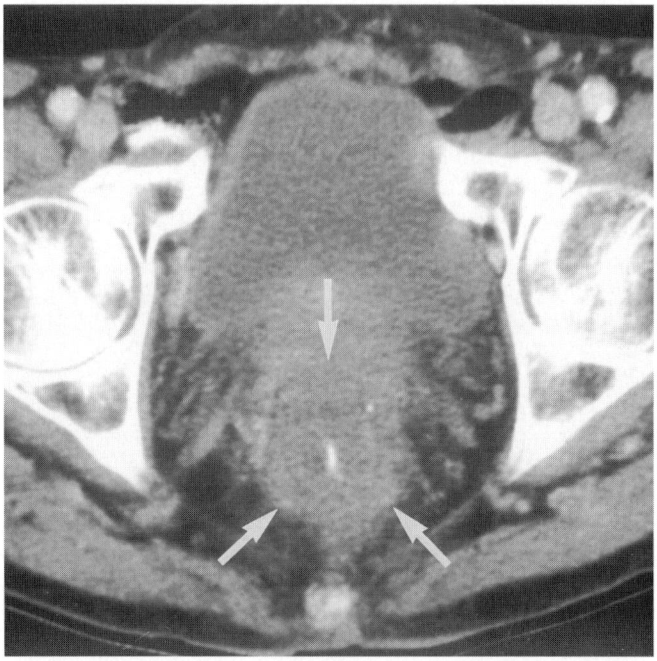

FIGURE 13.31 Lymphogranuloma venereum. Contrast-enhanced CT in a man with a history of long-standing lymphogranuloma venereum shows circumferential rectal wall thickening *(arrows)*. Rectal contrast is present within the strictured lumen, which necessitated colostomy placement. Note soft tissue infiltration of perirectal fat.

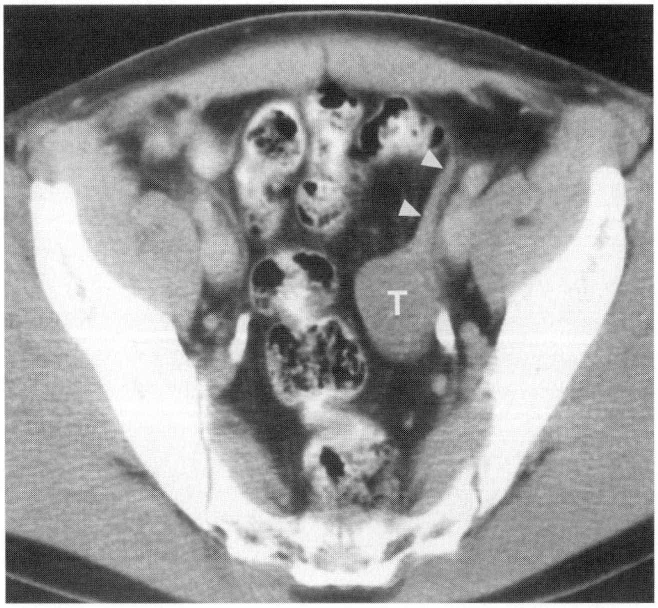

FIGURE 13.32 Seminoma in an undescended testis. Contrast-enhanced CT in a 34-year-old man demonstrates an ovoid mass in the extraperitoneal pelvis representing an undescended testis (T). Retroperitoneal lymphadenopathy was also present (not shown). Pathologic examination of the undescended testis revealed a seminoma. Note the gubernaculum *(arrowheads)*, which is a structure homologous to the round ligament in females and passes through the inguinal canal.

- **Undescended testes** are more common in premature infants, since gonadal descent to the inguinal ring occurs late in fetal development. Undescended testes are seen in less than 5 percent of full-term boys compared with 30 percent of premature infant boys at birth. In most cases, CT can successfully localize the undescended testis. The majority of undescended testes are present within the inguinal canal, but they are occasionally seen within the extraperitoneal pelvis or retroperitoneum **(Fig. 13.32).** The increased risk of malignancy within an undescended testis underscores the need for evaluation.

- **Rhabdomyosarcoma** is the most common pelvic malignancy in children and is usually of the embryonal histologic subtype. The tumor can arise from the prostate in boys and from the uterus or vagina in girls **(Fig. 13.33).** Tumors may also arise from the urinary bladder. These polypoid tumors often resemble a cluster of grapes on gross examination, hence the term *sarcoma botryoides*.

13.7

PRESACRAL MASS

Teratoma—sacrococcygeal
Chordoma
Neurogenic tumor—schwannoma, neurofibroma
Primary bone tumor
    Chondrosarcoma, giant cell tumor, aneurysmal bone cyst
Lymphadenopathy
Abscess
Hematoma
Duplication cyst
Anterior sacral meningocele

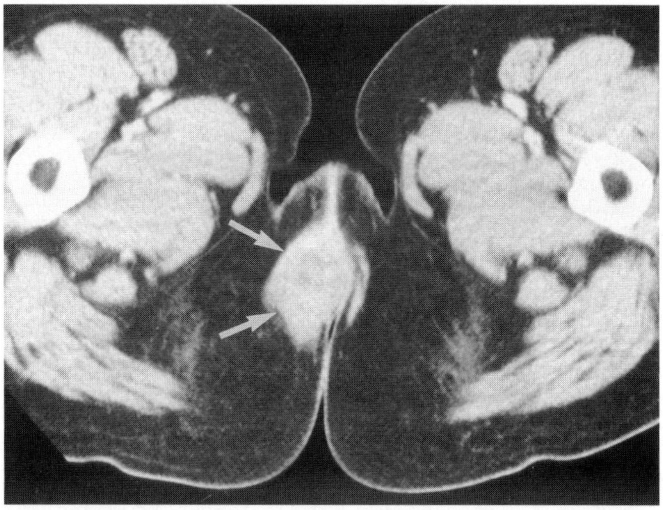

FIGURE 13.33 Pelvic rhabdomyosarcoma. Contrast-enhanced CT in a 21-year-old woman demonstrates a vulvar soft tissue mass *(arrows)* that proved to be rhabdomyosarcoma.

- CT can depict a wide variety of pathologic entities within the **presacral space (Differential 13.7).** The presacral space forms part of the extraperitoneal pelvis and as such is generally excluded from peritoneal disease processes. Retroperitoneal pathology, however, can involve the presacral region by direct extension along predetermined fascial planes. Lesions within the presacral space can arise from adjacent structures such as the sacrum or rectum or may represent a primary process. CT is useful for characterizing lesions as solid or cystic, determining the source, and evaluating for other sites of disease. The patient's age will alter the differential considerations, since some lesions, such as sacrococcygeal teratomas and duplication cysts, will present early in life, whereas presacral extension of a chondrosarcoma or rectal cancer will occur much later.

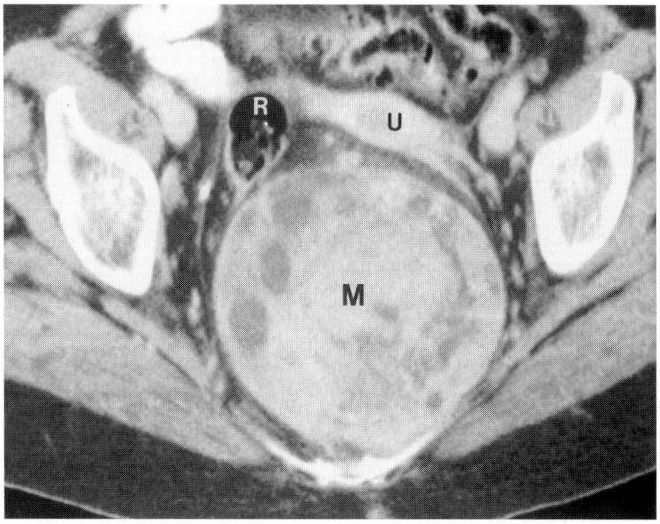

FIGURE 13.34 Presacral schwannoma. Contrast-enhanced CT in a 73-year-old woman demonstrates a large but well-defined heterogeneous presacral mass (M) that displaces the rectum (R) and uterus (U) anteriorly.

Neurogenic tumors such as neurofibromas and schwannomas can be isolated findings or may occur in the setting of neurofibromatosis **(Fig. 13.34).**

Bibliography

Forman HP, Heiken JP, Brink JA, Glazer HS, Fox LA, McClennan BL. CT screening for comorbid disease in patients with prostatic carcinoma: Is it cost-effective? *AJR* 1994;162:1125–1128.

Forstner RF, Hricak H, Occhipinti KA, Powell CB, Frankel SD, Stern JL. Ovarian cancer: Staging with CT and MR imaging. *Radiology* 1995;197:619–626.

Foshager MC, Walsh JW. CT anatomy of the female pelvis: A second look. *Radiographics* 1994;14:51–66.

Kimura I, Togashi K, Kawakami S, Takakura K, Mori T, Konishi J. Ovarian torsion: CT and MR imaging appearances. *Radiology* 1994;190:337–341.

Lee JKT, Willms AB, Semelka RC. Pelvis. In: Lee JKT, Sagel SS, Stanley RJ, Heiken JP, eds. *Computed Body Tomography with MRI Correlation,* 3rd ed. Philadelphia: Lippincott-Raven; 1998:1209–1274.

Meyer JI, Kennedy AW, Friedman R, Ayoub A, Zepp RC. Ovarian carcinoma: Value of CT in predicting success of debulking surgery. *AJR* 1995; 165:875–878.

Occhipinit KA. Computed tomography and magnetic resonance imaging of the ovary. In: Anderson JC, ed. *Gynecologic Imaging.* New York: Churchill Livingstone; 1999:345–360.

Rooholamini SA, Au AH, Hansen GC, et al. Imaging of pregnancy-related complications. *Radiographics* 1993;13:753–770.

Wong-You-Cheong JJ, Wagner BJ, Davis CJ. Transitional cell carcinoma of the urinary tract: Radiologic-pathologic correlation. *Radiographics* 1998;18:123–142.

Chapter 14

BODY WALL

Richard M. Slone and Andrew J. Fisher

14.1 Anatomy and Technique
14.2 Soft Tissues
14.3 Breast
14.4 External Hernias
14.5 Soft Tissue Tumors
14.6 Skeleton
14.7 Bone Tumors

14.1 ANATOMY AND TECHNIQUE

Anatomy

- The body wall is often overlooked during image interpretation, but it is a significant structure, composed of an array of tissues including bone, muscle, fat, vessels, and lymphatics. Disease processes can arise within or spread to involve these tissues **(Differential 14.1).**
- The **supraclavicular fossa** represents the thoracic outlet at the base of the neck. It contains the scalene muscles, subclavian vessels, and supraclavicular lymph nodes. The **brachial plexus** is a complex structure formed by the C5 through T1 nerve roots; these join and divide to form the trunks, divisions, cords, branches, and ultimately the nerves. The brachial plexus passes between the anterior and middle scalene muscles and is bordered along its lateral margin by the axillary artery and vein within the axillary sheath.

14.1

BODY WALL MASS

Sebaceous cyst
Hematoma
Scar or keloid
Tumors—**lipoma, fibroma,** hemangioma, desmoid, neurofibroma, schwannoma, osteochondroma, multiple myeloma, metastases, sarcoma, lymphoma, melanoma
Infection/abscess
Bacteria—*Actinomyces, Nocardia, Staphylococcus*
Fungus—blastomycosis, aspergillosis
Tuberculosis

- The **axilla** contains the axillary artery and vein, the brachial plexus, and lymph nodes. The anterior axillary fold is made up of the pectoralis major and minor muscles. The posterior axillary fold is created by the subscapularis, latissimus dorsi, and teres major muscles. The serratus anterior lines the lateral chest wall immediately deep and anterior to the latissimus dorsi. The long thoracic (serratus) and thoracodorsal (latissimus) nerves as well as the lateral thoracic (serratus) and thoracodorsal (latissimus) vessels course lateral to the muscles they supply.
- The external, internal, and innermost **intercostal** muscles insert between ribs, and the subcostal muscles course from the rib angle to the internal surface of the next lower rib. The intercostal nerve, artery, and vein run between the internal and innermost muscles, along the undersurface of the rib. The transverse thoracic muscle is seen as a thin soft tissue slip behind the sternum. The internal thoracic arteries, arising from the subclavian artery, are the primary blood supply to the anterior chest wall. A lymph node chain is found adjacent to these.
- The **breast** is demonstrated on computed tomography (CT), although intramammary processes are best evaluated with low-dose film-screen mammography. Further evaluation can be performed with ultrasound (US) in assessing for cystic lesions or magnetic resonance imaging (MRI) in evaluating breast implants or chest wall extension of tumor. CT shows fibroglandular parenchyma as strands of soft tissue with variable amounts of fat. Men should have no significant parenchymal tissue.
- The principal muscles of the **anterior abdominal wall** include the two bellies of the rectus abdominis separated by the linea alba. The linea semilunaris defines the lateral margin, separating the rectus from the more lateral external oblique, internal oblique, and transversus abdominis muscles. Above the umbilicus, the aponeurosis of the internal oblique divides around the rectus; however, below the umbilicus, the fibers pass anterior to the rectus, allowing communication of the rectus compartments across the midline. The transversalis fascia lines the inside of the abdominal wall immediately anterior to the peritoneum.

  The anterior abdominal wall is principally supplied by the superior epigastric vessels, continuations of the internal thoracic arteries, that course posterior to the rectus muscle. They anastomose with the inferior epigastric vessels arising from the external iliac arteries. Lymph nodes are present in the inguinal and periumbilical regions.
- The **posterior abdominal wall** is formed by the psoas major and minor and quadratus lumborum muscles, lying lateral to the lumbar

spine. The iliacus muscle lines the anterior aspect of the ilium. The **back muscles** include superficial (trapezius, latissimus dorsi, levator scapula, and rhomboids), intermediate (inferior and superior serratus), and deep (erector spinae: longissimus, iliocostalis, multifidus, and spinalis) groups.

- In the **pelvis,** at the level of the sacroiliac joint, the glutei minimus, medius, and maximus are seen posterior to the iliac. At the level of the acetabulum, the piriformis is seen adjacent to the posterior acetabulum as it spans from the greater trochanter to the sacrum, and the obturator internus rides against the medial acetabulum, inserting on the ischium. The **pelvic floor,** providing support for the rectum and bladder, is formed by the levator ani and deep transverse perinei muscle. The **sacral plexus,** formed by the fourth and fifth lumbar and first through third sacral nerve roots, lies between the piriformis and internal iliac vessels. The largest branch, the sciatic nerve, exits the pelvis through the sciatic foramen and is seen anterior to the piriformis muscle.

Technique

- **CT** readily displays the individual components of the body wall in cross section and can assess associated pathology. In addition to depicting soft tissues, CT is optimal for demonstrating cortical bone destruction. **Intravenous contrast** can be helpful in defining the relation of tumors to neurovascular structures, identifying areas of necrosis, and evaluating vascular abnormalities. Standard 5- to 10-mm collimation is used, with thinner sections acquired as needed.
- **MRI** allows direct multiplanar imaging, better soft tissue and bone marrow characterization, and improved assessment of vascular flow; consequently, it is the modality of choice for evaluating soft tissue tumors and the brachial and sacral plexus in patients with pain, neurologic deficit, muscular atrophy, or neoplastic involvement.

14.2 SOFT TISSUES

- **Muscular atrophy** is common adjacent to surgical incisions as a result of denervation. Stroke and other causes of central neurologic deficiency with associated paralysis commonly produce asymmetrical muscular atrophy **(Fig. 14.1).** Fatty replacement is obvious in comparison with the contralateral side. Symmetrical atrophy is more difficult to detect except when advanced. Common causes include quadriplegia, multiple sclerosis, and muscular dystrophy **(Fig. 14.2).**
- Enlarged **collateral vessels** in the body wall suggest occlusion of a major artery or vein within the thorax or abdomen. These vessels appear on CT as round or tubular structures that enhance in concert with other vessels after intravenous contrast administration **(see Fig. 4.11).** Transient venous enhancement on the side of the contrast injection, particularly in the periscapular and supraclavicular regions, can be seen because of retrograde flow caused by compression of the subclavian veins during hyperabduction of the arms and the increased flow rates produced by a power injector. Thoracic collaterals are most commonly the result of superior vena cava occlusion, and the **"caput medusae"** of periumbilical venous collaterals results from portal hypertension or thrombosis. Extra-anatomic arterial grafts, such as axillary-femoral bypass grafts, are readily demonstrated in the superficial soft tissues.
- CT depicts both superficial and deep **adenopathy.** It is consequently important to include the axillary soft tissues and supraclavicular fossa in the field of view, particularly in evaluating patients with lymphoma or breast cancer. Axillary lymph nodes drain the arm, breast, and body wall **(Fig. 14.3).** Nodes lateral to the pectoralis minor are designated level I, those under the muscle as level II, and those medial to it as level III. Axillary lymph nodes larger than 1 cm in short-axis diameter are abnormal unless they have a fatty center. Supraclavicular nodes are infrequently enlarged and usually less than 5 mm in diameter. They can be enlarged due to infection or cancer of the neck, lung, breast, or esophagus. The left supraclavicular chain can be involved from gastric cancer **(Virchow node).**

  Inguinal lymph nodes are often identified and should be considered enlarged if they are greater than 1 cm in short-axis

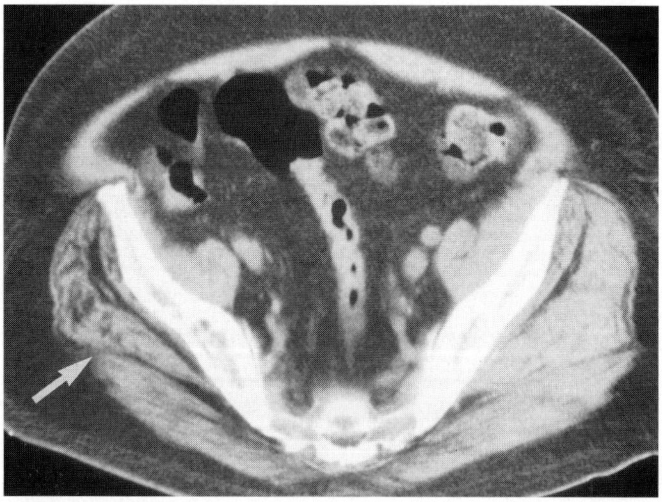

FIGURE 14.1 Skeletal muscle atrophy. Noncontrast CT showing fatty replacement of the right glutei minimus, medius, and maximus *(arrow)* muscles in a 67-year-old man following left cerebral infarction.

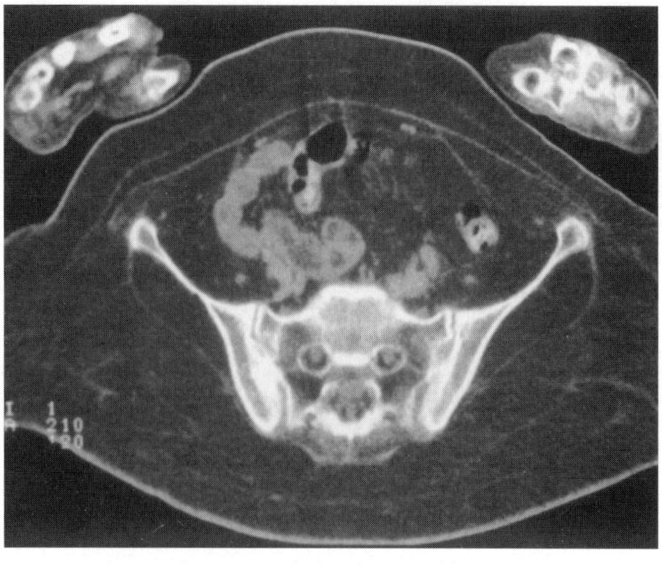

FIGURE 14.2 Muscular dystrophy. CT in a 32-year-old woman shows complete fatty replacement of skeletal muscle.

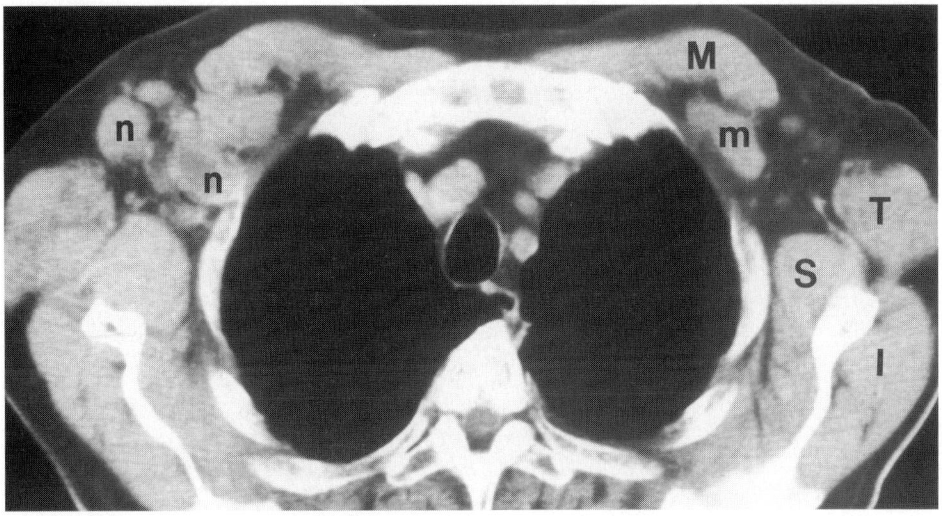

FIGURE 14.3 Axillary adenopathy. Chest CT shows right axillary adenopathy (n) in a 61-year-old man with an upper extremity melanoma. Note the necrotic center in the deeper node. M, pectoralis major; m, pectoralis minor; S, subscapularis; I, infraspinatus; T, teres major and latissimus major.

diameter. Intra-abdominal infections and neoplasia, lymphoma, and pelvic or lower extremity processes can pathologically enlarge inguinal lymph nodes. Lymphomatous nodes are often large, bulky, and homogeneously enhancing. Rarely, the periumbilical, **Sister Mary Joseph node** (not a true lymph node) can be identified with intra-abdominal malignancies, especially gastric cancer **(Fig. 14.4).**

- Primary **infections** of the body wall—such as cellulitis, fasciitis, or abscesses—are uncommon. More frequently, they are secondary to surgery, trauma, or direct extension from abdominal, thoracic **(Fig. 14.5),** or osseous infections. Fungus, mycobacteria, and bacteria (particularly *Nocardia* and *Actinomyces)* are the most frequent pathogens. Risk increases with age, diabetes, surgery, trauma, and diminished immunity.

  Infection is typically manifest as inflammation with edema in adjacent fat; however, infection can appear as an ill-defined infiltrating mass indistinguishable from a neoplastic process. An **abscess** appears as a localized fluid collection, often with peripheral enhancement following intravenous contrast administration **(Fig. 14.6).** Internal gas confirms the diagnosis. Fistulas, air-fluid levels, and bone destruction can be seen in advanced infection.

  Radiation therapy can produce localized skin thickening up to 1 cm. Inflammatory changes and increased attenuation in the subcutaneous fat is usually seen in the first few months, resolving on follow-up. The thickening should be confined to the radiation port.

- **Hemorrhage** into the body wall can result from trauma or surgery, or it can occur spontaneously in patients with a coagulopathy. Blood often dissects along fascial planes or produces diffuse enlargement when it is intramuscular. Localized hemorrhage leads to the development of a hematoma that can displace adjacent structures **(see Figs. 10.21 to 10.23).** Intravenous contrast is not necessary in assessing for hematomas, including retroperitoneal hemorrhage. An acute hematoma is isodense with intravascular blood on noncontrast CT. As the blood coagulates, it separates into low-density plasma and higher-density cellular components, forming a fluid-debris level **(Fig. 14.7).** With time, the entire collection becomes a uniformly low-density **seroma.**

  Infection is a common complication, and large hematomas can be evacuated to prevent this sequela. Depending on size and location, a seroma can be difficult to distinguish from an abscess, and diagnostic aspiration can be required to exclude infection. In rare cases, a subacute hematoma can simulate a tumor, although only a tumor will enhance after intravenous contrast injection. The wall of a chronic seroma can calcify **(see Fig. 8.6).**

- **Soft tissue calcification** is most commonly a result of connective tissue disease **(Fig. 14.8)**, posttraumatic myositis ossificans, vascular disease, calcified lymph nodes, and injection granulomas **(Differential 14.2).** Location, history, and CT appearance can be helpful in narrowing the differential diagnosis.

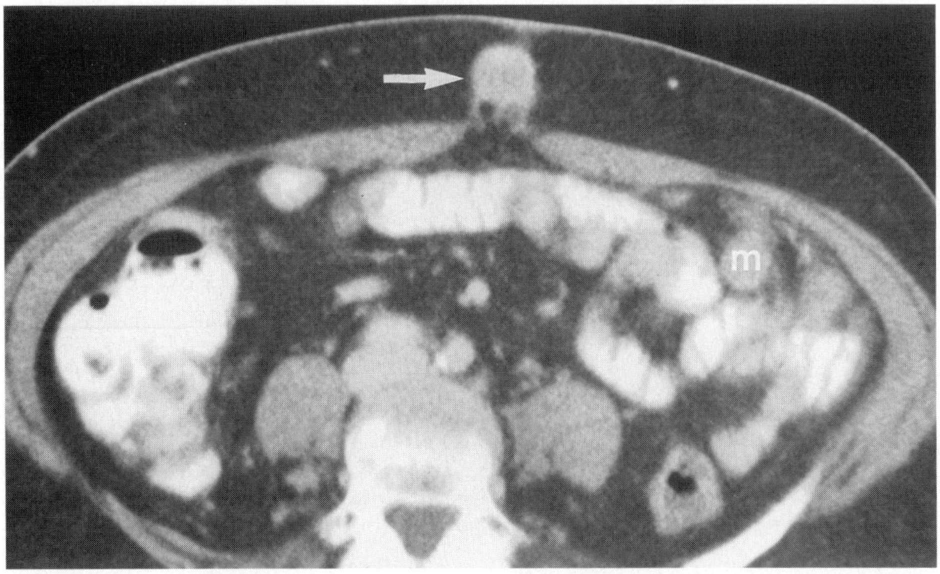

FIGURE 14.4 Sister Mary Joseph node. Contrast-enhanced CT in a 69-year-old woman with metastatic ovarian carcinoma shows an enlarged periumbilical lymph node *(arrow)* and peritoneal implant (M).

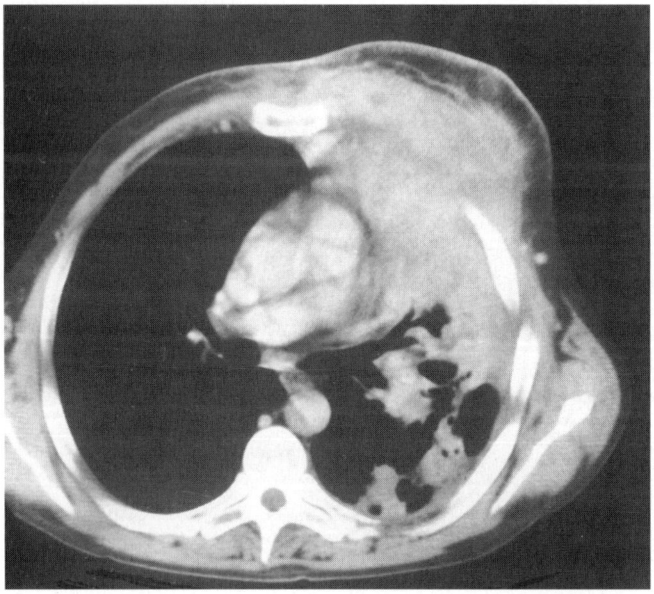

FIGURE 14.5 Actinomycosis. CT shows extensive pulmonary consolidation with contiguous chest wall invasion. [Figure courtesy of Jonathan Root, M.D., from Sagel SS, Slone RM. The lung. In: Lee JKT, Sagel SS, Stanley RJ, Heiken JP (eds.) *Computed Body Tomography with MRI Correlation,* 3rd ed. Philadelphia: Lippincott-Raven; 1998. With permission.]

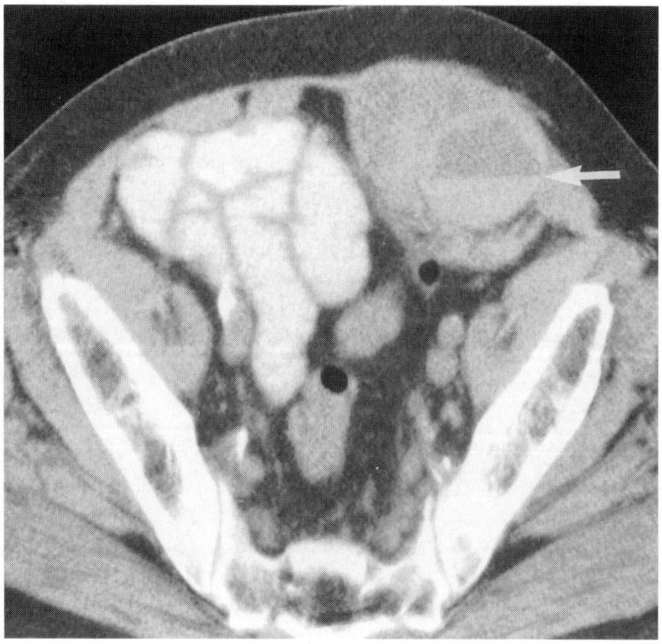

FIGURE 14.7 Rectus hematoma and fluid-debris level. A 76-year-old man on heparin. There is asymmetrical enlargement of the left rectus abdominis muscle with a well-defined fluid-debris level *(arrow)*. This is classic for a subacute hematoma with separation of plasma and cellular elements.

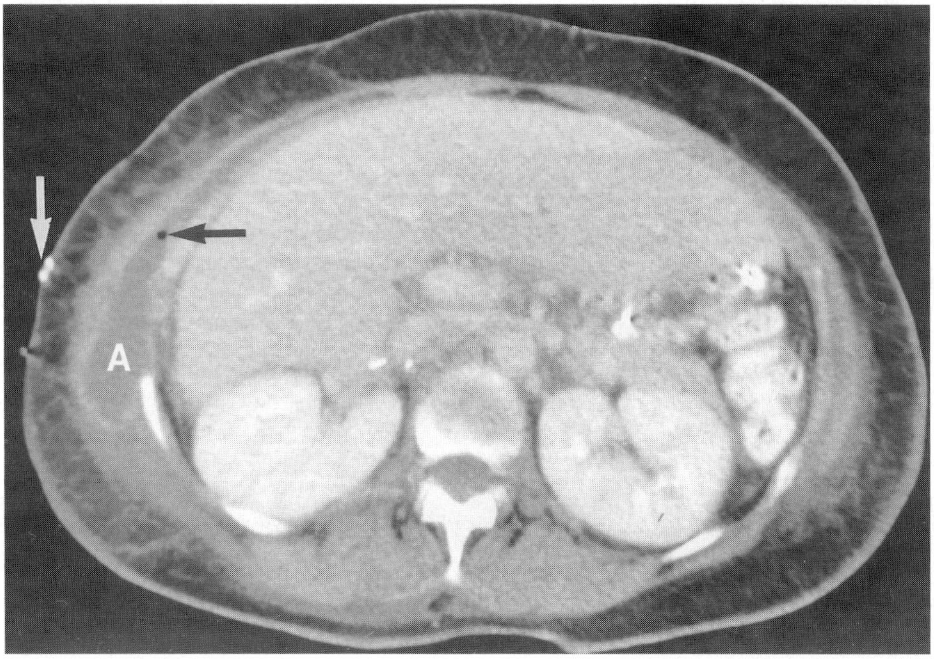

FIGURE 14.6 Abdominal wall abscess. There is a fluid-attenuation collection (A) in the right abdominal wall musculature in this patient who recently underwent laparotomy for pheochromocytoma. The focus of gas within the collection *(black arrow)* confirms the diagnosis. Surgical staples are present *(white arrow)*.

- **Subcutaneous nodules** and skin thickening are common observations on CT. Although often incidental and of little clinical concern, a subcutaneous nodule can be the result of **metastatic disease (Fig. 14.9)** or may represent a primary malignant soft tissue tumor. Most benign lesions are scars, keloids, sebaceous cysts, or mesenchymal tumors **(Section 14.5).**
- **Subcutaneous emphysema,** which appears as linear lucencies tracking along tissue planes, is common following surgery, drainage tube placement, or pneumothorax **(see Fig. 3.4).** Uncommonly, it can be the result of necrotizing fasciitis or infection.

14.3 BREAST

- **Gynecomastia** is a nonspecific symmetrical enlargement of the glandular tissue, typically in the male breast **(Differential 14.3).** Asymmetrical enlargement suggests breast cancer or inflammation.
- **Breast cancer** is the second leading cause of cancer death in women.

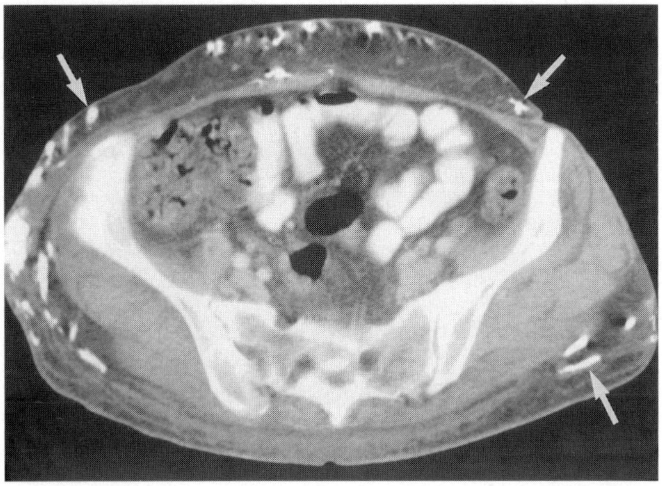

FIGURE 14.8 CREST syndrome. A 45-year-old woman with scleroderma. There are numerous calcific foci *(arrows)* within the subcutaneous soft tissues. This patient also had Raynaud syndrome and the other features of CREST syndrome.

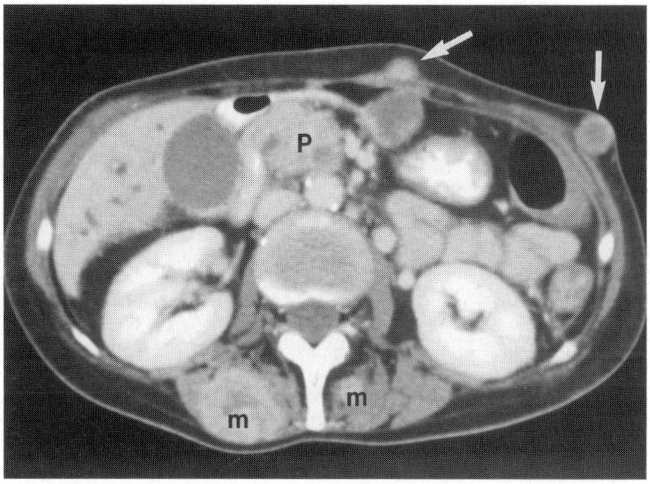

FIGURE 14.9 Metastatic pancreatic cancer. CT in a 52-year-old woman with pancreatic cancer (P) shows metastatic deposits within subcutaneous fat *(arrows)* and skeletal muscle (m).

Survival is increased by early detection. The incidence in men is 1 percent that in women **(Fig. 14.10).** Mammography is the mainstay in the detection and diagnosis of breast cancer; however, **CT** is helpful for staging breast cancer, particularly if chest wall invasion, adenopathy, or distant metastases are suspected **(Fig. 14.11).** Internal thoracic adenopathy can occur without axillary nodal involvement. Metastases are most common in the lung, liver, and skeleton. An incidental breast mass can be discovered on CT, but the appearance usually is nonspecific and mammography or biopsy is required for further evaluation **(Fig. 14.12).**

- **Mastitis,** inflammatory breast cancer, and radiation therapy can have the same CT appearance. There is edema, skin thickening, lymphadenopathy, and often ipsilateral arm swelling. Clinical history and skin punch biopsy identify the correct etiology.

14.2 SOFT TISSUE CALCIFICATIONS

Connective tissue diseases—scleroderma, dermatomyositis, CREST syndrome (calcinosis, Raynaud, esophageal dysmotility, sclerodactyly, telangiectasia)
Trauma—myositis ossificans, thermal and electrical injuries, fat necrosis
Injection granuloma
Vascular—atherosclerosis, venous phleboliths, diabetes
Calcified lymph nodes
Hypercalcemia/metabolic disease—hyperparathyroidism, renal osteodystrophy, widespread osseous metastases, excess vitamin D, CPPD, gout, sarcoid
Hemangioma—small phleboliths
Degenerating fibroadenoma of the breast
Parasites—cysticercosis, other worms

Key: CPPD, calcium pyrophosphate dihydrate deposition disease.

- **Radiation therapy** can produce skin thickening, inflammatory changes, and increased attenuation in the residual breast tissue and subcutaneous fat. Radiation ports used to treat the breast are tangential to the chest wall so as to minimize radiation to the lung, but it is common to see radiation pneumonitis or pulmonary fibrosis in the peripheral lung adjacent to the chest wall **(see Fig. 2.67).** The fibrosis can have a nodular appearance, simulating metastases or lymphangitic spread of tumor.
- **Deformities and scarring** from surgery or radiation complicate the evaluation of postoperative examinations. There is asymmetrical parenchyma and adipose tissue. Depending on the type of surgery performed (lumpectomy, radical or modified mastectomy), adjacent muscles and lymph nodes can be absent. Hematomas and seromas are occasionally present, and residual portions of muscle remaining at the sternal or costal attachment can mimic recurrent tumor. The overlying skin should be less than 5 mm thick following surgery.
- **Breast reconstruction** has become an important component of breast cancer treatment, and these surgical changes complicate the postmastectomy CT appearance. The transverse rectus abdominis musculocutaneous (TRAM) flap is a common reconstruction technique and involves transfer of fat, skin, and the rectus abdominis muscle onto the chest wall **(Fig. 14.13).** This is evident on CT as

14.3 GYNECOMASTIA

Drugs—estrogen, digitalis, marijuana, tricyclic antidepressants, reserpine, thiazides
Cirrhosis
Chronic renal failure with hemodialysis
Decreased serum testosterone—senile, hypogonadism, hypopituitarism
Tumor—adrenal, testicular or pituitary with hormonal activity
Chronic lung disease—especially emphysema

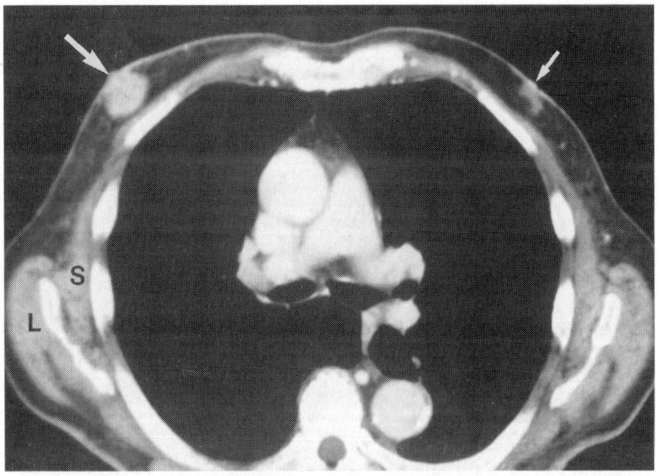

FIGURE 14.10 Male breast cancer. Contrast-enhanced chest CT in a 68-year-old man shows an enhancing soft tissue mass in the right breast *(large arrow)*. Note normal rudimentary left breast tissue *(small arrow)*. S, serratus anterior; L, latissimus dorsi.

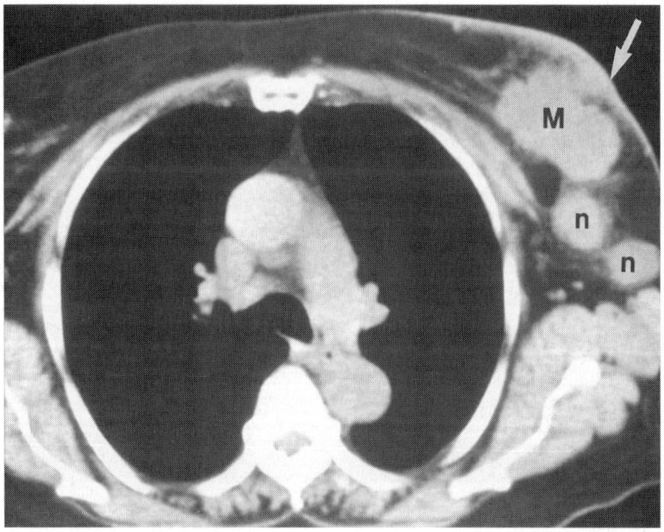

FIGURE 14.11 Advanced breast cancer. Contrast-enhanced CT in a 67-year-old woman shows a large left breast mass (M) with associated skin thickening *(arrow)* and axillary adenopathy (n).

asymmetrical breast size, with the reconstructed breast lacking parenchymal tissue. Usually, the ipsilateral rectus is surgically absent, although either side can be harvested.

- **Local recurrence** of breast cancer occurs within 5 years in up to 30 percent of patients, depending on the initial tumor type and treatment. Tumor can recur in the subcutaneous tissues, axilla, pectoral muscles, or internal mammary nodes **(Fig. 14.14)** and subsequently invade the chest wall, mediastinum, or sternum. CT is valuable in documenting and assessing the extent of recurrent breast carcinoma.
- **Breast implants** are common. CT demonstrates water-attenuation, encapsulated implants that can be either subglandular or subpectoral in position. MRI, ultrasound, and mammography are more sensitive for evaluating breast implant rupture.

14.4 EXTERNAL HERNIAS

- **Internal hernias** are discussed in **Section 6.4, diaphragmatic hernias** in **Section 3.9,** and **traumatic diaphragm rupture** in **Section 15.3.**
- Most **external hernias** are reducible and often asymptomatic. Others present as a palpable mass. The hernia sac can contain any abdominal contents, but mesenteric fat and bowel are most common. Hernias are more common and also more difficult to detect by physical exam in obese individuals. Complications include incarceration, strangulation, and bowel obstruction. **Incarceration** refers to a hernia that cannot be manually reduced. **Strangulation** is occlusion of the vascular supply to the bowel, leading to

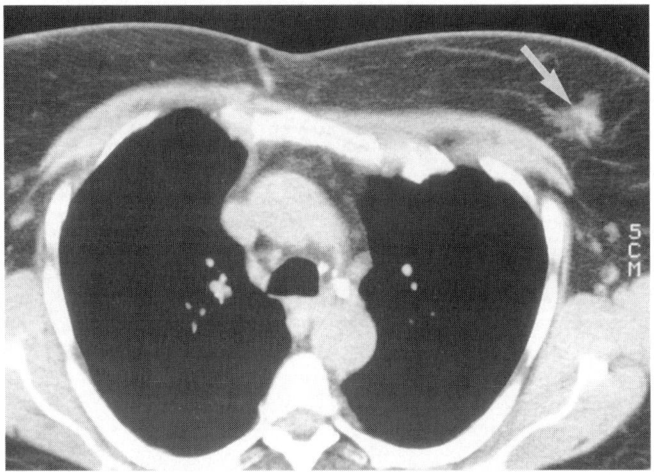

FIGURE 14.12 Subtle breast cancer. Chest CT in a 65-year-old woman with breast cancer *(arrow)*.

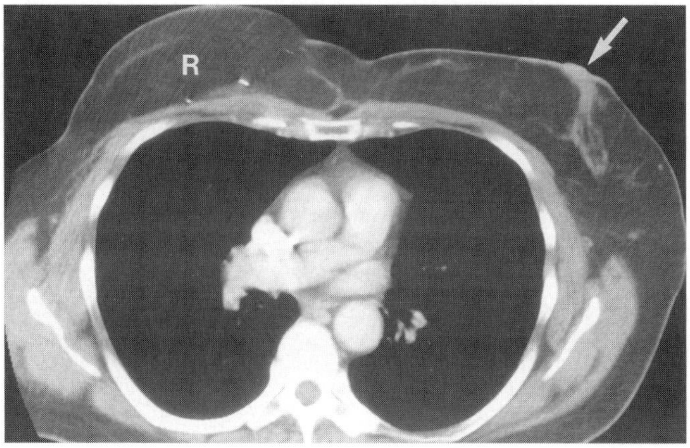

FIGURE 14.13 Mastectomy with TRAM (transverse rectus abdominis musculocutaneous) flap reconstruction. Contrast-enhanced CT shows a normal left breast and nipple *(large arrow)* and a right breast reconstruction (R) performed by mobilizing a musculocutaneous flap, which included the left rectus muscle.

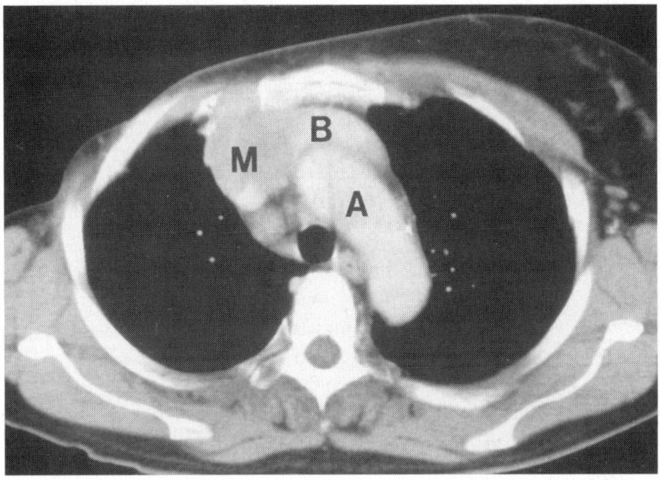

FIGURE 14.14 Recurrent breast cancer. Contrast-enhanced CT in a 69-year-old woman who has undergone right mastectomy for breast cancer. There is massive right internal thoracic adenopathy (M) with mediastinal invasion. B, left brachiocephalic vein; A, aorta.

infarction. Findings include bowel wall thickening, hemorrhage, and pneumatosis as well as venous engorgement and mesenteric edema. **Obstruction** is more frequent when the defect through which bowel contents protrude is small. CT signs of obstruction are proximal bowel dilatation and distal collapse. A **Richter hernia** contains only a single wall of a bowel loop but can still produce clinically important obstruction.

- **Ventral hernias** are very frequent; they are evident on CT as omentum or bowel herniating through a defect in the linea alba. **Incisional hernias** occur most commonly at the linea alba following laparotomy. **Parastomal hernias** occur adjacent to colonic or ileal ostomies and occasionally cause obstruction. A **Spigelian hernia** is herniation of abdominal contents through the hiatus semilunaris at the lateral edge of the rectus muscle **(Fig. 14.15).** Since a Spigelian hernia protrudes beyond the transverse abdominis and internal oblique muscles but is contained by the external oblique, it can be difficult to detect on physical examination. Strangulation is relatively common.

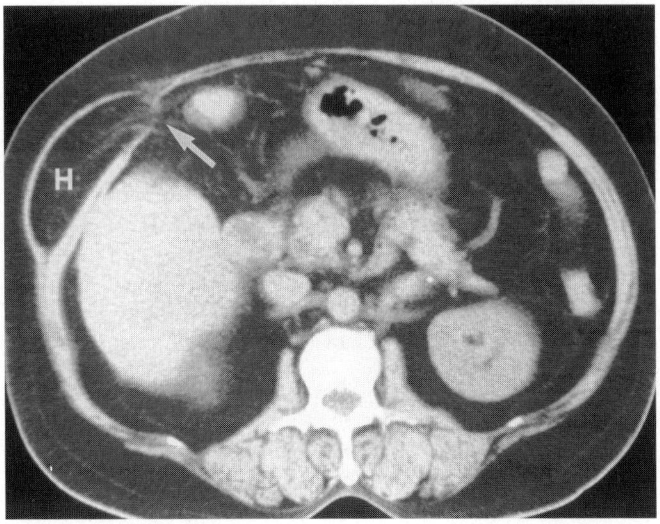

FIGURE 14.15 Spigelian hernia. Contrast-enhanced CT in a 28-year-old woman shows herniation of intra-abdominal fat (H) through the hiatus semilunaris *(arrow)* into the space between the internal and external oblique muscles.

- **Indirect inguinal hernias** are the most common external hernias. They allow protrusion of abdominal contents through the inguinal canal into the scrotum or labia **(Fig. 14.16).** The inguinal canal normally contains the spermatic cord in men and the round ligament in women. Indirect inguinal hernias occur lateral to the inferior epigastric vessels. **Direct inguinal hernias** occur through a weakening in the transversalis fascia medial to the inferior epigastric vessels. **Femoral hernias** occur through the femoral canal immediately adjacent to the femoral vessels. They are more common in women and pose a high risk of strangulation. CT shows the hernia sac lateral to the inguinal canal.
- **Obturator hernias** occur through the obturator canal, adjacent to the obturator externus muscle (see **Fig 6.19**). **Sciatic hernias** are quite rare and represent herniation through the greater or lesser sciatic notch. **Lumbar hernias** occur through either the superior (Grynfelt) or inferior (Petit) lumbar triangle. The superior lumbar triangle is formed by the twelfth rib, internal oblique, serratus posterior, and erector spinae muscles. The inferior lumbar triangle is formed by the iliac crest, latissimus dorsi, and external oblique muscles. The inferior triangle is a site of laparoscopic nephrectomy ports.

14.5 SOFT TISSUE TUMORS

- **CT** can identify the presence and extent of soft tissue infiltration and assess osseous involvement by soft tissue tumors. Masses with heterogeneous attenuation and irregular, infiltrative margins are suspicious for a malignancy, but infections and hematomas can have similar findings. Rapid growth, invasion of adjacent structures, and metastases support a diagnosis of malignancy. Benign tumors are more likely to appear homogeneous, smoothly marginated, and encapsulated. Biopsy is usually required for definitive diagnosis.
- Metastases are more common than primary malignancies, and almost any primary can metastasize to soft tissue. Primary soft tissue tumors, are more common than primary bone tumors, and most are malignant. Common benign lesions include lipomas and desmoid tumors, and common malignancies include malignant fibrous histiocytoma (MFH) and rhabdomyosarcoma.
- Tumors can involve the body wall by direct extension. In cases of peripheral lung pathology, the chest wall should be carefully examined for evidence of involvement. Bone destruction is a definitive observation; soft tissue infiltration, fat stranding, and pleural thickening are less reliable indications of body wall invasion. Pain indicates parietal pleural involvement. Advances in reconstructive surgery have facilitated extensive curative resections of malignant neoplasms involving the body wall, including both primary lesions and invasion by adjacent tumor.

Benign Tumors

- **Primary soft tissue tumors** are typically of mesenchymal origin, arising from the fat, fibrous, vascular, neural, muscular, or dermal tissues and include hemangiomas, lipomas, fibromas, and desmoid tumors.

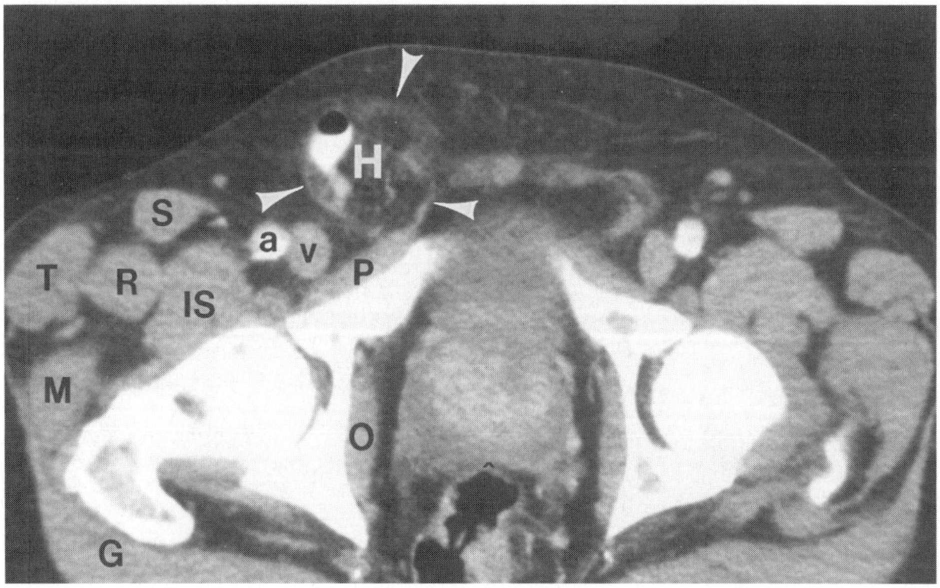

FIGURE 14.16 Inguinal hernia. Pelvic CT shows an indirect inguinal hernia (H) with fat and small bowel containing air and contrast material within an enlarged right inguinal canal *(arrowheads).* S, sartorius; T, tensor fascia lata; R, rectus femoris; IS, iliopsoas; a, femoral artery; v, femoral vein; P, pectineus muscle; M, gluteus medius; G, gluteus maximus; O, obturator internus.

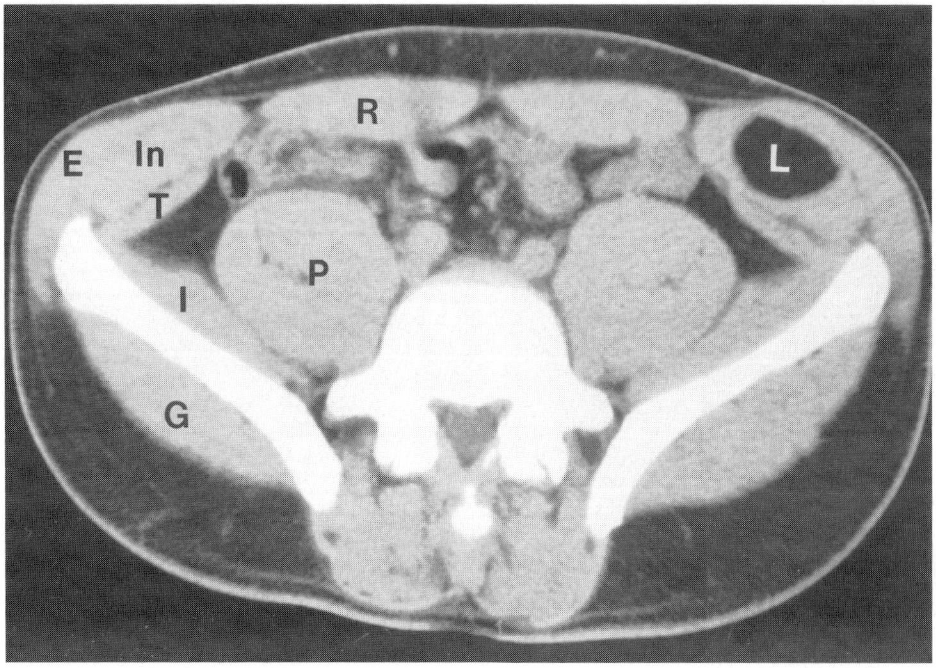

FIGURE 14.17 Abdominal wall lipoma. Noncontrast CT demonstrates a discrete fat attenuation mass (L) arising within the left internal oblique muscle. There are no internal septations or findings to suggest liposarcoma. E, external oblique; In, internal oblique; T, transverse abdominis; R, rectus abdominis; P, psoas; I, iliacus; G, gluteus maximus muscles.

- A **lipoma** is the most common soft tissue tumor. It can be subcutaneous, intramuscular, or extrapleural; in the last case, it can displace the pleura and mimic a pleural or pulmonary mass. Lipomas usually have sharp margins, minimal internal architecture except for a thin capsule or septations, and occasionally small calcifications **(Fig. 14.17).** They are easily diagnosed on CT by their characteristic homogeneous fat content. Lipomas have no malignant potential but can be resected for cosmetic reasons.

- **Neurogenic tumors**—including schwannomas and neurofibromas—can arise from the intercostal nerves, brachial and sacral plexuses, or other nervous system structures. They often have homogeneous low attenuation on CT because of their abundant lipid content, myxoid matrix, hypocellularity, and regions of cystic degeneration. Plexi-form neurofibromas in patients with neurofibromatosis can infiltrate the body wall, and malignant degeneration of neurofibromas can occur in patients with neurofibromatosis (usually associated with large nerves such as the sciatic nerve).

- **Hemangiomas** are benign vascular tumors found in the skin, soft tissues, and bones. They contain tortuous vessels that enhance following intravenous contrast administration and may contain phleboliths. **Arteriovenous malformations** appear as a collection of densely enhancing tubular structures.

- **Desmoid tumors** are benign fibrous tumors that typically appear at fascial aponeuroses. They are most common in the abdominal wall, and there is an association with Gardner syndrome and pregnancy. Desmoids are homogeneously of soft tissue or higher attenuation **(Fig. 14.18).** They extensively infiltrate adjacent structures and frequently recur when inadequately excised.

- **Localized lymphangioma** is a cystic mass of sequestered lymphatic tissue that can be confused with a hemangioma. These lesions usually present in the neck but can extend into the mediastinum, chest wall, or axilla **(see Fig. 4.13).** CT or MRI can define the extent of infiltration of adjacent tissues, which is important, since

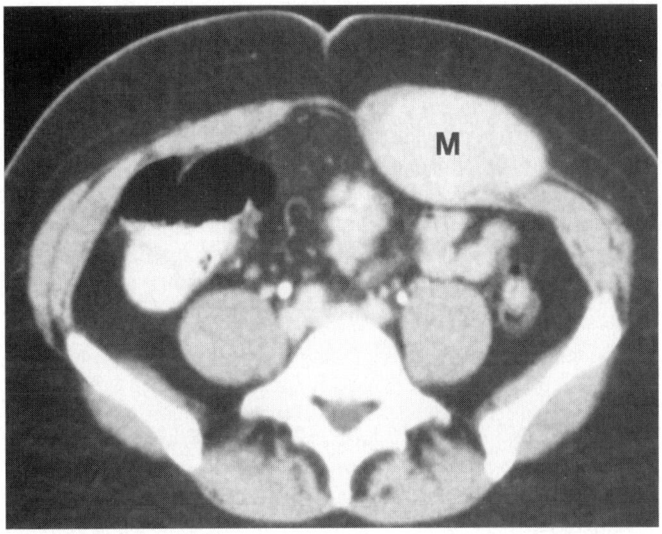

FIGURE 14.18 Desmoid tumor (fibromatosis). A 32-year-old woman with a palpable abdominal mass. Contrast-enhanced CT shows a well-defined, enhancing soft tissue mass (M) arising in the right rectus muscle at the level of the umbilicus.

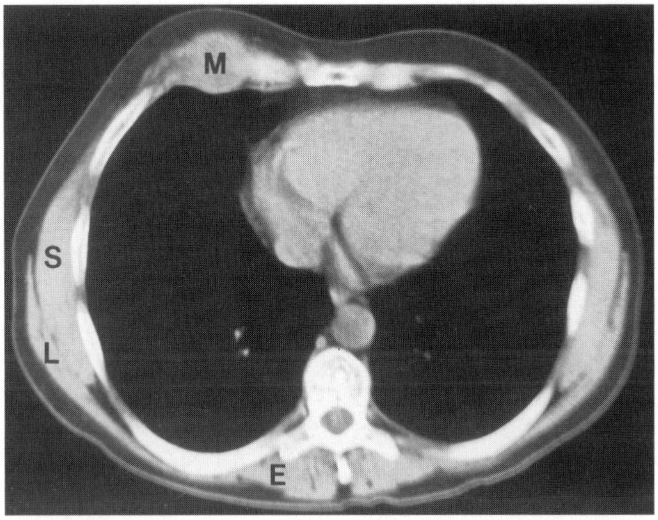

FIGURE 14.19 Chest wall lymphoma. Noncontrast chest CT shows a soft tissue mass (M), proven to be primary non-Hodgkin lymphoma. S, serratus anterior; L, latissimus dorsi; E, erector spinae.

recurrence is common following incomplete excision. Internal septations are frequent.

Malignant Tumors

- **Malignant fibrous histiocytoma (MFH)** is a primary soft tissue tumor seen in older adults. It typically appears as a lobulated soft tissue mass with indistinct and infiltrative margins. There is mild enhancement following intravenous contrast administration. It has a poor prognosis.
- **Lymphoma** involves the body wall by extension from adjacent lymph nodes in non-Hodgkin lymphoma or from the thymus in Hodgkin lymphoma **(Fig. 14.19).** Primary dermal involvement is uncommon. Sézary syndrome is an uncommon primary form of cutaneous T-cell lymphoma. CT demonstrates multiple soft tissue nodules within the body wall or more focal involvement **(Fig. 14.20).** Concurrent adenopathy is readily demonstrated.
- **Liposarcomas** are typically inhomogeneous fatty tumors that contain soft tissue components. They are generally large and infiltrating, allowing differentiation from benign lipoma, although a well-differentiated liposarcoma might appear similar. Other malignancies affecting the soft tissues **(Fig. 14.21)** include rhabdomyosarcoma, leiomyosarcoma, neurofibrosarcoma, primitive neuroectodermal tumor (PNET), and other sarcomas.

14.6 SKELETON

- Portions of the axial and appendicular skeleton are seen on all body CTs, and images windowed for bone detail should be reviewed in patients suspected of having osseous disease. **Degenerative changes** are common with advancing age and can develop prematurely as a consequence of overuse or trauma. Osteophyte formation, geodes, and sclerosis are common in osteoarthritis. A benign vacuum phenomenon is occasionally observed within the intervertebral disks or the sternoclavicular joints.
- **Congenital chest wall deformities** include scoliosis, pectus carinatum, and pectus excavatum. **Thoracoplasty** is surgical resection or collapse of the upper chest wall, originally devised as a treatment for tuberculosis by compressing underlying lung and creating a pulmonary environment unsuitable for the pathogen. The appearance can be bizarre and may mimic massive thoracic trauma **(Fig. 14.22).** Calcification and contralateral lung hyperexpansion are frequent associated findings.

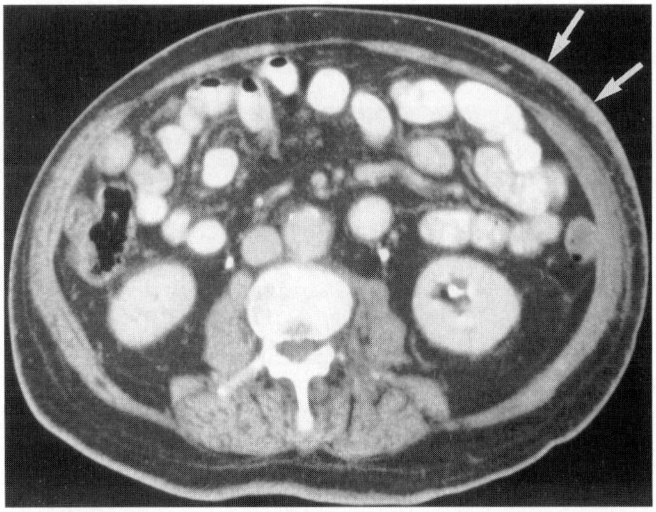

FIGURE 14.20 Cutaneous lymphoma. CT shows diffuse skin thickening *(arrows)* and mild soft tissue infiltration of the underlying subcutaneous fat in this 76-year-old man. Skin biopsy revealed Sézary syndrome of cutaneous T-cell lymphoma.

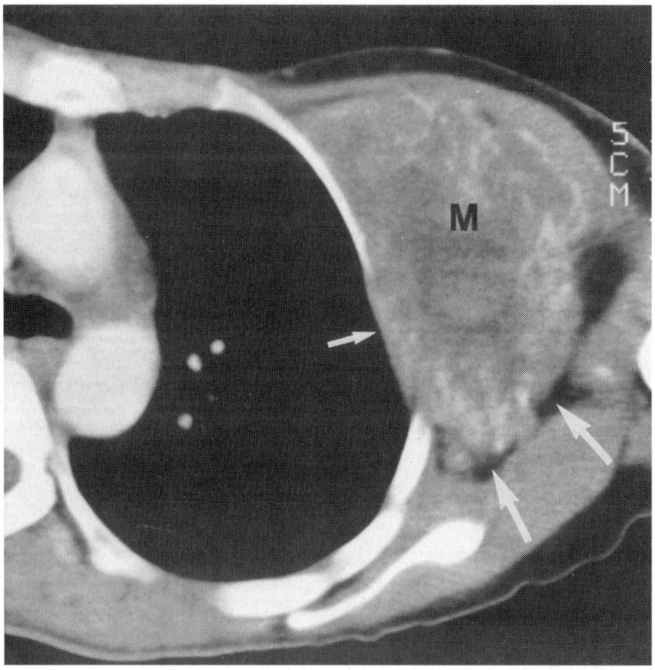

FIGURE 14.21 Epithelioid sarcoma. A vascular soft tissue mass (M) arising in the axilla. Note the irregular infiltrating margins *(large arrows)* and invasion of the extrapleural space *(small arrow)*. [From Slone RM, Gierada DS. Pleura, chest wall, and diaphragm. In: Lee JKT, Sagel SS, Stanley RJ, Heiken JP (eds.) *Computed Body Tomography with MRI Correlation,* 3rd ed. Philadelphia: Lippincott-Raven, 1998.]

- **Sternocostoclavicular hyperostosis,** sometimes accompanied by chronic pain and anterior chest swelling, is characterized by hyperostosis and soft tissue ossification between the clavicle, sternum, and upper ribs. Bone overgrowth can lead to a thick, wide sternum sometimes simulating Paget disease or chronic osteomyelitis. These sclerotic foci can simulate pulmonary nodules on plain films, but CT correctly demonstrates their intraosseous nature.

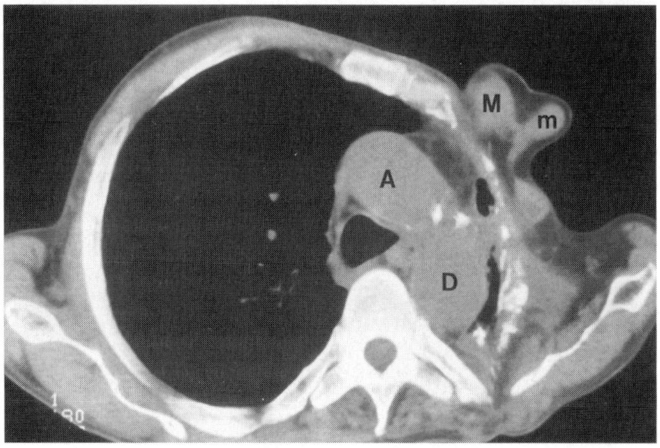

FIGURE 14.22 Thoracoplasty. Chest CT in a 68-year-old man shows a collapsed left chest wall nearly obliterating the pleural space. Note protrusion of the pectoralis major (M) and minor (m) muscles. A, ascending aorta; D, descending aorta.

- **Fractures** are a common consequence of trauma, often accompanied by an adjacent hematoma. Pathologic fractures from underlying metastasis or mutiple myeloma should be suspected when acute fracture margins are indistinct or there is an associated soft tissue mass. When a fracture is identified, associated injuries such as pneumothorax, pulmonary contusion, or visceral injury should be excluded. **Spinal compression fractures** in elderly adults occur as a consequence of osteopenia, typically osteoporosis, and are a common cause of back pain. Multiple fractures can cause a kyphotic deformity leading to atelectasis and pneumonia.
- **Costochondritis** (Tietze syndrome) is chest pain, tenderness, and swelling of the costal cartilage. Clinically, a mild focal cartilaginous enlargement can sometimes mimic a chest wall mass. **Osteomyelitis** or septic arthritis of the sternum or sternoclavicular joint is a rare complication of median sternotomy. Separation or bone destruction on CT is usually evident. **Mediastinitis (Sec. 4.3)** is an uncommon complication but carries a high mortality if untreated. CT is required, as it is difficult to diagnose this condition radiographically. Treatment consists of antibiotics, debridement, and drainage. Retrosternal air should not be present beyond 1 week following uncomplicated sternotomy, and mediastinal fluid should resorb by 3 weeks.
- **Diskitis** resulting from hematogenous spread of infection to the intervertebral disk can lead to loss of disk height and end-plate destruction. The vertebrae become sclerotic and can fuse after the infection heals. **Tuberculosis** (Pott disease) can involve the spine and classically destroys the vertebra and intervertebral disk. Other findings of disseminated tuberculosis may be present.
- **Diffuse skeletal sclerosis** can be caused by widespread metastases, particularly breast and prostate cancer, but also by metabolic bone disease, **(Differential 14.4). Radiation therapy** can result in localized sclerosis, osteoporosis, or even avascular necrosis of the bones contained in the radiation port. Modern three-dimensional treatment planning has greatly reduced the incidence of this complication.

14.7 BONE TUMORS

- Radiography and radionuclide bone scintigraphy are used for detecting fractures and bone tumors, but **CT** is useful for evaluating solitary, aggressive bone lesions and bone involvement by adjacent

14.4 DIFFUSE SCLEROSIS

Widespread metastases—breast or prostate
Sickle cell disease
Renal osteodystrophy and metabolic bone disease
Paget disease
Osteopetrosis
Mastocytosis—hepatomegaly, adenopathy
Myelofibrosis—splenomegaly, extramedullary hematopoiesis
Melorrheostosis
Neurocutaneous syndromes—neurofibromatosis, tuberous sclerosis
Fluorosis—more commonly ligamentous calcification
Pyknodysostosis

tumors. MRI is more sensitive for evaluating soft tissue and bone marrow involvement. Both benign and malignant tumors can involve the bones of the body wall. Metastases are more common than primary malignancies, and almost any primary can metastasize to bone. Common benign lesions include bone islands, osteochondromas, and fibrous dysplasia, and common malignancies include chondrosarcoma, osteosarcoma, and Ewing sarcoma.

- **Bone metastases** from lung, breast **(Fig. 14.23)**, renal, or thyroid carcinomas and multiple myeloma are the most common cause of destructive, lytic bone lesions **(Differential 14.5).** Prostate and breast cancer are the most common source for blastic metastases **(Fig. 14.24).** Skeletal metastases appear as multiple areas of lytic, mixed, or blastic destruction **(Differential 14.6).** Thyroid, renal cell carcinoma, and myeloma can have accompanying soft tissue masses. Pathologic fractures are common.
- **Benign bone tumors** include bone islands, simple bone cysts, enchondromas, giant-cell tumors, fibrous dysplasia, hemangiomas, osteochondromas, aneurysmal bone cysts, and eosinophilic granuloma. **Primary malignant tumors**—such as a chondrosarcoma, osteosarcomas, plasmacytoma, lymphoma, or Ewing sarcoma—are much less common. Lymphoma and mesothelioma can invade bone directly, as can bronchogenic and breast carcinomas.
- **Diffuse sclerosis** can be due to widespread bone metastases, typically prostate cancer in men or breast cancer in women. Myelofibrosis, mastocytosis, and osteopetrosis can have a similar appearance. **Paget disease** can involve the thoracic spine, clavicles, or humerus. It is characterized by sclerosis, thickened trabeculae, and enlargement of the involved bone.
- **Bone islands** (enostosis) appear as focal and discrete sclerotic foci, most commonly in the ribs, pelvis, and spine. Although they are the most common cause of a focal sclerotic lesion, bone islands must be differentiated from **sclerotic metastases,** typically due to prostate or breast cancer.

14.5

LYTIC BONE LESION

Malignancy
- **Hematogenous metastasis—**renal cell, thyroid cancer, lung cancer, lymphoma, neuroblastoma
- **Multiple myeloma** or plasmacytoma
- Direct extension
- Primary tumor—Ewing sarcoma, chondrosarcoma, fibrosarcoma

Osteomyelitis—can form Brodie abscess, sequestrum

Benign tumor—fibrous dysplasia, nonossifying fibroma, enchondroma, Langerhans cell histiocytosis, giant-cell tumor, osteoblastoma, brown tumor, chondroblastoma, chondromyxoid fibroma, intraosseous lipoma

Paget disease

Cysts—subchondral geodes, aneurysmal bone cyst, unicameral cyst

Fracture

- **Osteochondromas** (exostoses) are the most common benign tumors. They present as lobulated exophytic projections of cortical bone with a cartilaginous cap **(Fig. 14.25)**. Rapid growth or pain suggests malignant degeneration. **Enchondromas** (chondromas) are benign cartilaginous bone lesions that are typically well defined and lobulated, cause endosteal scalloping, and contain diffuse or stippled calcification.
- **Fibrous dysplasia** is the second most common benign bone tumor. Typically discovered in adulthood, fibrous dysplasia is most often seen in the ribs, pelvis, and proximal femur. It typically appears as a central, expansile, fusiform lytic lesion with cortical thinning. The "woven bone" matrix produces a "ground-glass" appearance **(Fig. 14.26).**

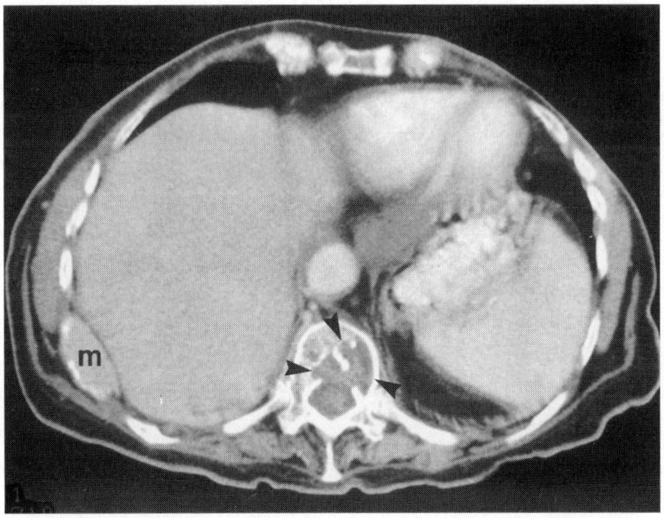

FIGURE 14.23 Metastatic breast cancer. A 74-year-old woman with a destructive lesion seen arising in the vertebral body *(arrowheads)* and extending into the spinal canal. A second lesion is seen in the posterolateral aspect of a right rib (m), also with an extraosseous soft tissue component.

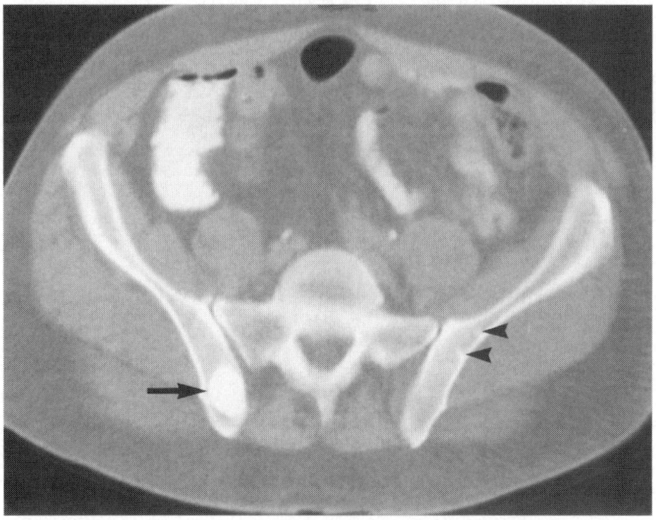

FIGURE 14.24 Sclerotic bone metastases from prostate cancer. There is a dominant sclerotic metastasis in the posterior aspect of the right iliac crest *(arrow)*. Two tiny additional metastatic foci *(arrowheads)* were evident only by using bone windows.

14.6

SCLEROTIC BONE LESION

Bone island
Metastasis—breast or prostate cancer, lymphoma; treated lytic lesion
Osteonecrosis/infarct—idiopathic, steroids, alcohol, sickle cell, vasculitis, trauma, caisson disease
Healing fracture
Benign lesion—fibrous dysplasia, osteochondroma, osteoma, healing nonossifying fibroma, ossifying fibroma, enchondroma, osteoid osteoma, infarct
Infection—chronic osteomyelitis
Primary malignancy—osteosarcoma, Ewing sarcoma, uncommonly myeloma
Paget disease—often polyostotic

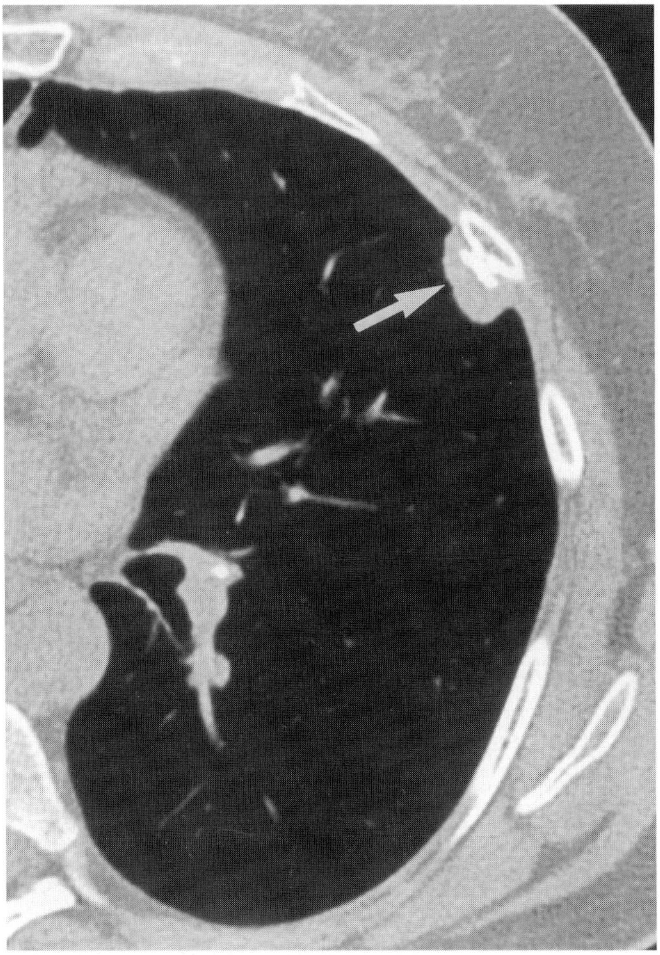

FIGURE 14.25 Osteochondroma. Thin-section CT shows an osseous and soft tissue tumor *(arrow)* arising from the cortical surface of a rib. The lesion remained unchanged over a 6-year period.

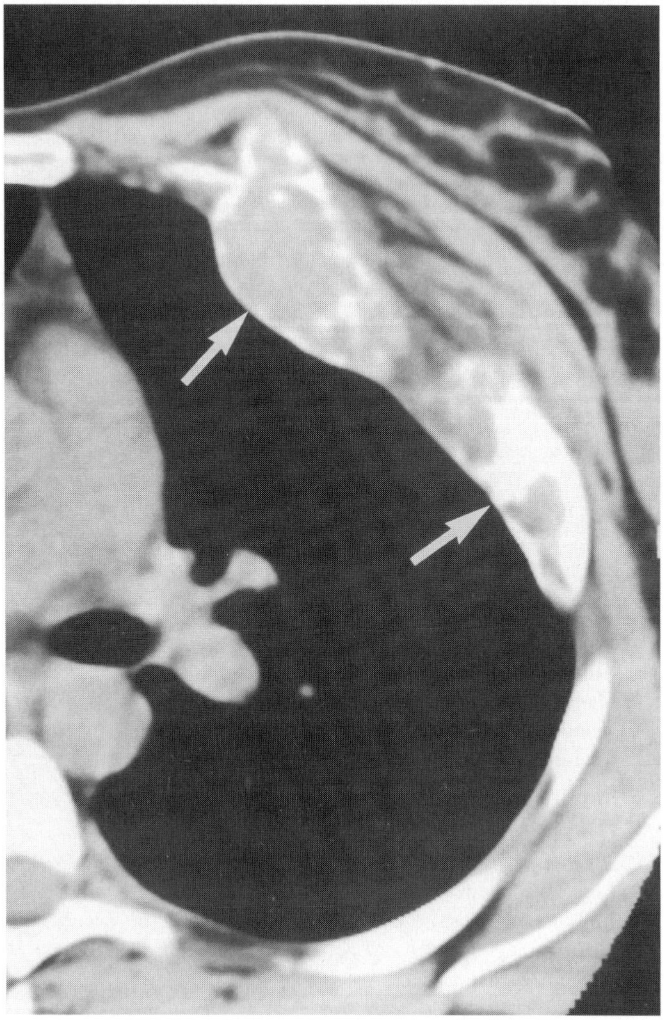

FIGURE 14.26 Fibrous dysplasia. CT shows an expansile lytic lesion involving two contiguous left ribs *(arrows)*. There is no cortical disruption or extraosseous soft tissue component. Two normal ribs are seen posteriorly. (From Slone RM, Gierada DS. Pleura, chest wall, and diaphragm. In: Lee JKT, Sagel SS, Stanley RJ, Heiken JP, eds. *Computed Body Tomography with MRI Correlation,* 3rd ed. Philadelphia: Lippincott-Raven, 1998.)

- **Aneurysmal bone cysts** present as expansile lytic lesions, sharply demarcated by a thin shell of periosteum. Most are seen in patients below age 20 and are likely to occur as a result of trauma to a preexisting bone lesion. **Hemangiomas,** which are benign, present as lytic lesions with coarse internal trabeculations and intact cortical margins. Pathologic fractures, which occur most frequently within a vertebral body, may lead to an acute presentation. **Hematopoietic disorders**—including thalassemia (**Fig. 14.27**), hereditary spherocytosis, and myelosclerosis—can produce enlargement of the medullary cavity. **Extramedullary hematopoiesis** can result in a paraspinal mass and splenomegaly.

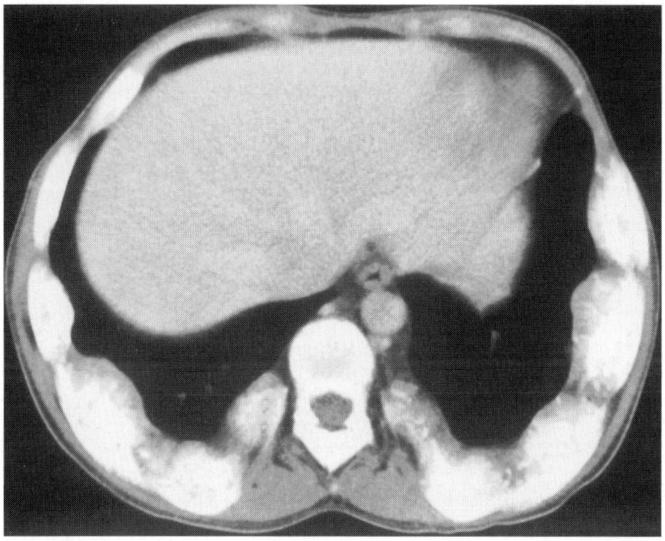

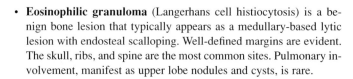

FIGURE 14.27 Thalassemia. Chest CT shows marked expansion of the ribs and extramedullary hematopoiesis as a result of chronic anemia.

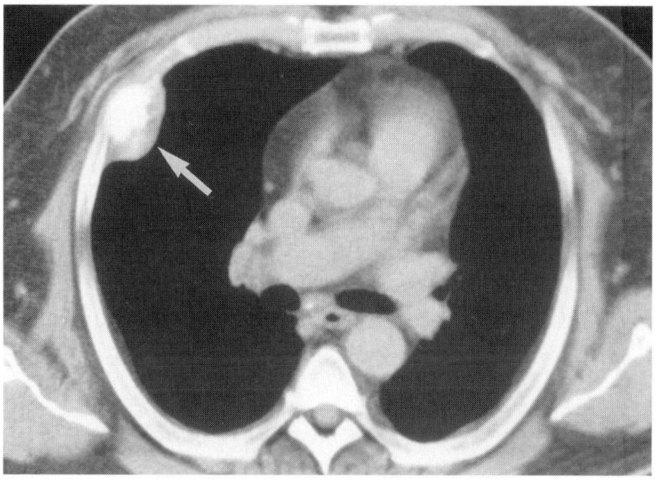

FIGURE 14.28 Osteosarcoma of rib. Chest CT in a 63-year-old man presenting with chest pain shows a sclerotic bone lesion *(arrow)* with an extraosseous soft tissue component and aggressive features.

- **Eosinophilic granuloma** (Langerhans cell histiocytosis) is a benign bone lesion that typically appears as a medullary-based lytic lesion with endosteal scalloping. Well-defined margins are evident. The skull, ribs, and spine are the most common sites. Pulmonary involvement, manifest as upper lobe nodules and cysts, is rare.
- **Osteosarcoma** is the most common primary malignancy of bone in the pediatric population. There are numerous subtypes; osteogenic osteosarcoma is the most common form, presenting with pain or mass. CT depicts a dense, poorly defined blastic lesion with periosteal reaction **(Fig. 14.28). Chondrosarcoma** often presents as a large, lobulated mass with poorly defined margins and associated cortical bone destruction. Chondrosarcomas typically have a chondroid internal matrix and potentially an associated soft tissue mass. **Ewing sarcomas** present with predominantly lytic bone destruction and a soft tissue mass. They are most common in children and young adults.

Bibliography

Jafri SZH, Roberts JL, Bree RL, Tabor HD. Computed tomography of chest wall masses. *Radiographics* 1989;9:51.

Kuhlman JE, Bouchardy L, Fishman EK, Zerhount EA. CT and MR imaging evaluation of chest wall disorders. *Radiographics* 1994;14:571–595.

Sharif HS, Clark DC, Aabed MY, Aideyan OA, Haddad MC, Mattson TA. MR imaging of thoracic and abdominal wall infections: Comparison with other imaging procedures. *AJR* 1990;154:989–995.

Slone RM, Fisher AJ. *Pocket Guide to Body CT Differential Diagnosis.* New York: McGraw-Hill; 1999.

Slone RM, Gierada DS. Pleura, chest wall, and diaphragm. In: Lee JKT, Sagel SS, Stanley RJ, Heiken JP, eds. *Computed Body Tomography with MRI Correlation,* 3rd ed. Philadelphia: Lippincott-Raven, 1998.

Slone RM, Gutierrez FR, Fisher AJ. *Thoracic Imaging: A Practical Approach.* New York: McGraw-Hill; 1998.

Wechsler RJ. *Cross-Sectional Analysis of the Chest and Abdominal Wall.* St. Louis: Mosby; 1989.

Zarvan NP, Lee FT, Yandow DR, Unger JS. Abdominal hernias: CT findings. *AJR* 1995;164:1391–1395.

Chapter 15

THORACIC AND ABDOMINAL TRAUMA

Andrew J. Fisher

15.1 Epidemiology and Technique
15.2 Acute Traumatic Aortic Injury
15.3 Thoracic Trauma
15.4 Hemoperitoneum
15.5 Abdominal Trauma
15.6 Genitourinary Trauma

15.1 EPIDEMIOLOGY AND TECHNIQUE

- It is essential to understand the pathophysiology and CT appearances of thoracoabdominal trauma. This is because of both the increasing prevalence of trauma and the significant impact accurate image interpretation has on patient care.
- The **epidemiology** of trauma is age-dependent. Trauma occurs with the highest frequency between age 15 and 34, is more common in men than in women, and has a disproportionately high frequency in minority populations. Trauma, including homicides and suicides, is the leading cause of death in patients under the age of 45 years and is the fourth overall cause of death in all age groups. Blunt trauma accounts for more lost life years than cardiovascular disease and cancer combined. Estimated medical, morbidity, and mortality costs exceed $250 billion per year.

  The majority of blunt thoracic and abdominal trauma is caused by motor vehicle collisions (MVCs). Less frequent yet nonetheless significant etiologies include homicides, suicides, falls, and burns. **Thoracic trauma** is a contributing factor in approximately half of blunt trauma patients and the cause of death in one-third. Three-quarters of patients with severe thoracic injuries have injuries to other organ systems. Blunt trauma accounts for 80 percent of all cases of abdominal trauma. Penetrating trauma, while often more dramatic, is imaged less frequently. This is attributable to the fact that 80 percent of abdominal gunshot injuries enter the peritoneum and the vast majority of these patients undergo surgical exploration because of the high likelihood of damage to intraperitoneal organs.

  As with all trauma patients, rapid evaluation is important. The first goal is to assess airway, breathing, and circulatory concerns and treat life-threatening injuries, including life-sustaining interventions such as fluid resuscitation and endotracheal or thoracostomy tube placement. When the patient is stabilized, radiographic evaluation and a systematic search for less critical injuries and complications begins. The radiographic evaluation varies depending on the site and mechanism of injury. Typically, limited views of the spine, chest, and pelvis are obtained before the appendicular skeleton is assessed.

- **Thoracic trauma CT technique** generally involves spiral CT scanning. Noncontrast examination of the head and spine can be performed as warranted. Following repositioning of tubing (which can generate troublesome artifacts), the patient's arms are placed above his or her head. Unless contraindicated, 100 to 150 ml of iodinated intravenous (IV) contrast is administered by power injector at 1.5 to 2 ml/s. Imaging begins after a 20- to 30-second delay to allow time for contrast circulation through the heart and lungs. For evaluation of the thoracic aorta, contiguous 5- to 8-mm-thick images can be obtained using a pitch of 1 to 1.5. General thoracic screening can be obtained using wider collimation. Spiral CT imaging of the abdomen can be obtained without the use of additional IV contrast. With conventional CT, it may be necessary to use additional contrast for the abdominal images. Lung, soft tissue, and bone windows should be evaluated.

- **Abdominal trauma CT technique** usually entails initial gastric decompression via a nasogastric tube. This eliminates air-fluid interfaces and consequent linear streak artifacts. Water-soluble oral contrast should be routinely given by nasogastric tube. This is safe in both intubated and neurologically impaired patients. While a 30- to 45-minute delay is optimal to allow for intestinal transit, more emergent situations may limit opacification to only the stomach and duodenum. Finally, overlying objects should be repositioned, the urinary catheter should be clamped to obtain bladder distention, and the nasogastric tube should be withdrawn into the distal esophagus for the period during which abdominal scans are obtained.

  IV contrast is required to maximally enhance abdominal visceral organs and exclude parenchymal injuries. 100 to 150 ml of IV contrast should be administered at a rate of 1.5 to 2 ml/s; imaging is performed after a 60- to 80-second delay. In pediatric patients, the total dose can be calculated using 2 mg/kg as a guide, and the rate of injection should allow for the total dose to be administered in 60 seconds.

  Conventional CT scanning can be employed using 5-mm collimation at 5- to 8-mm intervals. Spiral CT markedly reduces the study time required for emergent patients who have limited breath-hold capability. A pitch of 1 to 2 can be employed. The entirety of the abdomen and pelvis should be imaged to help identify secondary signs of trauma. In addition to reviewing images on soft tissue settings, lung windows prove helpful in identifying subtle pneumatosis or pneumoperitoneum. Likewise, bone windows are required for proper identification of fractures and dislocations.

- **CT cystography** can be used to exclude bladder injury. Typically, 10 to 15 ml of 60 percent iodinated IV contrast is diluted in 500 ml of saline; 300 ml of this mixture is introduced by Foley catheter and the pelvis is scanned. This provides for adequate bladder distention and opacification to exclude bladder injuries. In less emergent instances, delayed images obtained with the urinary catheter clamped for 15 to 20 minutes can replace contrast cystography. The sensitivity of CT cystograms is equivalent to that of conventional cystography. A Foley catheter should not be placed in a trauma setting until the urethra has been evaluated and is known to be free of injury **(Fig. 15.1).**

15.2 ACUTE TRAUMATIC AORTIC INJURY

- **Acute traumatic aortic injury (ATAI)** is a common cause of mortality following MVCs. The typical mechanism of injury is rapid deceleration with rotation and torsion of the relatively mobile aortic arch, tethered by the ligamentum arteriosum, diaphragm, and aortic root. A direct blow with compression of mediastinal structures against the spine is another potential mechanism. ATAI can be catastrophic, accounting for 15 percent of all MVC fatalities; 85 percent of these patients die before any intervention is possible. Clinical findings include shock, systolic murmur from turbulent flow, and acute coarctation syndrome with differential upper and lower extremity pressures.

  ATAI occurs at sites where the aorta is fixed. More than 90 percent occur at the aortic isthmus adjacent to the ligamentum arteriosum and the remainder at the aortic root or descending aorta near the diaphragmatic hiatus. Patients with complete transection of the aorta generally die. Those with a contained rupture (pseudoaneurysm) or intimal injury of the aorta may survive the "golden hour" following trauma. These patients invariably have concomitant small vessel mediastinal bleeding, which accounts for many of the radiologic manifestations.

  Mediastinal blood obscures adjacent structures such as the aortic knob, and mass effect from the hematoma causes displacement of anatomic landmarks such as the trachea and left main bronchus. The most discriminating radiographic findings include obscuration of the aortic contour, a widened right or left paraspinal stripe (when no spinal fracture is present), rightward displacement of a nasogastric tube, and opacification of the aorticopulmonary window. Radiographic findings vary in their sensitivity and specificity, and a normal frontal chest radiograph has a 98 percent negative predictive value for ATAI. Sensitivity for aortic injury exceeds 85 percent, yet specificity is low.

- **Further evaluation with CT** is performed in cases where the chest radiograph is equivocal or suggestive of ATAI and the patient is hemodynamically stable. The scan should be performed with IV contrast but without oral contrast. IV contrast enhances evaluation of the vascular structures, definition of the aortic lumen, and detection of wall irregularities, and it is valuable for evaluating the involvement of visceral organs. Spiral technique allows more rapid scanning and makes possible the creation of multiplanar reconstructions, which may be helpful in demonstrating ATAI in a fashion similar to that of conventional angiography. CT angiography is beginning to replace aortography at some centers.

  The initial purpose of CT is to detect or exclude a mediastinal hematoma. Absence of a mediastinal hematoma confidently excludes ATAI. A hematoma appears as a soft tissue density adjacent to the aorta and is usually due to venous bleeding, but it can be due to fractures or other mediastinal injuries. Therefore, a hematoma from ATAI should abut the aorta and at least partially encase it **(Fig. 15.2).** Pericardial fluid in the anterior and posterior aortic

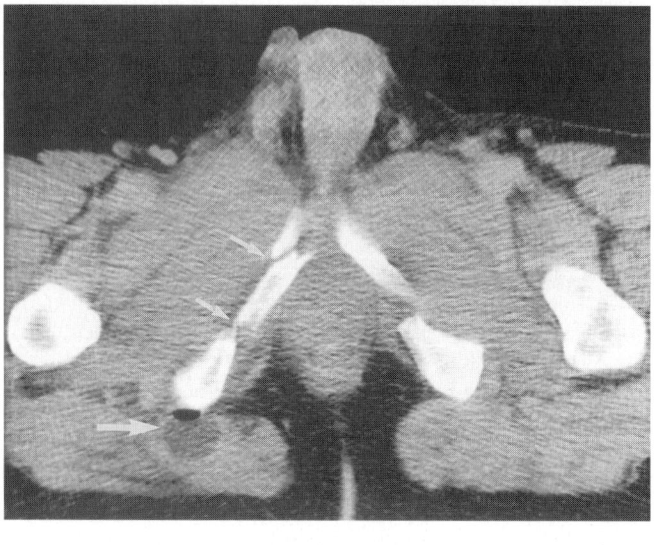

FIGURE 15.1 Misplaced urinary catheter. Following urinary catheter placement, there was no urinary output in this motor vehicle collision (MVC) victim. The urinary catheter balloon *(large arrow)* tracked through a complete urethral tear into the pelvic muscles and now is present adjacent to the right ischial tuberosity. There is a segmental fracture of the right inferior pubic ramus *(small arrows).*

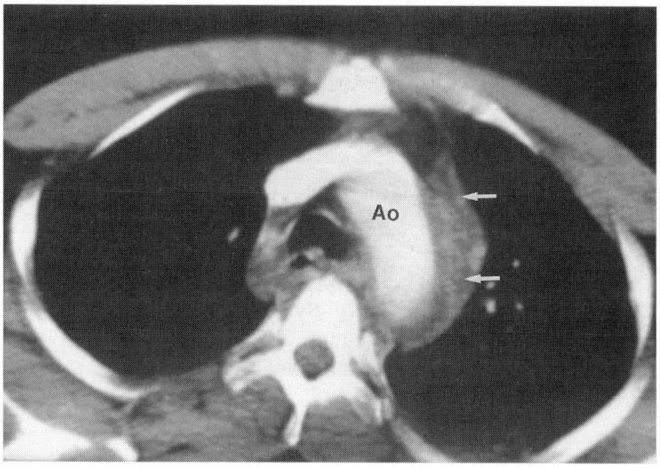

FIGURE 15.2 Mediastinal hematoma, acute traumatic aortic injury (ATAI). There is soft tissue attenuation blood *(arrows)* adjacent to the aortic arch (Ao). No fat plane is interposed between the hematoma and the aorta. An aortogram showed ATAI at the aortic isthmus.

recesses is normal and should not prompt alarm. The thymus may pose a diagnostic challenge in young victims; symmetry, distribution, and a preserved aortic fat plane are helpful differentiating features.

Improved CT angiography techniques may demonstrate the ATAI itself. This can be apparent as focally decreased vessel size, focal enlargement or wall irregularity, contrast extravasation, an intraluminal flap, or a pseudoaneurysm **(Fig. 15.3).** When present, these findings are diagnostic of ATAI and the patient should proceed to surgical intervention.

A CT that either shows no hematoma or shows a mediastinal hematoma but a preserved aortic fat plane requires no further evaluation. Those that demonstrate periaortic hematoma but no definite ATAI should progress to angiography. Patients with a radiograph strongly suggestive of ATAI should proceed directly to angiography. By this algorithm, 50 percent or more of patients can be spared angiography.

- **Other vessels** may be injured in chest trauma. Almost 20 percent of thoracic arterial injuries from trauma affect the great vessels. The left subclavian artery is most commonly injured, followed by the brachiocephalic, right subclavian, left common carotid, and vertebral arteries. Over 70 percent are unsuspected by physical examination. While CT may demonstrate perivascular hematoma, angiography is often required. Fractures of the distal third of the clavicle can injure the subclavian or axillary vessels, as can traumatic insertion of a central line. These injuries appear as an extrapleural density in the subclavicular area; if the pleura is violated, a hemothorax develops over time. The vena cava is the most frequently injured vein in thoracic trauma. Caval injuries may be difficult to repair and are often fatal. They are manifest as a right-sided mediastinal hematoma.

15.3 THORACIC TRAUMA

- In all patients with thoracic trauma, the first order of business is to assess the airway. Evaluation of the airway at the trauma center usually involves auscultation, physical examination, and chest radiography. An **endotracheal tube** placed hurriedly can be malpositioned within a main bronchus, usually the right, owing to its relatively shallow angle of takeoff from the trachea. In such cases, CT will demonstrate limited contralateral lung aeration. Esophageal intubation is another frequent type of malposition. CT will demonstrate bilaterally decreased pulmonary volumes with associated gastric distention. Likewise, **nasogastric tubes** may be placed incorrectly within the airway and cause pneumothorax, aspiration, or collapse.

Air Collections

- **Pneumothorax** is a common sequela of thoracic trauma and is often associated with rib fractures. Although apical pneumothoraces can be detected on upright radiographs, they are more difficult to detect on supine films. CT is more sensitive than radiography for detecting small pneumothoraces. Lung windows demonstrate air interposed between the lung and chest wall and often show subcutaneous emphysema. The size of the pneumothorax is readily demonstrated, and when contralateral mediastinal shift is present, the specific diagnosis of tension pneumothorax is easily made. The presence of an air-fluid level strongly suggests a hemopneumothorax.
- Although **chest tube placement** is routinely confirmed radiographically, malpositioned tubes are sometimes not detected. A malpositioned chest tube may reside in the chest wall, in the pulmonary parenchyma, within an interlobar fissure, or with its tip against the mediastinum **(Fig. 15.4).**
- **Subcutaneous emphysema** is often seen in conjunction with a pneumothorax. It may also be the sequela of soft tissue laceration or pneumomediastinum. The condition is itself innocuous but should prompt a search for the underlying etiology. CT demonstrates air tracking along fascial and intramuscular planes **(Fig. 15.5).**

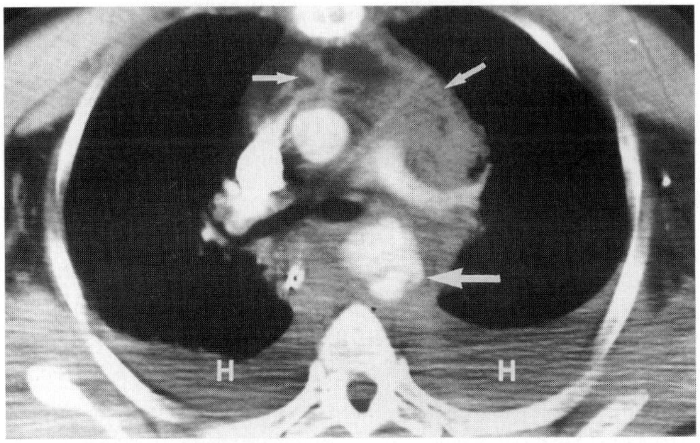

FIGURE 15.3 Acute traumatic aortic injury. Contrast-enhanced CT in a patient following an MVC demonstrates a mediastinal hematoma *(small arrows)* and an enlarged, deformed aortic isthmus *(large arrow)* with a pseudo-aneurysm present anteriorly. These findings are diagnostic, and no further imaging is warranted prior to surgical repair. Bilateral hemothoraces (H) are identified.

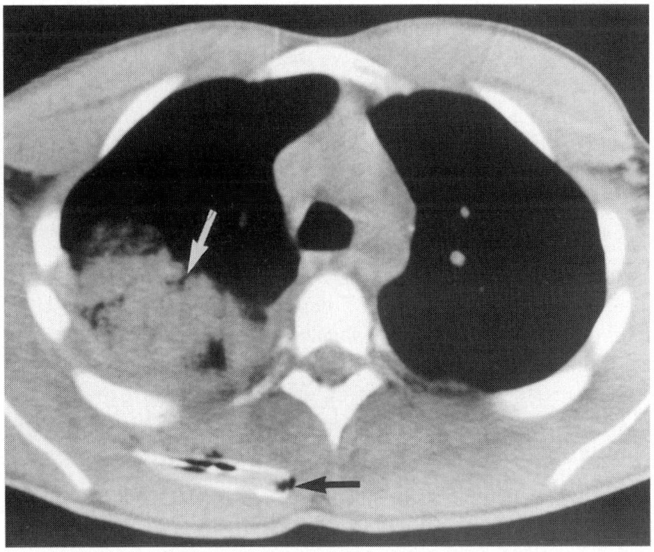

FIGURE 15.4 Malpositioned thoracostomy tube. This 16-year-old youth sustained a gunshot wound to the right chest. The thoracostomy tube tip *(black arrow)* is malpositioned within the paraspinal musculature. A pulmonary contusion *(white arrow)* and hemothorax are also present.

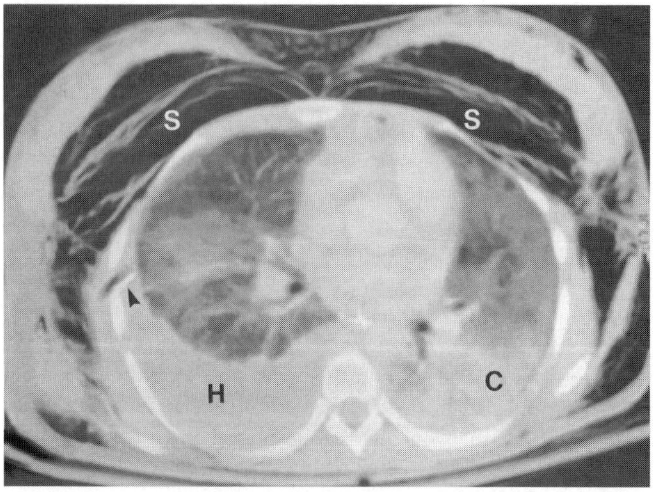

FIGURE 15.5 Subcutaneous emphysema. There is extensive subcutaneous emphysema (S) throughout the chest wall musculature in this 23-year-old MVC victim. A thoracostomy tube *(arrowhead)*, right hemothorax (H), and left pulmonary contusion with air bronchograms (C) are present.

- **Pneumomediastinum** can be seen in the setting of penetrating or blunt injury. In the latter, airway or esophageal injury must be excluded. Pneumomediastinum can extend cephalad to the aortic knob, where it decompresses into the cervical soft tissues or caudally through the diaphragmatic hiatus into the peritoneum or retroperitoneum.
- **Pneumoperitoneum** in a patient with blunt trauma requires careful evaluation of the abdomen and pelvis. It is usually due to injury to an abdominal hollow viscus or inferior extension of a pneumomediastinum.

Airway Injury

- **Tracheobronchial injuries** are rare yet serious results of thoracic trauma. They have a 30 percent mortality and cause 3 percent of deaths due to blunt trauma, partly because of delayed detection or associated injuries. The injury can be intra- or extrathoracic, the latter resulting from direct trauma to the neck. Physical findings include cervical crepitus, hoarseness, and dyspnea. When correctly diagnosed, these injuries can be successfully treated with flexible bronchoscopy and intubation. Undiagnosed, they are fatal.
- **Intrathoracic tracheobronchial fractures** typically occur close to the carina. They are difficult to detect radiographically and delayed diagnosis is common. They should be suspected whenever a pneumothorax fails to resolve despite adequate thoracostomy tube decompression. CT shows disruption of the lumen of the trachea or bronchus and mediastinal or deep cervical emphysema. Thin-collimation spiral technique should be employed if a tracheobronchial fracture is suspected. Airway scarring and stenosis are late complications.
- **Esophageal injury** is generally the result of penetrating trauma but can also be iatrogenic or the result of violent retching (Boerhaave disease). CT manifestations include pneumomediastinum, pneumothorax, pleural effusions, and—when evaluation is delayed—mediastinitis and abscess. Occasionally, the mural defect can be identified following administration of water-soluble oral contrast.

Posttraumatic Fluid Collections and Cardiac Injury

- **Hemorrhage** is a common result of thoracic trauma. Blood may collect in any space, including the subcutaneous tissues, pleural or pericardial spaces, mediastinum, or pulmonary parenchyma.
- **Hemothorax** may be due to intercostal, internal thoracic, subclavian, or other chest wall vascular injury as well as cardiac, parenchymal, or mediastinal injuries. It is considered massive when its volume exceeds 1500 ml. The appearance of hemothorax on plain films is indistinguishable from that of other effusions, but CT can show characteristic findings of high attenuation or heterogeneity in the effusion. To prevent fibrothorax, a hemothorax should be evacuated once the bleeding has stopped.
- **Chylothorax,** or accumulation of lymph in the pleural space, has a different prognosis and treatment than hemothorax. While chylothorax has nontraumatic etiologies, traumatic chylothorax is due to **thoracic duct injury.** There is a 7- to 10-day latent period following duct disruption before a significant chylothorax develops. Chylothorax is indistinguishable from other pleural fluid collections on CT. Diagnosis is made when aspiration of the effusion yields chylous fluid. A right chylothorax usually occurs with thoracic duct disruption below T4-T6 and a left chylothorax occurs when the injury is above T4.
- **Hemopericardium** can result from direct cardiac injury or retrograde dissection from a vascular injury. On chest radiographs, it may be manifest as globular cardiomegaly. CT demonstrates fluid within the pericardium. Penetrating trauma may lead to a hemopneumopericardium seen as an air-fluid level limited to this space. **Cardiac tamponade** can result from hemopericardium and must be urgently addressed. Clinical features of tamponade are muffled heart sounds, pulsus paradoxus, and distended neck veins. It is not a radiologic diagnosis but a clinical diagnosis supported by imaging findings of hemopericardium.
- **Myocardial injuries** are uncommon. They include cardiac contusion, pericardial and myocardial rupture, and injuries to valves or septa. The aortic valve is the most frequently injured. Radiographic findings are not specific, showing only hemopericardium. CT can demonstrate areas of pericardial discontinuity or myocardial thinning. A sternal fracture is often present and can directly cause contusions or lacerations. Arrhythmias are a dangerous complicating factor in cardiac contusions.

Pulmonary Injuries

Parenchymal injuries are common following blunt and penetrating trauma and should be recognized. Moderate injuries may compromise oxygenation. Failure of these injuries to resolve after 3 to 4 days should suggest superimposed aspiration or infection.

- **Pulmonary contusion** represents a parenchymal bruise and can be immediately deep to the site of direct trauma or distributed in a contrecoup location. Associated with interstitial and alveolar edema and blood, which locally limit oxygenation, it appears on plain films within 6 hours of injury and resolves within 3 to 6 days. Hence, initial radiographs may be normal. Pulmonary contusion is seen on CT as an infiltrate with interstitial and alveolar components, and is often associated with an adjacent hemothorax or rib fracture (see **Fig. 15.4**).

- A **pulmonary laceration** is due to a shearing or penetrating force that produces cystic spaces which fill with blood and air **(Fig. 15.6).** These injuries are more common in young patients and pose a risk of air embolism, a frequently fatal complication. A laceration filled with blood is a **pulmonary hematoma.** It is a fairly homogeneous parenchymal mass that becomes more obvious as the overlying contusion resolves. Pulmonary hematomas can persist for several months. They become smaller, better defined, and of lower attenuation on CT over time.
- **Traumatic pneumatoceles** are unilocular or multilocular air cavities within the parenchyma that appear within the first 2 days following thoracic trauma. They have the imaging appearance of a bulla or bleb and generally resolve within several weeks.
- **Aspiration** due to altered consciousness, or increased intra-abdominal pressure is fairly common following trauma. Location depends upon the positioning of the victim at the time the aspiration occurs. The lower lobes (particularly the right) and middle lobe are commonly affected in patients who are erect. The posterior segment of the upper lobes and superior segment of the lower lobes are common sites in supine victims. Aspiration has a radiographic appearance similar to that of a contusion, showing air-space infiltrate and air bronchograms, but it is slower to resolve.
- **Fat embolism** generally occurs as a subclinical event and results from fractures of the pelvis or long bones. Fat droplets from bone marrow gain intravascular access and cause injury by inducing thrombosis and vasculitis. The more dramatic "fat embolism syndrome" is distinctly uncommon and is the result of thrombosis or vasculitis in the lungs, brain, kidneys, or skin. There is a latent period of 12 to 48 hours before the onset of symptoms. Chest CT may be normal or may show multiple alveolar infiltrates or pulmonary edema. Pleural effusions are uncommon.

Chest Wall Injuries

- After trauma, **chest wall injuries** are the most common finding. Thoracic fractures may be subtle; consequently, the presence of dramatic findings elsewhere should not limit the search for other injuries or the potential complications of various fractures.

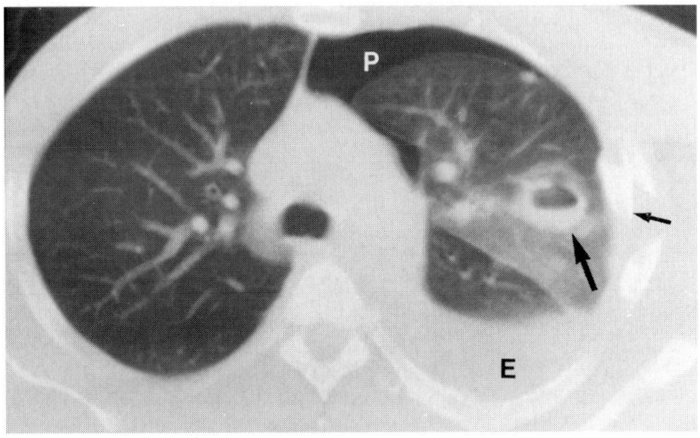

FIGURE 15.6 Pulmonary laceration with hematoma. Chest CT 1 week following an MVC shows a persistent left pneumothorax (P) and a cavitary pulmonary lesion *(large arrow)* adjacent to a displaced rib fracture *(small arrow).* E, pleural effusion.

- **Rib fractures** are very common and can be the result of even minor trauma, particularly in osteopenic patients. The complications of these fractures, particularly pneumothorax, can cause significant morbidity and warrant surveillance. First- and second-rib fractures imply significant energy transfer and are associated with ATAI, while posterior lower rib fractures are associated with visceral injury. CT readily demonstrates cortical disruption and displacement. A **flail chest** is paradoxical movement of a segment of the thoracic cage from multiple rib fractures. Usually this requires segmental rib fractures at three contiguous levels or single fractures at five adjacent levels.
- **Vertebral fractures** result from hyperflexion in the mid- to lower thoracic spine and axial loading at the thoracolumbar junction. They may occur at discontinuous levels; 10 percent are multiple. Vertebral fractures present with clinical findings of focal pain or spinal cord injury, although some are nearly asymptomatic. Radiographs may show focal scoliosis, kyphosis, loss of vertebral body height, or a widened interpedicular distance; an associated hematoma causes paraspinal widening. CT directly assesses osseous detail, facet dislocations, fragmentation, and spinal canal encroachment. MRI is useful in detecting cord, marrow, or soft tissue injuries.
- **Sternal fractures,** seen in up to 8 percent of victims of blunt thoracic trauma, are due to direct blows, often against the steering wheel in a MVC. They are associated with cardiac contusions in 20 percent of cases. Displaced sternal fractures can cause pericardial or cardiac laceration. Lateral chest radiographs best demonstrate the fracture line. CT can fail to show transverse sternal fractures that occur in the plane of imaging. Sagittal fractures and mediastinal hematomas are easily identified on CT.
- **Sternoclavicular dislocations** are rare and difficult to detect on radiographs. CT is more sensitive. Anterior dislocations are more common and easily detected clinically. Posterior dislocations can be associated with severe vascular and airway injury **(Fig. 15.7). Clavicular fractures** commonly occur and are readily identified on both radiographs and CT.
- The **glenohumeral joint** dislocates anteriorly in over 90 percent of cases, resulting in malposition of the humeral head in a subcoracoid or subglenoid location. **Posterior dislocations** are uncommon and often difficult to identify on radiographs; CT readily identifies the posterior position of the humeral head, which can be impacted in the posterior glenoid lip. Inferior dislocations are rare.
- **Scapular fractures** generally indicate significant trauma and are difficult to detect on plain films (more than 40 percent are missed on trauma chest radiographs). Scapular fractures often occur at the glenoid and scapular neck. CT demonstrates the fracture line and can assess for the presence of articular extension.

Diaphragmatic Injuries

- **Traumatic diaphragmatic rupture** results from penetrating or blunt injury that produces elevation of intra-abdominal pressure. Up to 4 percent of blunt trauma patients have diaphragmatic tears; this figure increases to 15 percent in victims of penetrating thoracic trauma, and to 30 percent when the injury is inframammary. This accounts for less than 5 percent of all diaphragmatic hernias but 90 percent of those that become strangulated. The left hemidi-

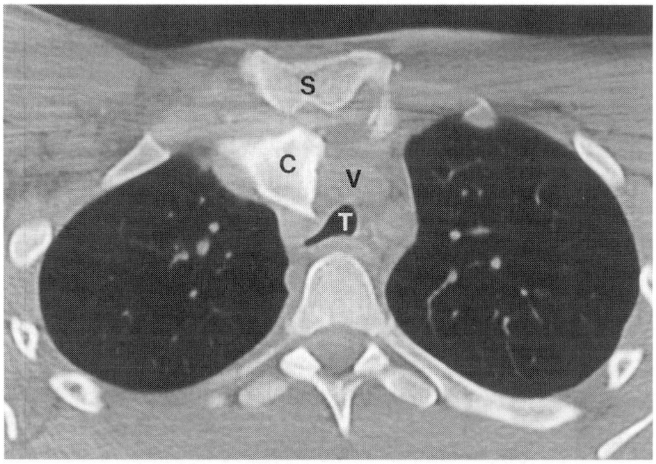

FIGURE 15.7 Posterior sternoclavicular dislocation. A chronic posterior dislocation of the medial clavicle (C) is present. There is a large spur along the posterior aspect, which further compresses the trachea (T). The left brachiocephalic vein (V) is also compressed by this dislocation. S, sternum. (Case courtesy of Dr. David Rubin, St. Louis, MO.)

aphragm is more often affected and better visualized. Abdominal organs that enter traumatic hernias include the stomach, large or small bowel, omentum, or spleen. Traumatic diaphragmatic rupture can enlarge over time, particularly after cessation of positive-pressure ventilation.

Approximately 60 percent of diaphragmatic injuries are overlooked on initial **radiographs;** therefore a high index of suspicion must be maintained. Suggestive findings include an indistinct or elevated hemidiaphragm, pleural effusion, or basilar consolidation. Intrathoracic bowel or the presence of a nasogastric tube above the diaphragm are confirmatory signs.

CT findings include discontinuity or complete lack of visualization of the diaphragm (absent diaphragm sign), abdominal organs or peritoneal fat above the diaphragm, or gastric narrowing (collar or hourglass sign) at the diaphragmatic defect. Thin-section spiral CT with sagittal reformations can improve depiction of the disruption **(Fig. 15.8).** The multiplanar capability of MRI can be helpful in assessing the diaphragm, as traumatic hernias may be more readily recognized in coronal or sagittal planes.

15.4 HEMOPERITONEUM

- **Hemoperitoneum** is a common ancillary finding in patients who have sustained injury to abdominal parenchymal organs. Its location and attenuation can prove helpful in identifying the site of injury.
- **Hemorrhage that is actively occurring** at the time of scanning is denser than either the hepatic or splenic parenchyma **(Fig. 15.9)** and is best appreciated on noncontrast images. Following IV contrast administration, hemoperitoneum appears less dense than the adjacent parenchymal organs. Active hemorrhage measures 80 HU or more; retracted clot and lysed blood measure between 30 and 80 HU. Water-attenuation (0 to 20 HU) intraperitoneal fluid suggests bile, urine, or bowel secretions; however, 10 percent of acute

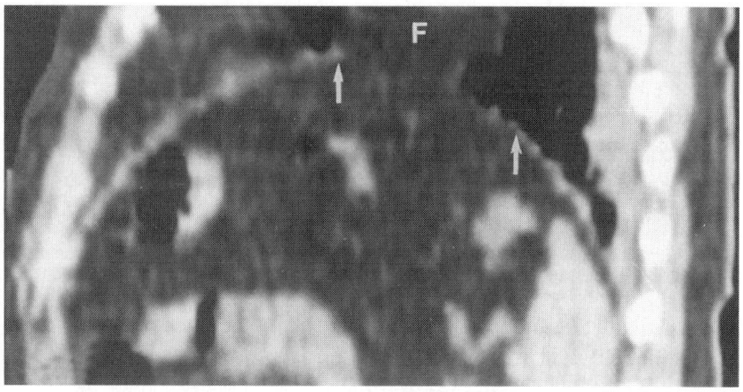

FIGURE 15.8 Traumatic diaphragmatic rupture. Sagittal reconstruction shows discontinuity of the left hemidiaphragm *(arrows)* with herniation of omental fat (F) in this victim of blunt abdominal trauma. [From Slone RM, Gutierrez FR, Fisher AJ (eds.) *Thoracic Imaging: A Practical Approach.* New York: McGraw-Hill; 1999. With permission.]

hemoperitoneum may be of water attenuation. Hemorrhage near the site of injury is typically of higher attenuation and has been termed the "sentinel clot-sign."

- The location of a hemoperitoneum can be diagnostically useful. Morison's pouch, a peritoneal reflection lying between the right kidney and posterior segment of the right hepatic lobe, is the most dependent portion of the upper abdomen. Fluid is seen in this location in the majority of patients with splenic lacerations. Hemoperitoneum also tends to collect in the paracolic gutters, resulting in

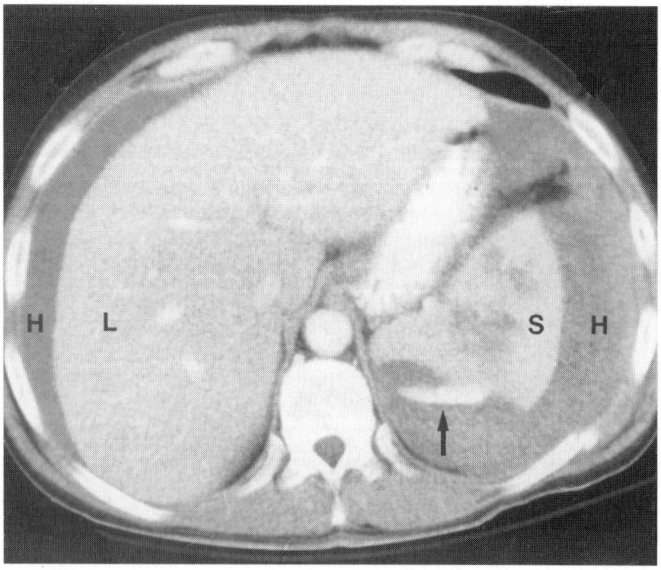

FIGURE 15.9 Active hemorrhage, splenic fracture. High attenuation *(arrow)* at the margin of a splenic fracture represents active hemorrhage in this victim of blunt trauma. Low-attenuation intrasplenic hematoma is seen, and there is a hemoperitoneum (H) adjacent to the spleen (S) which is of higher attenuation than the liver (L), signifying that it is more acute. There is a left rib fracture.

medial displacement of the colon. The pelvis is the most dependent portion of the peritoneal cavity and often collects significant amounts of intraperitoneal fluid.

- **Localization of retroperitoneal hematomas** can provide clues to the organ of injury. Collections within the anterior pararenal space/retromesenteric plane are generally attributable to duodenal or pancreatic injuries. Collections within the perinephric space are due to renal injuries, although other causes include adrenal, aortic, or inferior vena caval trauma. Finally, posterior pararenal space/retrorenal plane collections may be demonstrable in cases of vertebral or paraspinal muscle injury.

  Although hemodynamic compromise is evident to the trauma physician, **CT findings of shock** serve as clues to the radiologist. Because of hypovolemia, there is flattening of the inferior vena cava (IVC), which measures less than 9 mm in anteroposterior dimension at the level of the left renal vein. With more significant volume depletion, the aorta and other abdominal vessels are decreased in caliber. Renal underperfusion is associated with a dense and persistent nephrogram. **Shock bowel** is evident as fluid-filled, dilated loops of small bowel with striking enhancement of the bowel wall **(Fig. 15.10).** The exact etiology is uncertain, although it is postulated that this is related to ischemia that produces slowing of mucosal flow due to capillary arteriolar changes. Anemia can be identified on a noncontrast study when a noncalcified arterial wall is higher in attenuation than intravascular blood.

- **Terms** applied to describe the severity of organ trauma include *contusion, laceration, fracture,* and *shatter.* An organ **contusion** is a focal bruise or injury without disruption of the parenchymal surface. A **laceration** represents disruption of the parenchyma extending to a capsular margin (the organ capsule may be either disrupted or intact). An organ **fracture** represents disruption of both surfaces of the organ. Finally, a **shatter** represents multiple fracture planes within a single organ.

15.5 ABDOMINAL TRAUMA

- **Hepatic injury** is rather common (15 percent) in patients who have sustained blunt abdominal trauma. The morbidity and mortality of hepatic trauma depends on the degree of injury and the presence of comorbid factors. The right hepatic lobe is most commonly injured, and 50 percent of these patients have right lower rib fractures. Injuries to the left hepatic lobe often occur deeper in the parenchyma or are complex fractures. Left lobe injuries generally result from an anteriorly applied force compressing abdominal structures against the spine; consequently, left hepatic injuries are associated with pancreatic and retroperitoneal trauma.

  CT is helpful in assessing patients with hepatic trauma: It displays the hepatic injury and defines its overall extent. Injuries to other organs are readily demonstrated. CT is also valuable in following patients (whether they are managed conservatively or surgically) to document healing and to detect posttraumatic complications.

  Hepatic injuries vary widely in extent. Limited injury produces a small perihepatic collection; more substantial forces produce lacerations or fractures; and massive trauma can cause burst injuries or portal transection. Bile slows resorption of intraparenchymal hematomas, which generally take several months to resolve. Subcapsular hematomas lack bile and resolve within 2 months. **Periportal tracking** is identified as low attenuation adjacent to the portal vein and its branches. This is distinguished from biliary dilatation, which would be present on only one side of the portal vein **(Fig. 15.11).** Periportal tracking can have several etiologies: free intra-abdominal fluid, hepatic parenchymal injury, or elevated central venous pressure.

  Subcapsular hematomas appear as low-density lenticular collections adjacent to the hepatic margins **(Fig. 15.12).** These deform the hepatic contour, since they are contained by the overlying, intact capsule. Hemoperitoneum is not present in purely subcapsular

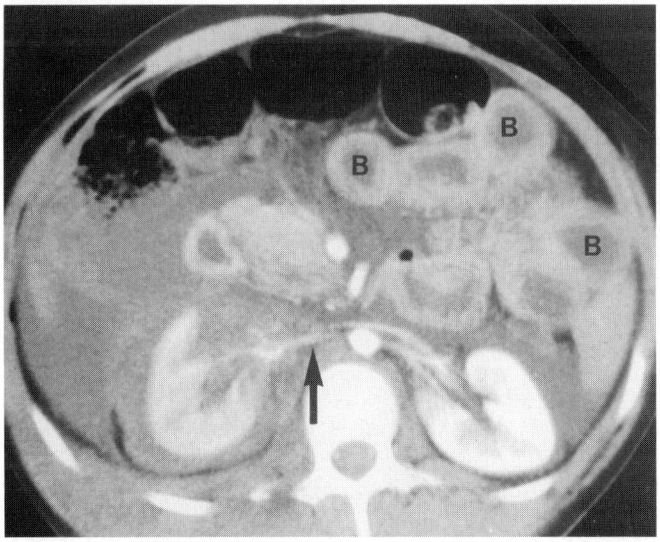

FIGURE 15.10 Shock bowel. In this patient with hemoperitoneum from a splenic injury, there is dilatation and enhancement of the small bowel (B) and perinephric blood from a renal laceration. Hypovolemia is evidenced by a flattened IVC *(arrow)* and a small aorta and renal arteries.

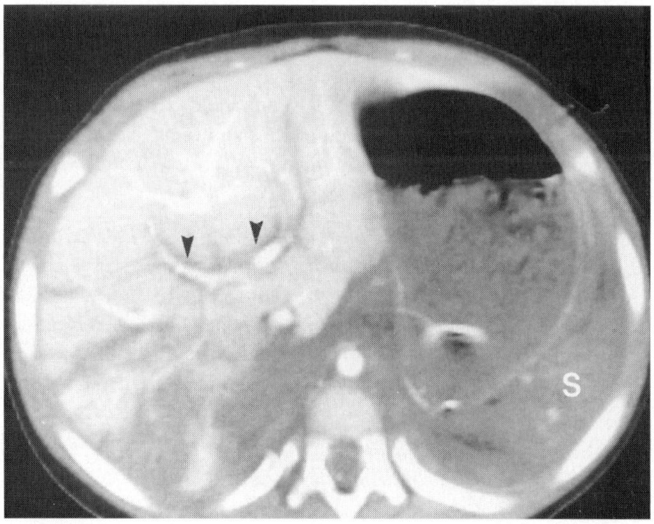

FIGURE 15.11 Shattered posterior segment of the liver. Multiple fractures of the right hepatic lobe are present with regions of absent perfusion. There is periportal tracking of fluid *(arrowheads),* as well as an injury of the splenic pedicle (S).

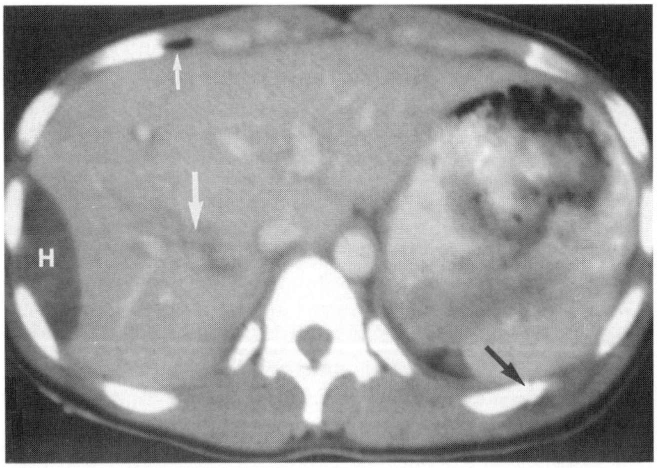

FIGURE 15.12 Intrahepatic laceration and subcapsular hematoma. A linear, low-attenuation laceration *(large white arrow)* traverses the right hepatic lobe and a crescentic, well-marginated subcapsular hematoma (H) indents the hepatic margin. The tiny focus of air anteriorly *(small arrow)* is the anterior pulmonary sulcus. There is a left rib fracture *(large black arrow)*. [From Slone RM, Gutierrez FR, Fisher AJ (eds.) *Thoracic Imaging: A Practical Approach*. New York: McGraw-Hill; 1999. With permission.]

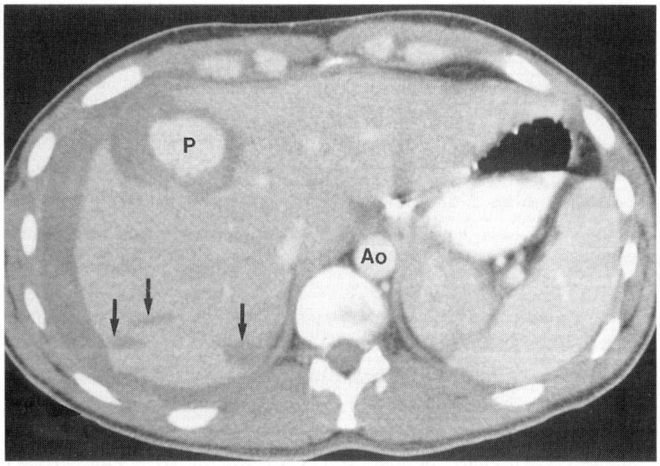

FIGURE 15.13 Hepatic pseudoaneurysm. This 34-year-old man has hepatic lacerations *(arrows)* and a pseudoaneurysm (P) following an MVC. The pseudoaneurysm enhances as densely as the aorta (Ao).

hematomas; however, lacerations of the liver that disrupt the capsule lead to perihepatic and free peritoneal fluid. Lacerations are depicted as low-density, irregularly marginated bands traversing hepatic parenchyma. They heal within several weeks and nonoperative, supportive management is preferred in hemodynamically stable patients. More complex injuries include multiple lacerations in a "bear claw" configuration. There can be fragmentation of the hepatic parenchyma, producing avascular regions of nonenhancing parenchyma (see **Fig. 15.11**). Avulsion of the hepatic vasculature is much less common and is associated with global hepatic hypoperfusion.

Pseudoaneurysms can be identified along the hepatic fracture line **(Fig. 15.13).** These are detected as densely enhancing, well-circumscribed round or ovoid foci. They are important to identify since they have a high propensity to rupture. Most are treated with catheter embolization, although some require operative intervention. Other **posttraumatic complications** include bilomas and biliary strictures.

- **Splenic trauma** is common. Clinical findings include hemodynamic instability, an expanding left-upper quadrant mass, or left flank pain. Referred pain to the left shoulder may be present (Kehr sign) due to diaphragmatic irritation. Any pathologic condition involving the spleen, particularly mononucleosis or lymphoma, predisposes it to injury with relatively minor trauma. Conservative therapy is favored (because of an increased incidence of pneumococcal infections following splenectomy), although splenic resection is required in cases of persistent hemodynamic instability.

Splenic injury caused by a blunt force to the left upper quadrant is associated with other injuries. Some 40 percent of patients with splenic injury have a left-sided rib fracture (although only 20 percent of those with left lower rib fractures have a splenic injury). Up to 25 percent of patients who have left renal injury also have demonstrable splenic injuries.

- **CT findings of splenic trauma** include subcapsular hematomas deforming the splenic margin, low-attenuation fracture planes **(Fig. 15.14),** and regions of devascularized, nonenhancing parenchyma. Hemoperitoneum is present in cases of capsular disruption. A vascular pedicle injury is manifest as absence of splenic enhancement after IV contrast administration (see **Figs. 15.12 and 15.15**).

- **Delayed splenic rupture** is an uncommon entity that may actually represent a missed initial diagnosis. Delayed splenic rupture generally occurs up to several weeks following the traumatic event.

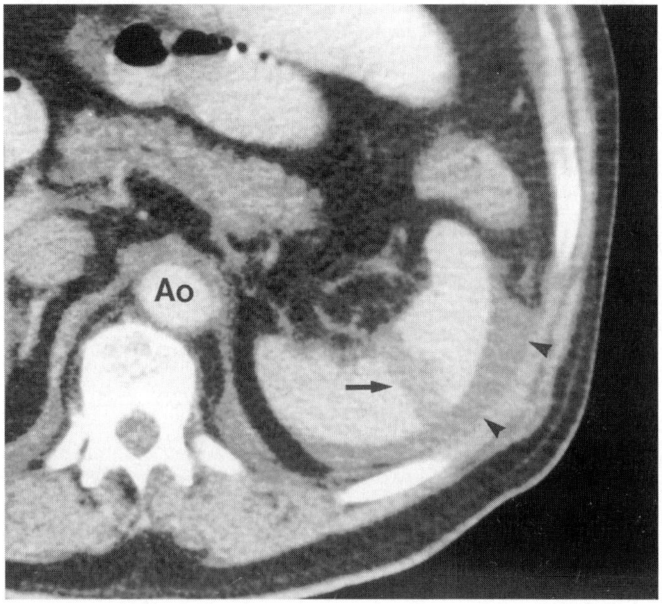

FIGURE 15.14 Splenic fracture. A band of low attenuation traverses the splenic parenchyma and represents a fracture *(arrow)*. Adjacent hematoma is present *(arrowheads)*. Ao, Aorta.

Consequently, reimaging should be performed whenever the clinical symptomatology suggests splenic injury.

- **Pancreatic trauma** is relatively uncommon, accounting for less than 5 percent of complications following blunt abdominal trauma. The mortality rate is high (up to 25 percent of affected patients) and significant complications occur in one-third of survivors. Clinically, significant retroperitoneal hemorrhage may be due to pancreatic injury detected as periumbilical ecchymosis (Cullen sign) or flank ecchymosis (Grey Turner sign). An elevated serum amylase level is not helpful: only 10 percent of patients with an elevated serum amylase have a pancreatic injury, but up to 40 percent of those with pancreatic injury have a normal amylase level.

  Abdominal CT may be normal in the first 12 hours following injury. Positive CT findings include mild enlargement of the pancreas, peripancreatic stranding, or hematoma within the anterior pararenal space. As the pancreas is normally lobulated, subtle lacerations of the surface can be difficult to detect. Fractures of the pancreas in the region of the pancreatic neck are depicted as linear low-attenuation bands traversing this region **(Fig. 15.15).** A helpful associated finding is the interposition of fluid between the pancreas and splenic vein, representing associated hematoma. Mild pancreatic injuries—including contusions, hematomas, and mild lacerations—are generally treated conservatively. Significant lacerations, defined as those that extend through more than half of the gland's thickness or cause gross disruption of the pancreatic duct, are treated with pancreatic stenting via endoscopic retrograde cholangiopancreatography (ERCP) or surgical intervention. Posttraumatic complications include pseudoaneurysms, pancreatic duct strictures, and pseudocysts **(Fig. 15.16).**

- **Bowel trauma** is infrequent, accounting for less than 5 percent of blunt intra-abdominal injuries. At least half of these injuries occur in the second or third portions of the duodenum, and the majority are associated with injuries to other organs, particularly the liver and pancreas. Most injuries are manifest as intramural hematomas, with full-thickness tears uncommon. Full-thickness injuries, however, are treated surgically, while hematomas are frequently treated expectantly.

  CT is not as reliable for bowel injury as it is for injury to other abdominal organs. Intraperitoneal fluid is almost always present on CT, but pneumoperitoneum is an insensitive finding, seen in only one-third of cases involving duodenal rupture. CT demonstrates bowel wall thickening in at least half the cases **(Fig. 15.17).** However, CT may be normal in up to 30 percent of cases of duodenal rupture; consequently, a high index of suspicion must be maintained.

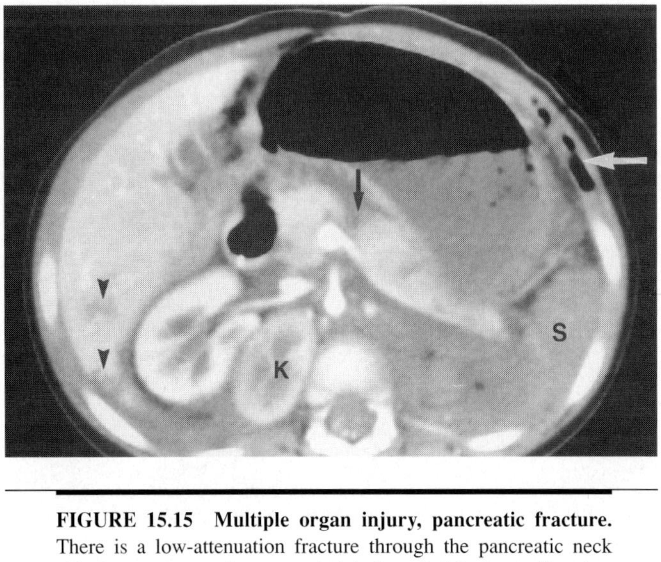

FIGURE 15.15 Multiple organ injury, pancreatic fracture. There is a low-attenuation fracture through the pancreatic neck *(black arrow)* as well as several right hepatic lobe lacerations *(arrowheads)*, a devascularized and nonenhancing spleen (S), and subcutaneous emphysema *(white arrow)* from a pneumothorax. There is unfused crossed renal ectopy, with the anatomic left kidney (K) hypoperfused from vascular injury.

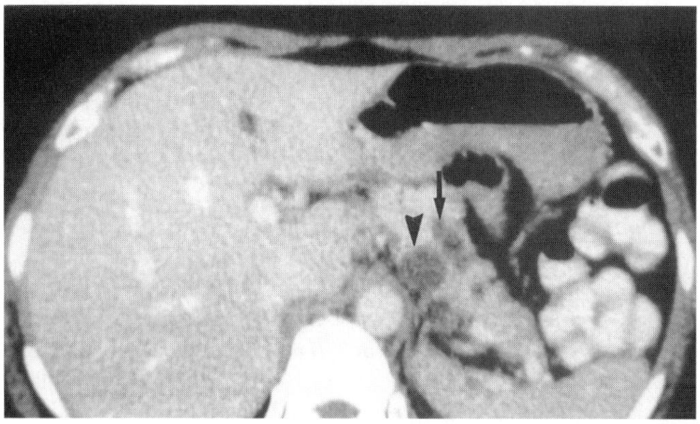

FIGURE 15.16 Posttraumatic pancreatic pseudocyst. There is a 2-cm cyst *(arrowhead)* along the posterior aspect of the pancreatic body and a dilated pancreatic duct *(arrow)* due to a posttraumatic stricture.

15.6 GENITOURINARY TRAUMA

- **The kidney** is the most frequently injured organ in blunt abdominal trauma, although the spleen is the organ that most frequently ne-

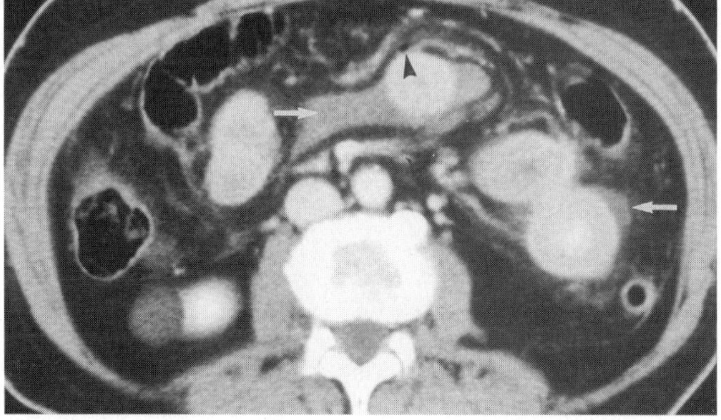

FIGURE 15.17 Jejunal perforation. A 45-year-old woman following a MVC. Contrast-enhanced CT demonstrates thickened loops of jejunum in the left midabdomen with adjacent intraperitoneal fluid *(arrows)* and a tiny focus of free air *(black arrowhead)*.

cessitates operative intervention. Most trauma-related renal damage is minor and heals with supportive therapy. Gross hematuria is present in over 95 percent of renal injuries; however, it is a nonspecific finding, since only 25 percent of patients with hematuria have significant renal injury. Moreover, 25 percent of patients with severe pedicle injuries lack hematuria.

Direct force causes renal lacerations, contusions, and fractures. Deceleration or rotational injuries can cause an arterial intimal tear or disruptions of the ureteropelvic junction. Underlying renal disease should be suspected if the inciting trauma and the apparent extent of the injury are discordant. Neoplasms or cysts can hemorrhage readily, and enlarged or hydronephrotic kidneys, as seen in congenital obstruction of the ureteropelvic junction, can be injured with only minor trauma (**Fig. 15.18**). The pediatric kidney is more vulnerable to traumatic injury than the adult kidney.

- **The classification and management of renal injuries** is divided into four categories. **Minor injuries** constitute 85 percent of all injuries and include superficial cortical lacerations and small perinephric hematomas; they are treated conservatively. **Major renal injuries** constitute 10 percent of all cases and involve deep corticomedullary lacerations or fractures that extend to the collecting system. Therapy depends upon the clinical status, extent of bleeding, amount of urine extravasated, and amount of viable residual tissue. The remaining 5 percent of injuries include **catastrophic injuries** (vascular pedicle injuries and shattered kidneys) and **injuries to the renal pelvis and ureteropelvic junction.** These patients are treated surgically.

The **CT appearance** depends on the class of renal injury. Minor injuries are usually heralded by the presence of infiltration of the perinephric fat or by adjacent fluid collections reflecting hematomas (**Fig. 15.19**). If a hematoma is subcapsular, it produces deformity of the renal contour. Disruption of the capsule leads to fluid tracking along the connective tissue septa of the perinephric fat. Lacerations and fractures are demonstrated as linear regions of low-attenuation, nonenhancing parenchyma. Areas of nonviable renal parenchyma fail to demonstrate enhancement after IV contrast administration.

Vascular pedicle injuries should be suspected when there is global nonenhancement after IV contrast administration (**Fig. 15.20**). Arterial occlusion can be caused by traumatic dissection of the renal artery, avulsion of the pedicle, or an embolus. Contrast extravasation adjacent to the kidney can arise from deep lacerations involving the collecting system or disruption of the ureteropelvic junction.

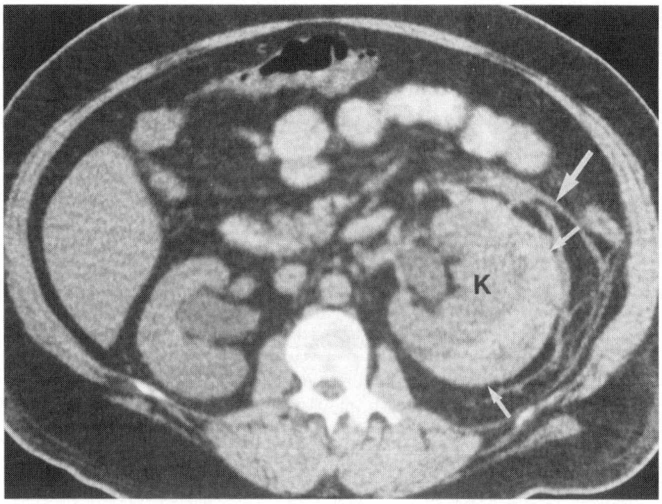

FIGURE 15.19 Renal subcapsular hematoma. There is high-attenuation blood *(small arrows)* surrounding the left kidney (K) and deforming its contour. Gerota's fascia *(large arrow)* is thickened and there is stranding in the perinephric fat.

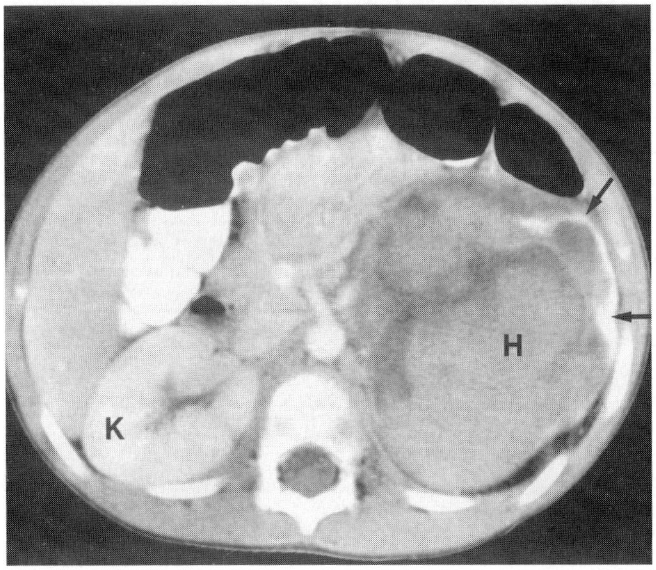

FIGURE 15.18 Hemorrhage into a congenital ureteropelvic junction obstruction. This 6-year-old boy had flank pain and hematuria following a fall. There is a large, heterogeneous hematoma (H) filling a distended left renal collecting system. A thin rim of enhancing renal parenchyma *(arrows)* is present. The right kidney (K) is normal.

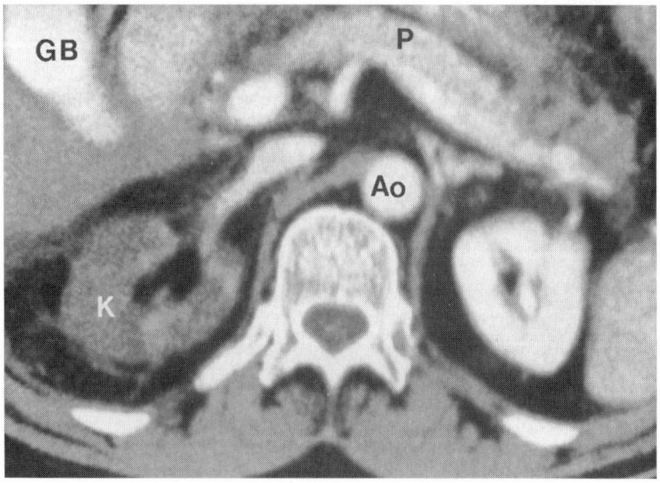

FIGURE 15.20 Renal pedicle injury. This young trauma victim had no hematuria. There is essentially complete lack of enhancement of the right kidney (K) despite dense aortic, left renal, and pancreatic (P) enhancement. Contrast is present within the gallbladder (GB) lumen.

- **Bladder trauma** is readily demonstrated on CT. Subtle bladder perforations are best depicted by distending the bladder with contrast material **(Section 15.1).** Urethral injuries are much more difficult to identify and are best assessed by retrograde urethrograms. Bladder injuries are classified according to the location of urine leakage—namely, intraperitoneal or extraperitoneal.

- **Extraperitoneal bladder rupture** is the more common form of bladder rupture, occurring in 80 percent of cases of bladder perforation. Etiologies include pelvic fractures associated with bladder puncture by bone fragments or avulsive tears at the fixation point of the puboprostatic ligament. Extraperitoneal bladder rupture typically occurs at the anterolateral bladder base and is managed by catheter drainage.

  On **CT,** urinary contrast is easily detected within the space of Retzius. Extraperitoneal fluid can extend cephalad into the abdominal wall or laterally into the perineum, scrotum, or thigh. The characteristic appearance of fluid within the space of Retzius has been termed the "molar tooth sign" **(Fig. 15.21).**

- **Intraperitoneal bladder rupture** accounts for the remaining 20 percent of cases. The etiology is blunt trauma to a distended bladder with a concurrent sudden increase in the intravesical pressure. This causes rupture of the relatively weak bladder dome and urine spills into the peritoneal space. Owing to consequent electrolyte imbalances, intraperitoneal bladder rupture can mimic renal failure clinically. The treatment is operative repair.

  CT findings of intraperitoneal bladder rupture are those of free intra-abdominal fluid. In order to differentiate hemoperitoneum from intraperitoneal bladder rupture, CT cystography is necessary **(Fig. 15.22).**

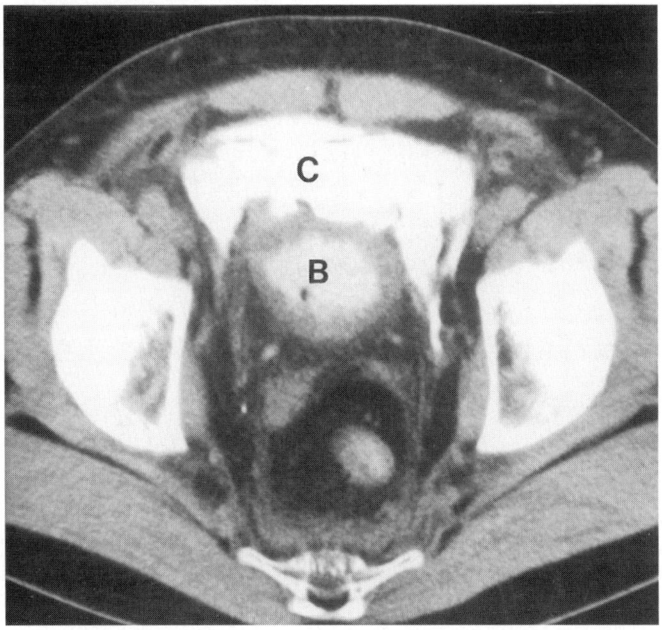

FIGURE 15.21 Extraperitoneal bladder rupture. This CT cystogram shows high-attenuation contrast (C) in the space of Retzius with a characteristic "molar tooth" appearance. The bladder (B) is decompressed and thick-walled despite infusion of 300 ml of contrast.

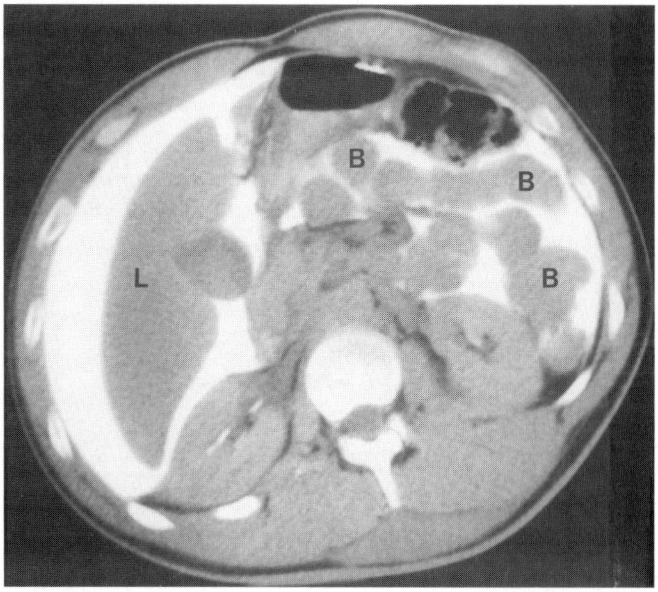

FIGURE 15.22 Intraperitoneal bladder rupture. CT following excessive administration of cystographic contrast demonstrates a large amount of free intraperitoneal fluid outlining the bowel (B) and liver (L).

Bibliography

Federle MP, Peitzman A, Krugh J. Use of oral contrast material in abdominal trauma CT scans: Is it dangerous? *J Trauma* 1995;38:51–53.

Gavant ML, Menke PG, Fabian T, Flick PA, Graney MJ, Gold RE. Blunt traumatic aortic rupture: Detection with spiral CT of the chest. *Radiology* 1995;197:125–133.

Gavant ML, Schurr M, Flick PA, Croce MA, Fabian TC, Gold RE. Predicting clinical outcome of nonsurgical management of blunt splenic injury: Using CT to reveal abnormalities of splenic vasculature. *AJR* 1997;168:207–212.

Lane MJ, Katz DS, Shah RA, Rubin GD, Jeffrey RB Jr. Active arterial contrast extravasation on spiral CT of the abdomen, pelvis, and chest. *AJR* 1998;171:679–685.

Lane MJ, Mindelzun RE, Jeffrey RB. Diagnosis of pancreatic injury after blunt abdominal trauma. *Semin Ultrasound CT MR* 1996;17:177–182.

Levine CD, Patel UJ, Silverman PM, Wachsberg RH. Low attenuation of acute traumatic hemoperitoneum on CT scans. *AJR* 1996;166:1089–1093.

Mirvis SE, Bidwell JF, Buddemeyer EU, Diaconis JN, Pais SO, Whitley JE, Goldstein LD. Value of chest radiography in excluding traumatic aortic rupture. *Radiology* 1987;163:487–493.

Mirvis SE, Shanmuganathan K, Erb R. Diffuse small-bowel ischemia in hypotensive adults after blunt trauma (shock bowel): CT findings and clinical significance. *AJR* 1994;163:1375–1379.

Murray JG, Caoili E, Gruden JF, Evans SJJ, Halvorsen RA Jr, Mackersie RC. Acute rupture of the diaphragm due to blunt trauma: Diagnostic sensitivity and specificity of CT. *AJR* 1996;166:1035–1039.

Roberts JL, Dalen K, Bosanko CM, Jafir SZH. CT in abdominal and pelvic trauma. *Radiographics* 1993;13:735–752.

Shanmuganathan K, Mirvis SE, Amoroso M. Periportal low density on CT in patients with blunt trauma: Association with elevated venous pressure. *AJR* 1993;160:279–283.

Shuman WP. CT of blunt abdominal trauma in adults. *Radiology* 1997;205:297–306.

Van Hise ML, Primack SL, Israel RS, Müller NL. CT in blunt chest trauma: Indications and limitations. *Radiographics* 1998;18:1071–1084.

Vu Nghiem H, Jeffrey RB Jr, Mindelzun RE. CT of blunt trauma to the bowel and mesentery. *AJR* 1993;160:53–58.

INDEX

INDEX

Note: Page numbers followed by *f* indicate figures; page numbers followed by *t* indicate tables.

A

AAA. *See* Abdominal aortic aneurysm
Abdomen
  and pelvis protocols, 4, 6
  protocol, 4
  trauma. *See* Thoracic and abdominal trauma
Abdominal abscess, 164*f*
  differential diagnosis, 164
Abdominal aortic aneurysm (AAA), 86
  leak or rupture, 169, 169*f*, 171*f*
    differential diagnosis, 169
  protocol, 6
Abdominal wall abscess, 225, 226*f*
Acalculus cholecystitis, 129
Achalasia, 71
  differential diagnosis, 71
Acinar cell carcinoma, 157
Acquired pulmonary hypoplasia, 31
Actinomycosis, 15, 15*f*, 218*f*, 226*f*
Acute chest syndrome, 33
Acute cortical necrosis, 192, 193*f*
Acute eosinophilic pneumonia, 40
Acute pericarditis, 76, 77*f*
Acute respiratory distress syndrome (ARDS), 11*f*, 23
  differential diagnosis, 11
Acute traumatic aortic injury (ATAI), 238–239, 238*f*–239*f*
Acute upper airway obstruction, 23
Addison disease, 182
Adenocarcinoma, 24*f*, 27–28, 97
  colon and rectum, 109–110
    differential diagnosis, 109
  differential diagnosis, 97–98, 106
  gastric, 98*f*
    differential diagnosis, 98
  interstitial spread of, 21*f*
  pancreas, 154*f*
  prostate, 217–218
  small bowel, 102, 103*f*
Adenoid cystic carcinoma, 27–28
  differential diagnosis, 70
Adenomas, 58
  adrenal glands, 182, 183*f*
    differential diagnosis, 182
  liver, 121–122, 122*f*
  microcystic, 151, 151*f*
  renal, 199
Adenomyomatosis, 130
  differential diagnosis, 131
Adenopathy
  differential diagnosis, 71
Adenovirus, 16
Adhesions, 104
  differential diagnosis, 103
Adhesive atelectasis, 13
ADPCKD (autosomal dominant polycystic kidney disease), 197, 197*f*
Adrenal glands
  anatomy and physiology, 179, 180*f*
  calcification, 181, 181*f*
    differential diagnosis, 181
  congenital abnormalities, 179–180, 180*f*
  CT technique, 179
  endocrine abnormalities, 181–182
  hemorrhage, 181, 181*f*
  hyperplasia, 180–181, 180*f*
  infection, 181, 181*f*
  masses
    benign, 182–185, 182*f*–185*f*
    differential diagnosis, 182
    malignant, 185–187, 187*f*
    metastases, 185–186, 186*f*
  protocol, 4, 7
Adynamic ileus
  differential diagnosis, 103
AIDS patients
  lymphadenopathy, 174
  pulmonary infections and tumors in, 20
Airspace disease, 10–11
  differential diagnosis, 11

Air trapping, 11–12
Alimentary tract
  anatomy, 95–96, 96*f*
  colon and rectum, 104–110, 106*f*–110*f*
  congenital abnormalities, 96–97, 97*f*
  Crohn disease, 111, 111*f*. *See also* Crohn disease
  CT technique, 95–96
  intussusception, 111, 111*f*
  pneumatosis, 112, 112*f*
  small bowel, 99–104, 101*f*–105*f*
  stomach, 97–99, 98*f*–100*f*
Allergic bronchopulmonary aspergillosis (ABPA), 16–17
Alport syndrome, 192
Alveolar microlithiasis, 39–40
Alveolar proteinosis, 39
Alveolar sarcoidosis, 41, 41*f*
Amebic liver abscesses, 119
Amiodarone
  deposition in liver, 115–116, 117*f*
  lung disease and, 39
Amyloidosis, 69*f*, 116, 169
Androgenital syndrome, 182
Aneurysm
  aortic. *See* Aortic aneurysm
  inflammatory, differential diagnosis, 170
Aneurysmal bone cysts, 234
Aneurysmal rupture protocol, 6
Angiomyolipomas (AMLs), 198, 199*f*
  differential diagnoses, 199
Angiosarcoma, 80, 82*f*, 123–124
  spleen, 142
Ankylosing spondylitis, 23
Anterior mediastinal mass
  differential diagnosis, 64
  protocol, 5
Aorta, 84–87
  acquired conditions, 85–87, 85*f*–88*f*
  anomalies of aortic arch, 85
  normal anatomy, 85
  penetrating atherosclerotic ulcer of, 87, 88*f*
  protocols, 4, 6
Aortic aneurysm, 85–86, 85*f*
  abdominal. *See* Abdominal aortic aneurysm
  differential diagnosis, 67
Aortic branch occlusion, 87
Aortic dissection, 86, 86*f*–87*f*, 90
  protocol, 6
Aortic drape sign, 86
Aortic stenosis, 80
Aortic transection, traumatic, 90
Appendicitis, 96, 104, 105*f*
  differential diagnosis, 105
ARDS (acute respiratory distress syndrome), 11*f*, 23
  differential diagnosis, 11
ARPCKD (autosomal recessive polycystic kidney disease), 197
Arteriovenous malformations (AVMs), 32, 33*f*, 230
  protocol, 6
Artifacts, 2
Asbestos
  exposure, 10*f*, 51
    differential diagnosis, 51
  pleural plaques, 51–52, 52*f*
Asbestosis, 21, 22*f*, 38, 51
  protocol, 6
Ascites, 160–161, 162*f*–163*f*
  differential diagnosis, 131, 162
Aspiration, 241
Aspiration pneumonia, 15, 16*f*
Asplenia, 137
Asthma, 36
ATAI (acute traumatic aortic injury), 238–239, 238*f*–239*f*
Atelectasis, 48, 48*f*
  pulmonary collapse and, 13–14, 13*f*–14*f*
Atrial septal defect
  differential diagnosis, 70
Autoimmune and connective tissue disease, 22–23
Autosomal dominant polycystic disease, 150
Autosomal dominant polycystic kidney disease (ADPCKD), 197, 197*f*
Autosomal recessive polycystic kidney disease (ARPCKD), 197
Axillary adenopathy, 224, 225*f*
Azygos vein enlargement, 55

B

BAC (bronchoalveolar cell carcinoma), 11*f*, 27–28, 29*f*
Back-projection, 1
Bacterial pneumonia, 15–16, 15*f*–16*f*
BALT (bronchus-associated lymphoid tissue), 27
Bare-area sign, 49
Barotrauma
  differential diagnosis, 47
Beaded-septum sign, 20
Beak sign, 197
Beam-hardening artifact, 2
Behçet disease, 98*f*
Behçet syndrome, 84
Belsey fundoplication, 74
Benign prostatic hypertrophy (BPH), 216–217
Bental procedure, 90
Bertin, column of differential diagnoses, 199

Biliary obstruction, 149–150
  differential diagnosis, 130
Biliary sludge, 129
Biliary system. *See* Gallbladder and biliary system
Bilomas, 129, 165, 166*f*
Bird-fancier's lung, 39
Bladder, 207–210, 207*f*–210*f*
  air in bladder wall or lumen, 209
    differential diagnosis, 210
  cancer protocol, 7
  focal bladder lesion or filling defect, 207
    differential diagnosis, 208
  wall thickening, 207
    diffuse, differential diagnosis, 209
Bland thrombus
  differential diagnosis, 80
Blastomycosis, 18*f*
Blebs, 12
  differential diagnosis, 12
Bochdalek hernia, 55, 55*f*
Body wall
  anatomy, 223–224
  bone tumors, 232–235, 233*f*–235*f*
    lytic bone lesion, differential diagnosis, 233
    sclerotic bone lesions, differential diagnosis, 234
  breast, 226–228, 228*f*–229*f*
  CT technique, 224
  external hernias, 228–229, 229*f*–230*f*
  mass, differential diagnosis, 223
  skeleton, 231–232, 232*f*
  soft tissues, 224–226, 224*f*–227*f*
    calcifications, differential diagnosis, 227
  soft tissue tumors
    benign, 229–231, 230*f*–231*f*
    malignant, 231, 231*f*–232*f*
    overview, 229
Bone islands, 233
  differential diagnosis, 234
BOOP (bronchiolitis obliterans with organizing pneumonia), 37, 37*f*
Bosniak cortical renal cyst classification, 197
Bowel obstruction protocol, 6
Bowel perforation
  differential diagnosis, 164
Bowel trauma, 245
BPH (benign prostatic hypertrophy), 216–217
Breast, 226–228, 228*f*–229*f*
  cancer, 226–227, 228*f*
    metastatic, 25*f*
    protocol, 5
  implants, 228
  mastitis, 227
  reconstruction, 227–228, 228*f*
Bronchial atresia, 34, 34*f*
Bronchial carcinoids, 26, 26*f*
Bronchial wall thickening, 34
Bronchiectasis, 33–36, 36*f*
  differential diagnosis, 12
  protocol, 6
Bronchiolitis, 36, 36*f*
Bronchiolitis obliterans, 36–37
Bronchiolitis obliterans with organizing pneumonia (BOOP), 37, 37*f*
Bronchitis, 34
Bronchoalveolar cell carcinoma (BAC), 11*f*, 27–28, 29*f*
Bronchoalveolar lavage, 42
Bronchocele, 34, 34*f*
Bronchogenic carcinoma, 27–31, 28*f*–32*f*, 51, 60*f*
  differential diagnosis, 24–25, 67, 70
  paraneoplastic syndromes, 29–30
  staging, 30, 31*f*–32*f*
  treatment, 30–31, 32*f*
Bronchogenic cysts, 62
Bronchopleural fistula, 42, 47
Bronchopneumonia, 15
  differential diagnosis, 26
Bronchopulmonary sequestration, 33*f*
Bronchovascular disease
  differential diagnosis, 10
Bronchus-associated lymphoid tissue (BALT), 27
Budd-Chiari syndrome, 126, 127*f*
  protocol, 6
Bullae, 12
  differential diagnosis, 12

C

Calcific pericarditis, 77*f*
Calcified lymph nodes, 175
  differential diagnosis, 175
Cancer staging protocol, 6
Caplan syndrome, 23
Caput medusae, 224
Carcinoid syndrome, 26, 81, 83*f*
Carcinoid tumor, 102, 103*f*
  differential diagnoses, 102, 166
Carcinoma
  adrenocortical, 186, 187*f*
  colon, 109*f*–110*f*
  endometrial, 210
  ovaries, 215, 216*f*
  peritoneum, 166, 168
  prostate, 217–218, 217*f*
  rectal, 109*f*
  renal, 200–201, 200*f*–201*f*, 204
    differential diagnoses, 199
  thyroid, 58
  trachea, 70*f*

Carcinomatosis
differential diagnosis, 162
Cardiac enlargement
differential diagnosis, 78
Cardiac mass
differential diagnosis, 80
Cardiac tamponade, 240
Cardiac trauma, 240
Cardiomyopathy
differential diagnosis, 70
restrictive
constrictive pericarditis, differentiating from, 77
Cardiovascular CT
aorta, 84–87
acquired conditions, 85–87, 85*f*–88*f*
anomalies of aortic arch, 85
normal anatomy, 85
cardiovascular intervention and surgery, 90–92, 92*f*
caval system
inferior vena cava, 89, 89*f*–91*f*
superior vena cava, 87, 89, 89*f*
heart
anatomy, 78
cardiac neoplasms, 80, 81*f*–82*f*
CT technique, 78
ischemic heart disease, 78–79, 79*f*–80*f*
valvular heart disease, 80–81, 82*f*–83*f*
pericardium
acquired pericardial disease, 76–78, 77*f*–78*f*
anatomy and function, 75, 75*f*
congenital anomalies, 76, 76*f*
CT, 75–76
pulmonary vessels
anatomy, 81–83
thromboembolism, 83–84, 83*f*-84*f*
veins, 84
Caroli disease, 128, 128*f*
Castleman disease, 59–60, 169, 173, 174*f*
Cavernous hemangioma, 120, 121*f*
Cavitary lung lesion
differential diagnosis, 25
Cavitation, 14, 25
CCAMs (congenital cystic adenomatoid malformations), 31–32, 33*f*
Central airway protocol, 4
Centrilobular emphysema, 37, 38*f*
Cervical cancer, 210, 211*f*
CF. *See* Cystic fibrosis
Chagas disease, 71, 110
Chamberlain procedure, 42
Chest, abdomen, and pelvis protocol, 5
Chest protocols, 4–5
Chest radiography
lung disease, 9
Chest wall deformities, congenital, 231
Chest wall injuries, 241, 242*f*
CHF (congestive heart failure)
differential diagnosis, 48, 70
Cholangiocarcinoma, 125*f*, 130
protocol, 6
Cholecystitis, 129, 130*f*–131*f*
differential diagnosis, 131
Choledocholithiasis, 129, 130*f*
Cholelithiasis and biliary obstruction, 128–129, 130*f*
differential diagnosis, 130, 146
Chondrosarcoma, 235
Choriocarcinoma, 212
Chronic cholecystitis, 129
Chronic eosinophilic pneumonia, 40
Chronic pancreatitis, 149, 150*f*, 157
differential diagnosis, 150
Chylothorax, 240
Cicatrizing atelectasis, 13
Cirrhosis, 116–118, 118*f*–119*f*
differential diagnosis, 162, 227
protocol, 6
Clagett window, 47, 47*f*
Clavicular fractures, 241
CMV colitis, 106*f*
Coal worker's pneumoconiosis, 38
differential diagnosis, 26
Coccidiomycosis, 18
Colitis, 105–107, 106*f*–107*f*
Collagen vascular diseases, 22–23
differential diagnosis, 227
Colon and rectum, 104–110, 106*f*–110*f*
colonic dilatation, 110
colonic diverticulitis, 107–108, 108*f*
colonic mass, 108, 109*f*
differential diagnosis, 109
lipomas, 108, 109*f*
Common bile duct stones protocol, 6
Compensatory emphysema, 37
Compressive atelectasis, 13
Computed tomography. *See* CT
Congenital airway disorders, 33
Congenital and vascular pulmonary lesions, 31–33, 33*f*–34*f*
Congenital bronchiectasis, 35
Congenital cystic adenomatoid malformations (CCAMs), 31–32, 33*f*
Congenital lobar emphysema, 31
Congenital tracheobronchomegaly, 69
Congestive heart failure (CHF)
differential diagnosis, 48, 70
Conn syndrome, 182
Connective tissue disease, 22–23
Constrictive pericarditis, 76, 77*f*

Contrast
intravenous, 3
oral, 3–4
Contrast resolution, 2
Contusion (organ trauma), definition of, 243
Coronary artery aneurysms, 79
Coronary artery bypass grafts, assessing patency with CT, 79, 79*f*
Coronary artery calcification, 78, 79*f*
Coronary artery bypass surgery, 91
Cor pulmonale
differential diagnosis, 70
Cortical nephrocalcinosis, 192
differential diagnosis, 193
Costochondritis, 232
Creeping fat, 111
CREST syndrome, 23
Crohn disease, 101, 107, 111, 111*f*
differential diagnosis, 105–106
Cryptococcosis, 17–18
CT (computed tomography)
contrast
intravenous contrast, 3
oral contrast, 3–4
CT colonography, 96
CT cystography, 238
CT-guided lung biopsy, 28*f*, 41–43, 41*f*
expiratory high-resolution computed tomography (HRCT), 12, 12*f*
general description, 1
high-resolution. *See* HRCT (high-resolution computed tomography)
image reconstruction, 1
physics, 1–3
artifacts, 2
image display, 2
resolution, 2
Cushing syndrome, 26, 180, 182
Cylindrical bronchiectasis, 35, 35*f*
Cystadenocarcinoma
biliary, 132
differential diagnosis, 216
ovaries, 215, 215*f*
Cystadenomas
biliary, 132
ovaries, 214, 215*f*
differential diagnosis, 213
Cystic bronchiectasis, 35, 35*f*
Cystic fibrosis (CF), 36, 36*f*, 151
differential diagnosis, 47, 157
Cystic lung disease, 12
Cystic mesothelioma, 166, 166*f*
Cystitis, 209, 209*f*

D

Decortication of the lung, 42
Dependent atelectasis, 21, 22*f*
Dermatomyositis, 23
Desmoid tumors, 167
body wall, 230, 231*f*
Desmoplastic small round cell tumor (DSRT), 168, 168*f*
Diabetes mellitus
differential diagnosis, 192
Diaphragm, 55–56
hernias, 55–56, 55*f*–56*f*
injuries, 56, 241–242, 242*f*
tumors, 55
Diaphragm sign, 49
Diffuse lung disease, 9
differential diagnosis, 10, 47
Diffuse panbronchiolitis, 37
Diffuse skeletal sclerosis, 232–233
differential diagnosis, 232
Dilated bowel
differential diagnosis, 103
Dilated common bile duct without obstruction
differential diagnosis, 129
Dilated esophagus
differential diagnosis, 71
Direct inguinal hernias, 229
Diskitis, 74, 232
Displaced crus sign, 49
Disseminated histoplasmosis, 20
Diverticulitis, 107–108, 108*f*
differential diagnosis, 106
protocol, 6
Dressler syndrome, 77
Dromedary hump
differential diagnoses, 199
Ductal adenocarcinoma, 152, 153*f*
differential diagnosis, 153
Duct-ectatic mucinous tumor, 152, 152*f*
Duodenal obstruction, 150
Duodenal trauma, 245, 245*f*
Duplication cyst, 63, 63*f*
peritoneum and retroperitoneum, 165
Dysmotile cilia syndrome, 35

E

Echinococcal cysts, 119–120, 119*f*, 138, 138*f*
Echocardiography
pericardium, 75
Ectopic goiter, 58*f*
Ectopic parathyroid mass, 67
protocol, 5
Edematous pancreatitis, 147, 147*f*

EG (eosinophilic granuloma), 40, 40*f*, 235
Eisenmenger syndrome, 83
Emphysema, 10*f*, 47*f*, 239
Emphysematous cholecystitis, 129–130
Emphysematous cystitis, 209, 209*f*
Emphysematous pyelonephritis, 195
Empyema necessitans, 50, 51*f*
Empyemas, 15, 49–50, 50*f*–51*f*
  differential diagnosis, 52
  protocol, 6
Enchondromas, 233
Endobronchial mass
  differential diagnosis, 70
  metastases, 26
Endometrial cancer, 211*f*
  differential diagnosis, 210
Endometriomas, 213, 214*f*
Endometriosis, 165, 213
Enhancing lymph nodes, 59
Enterocolitis, necrotizing
  differential diagnosis, 112
Environmental, occupational, and iatrogenic lung disease, 38–39, 38*f*–39*f*
Eosinophilic granuloma (EG), 40, 40*f*, 235
Eosinophilic pneumonia, 40
Epiploic appendagitis, 165
Epithelioid hemangioendothelioma, 124
Esophageal cancer, 72–73, 72*f*–73*f*
  CT staging, 73*t*
  differential diagnosis, 71
  protocol, 6
Esophageal diverticulum, 71
Esophageal duplication cysts, 63
Esophageal injury, 61*f*, 240
Esophageal varices, 71
Esophagectomy, 74
Esophagopleural fistula, 51*f*
Esophagus, 71
Ewing sarcomas, 235
Expiration, 2
Expiratory high-resolution computed tomography (HRCT), 12, 12*f*
External hernias, 104, 228–229, 229*f*–230*f*
Extralobar sequestration, 32
Extramedullary hematopoiesis, 74
Extrapleural fat deposition
  differential diagnosis, 51
Extrapleural hematoma, 49*f*
Extrapleural lesion
  differential diagnosis, 46
  lipoma, 52*f*
Extrinsic allergic alveolitis, 38
Exudates, 48

F

False aneurysms, 79, 85
Farmer's lung, 39
Fat embolism, 33, 241
Fatty infiltration, 116–117, 117*f*
  differential diagnosis, 114–115
Fatty replacement (pancreas), 157, 158*f*
Femoral hernias, 229
Ferruginous bodies, 38
Fiberoptic bronchoscopy, 42
Fibrolamellar carcinoma, 122–123
Fibrosing alveolitis
  differential diagnosis, 10
Fibrosing mediastinitis, 61
Fibrosis with honeycombing
  differential diagnosis, 12
Fibrothorax, 50
Fibrous dysplasia, 233, 234*f*
Fibrous pleural tumors, 52, 53*f*
Field of view (FOV), 2
Filtering, 1–2
FNH (focal nodular hyperplasia), 121, 121*f*
Focal eventration, 55
Focal fat sparing (liver), 118*f*
  differential diagnosis, 114
Focal fatty infiltration
  differential diagnosis, 117
Focal lung disease
  differential diagnosis, 47
Focal nodular hyperplasia (FNH), 121, 121*f*
Focal pyelonephritis, 195
Follow-up pulmonary nodule protocol, 6
Fournier gangrene, 219, 219*f*
Fourth-generation scanners, 1
FOV (field of view), 2
Fracture (organ trauma), definition of, 243
Fungal infections, 16–18, 16*f*–18*f*
  fungus ball, 16, 17*f*
  liver abscess, 119
  splenic microabscesses, 139, 141*f*

G

Gallbladder and biliary system
  anatomy and physiology, 128
  cancer, 131, 131*f*
    differential diagnosis, 131
  cholelithiasis and biliary obstruction, 128–129, 130*f*
  congenital abnormalities, 128, 128*f*
  CT technique, 128
  enlarged
    differential diagnosis, 130

Gallbladder and biliary system (*Cont.*)
inflammation, 129–130, 131*f*
neoplasia, 130–132, 131*f*
wall thickening
differential diagnosis, 131
Ganglioneuroblastomas, 73–74, 184*f*
Ganglioneuromas, 73–74, 184, 184*f*
Gardner syndrome, 167
Gastric bezoars, 99, 100*f*
Gastric interposition
differential diagnosis, 71
Gastric mass, 97
differential diagnosis, 98
Gastric metastatic disease, 99, 100*f*
Gastric polyps, 99
Gastric ulcer, benign, 97, 98*f*
Gastric varices, 99, 100*f*
Gastric wall thickening, 97, 98*f*
differential diagnosis, 97
Gastrinomas, 155
Gastritis, 97
differential diagnosis, 97
Gastroesophageal reflux, 74
General abdomen and pelvis protocols, 6
Genitourinary trauma, 245–247, 246*f*–247*f*
Germ-cell tumors, 67
differential diagnosis, 64, 216
Gestational trophoblastic disease (GTD), 212, 212*f*
Ghon complex, 18
Glenohumeral joint, 241
Glomerulonephritis
differential diagnosis, 191–193
Glucagonoma, 155
Goiter
differential diagnosis, 58
Goodpasture disease, 11
Graft-*versus*-host disease, 101
Gram-negative pneumonias, 15
Granulomas
differential diagnosis, 24
Granulomatous disease, 181
differential diagnosis, 10, 25–26, 71
healed, 26
differential diagnoses, 119, 138, 175
Ground-glass appearance, 10, 20*f*
differential diagnosis, 10
GTD (gestational trophoblastic disease), 212, 212*f*
Gynecomastia, 226
differential diagnosis, 227

H

Halo sign, 16, 16*f*, 24
Hamartomas, 24*f*, 26, 139
Heart. *See also* Cardiac entries
anatomy, 78
cardiac neoplasms, 80, 81*f*–82*f*
CT technique, 78
failure, differential diagnosis, 115
ischemic heart disease, 78–79, 79*f*–80*f*
valvular heart disease, 80–81, 82*f*–83*f*
Heller esophagomyotomy, 74
Hemangioendothelioma, 124
Hemangiomas, 138–139, 168
body wall, 230, 234
differential diagnoses, 114, 117–118, 139
retroperitoneal, 171
spleen, 140*f*
Hematopoietic disorders, 234
Hematuria protocol, 7
Hemochromatosis, 115, 116*f*
Hemolytic anemia
differential diagnosis, 137
Hemopericardium, 240
Hemoperitoneum, 242–243, 242*f*–243*f*
Hemosiderosis, 115
Hemothorax, 48, 240
Hepatectomy, 132, 132*f*
Hepatic abscess, 119*f*
Hepatic calcifications, 114
differential diagnosis, 115
Hepatic congestion
differential diagnosis, 115–116
Hepatic infarction, 127
Hepatic veno-occlusive disease, 126
Hepatitis, 118
Hepatoblastoma, 124, 126*f*
Hepatocellular carcinoma, 122, 124*f*–125*f*
differential diagnosis, 114–115
Hepatomegaly
differential diagnosis, 115
Hernias
diaphragm, 55–56, 55*f*–56*f*
differential diagnosis, 103
hiatal, 56, 56*f*, 71
differential diagnosis, 71
High-altitude edema, 23
High-attenuation bile
differential diagnosis, 130
High-density liver precontrast
differential diagnosis, 115
High-output heart disease
differential diagnosis, 70
High-resolution computed tomography. *See* HRCT
Hilar enlargement, 60*f*, 70
bilateral, differential diagnosis, 71
unilateral, differential diagnosis, 71
Histoplasmosis, 17, 17*f*, 173*f*

Hodgkin disease, 59, 64, 64*f*, 102, 175
Honeycomb cysts, 12
Honeycomb pattern, 21
Hounsfield units (HU), 2
HRCT (high-resolution computed tomography), 2, 3*f*
  bronchiectasis, 34
  expiratory, 12, 12*f*
  ground glass opacities, 10
  interstitial lung disease, 20–21
  lung disease, 9
  protocol, 4
  pulmonary emphysema, 37
HU (Hounsfield units), 2
Hydronephrosis, 192*f*
  differential diagnosis, 192
Hydrosalpinx, 218, 218*f*
Hydrostatic edema, 23
Hyperaldosteronoma, 182*f*
Hypercalcemia, 192
Hyperparathyroidism
  differential diagnosis, 193
Hyperplasia
  differential diagnosis, 182
Hypersensitivity pneumonitis, 38, 39*f*
Hypertrophic osteoarthropathy, 29
Hypervascular liver lesions
  differential diagnosis, 114
Hypervascular lymph nodes
  differential diagnosis, 175
Hypogenetic lung, 31

I

Iatrogenic injuries
  chest trauma
    differential diagnosis, 47
  lung disease. *See* Environmental, occupational, and iatrogenic lung disease
  retroperitoneal hemorrhage, 169
Idiopathic pulmonary fibrosis (IPF), 21–22
Ileocecal region, thickened
  differential diagnosis, 105
Image display, 2
Image reconstruction, 1
Immotile cilia syndrome, 35
Incisional hernias, 229
Indirect inguinal hernias, 229, 230*f*
Infantile hemangioendothelioma, 125
Inferior vena cava, 89, 89*f*–91*f*
Influenza, 16
Injection granulomata
  differential diagnosis, 227
Insulinomas, 155, 155*f*
Intensive care unit screening protocol, 5
Interface sign, 49
Internal hernias, 104
Interpretation. *See* Techniques and interpretation
Interstitial lung disease, 9
  acute respiratory distress syndrome (ARDS), 23
  autoimmune and connective tissue disease, 22–23
  differential diagnosis, 10
  malignancy, 23
  overview, 20–21, 20*f*–21*f*
  protocol, 6
  pulmonary edema, 23
  pulmonary fibrosis, 21–22, 21*f*–22*f*
Interstitial pneumonia, 15
Intestinal tuberculosis, 101*f*
Intrahepatic biliary dilatation, 129*f*
  differential diagnosis, 129
Intrahepatic cholangiocarcinoma, 123
Intralobar sequestration, 32
Intrathoracic stomach, 71
Intravenous contrast, 3
Intubation injuries, 239, 239*f*
Intussusception, 111, 111*f*
Invasive mole, 212
IPF (idiopathic pulmonary fibrosis), 21–22
Ischemic bowel protocol, 6
Ischemic colitis, 107, 107*f*
Ischemic heart disease, 78–79, 79*f*–80*f*
  differential diagnosis, 70
Islet-cell tumors, 154
  differential diagnosis, 155
Ivor-Lewis esophagectomy, 74

J

Jaundice (new-onset) protocol, 7
Jejunal perforation, 245

K

Kaposi sarcoma, 27, 124
Kartagener syndrome, 35
Kawasaki disease, 79
Kidneys. *See also* Renal *entries*
  anatomy and physiology, 189
  congenital abnormalities, 189–191, 191*f*–193*f*
    differential diagnoses, 191–195
  CT technique, 189, 190*f*
  cystic disease, 196–198, 197*f*–198*f*
    differential diagnosis, 196, 199
  infectious, inflammatory, and vascular conditions, 194–196, 194*f*–196*f*
  masses
    benign, 198–200, 199*f*–200*f*
    differential diagnoses, 199
    malignant, 200–204, 200*f*–204*f*

Kidneys (*Cont.*)
nephrocalcinosis and urolithiasis, 191–194, 193*f*–194*f*
differential diagnoses, 192–193
surgery, 204
trauma, 245–246, 246*f*
Krukenberg tumors, 215, 216*f*

L

Laceration (organ trauma), definition of, 243
LAM (lymphangioleiomyomatosis), 13*f*, 14, 40, 175, 175*f*
Langerhans cell histiocytosis, 40
Large airway disease, 33–36, 34*f*–36*f*
Large cell undifferentiated carcinoma, 28
Lead mass, 111
Left lobe collapse, 13, 14*f*
Left-to-right shunt
differential diagnosis, 82
Left ventricular aneurysmectomy, 91–92
Left ventricular reduction surgery, 92
Legionnaire disease, 15
Leiomyomas, 73, 99
small bowel
differential diagnosis, 102
uterus, 210, 211*f*
Leiomyosarcomas, 89, 99, 99*f*, 172, 172*f*
Leukemia, 54, 202*f*
Linitis plastica, 98
Lipoid pneumonia, 12*f*
Lipomas, 52, 108, 109*f*
body wall, 230, 230*f*
differential diagnosis, 46
retroperitoneal, 171
Lipomatous hypertrophy of interatrial septum, 80, 81*f*
Liposarcomas, 53–54
body wall, 231
retroperitoneal, 172*f*
Liver
anatomy and physiology, 113
benign masses, 120–122, 120*f*–122*f*
biopsy, 132, 132*f*
CT technique, 113
cysts, 120, 120*f*
differential diagnosis, 120
diffuse disease and cirrhosis, 113–118, 115*f*–118*f*
infection, 118–120, 119*f*
lesions
differential diagnoses, 114–115, 117–118
multiple, 114–115
malignant neoplasms, 114*f*, 122–125, 122*f*–126*f*
protocols, 4–6
surgery, 132–133, 132*f*
transplant
follow-up protocol, 6
pre-transplant protocol, 6
trauma, 243–244, 243*f*–244*f*
triple-phase protocol, 4–5
vascular phenomena, 125–127, 127*f*
Lobar pneumonia, 15
Lobectomy, 30, 42
Loculated ascites
differential diagnosis, 165
Loculated pleural effusion, 48*f*
differential diagnosis, 52
Lofgren syndrome, 40
Low-attenuation lymphadenopathy, 174
differential diagnosis, 175
Low-attenuation lymph nodes, 59
Low-attenuation mediastinal mass
differential diagnosis, 62
Low-density liver lesion postcontrast
differential diagnosis, 114
Low-density liver precontrast
differential diagnosis, 116
Lower lung disease
differential diagnosis, 10
Lumbar hernias, 229
Lungs. *See also* Pulmonary *entries*
abscess, 15, 50, 51*f*
differential diagnosis, 25
anatomy and physiology, 9
atelectasis and pulmonary collapse, 13, 13*f*–14*f*
bronchogenic carcinoma, 27–31, 28*f*–31*f*
paraneoplastic syndromes, 29–30
staging, 30, 31*f*–32*f*
treatment, 30–31, 32*f*
cancer, 10*f*, 28*f*, 30*f*-32*f*
differential diagnosis, 52
staging or follow-up protocol, 5
congenital and vascular pulmonary lesions, 31–33, 33*f*-34*f*
CT-guided biopsy, 41–43, 41*f*
CT technique, 9
environmental, occupational, and iatrogenic lung disease, 38–39, 38*f*–39*f*
chemotherapy, 39
radiation therapy, 39, 39*f*
idiopathic lung disease, 39–41, 40*f*-41*f*
interstitial lung disease. *See* Interstitial lung disease
large airway disease and bronchiectasis, 33–36, 34*f*–36*f*

Lungs (*Cont.*)
  patterns of disease, 9–13, 10*f*–13*f*
  protocols, 5–6
  pulmonary infections. *See* Pulmonary infections
  pulmonary neoplasms, 26–27, 26*f*–27*f*
  pulmonary nodules
    multiple, 25–26, 25*f*
    solitary, 24–25, 24*f*
  small airway and obstructive lung disease, 36–38, 36*f*–37*f*
    pulmonary emphysema, 37–38, 38*f*
  thoracic surgery, 41–43
  transplant protocol, 6
  volume reduction surgery evaluation protocol, 6
Lymphadenopathy, 55
  differential diagnosis, 67, 171, 173
  mediastinum, 58–61, 59*f*–62*f*
  peritoneum and retroperitoneum, 173–175, 173*f*–176*f*
    differential diagnosis, 166
Lymphangioleiomyomatosis (LAM), 13*f*, 14, 40, 175, 175*f*
Lymphangiomas, 63, 63*f*
  body wall, 230
  peritoneum and retroperitoneum, 165
  retroperitoneal, 171
  spleen, 141
Lymphangitic carcinomatosis, 21*f*, 23
Lymphocele, 165
Lymphogranuloma venereum, 219, 219*f*
Lymphomas
  adrenal glands, 186–187, 187*f*
  anterior mediastinum, 64, 64*f*
  body wall, 231, 231*f*
  colonic or rectal, 110, 110*f*
  differential diagnosis, 52, 64, 67, 97
  gastric, 98–99, 99*f*
    differential diagnosis, 98
  hepatic, 123
  liver, 126*f*
  pancreas, 156, 156*f*
  peritoneum
    differential diagnosis, 166
  peritoneum and retroperitoneum, 175–176, 176*f*
  pleura, 54
  protocol, 5–6
  renal, 202, 202*f*
  small bowel, 102*f*
    differential diagnosis, 102
  spleen
    differential diagnosis, 137, 139
Lytic bone lesion
  differential diagnosis, 233

M

Magnetic resonance imaging. *See* MRI
MAI. *See* Mycobacterium avium-intracellulare
Malignant effusion protocol, 6
Malignant fibrous histiocytoma (MFH), 168, 172, 231
MALT (mucosa-associated lymphoid tissue), 27
Mastocytosis, 101
Median sternotomy, 42
Mediastinitis, 60, 232
  protocol, 5
Mediastinoscopy, 42
Mediastinum
  anatomy, 57
  anterior, 63–67
    lymphoma, 64, 64*f*
    miscellaneous masses, 67, 67*f*
    thymus, 64–67, 65*f*–67*f*
  CT technique, 57
  hemorrhage, 62
  low-attenuation masses, 62–63
    cystic masses, 62–63, 63*f*
    fatty masses, 63, 64*f*
  lymphadenopathy and inflammatory changes, 58–61, 59*f*–62*f*
  middle, 67–71, 68*f*–70*f*
  pneumomediastinum, 61–62
  posterior, 71–74, 72*f*
    esophageal cancer, 72–73, 72*f*–73*f*
    neurogenic tumors, 73–74, 73*f*
  postoperative, 74
  protocols, 5–6
  thoracic inlet, 57–58, 58*f*
Medullary sponge kidney, 191–192, 193*f*
  differential diagnosis, 193
Meig syndrome, 215
Melanoma (peritoneal), 168*f*
MEN (multiple endocrine neoplasia) syndrome, 183
Ménétrier disease, 99
Mesenchymal hamartoma, 122
Mesenteric adenitis, 164
Mesenteric cysts, 165, 165*f*
Mesenteric hemangioma, 168*f*
Mesenteric ischemia, 100, 101*f*
  differential diagnosis, 112
Mesenteric lipodystrophy, 164
Mesenteric panniculitis, 164, 165*f*
Mesenteric teratomas, 166
Mesoblastic nephromas, 199–200, 200*f*
Mesothelial cysts, 165
Mesothelioma, 54, 54*f*
MFH (malignant fibrous histiocytoma), 168, 172, 231

Middle mediastinal mass
  differential diagnosis, 67
  protocol, 5
Miliary nodules, 26
  differential diagnosis, 26
Miliary pattern, 15
Miliary tuberculosis, 18
Minimally invasive cardiac surgery, 92
Mirrizi syndrome, 130
Mitral stenosis, 92
Mitral valve
  disease, 81, 82*f*
  repair, 92
  replacement, 92
Morgagni hernias, 55–56, 55*f*
Mosaic attenuation, 12
Mosaic perfusion, 12
Mounier-Kuhn syndrome, 36, 69, 69*f*
MRI (magnetic resonance imaging)
  adrenal adenomas, 183, 186
  brachial and sacral plexus, 224
  diaphragm, 55
  lung carcinoma, 29
  MRI angiography
    pulmonary emboli, 83
  pericardium, 76
  pleura, 46
Mucinous cystic neoplasm, 152, 152*f*
Mucocele of the appendix, 104, 106*f*
Mucoepidermoid carcinoma, 28
Mucoid impaction, 34, 35*f*
Mucormycosis, 20
Mucosa-associated lymphoid tissue (MALT), 27
Mucus, 69
  differential diagnosis, 70
Multicystic dysplastic kidney, 191, 193*f*
Multilocular cystic nephromas, 199, 200*f*
Multiple endocrine neoplasia (MEN) syndrome, 183
Multiple myeloma
  differential diagnosis, 233
Multiple pulmonary nodules
  differential diagnosis, 26
  protocol, 6
Murphy sign, 129
Muscular dystrophy, 224*f*
Mycobacterial infections, 18, 18*f*–19*f*
Mycobacterium avium-intracellulare (MAI), 18–19, 19*f*
  retroperitoneum, 174, 174*f*
  spleen, 140, 141*f*
Mycoplasmal pneumonia, 15
Myelolipomas, 184, 185*f*
Myeloma
  differential diagnosis, 46
Myocardial injuries, 240
Myxomas, 80, 81*f*

N

Nasopharyngeal tumor, 58*f*
Necrobiotic nodules, 232
Necrotizing pancreatitis, 147, 147*f*–148*f*
Necrotizing pneumonia
  differential diagnosis, 25
Nephrectomy, 204
  follow-up protocol, 7
Nephroblastomatosis, 203
Nephrocalcinosis and urolithiasis, 191–194, 193*f*–194*f*
Nephrolithiasis protocol, 7
Nerve-sheath tumors, 73
  retroperitoneal, 171
Neurilemmomas, 73
Neuroblastomas, 73–74
  adrenal glands, 187, 187*f*
  differential diagnosis, 182
Neuroenteric cysts, 63
Neurofibromas, 73
  retroperitoneal, 172*f*
Neurofibromatosis, 40
Neurogenic edema, 23
Neurogenic tumors, 73*f*
  body wall, 230
  differential diagnosis, 71
  posterior mediastinum, 73–74, 73*f*
Neutropenic colitis, 107, 107*f*
NHL (non-Hodgkin lymphoma), 64, 99, 176, 176*f*
Nissen fundoplication, 74
Nocardia, 19*f*
Nodular pattern (lungs), 11
Nodular sclerosing, 175
Nodule characterization protocol, 4
Noncardiogenic edema, 23
  differential diagnosis, 11
Non-Hodgkin lymphoma (NHL), 64, 99, 176, 176*f*
Nonseminomatous germ-cell tumors, 67
Non-small cell carcinoma staging, 30
North American blastomycosis, 17
Noxious gas inhalation, 39

O

Obstruction, 229
Obstructive atelectasis, 13
Obstructive lung disease, 36–38, 36*f*–38*f*
Obturator hernias, 105*f*, 229
Occult lung cancer, 28*f*
Occupational lung disease. *See also* Environmental, occupational, and iatrogenic lung disease

protocol, 6
Octreotide nuclear scintigraphy, 26
Ogilvie syndrome, 110
Omental caking, 167
Omental fat, 63
Oncocytomas, 198–199
Open-window thoracotomy, 47
Oral contrast, 3–4
Osler-Weber-Rendu syndrome, 32–33
Osteochondromas, 233, 234*f*
Osteomyelitis of sternum or sternoclavicular joint, 232
Osteosarcoma, 235, 235*f*
Ovaries, 213–216, 214*f*–217*f*
ovarian vein thrombophlebitis, 218, 219*f*
predominately cystic adnexal lesion
differential diagnosis, 213
predominately solid adnexal mass
differential diagnosis, 216
torsion, 216, 217*f*
Oxalosis, primary, 192

P

Paget disease, 233
Pancoast tumor, 29
Pancreas
anatomy and physiology, 145
calcification
differential diagnosis, 150
congenital abnormalities, 146, 146*f*
CT technique, 145–146
cystic lesions, 150–152, 151*f*–153*f*
dual-phase protocol, 5
fatty change
differential diagnosis, 157
fatty replacement, 157, 158*f*
fistulas, 150
lesions, cystic
differential diagnosis, 151
mass, hypervascular
differential diagnosis, 155
mass, solid
differential diagnosis, 153
pancreatitis, 146–150, 147*f*–150*f*
protocol, 7
pseudocysts, 63, 149, 149*f*
solid tumors, 152–157, 153*f*–156*f*, 157*t*
surgery, 157–158
transplantation, 158
trauma, 245, 245*f*
Pancreaticoblastoma, 156, 156*f*
Pancreatitis, 97, 146–150, 147*f*–150*f*
differential diagnosis, 146, 164
protocol, 7
Panlobular emphysema, 37
Paracicatricial ("scar") emphysema, 37–38
Paraesophageal hernias, 71
Paragangliomas, 73, 171, 172*f*, 184, 184*f*
Paraneoplastic syndromes, 29–30
Parapelvic cysts, 197, 197*f*
Parapneumonic inflammation
differential diagnosis, 48
Parapneumonic pleural effusions, 49–50
Paraseptal emphysema, 37, 38*f*
Parastomal hernias, 229
Parenchymal bands, 21
Parenchymal high attenuation, 13
Parenchymal injury. *See entry under* Thoracic and abdominal trauma
Partial-volume artifact, 2
Peliosis hepatis, 127
Pelvis
anatomy, 205–206, 206*f*–207*f*
bladder, 207–210, 207*f*–210*f*
inflammatory diseases, 218–219, 218*f*–219*f*
masses, 219–220, 220*f*
female patients, protocol, 6
presacral, differential diagnosis, 220
ovaries, 213–216, 214*f*–217*f*
prostate, 216–218, 217*f*–218*f*
protocol, 4
technique, 206–207
uterus, 210–213, 211*f*–213*f*
Percutaneous transluminal coronary angioplasty (PTCA), 90–91
Pericardial diverticula, 62
Pericardial effusion, 76
differential diagnosis, 76
Pericarditis, infectious
differential diagnosis, 76
Pericardium
acquired pericardial disease, 76–78, 77*f*–78*f*
anatomy and function, 75, 75*f*
congenital anomalies, 76, 76*f*
CT, 75–76
cysts, 62, 76, 76*f*
Peridiverticular abscess, 108*f*
Perihepatic abscess, 164*f*
Perihilar lung disease
differential diagnosis, 10
Perinephric lesions
differential diagnosis, 202
Perinephric lymphoma, 202, 203*f*
Peripheral lung disease
differential diagnosis, 10

Periportal tracking, 243
Peritoneal carcinomatosis, 166, 167*f*
  differential diagnosis, 165–166
Peritoneum and retroperitoneum
  anatomy, 159–160, 160*f*–162*f*
  ascites, 160–161, 162*f*–163*f*
  CT technique, 160
  cystic peritoneal lesions, 165–166, 165*f*–166*f*
    differential diagnosis, 165
  lymphadenopathy, 173–175, 173*f*–176*f*
  lymphoma, 175–176, 176*f*
  peritoneal inflammation and abscess, 161–165, 164*f*–165*f*
  pneumoperitoneum, 161, 163*f*–164*f*
  retroperitoneal fibrosis, 170, 170*f*–171*f*
    differential diagnosis, 170
  retroperitoneal hemorrhage, 169–170, 169*f*–170*f*
    differential diagnosis, 169
    protocol, 6
  retroperitoneal masses, 170–173, 171*f*–173*f*
    differential diagnosis, 171
  retroperitoneal teratoma, 171*f*
  solid peritoneal masses, 166–169, 167*f*–168*f*
Peritonitis, 161, 163*f*
PET (positron emission tomography)
  esophageal cancer, 73
Peustow procedure, 158
Pheochromocytomas, 183, 184*f*
Phlegmon, 163
Pigeon breeder's lung, 39
Pitch, 1
Pixel size, 2
Pleura
  anatomy, 45–46, 45*f*–46*f*
  effusion, 47–49, 48*f*–49*f*
    differential diagnosis, 48
    fluid location, 49, 49*f*
    malignant, 53*f*
    parapneumonic, 49–50
  evaluating pleural lesions, 46
  imaging, 46
  infections, 49–50, 50*f*–51*f*
  mass
    differential diagnosis, 52
    protocol, 6
  metastases, 54*f*
    differential diagnosis, 48, 52
    protocol, 6
  plaques, 50–52, 52*f*
    differential diagnosis, 52
    protocols, 6
  pneumothorax, 47, 47*f*
  thickening, 48, 50
    differential diagnosis, 51–52
  trauma. *See entry under* Thoracic and abdominal trauma
  tumors
    benign, 52, 52*f*–53*f*
    malignant, 53–54, 54*f*
    metastases, 52–53, 53*f*–54*f*
    overview, 52
Pleural tags, 24, 24*f*
PNET (primitive neuroectodermal tumors), 74
Pneumatoceles, 13
  traumatic, 241
Pneumatosis, 112, 112*f*
  differential diagnosis, 112
Pneumobilia, 129
  differential diagnosis, 129
Pneumoconiosis, 38
Pneumocystis carinii pneumonia (PCP), 20, 20*f,* 120
  differential diagnosis, 47
  spleen, 140
Pneumomediastinum, 61–62, 240
Pneumonectomy, 42
Pneumonia, 14*f*
  differential diagnosis, 10–11
Pneumopericardium, 62
  differential diagnosis, 62
Pneumoperitoneum, 161, 163*f*–164*f,* 240
  differential diagnosis, 163
Pneumoretroperitoneum, 161, 164*f*
Pneumothorax, 42, 47, 47*f,* 239
  differential diagnosis, 47
Polyarteritis nodosa, 196
Polychondritis, relapsing, 69
Polycystic kidney disease
  differential diagnosis, 192
Polycystic liver disease, 120, 120*f*
Polyps
  differential diagnosis, 109
Porcelain gallbladder, 123*f,* 131
Portal hypertension, 126
Portal venous gas, 126
Positron emission tomography (PET)
  esophageal cancer, 73
Posterior mediastinal mass
  differential diagnosis, 71
  protocol, 5
Postobstructive pneumonia, consolidation, or abscess protocol, 5
Postpartum fever protocol, 6
Postpericardiotomy syndrome, 77
Posttransplantation lymphoproliferative disease (PTLD), 27, 27*f*

Presacral mass, 220–221, 220*f*
  differential diagnosis, 220
Primary mesothelioma, 167
Primary tuberculosis, 18
Primitive neuroectodermal tumors (PNET), 74
Projection, 1
Prostate, 216–218, 217*f*–218*f*
  enlarged, differential diagnosis, 208
Prostatitis, 218
Protocols. *See* Techniques and interpretation, protocols
Pseudoaneurysms, 85, 147, 148*f*, 150, 244, 244*f*
Pseudobronchiectasis, 34
Pseudocirrhosis, 123*f*
Pseudocyst
  differential diagnosis, 151
Pseudolymphoma, 27
Pseudomembranous colitis, 105, 106*f*
  differential diagnosis, 106
Pseudomyxoma peritonei, 104, 161, 163*f*
Pseudotumor, 49
  inflammatory, 122
  spleen, 141
PTLD (posttransplantation lymphoproliferative disease), 27, 27*f*
Pulmonary agenesis, 31
Pulmonary amyloidosis, 40
Pulmonary aplasia, 31
Pulmonary artery
  aneurysms, 83–84
  enlargement, 82
    differential diagnosis, 71, 82
  hypertension
    differential diagnosis, 82
  tumors, 84
Pulmonary aspergillosis, 16, 16*f*–17*f*, 19
Pulmonary blastoma, 30*f*
Pulmonary collapse, 13–14, 13*f*–14*f*
Pulmonary consolidation, 10–11
  differential diagnosis, 11
Pulmonary edema, 10*f*, 23
  differential diagnosis, 10–11
Pulmonary embolism
  differential diagnosis, 48
  protocol, 4
Pulmonary emphysema, 37–38, 38*f*
Pulmonary fibrosis, 21–22, 21*f*–22*f*
  differential diagnosis, 10
Pulmonary hemorrhage, 10–11, 11*f*
  differential diagnosis, 11
Pulmonary hemosiderosis, 40
Pulmonary hila, 69–70
  enlargement, 69–70
  hilar adenopathy, 70–71
Pulmonary hypoplasia, 31
Pulmonary infarction, 33, 90*f*
Pulmonary infections, 14–20, 14*f*
  bacterial pneumonia, 15–16, 15*f*–16*f*
  differential diagnosis, 10
  fungal infections, 16–18, 16*f*–18*f*
  mycobacterial infections, 18–19, 18*f*–19*f*
  opportunistic infections, 19–20, 19*f*–20*f*
  viral pneumonia, 16
Pulmonary injuries, 239*f*, 240–241, 241*f*
Pulmonary lymphoma, 27, 27*f*
Pulmonary metastases, 25, 25*f*
  differential diagnosis, 24–26
  protocol, 6
Pulmonary neoplasms, 26–27, 26*f*–27*f*
Pulmonary nodules
  multiple, 25–26, 25*f*
  protocols, 6
  solitary, 23–25, 24*f*
Pulmonary resection, 42
Pulmonary sequestration, 32
Pulmonary stenosis, 81, 82*f*
Pulmonary thromboembolism, 83*f*
Pulmonary thromboendarterectomy, 90
Pulmonary varices, 84
Pulmonary venolobar syndrome, 31
Pulmonary veno-occlusive disease, 84
Pulmonary venous anomalies, 84
Pulmonary venous hypertension
  differential diagnosis, 82
Pyelonephritis, 194–195, 194*f*–195*f*
  differential diagnosis, 192
Pyogenic abscess, 118–119
Pyogenic splenic abscesses, 139

Q

Quantum mottle, 2

R

Radiation enteritis, 101
Radiation fibrosis, 39, 39*f*
Radiation pericarditis, 77
Radiation pneumonitis, 39, 39*f*
Radiography, conventional
  pneumothorax, 47
Ray sum, 1
Rebound thymic hyperplasia, 65, 65*f*
Reconstruction interval, 1
Reexpansion pulmonary edema, 23, 47
Renal calcification
  differential diagnosis, 193
Renal calculi, 192

Renal cell carcinoma, 200, 200*f*–201*f*
metastatic, 61*f*
Renal infarct, 196, 196*f*
Renal osteodystrophy
differential diagnosis, 232
Renal protocols, 5
renal mass, 7
renal stone, 5
triple-phase, 5
Renal tubular acidosis, 191
differential diagnosis, 193
Resolution, 2
Resorptive atelectasis, 13
Retractile mesenteritis, 164
Retroperitoneum. *See* Peritoneum and retroperitoneum
Rhabdoid tumor, 204*f*
Rhabdomyoma, 80
Rhabdomyosarcoma
biliary tree, 132
bladder, 208
children, 220
retroperitoneal, 171*f*
Rheumatoid arthritis, 23
Ribs
fractures, 241
metastasis
differential diagnosis, 46
Richter hernia, 229
Right lobe collapse, 13, 13*f*–14*f*
Right ventricular failure
differential diagnosis, 70
Rigler triad, 104
Ring artifacts, 2
Robson staging classification, 201
Round pneumonia, 15
Rounded atelectasis, 13, 14*f*, 52
Rubeola, 16
Ruptured cystic airspace
differential diagnosis, 47

S

Saber-sheath trachea, 68, 68*f*
Sandwich sign, 176, 176*f*
Sarcoidosis, 21, 40, 60, 116
differential diagnosis, 10, 26, 71
spleen, 141, 142*f*
Sarcomas
body wall, 232*f*
kidney, 203
uterine, 212, 212*f*
Scan time, 1
Scapular fractures, 241
Schistosomiasis, 120
Schwannomas, 73
presacral, 220*f*, 221
Sciatic hernias, 229
Scimitar syndrome, 31
Scleroderma, 23
differential diagnosis, 227
Sclerosing cholangitis, 130
differential diagnosis, 129
protocol, 6
Secondary tuberculosis, 18
Segmental omental infarction, 165
Segmentectomy, 42
Seminomas, 67
Sentinel clot-sign, 242
Septic emboli, 33
Sex-cord stromal tumors, 215
Shatter (organ trauma), definition of, 243
Shock, 243
Shock bowel, 243, 243*f*
Sickle cell disease, 33, 137*f*
differential diagnosis, 138, 232
splenomegaly and, 137
Sigmoid diverticulitis, 108*f*
Silicosis, 38, 38*f*, 60*f*
differential diagnosis, 26
Silicotuberculosis, 38
Silo filler's disease, 39
Sister Mary Joseph node, 225, 225*f*
Sjögren syndrome, 23
Skeletal muscle atrophy, 224, 224*f*
Sliding hernias, 56, 71
Small airway disease, 36–38, 36*f*–37*f*
Small bowel, 99–104, 101*f*–105*f*
mass, 102
differential diagnosis, 102
obstruction, 103–104, 104*f*
carcinoma, 110
differential diagnosis, 103
hernias, 104, 104*f*–105*f*
thickened, 99–103, 102*f*
differential diagnosis, 101
Small cell carcinoma, 28, 29*f*
staging, 30
Solitary pulmonary nodule
differential diagnosis, 24
Somatostatinomas, 155
Spatial resolution, 2
Spigelian hernia, 229, 229*f*
Spinal compression fractures, 232
Spiral CT, 1–2
Spiral CT angiography (CTA)
aortic disease, 84–85

Spleen
anatomy and physiology, 135–136, 135*f*
CT technique, 136, 136*f*
diffuse disease, 136–137, 136*f*–137*f*
lesions
benign, 138–141, 139*f*–142*f*
differential diagnosis, 139
malignant, 141–143, 142*f*–143*f*
splenic cysts, 138, 138*f*
trauma, 244–245, 244*f*–245*f*
Splenomegaly, 136, 136*f*
differential diagnosis, 137
Splenosis, 53*f*
Split-pleura sign, 50
Spontaneous pneumothorax, 47
Squamous cell carcinoma, 25*f*, 27
bladder, 208
Staphylococcal pneumonia, 15
Sternal fractures, 241
Sternoclavicular disolcations, 241, 242*f*
Stomach, 97–99, 98*f*–100*f*
Strangulation, small bowel, 104, 228–229
Streak artifacts, 2
Streptococcal pneumonia, 15
Stromal tumors
ovaries, differential diagnosis, 216
small bowel, 99*f*, 102
Subpleural lines, 21
Superior sulcus tumor, 29
protocol, 5
Superior vena cava, 87, 89*f*
Swyer-James syndrome, 12*f*, 31
Systemic lupus erythematosus, 23

T

Table speed, 1
TB. *See* Tuberculosis
Techniques and interpretation
contrast, 3*f*
intravenous contrast, 3
oral contrast, 3–4
CT physics, 1–3
artifacts, 2
image display, 2
resolution, 2
problem-oriented approach to scanning
adrenal glands, 7
aorta, 6
general abdomen and pelvis, 6
liver, 6
lung and mediastinum, 5
mediastinum, 5–6
pancreas/biliary, 7
pleural process, 6
pulmonary, 6
urinary tract, 7
protocols, 4–5
abdomen, 4
abdomen and pelvis, 4
adrenal glands, 4
aorta, 4
central airway, 4
chest, 4
chest, abdomen, and pelvis, 5
dual-phase pancreas, 5
HRCT, 4
nodule characterization, 4
pelvis, 4
pulmonary emboli, 4
renal, 5
renal stone, 5
triple-phase liver, 4–5
triple-phase renal, 5
Tension pneumothorax, 47
Teratomas, 67
hepatic, 122
mature cystic (ovaries), 213–214, 214*f*
differential diagnosis, 213
pancreatic, 152
Testes, undescended, 220, 220*f*
Testicular neoplasms, 173–174, 174*f*
THAD (transient hepatic attenuation difference), 127, 127*f*
Thalassemia, 235*f*
Thickened colon
differential diagnosis, 106
Third-generation scanners, 1
Thoracentesis, 47
Thoracic and abdominal trauma
acute traumatic aortic injury (ATAI), 238–239, 238*f*–239*f*
CT technique, 237–238, 238*f*
duodenal trauma, 245, 245*f*
epidemiology, 237
genitourinary trauma, 245–247, 246*f*–247*f*
hemoperitoneum, 242–243, 242*f*–243*f*
hepatic trauma, 243–244, 243*f*–244*f*
pancreatic trauma, 245, 245*f*
parenchymal, pleural, and chest wall injury, 239
air collections, 239–240, 239*f*–240*f*
airway injury, 240
cardiac injury, 240
chest wall injuries, 241, 242*f*
diaphragmatic injuries, 241–242, 242*f*
intubations, 239, 239*f*

Thoracic and abdominal trauma, parenchymal, pleural, and chest wall injury (*Cont.*)
posttraumatic fluid collections, 240
pulmonary injuries, 239*f*, 240–241, 241*f*
splenic trauma, 244–245, 244*f*–245*f*
Thoracic aortic aneurysms, 90
protocol, 6
Thoracic goiters, 58
Thoracic inlet, 57–58, 58*f*
mass, differential diagnosis, 57
Thoracic splenosis, 52
Thoracic surgery, 41–43
Thoracoabdominal aneurysms, 90
Thoracoplasty, 231, 232*f*
Thorotrast, 114–115, 116*f*, 137
Thromboembolism, 83–84, 83*f*–84*f*
Thymolipomas, 66
Thymomas, 65, 66*f*
protocol, 5
Thymus, 64–67, 65*f*–67*f*
carcinoma, 66–67
cysts, 64, 65*f*
hyperplasia, 65
lymphoma, 66, 66*f*
tumor, differential diagnosis, 64
Thyroid lesions
differential diagnosis, 58
Thyroid mass
differential diagnosis, 57, 64
Thyroid tumors, 58
Tiny pulmonary nodules
differential diagnosis, 26
TMN cancer staging system, 30
TOP (tracheopathia osteochondroplastica), 68, 68*f*
Toupet fundoplication, 74
Toxic colitis, 106–107, 107*f*
Trachea, 67–68
mass
differential diagnosis, 70
protocol, 5
narrowing, 68
tumors, 69, 70*f*
Tracheobronchial papillomatosis, 70*f*
Tracheobronchial trauma, 240
differential diagnosis, 62
Tracheobronchomegaly, 35
Tracheomalacia, 68
Tracheomegaly, 69
Tracheopathia osteochondroplastica (TOP), 68, 68*f*
Traction bronchiectasis, 35
Transient hepatic attenuation difference (THAD), 127, 127*f*
Transitional cell carcinoma, 201, 202*f*
bladder, 207, 207*f*–208*f*
Transudates, 48
Tree-in-bud sign, 21
Tricuspid valve disease, 81
TS (tuberous sclerosis), 40, 198
Tuberculoma, 18
Tuberculosis (TB), 18–19, 18*f*–19*f*, 232
intestinal, 101*f*
spleen, 139
Tuberculous peritonitis, 169
Tuberous sclerosis (TS), 40, 198
Tubo-ovarian abscess, 218*f*
differential diagnosis, 213

U

Ulcerative colitis (UC), 106
differential diagnosis, 106
Ultrafast CT, 78
Ultrasound
pleural, 46
Undifferentiated embryonal sarcoma, 125
Upper lung disease
differential diagnosis, 10
Urachal carcinomas, 208, 209*f*
Ureteral dilatation
differential diagnosis, 194
Urinary tract
protocol, 7
Urolithiasis, 191–194, 193*f*–194*f*
Urothelial tumor
differential diagnosis, 208
Uterus, 210–213, 211*f*–213*f*
congenital anomalies, 212–213, 213*f*
enlarged, differential diagnosis, 210

V

Valvular heart disease, 81, 82*f*–83*f*
Varicella zoster, 16
Varicose bronchiectasis, 35
Vascular masses
diaphragm, 55
mediastinum, 58
Vasculidites, 23
Vasculitis, 101, 107
VATS (video-assisted thoracic surgery), 42–43
Venous thrombosis, 90*f*
Ventral hernias, 229
Ventricular aneurysms, 79
Vertebral fractures, 241

Vesicoureteral reflux
differential diagnosis, 194
VHL (von Hippel-Lindau disease), 150, 198, 198*f*
Video-assisted thoracic surgery (VATS), 42–43
VIPomas (vasoactive intestinal peptide tumors), 155, 156*f*
Viral pneumonia, 16
Virchow node, 224
Volvulus, colonic, 110, 110*f*
Von Hippel-Lindau (VHL) disease, 150, 198, 198*f*

W

Wandering spleen, 135
Waterhouse-Friderichsen syndrome, 181
Wegener granulomatosis, 11, 33, 34*f*, 69, 102*f*
differential diagnosis, 25
Whipple procedure, 158
Williams-Campbell syndrome, 35
Wilms tumor, 203, 203*f*
differential diagnoses, 199
Wilson disease, 115
Window center, 2
Window level, 2
Window width, 2
Wolfman disease, 181

X

Xanthogranulomatous pyelonephritis (XGP), 195–196, 196*f*
differential diagnoses, 199

Z

Zenker diverticulum, 72
Zollinger-Ellison syndrome, 99, 155

Notes

NOTES

NOTES

NOTES